# MEDICAL ASSISTING ADMINISTRATIVE SKILLS CD QUICK LOCATOR

This is your link to *Delmar's Medical Assisting Administrative Skills* CD-ROM, which is found on the inside back cover of this book.

| Text Chapter | Skills and Their Location on the CD-ROM |
|---|---|
| 7 | Legal Concepts |
| 10 | Patient Reception |
| 12 | Telephone Skills |
| 12 | Telephone Messages |
| 13 | Scheduling |
| 14 | Records Management |
| 15 | Parts of a Letter |
| 15 | Parts of the Envelope |
| 15 | Telephone Messages |
| 15 | Prescriptions |
| 15 | Medical Record |
| 17 | Patient Receipts |
| 17 | Purchase Orders |
| 17 | Payroll Procedures |
| 17 | Banking |
| 19 | Insurance Coding |
| 20 | Pegboard Accounting |
| 20 | Superbill, Ledger Card, Daily Log/Day Sheet |
| 25 | Résumé Writing |

# DELMAR'S ADMINISTRATIVE MEDICAL ASSISTING

# Delmar's ADMINISTRATIVE
# MEDICAL ASSISTING

## 2nd Edition

Wilburta Q. Lindh

Marilyn S. Pooler

Carol D. Tamparo

DELMAR

THOMSON LEARNING™    Australia    Canada    Mexico    Singapore    Spain    United Kingdom    United States

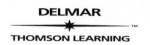

**DELMAR**
™
**THOMSON LEARNING**

**Delmar's Administrative Medical Assisting, 2nd Edition**
by Wilburta Q. Lindh, Marilyn S. Pooler, and Carol D. Tamparo

**Health Care Publishing Director:**
William Brottmiller

**Executive Marketing Manager:**
Dawn F. Gerrain

**Production Coordinator:**
John Mickelbank

**Acquisitions Editor:**
Rhonda Dearborn

**Executive Editor:**
Cathy L. Esperti

**Art/Design Coordinator:**
Mary Colleen Liburdi

**Senior Developmental Editor:**
Elisabeth F. Williams

**Project Editor:**
David Buddle

**Cover Design:**
The Drawing Board

**Editorial Assistant:**
Jill Korznat

**Technology Manager:**
Laurie Davis

**Technology Assistant:**
Sherry McGaughan

For permission to use material from this text or product, contact us by
Tel   800-730-2214
Fax  800-730-2215
www.thomsonrights.com

Library of Congress Cataloging-in-Publication Data

Lindh, Wilburta Q.
Delmar's administrative medical assisting / Wilburta Q. Lindh, Marilyn S. Pooler, Carol D. Tamparo.—2nd ed.
    p.   cm.
    Includes bibliographical references and index.
    ISBN 0-7668-2423-3
    1. Medical assistants.   2. Medical offices—Management.   I. Pooler, Marilyn S.   II. Tamparo, Carol D., 1940–   .   III. Title.
    R728.8 .L54 2001
    610.69'53—dc21

                                    2001047101

**NOTICE TO THE READER**

Publisher does not warrant or guarantee any of the products described herein or perform any independent analysis in connection with any of the product information contained herein. Publisher does not assume, and expressly disclaims, any obligation to obtain and include information other than that provided to it by the manufacturer.

The reader is expressly warned to consider and adopt all safety precautions that might be indicated by the activities herein and to avoid all potential hazards. By following the instructions contained herein, the reader willingly assumes all risks in connection with such instructions.

The publisher makes no representation or warranties of any kind, including but not limited to, the warranties of fitness for particular purpose or merchantability, nor are any such representations implied with respect to the material set forth herein, and the publisher takes no responsibility with respect to such material. The publisher shall not be liable for any special, consequential, or exemplary damages resulting, in whole or part, from the readers' use of, or reliance upon, this material.

# CONTENTS

Managing Authors                                  x

Acknowledgments                                   xi

Reviewers                                         xii

Contributors                                      xiii

List of Procedures                                xiv

Preface                                           xv

How to Use This Book                              xviii

How to Use the Medical
Assisting Administrative Skills
CD-ROM                                            xx


## SECTION I: GENERAL PROCEDURES                  1

Unit 1:    Introduction to Medical
           Assisting and Health
           Professions                            2

Chapter 1:  Medical Assisting as a
            Profession                            3

Personal Attributes of the
Professional . . . . . . . . . . . . . . 4
Empathy . . . . . . . . . . . . . . . . . 5
Attitude . . . . . . . . . . . . . . . . . 5
Dependability . . . . . . . . . . . . 5
Initiative . . . . . . . . . . . . . . 5
Flexibility . . . . . . . . . . . . . 5
Desire to Learn . . . . . . . . . . . . 6
Physical Attributes . . . . . . . . . 6
Ability to Communicate . . . . . . 7
Ethical Behavior . . . . . . . . . . . 7
Historical Perspective of
Medical Assisting . . . . . . . . . 7
American Association of
Medical Assistants . . . . . . . . . 8
Accreditation . . . . . . . . . . . . 8
Certification . . . . . . . . . . . . 8
Continuing Education . . . . . . . . 9

Registered Medical Assistant  . 9
Education of the Professional
Medical Assistant . . . . . . . . . . 9
Preparation for Externship . . . 10
Career Opportunities . . . . . . 11
Regulation of Health Care
Providers . . . . . . . . . . . . . . . 11
Scope of Practice . . . . . . . . . . 11

Chapter 2:  Health Care Settings and
            the Health Care Team      15

Ambulatory Health Care
Settings . . . . . . . . . . . . . . . 16
Individual and Group Medical
Practices . . . . . . . . . . . . . . . 16
Urgent Care Centers . . . . . . . . 17
Managed Care Operations . . . 17
The Impact of Managed Care
in the Health Care Setting . . 18
The Health Care Team . . . . 18
The Role of the Medical
Assistant . . . . . . . . . . . . . . 18
Health Care Professionals and
Their Roles . . . . . . . . . . . . . 19
Allied and Other Health
Professionals and Their Roles . 21
The Role of Integrative or
Alternative Health Care
Therapies . . . . . . . . . . . . . . 24
The Value of the Medical
Assistant to the Health Care
Team . . . . . . . . . . . . . . . . . 25

Chapter 3:  History of Medicine      29

Cultural Heritage in
Medicine . . . . . . . . . . . . . . 30
Medical Specialists . . . . . . . . 30
Medical Education . . . . . . . . . 31
Attitudes Toward Illness . . . 31
Medical Treatments . . . . . . . 32
Significant Contributions to
Medicine . . . . . . . . . . . . . . 33
New Frontiers in Medicine . . 34

(A) For practice activities, this icon tells you when to turn to *Delmar's Medical Assisting Administrative Skills* CD-ROM in the back of the book.

**Unit 2:    The Therapeutic
Approach    36**

**Chapter 4:    Therapeutic
Communication Skills    37**

Importance of
Communication . . . . . . . . . . 39
Cultural Influence on Thera-
peutic Communication . . . . . 39
Biases and Prejudices . . . . . . 40
The Communication Cycle . 40
The Sender . . . . . . . . . . . . . . 40
The Message . . . . . . . . . . . . . 40
The Receiver . . . . . . . . . . . . . 41
Feedback . . . . . . . . . . . . . . . . 41
Listening Skills . . . . . . . . . . . 41
Verbal Communication . . . . 41
The Five Cs of
Communication . . . . . . . . . . 41
Nonverbal Communication . 42
Facial Expression . . . . . . . . . 43
Territoriality . . . . . . . . . . . . . 43
Posture . . . . . . . . . . . . . . . . . 43
Position . . . . . . . . . . . . . . . . . 44
Gestures and Mannerisms . . 44
Touch . . . . . . . . . . . . . . . . . . 44
Congruency In
Communication . . . . . . . . . . 44
Perception . . . . . . . . . . . . . . . 45
Maslow's Hierarchy of Needs . 45
Technology and
Communication . . . . . . . . . . 45
Roadblocks to Therapeutic
Communication . . . . . . . . . . 45
Defense Mechanisms . . . . . . 46
Introjection . . . . . . . . . . . . . . 46
Denial . . . . . . . . . . . . . . . . . . 46
Compensation . . . . . . . . . . . 46
Regression . . . . . . . . . . . . . . . 46
Repression . . . . . . . . . . . . . . . 46
Sublimation . . . . . . . . . . . . . 46
Projection . . . . . . . . . . . . . . . 46
Displacement . . . . . . . . . . . . 46
Rationalization . . . . . . . . . . . 47
Interview Techniques . . . . . . 47
Telephone Techniques . . . . . 47

**Chapter 5:    Coping Skills for the
Medical Assistant    51**

What Is Stress? . . . . . . . . . . 52
Adaptation to Stress . . . . . . . 52
Coping with Stress . . . . . . . . 53
What Is Burnout? . . . . . . . . 54
Burnout in the Workplace . . 54
What to Do If You Are Burned
Out . . . . . . . . . . . . . . . . . . . . 55
Preventing Burnout . . . . . . . 55
Goal Setting as a Stress
Reliever . . . . . . . . . . . . . . . . 55

**Chapter 6:    The Therapeutic Approach
to the Patient with Life-
Threatening Illness    59**

Life-Threatening Illness . . . . 60
Cultural Perspective on Life-
Threatening Illness . . . . . . . . 60

Choices in Life-Threatening
Illness . . . . . . . . . . . . . . . . . 61
The Range of Psychological
Suffering . . . . . . . . . . . . . . . 62
The Therapeutic Response to
the Patient with Aids . . . . . . 62
The Challenge for the
Medical Assistant . . . . . . . . 63

**Unit 3:    Responsible Medical
Practice    66**

**Chapter 7:    Legal Considerations    67**
Ⓐ **Legal Concepts**
Civil and Criminal Law . . . . 69
Medical Practice Acts and the
Medical Assistant's Role . . . . 69
Patient Rights . . . . . . . . . . . 69
The Physician, the Medical
Assistant, and the Law . . . . . 69
Contracts . . . . . . . . . . . . . . . 69
Termination of Contracts . . . . 71
Standard of Care and the
4 Ds of Negligence . . . . . . . . 72
Torts . . . . . . . . . . . . . . . . . . . 72
Battery . . . . . . . . . . . . . . . . . 73
Defamation of Character . . . . . 74
Invasion of Privacy . . . . . . . . 74
Medical Records . . . . . . . . . . 74
Informed Consent . . . . . . . . . 74
Implied Consent . . . . . . . . . . 75
Consent and Legal
Incompetence . . . . . . . . . . . . 75
Subpoenas . . . . . . . . . . . . . . . 75
Confidentiality . . . . . . . . . . . 76
Statute of Limitations . . . . . . 76
Public Duties . . . . . . . . . . . . 76
Drug Screening . . . . . . . . . . . 76
AIDS . . . . . . . . . . . . . . . . . . 77
Abuse . . . . . . . . . . . . . . . . . . 77
Good Samaritan Law . . . . . . 77
Physician's Directives . . . . . 78
Americans with Disabilities
Act (ADA) . . . . . . . . . . . . . 78

**Chapter 8:    Ethical Considerations    83**
Ethics Defined . . . . . . . . . . . 84
Bioethics Defined . . . . . . . . . 85
Keys to the AAMA Code of
Ethics . . . . . . . . . . . . . . . . . 86
AMA Ethical Guidelines . . . 87
Advertising . . . . . . . . . . . . . . 87
Media Relations . . . . . . . . . . 87
Confidentiality . . . . . . . . . . . 87
Medical Records . . . . . . . . . . 88
Professional Fees and
Charges . . . . . . . . . . . . . . . . 88
Professional Rights and
Responsibilities . . . . . . . . . . 88
Abuse . . . . . . . . . . . . . . . . . . 88
Bioethical Dilemmas . . . . . . 89
Allocation of Scarce Medical
Resources . . . . . . . . . . . . . . . 89
Abortion and Fetal Tissue
Research . . . . . . . . . . . . . . . . 89

Genetic Engineering/
Manipulation . . . . . . . . . . . . 90
Artificial Insemination/
Surrogacy . . . . . . . . . . . . . . . 90
Dying and Death . . . . . . . . . . 90
HIV and AIDS . . . . . . . . . . . 90

**Chapter 9:    Emergency Procedures
and First Aid    93**
Recognizing an Emergency . . 95
Responding to an Emergency . 95
Primary Survey . . . . . . . . . . . 96
Using the 911 or Emergency
Medical Services System . . . . . 97
Good Samaritan Laws . . . . . . . 97
Blood, Body Fluids, and Disease
Transmission . . . . . . . . . . . . . 97
Preparing for an Emergency . 97
The Medical Crash Tray or
Cart . . . . . . . . . . . . . . . . . . . . 98
Common Emergencies . . . . . 99
Shock . . . . . . . . . . . . . . . . . . . 99
Wounds . . . . . . . . . . . . . . . . 100
Burns . . . . . . . . . . . . . . . . . . 101
Musculoskeletal Injuries . . . . 105
Heat- and Cold-Related
Illnesses . . . . . . . . . . . . . . . . 107
Poisoning . . . . . . . . . . . . . . . 107
Sudden Illness . . . . . . . . . . . 108
Cerebral Vascular Accident
(CVA) . . . . . . . . . . . . . . . . . 110
Heart Attack . . . . . . . . . . . . 110
Procedures for Breathing
Emergencies and Cardiac
Arrest . . . . . . . . . . . . . . . . . 111
Heimlich Maneuver
(Abdominal Thrust) . . . . . . . 111
Rescue Breathing . . . . . . . . . 112
Cardiopulmonary
Resuscitation (CPR) . . . . . . . 112

**SECTION II:
ADMINISTRATIVE
PROCEDURES    129**

**Unit 4:    Integrated Adminis-
trative Procedures    130**

**Chapter 10:    Creating the Facility
Environment    131**
Ⓐ **Patient Reception**
The Reception Area . . . . . . 132
Office Design and
Environment . . . . . . . . . . . 133
Americans with Disabilities
Act . . . . . . . . . . . . . . . . . . . 133
The Receptionist's Role . . . 134
Opening the Facility . . . . . . 134
Closing the Facility . . . . . . 135

**Chapter 11: Computers in the Ambulatory Care Setting**     **137**

Types of Computers . . . . . . 139
Components of a Computer
System . . . . . . . . . . . . . . . 139
Hardware . . . . . . . . . . . . . . 139
Power Outage, Electrical
Surge, and Static Discharge
Protection Devices . . . . . . . 141
Software . . . . . . . . . . . . . . . 141
Documentation . . . . . . . . . . 141
Common Software
Applications in the
Medical Office . . . . . . . . . . 141
Word Processing . . . . . . . . . 142
Graphics . . . . . . . . . . . . . . . 144
Spreadsheets . . . . . . . . . . . . 144
Databases . . . . . . . . . . . . . . 144
Virus Protection . . . . . . . . . 146
Patient Confidentiality in
the Computerized Medical
Office . . . . . . . . . . . . . . . 146
Computerizing the Medical
Office . . . . . . . . . . . . . . . 147
The Safe Use of
Computers . . . . . . . . . . . . 149

**Chapter 12: Telephone Techniques**     **155**

Ⓐ **Telephone Skills**
Ⓐ **Telephone Messages**
Basic Telephone
Techniques . . . . . . . . . . . . 157
Telephone Personality . . . . . 157
Telephone Etiquette . . . . . . . 158
Answering Incoming Calls . 159
Preparing to Take Calls . . . . 159
Answering Calls . . . . . . . . . 159
Screening Calls . . . . . . . . . . 159
Transferring a Call . . . . . . . . 160
Taking a Message . . . . . . . . . 160
Ending the Call . . . . . . . . . . 161
Types of Calls the Medical
Assistant Can Take . . . . . . 161
Types of Calls Referred to
the Physician . . . . . . . . . . 162
Special Consideration Calls 162
Referring Calls . . . . . . . . . . 162
Emergency Calls . . . . . . . . . 163
Angry Callers . . . . . . . . . . . 164
Elderly Callers . . . . . . . . . . 164
English as a Second Language
Callers . . . . . . . . . . . . . . . 164
Placing Outgoing Calls . . . . 165
Placing Long Distance
Calls . . . . . . . . . . . . . . . . 165
Placing Calls. . . . . . . . . . . . . 165
Time Zones . . . . . . . . . . . . . 165
Long-Distance Carriers . . . . . 166
Telephone Documentation . 166
Using Telephone
Directories . . . . . . . . . . . . 166
Legal and Ethical
Considerations . . . . . . . . . 167
Telephone Technology . . . . 167
Automated Routing Units . . 168

Answering Services and
Machines . . . . . . . . . . . . . 168
Facsimile (Fax) Machines . . . 168
Electronic Mail . . . . . . . . . . 168
Cellular Service . . . . . . . . . . 168
Paging Systems . . . . . . . . . . 169

**Chapter 13: Patient Scheduling**     **175**

Ⓐ **Scheduling**
Tailoring the Scheduling
System . . . . . . . . . . . . . . . 177
Types of Scheduling
Systems . . . . . . . . . . . . . . 177
Open Hours . . . . . . . . . . . . 177
Double Booking . . . . . . . . . 177
Clustering . . . . . . . . . . . . . 177
Wave . . . . . . . . . . . . . . . . . 177
Modified Wave . . . . . . . . . . 177
Stream . . . . . . . . . . . . . . . . 177
Practice-Based . . . . . . . . . . . 178
Analyzing Patient Flow . . . 178
Waiting Time . . . . . . . . . . . . 179
Flexibility . . . . . . . . . . . . . . 179
Legal Issues . . . . . . . . . . . . . 179
Interpersonal Skills . . . . . . 180
Guidelines for Scheduling
Appointments . . . . . . . . . . 180
Triage Calls . . . . . . . . . . . . . 180
Referral Appointments . . . . 180
Recording Information . . . . 180
Computer Scheduling . . . . . 181
Patient Check-In . . . . . . . . . 181
Patient Cancellation and
Appointment Changes . . . . 182
Computer Cancellations . . . . 182
Reminder Systems . . . . . . . . 183
Scheduling Representatives . 183
Scheduling Materials . . . . . 183
Appointment Books . . . . . . . 183
Appointment Sheets . . . . . . . 183
Daily Worksheets . . . . . . . . . 184
Computer Equipment . . . . . . 184
Appointment Cards . . . . . . . 184
Establishing an Appointment
Book . . . . . . . . . . . . . . . . 184
Informational Brochure . . . 186

**Chapter 14: Medical Records Management**     **191**

Ⓐ **Records Management**
The Importance of Accurate
Medical Records . . . . . . . . 193
Equipment and Supplies . . . 193
Vertical Files . . . . . . . . . . . . 193
Open-Shelf Lateral Files . . . . 193
Movable File Units . . . . . . . . 193
File Folders . . . . . . . . . . . . . 194
Identification Labels . . . . . . . 194
Guides and Positions . . . . . . 194
Out Guides . . . . . . . . . . . . . 195
Basic Rules for Filing . . . . . 195
Indexing Units . . . . . . . . . . . 195
Filing Patient Charts . . . . . . . 195
Filing Identical Names . . . . . 196
Filing Business and
Organizational Records . . . . 196

Steps for Filing Medical
Documentation in Patient
Files . . . . . . . . . . . . . . . . 198
Inspect . . . . . . . . . . . . . . . . 198
Index . . . . . . . . . . . . . . . . . 198
Code . . . . . . . . . . . . . . . . . . 198
Sort . . . . . . . . . . . . . . . . . . 198
File . . . . . . . . . . . . . . . . . . . 198
Filing Techniques and
Common Filing Systems . . . 198
Color Coding . . . . . . . . . . . . 198
Alphabetic Filing . . . . . . . . . 201
Numeric Filing . . . . . . . . . . 201
Subject Filing . . . . . . . . . . . 201
Choosing a Filing System . . 202
Filing Procedures . . . . . . . . 203
Cross-Referencing . . . . . . . . 203
Tickler Files . . . . . . . . . . . . . 204
Release Marks . . . . . . . . . . . 204
Check-Out System . . . . . . . . 204
Locating Missing Files or
Data . . . . . . . . . . . . . . . . 205
Filing Chart Data . . . . . . . . 205
Retention and Purging . . . . . 206
Correspondence . . . . . . . . . 207
Incoming Correspondence . . 207
Outgoing Correspondence . . 207
Filing Procedures for
Correspondence . . . . . . . . . 207
Computer Applications . . . 208
Databases . . . . . . . . . . . . . . 208
Archival Storage . . . . . . . . . 209
Transfer of Data . . . . . . . . . 210
Confidentiality . . . . . . . . . . 210

**Chapter 15: Written Communications**     **215**

Ⓐ **Parts of a Letter**
Ⓐ **Parts of the Envelope**
Ⓐ **Telephone Messages**
Ⓐ **Prescriptions**
Ⓐ **Medical Record**
Composing
Correspondence . . . . . . . . 217
Writing Tips . . . . . . . . . . . . 217
Spelling . . . . . . . . . . . . . . . 217
Proofreading . . . . . . . . . . . . 218
Components of a Business
Letter . . . . . . . . . . . . . . . 219
Date Line . . . . . . . . . . . . . . 219
Inside Address . . . . . . . . . . . 219
Salutation . . . . . . . . . . . . . . 219
Subject Line . . . . . . . . . . . . 219
Body of Letter . . . . . . . . . . . 220
Complimentary Closing . . . . 220
Keyed Signature . . . . . . . . . . 220
Reference Initials . . . . . . . . . 220
Enclosure Notation . . . . . . . 220
Carbon Copy Notation . . . . . 220
Postscripts . . . . . . . . . . . . . . 220
Continuation Page Heading . 220
Letter Styles . . . . . . . . . . . . 221
Full Block . . . . . . . . . . . . . . 221
Modified Block . . . . . . . . . . 222
Simplified . . . . . . . . . . . . . . 222

Supplies for Written
Communication . . . . . . . . . 224
Letterhead . . . . . . . . . . . . . . 224
Second Sheets . . . . . . . . . . . 225
Envelopes . . . . . . . . . . . . . . . 225
Other Types of
Correspondence . . . . . . . . . 226
Memoranda . . . . . . . . . . . . . 226
Meeting Agendas . . . . . . . . 226
Meeting Minutes . . . . . . . . . 227
Processing Incoming and
Outgoing Mail . . . . . . . . . 228
Incoming Mail and
Shipments . . . . . . . . . . . . . . 228
Outgoing Mail and
Shipments . . . . . . . . . . . . . . 228
Postal Classes . . . . . . . . . . . 228
Formats for Efficient
Processing . . . . . . . . . . . . . . 229
International Mail . . . . . . . . 229
Technologies . . . . . . . . . . . . 229
Facsimile (Fax) . . . . . . . . . . 229
Electronic Mail (E-Mail) . . . . 230
Legal and Ethical Issues . . . 231

**Chapter 16: Transcription            241**
History of the American
Association for Medical
Transcription . . . . . . . . . . . 243
AAMT Membership . . . . . . . 243
The Medical Transcription-
ist's Career . . . . . . . . . . . . . 243
Attributes of the Medical
Transcriptionist . . . . . . . . . . 243
Job Description . . . . . . . . . . 244
Employment Opportunities . . 244
Certification for Medical
Transcriptionists . . . . . . . . . 245
Transcription Tools . . . . . . 246
Equipment . . . . . . . . . . . . . . 246
Ergonomics . . . . . . . . . . . . . 246
Facsimile Machines . . . . . . . . 247
Photocopy Machines . . . . . . 247
Transcription Guidelines . . 247
Proofreading and Making
Corrections . . . . . . . . . . . . . 247
Proofreading Skills . . . . . . . 247
Where Errors Occur . . . . . . . 247
Editing . . . . . . . . . . . . . . . . . 248
Making Corrections . . . . . . . 248
Medical Reports . . . . . . . . . 248
Chart Notes and Progress
Notes . . . . . . . . . . . . . . . . . . 249
History and Physical
Examination Reports . . . . . . 249
Consultation Reports . . . . . . 249
Correspondence . . . . . . . . . . 249
Turnaround Time . . . . . . . . 249
Ethical and Legal Issues . . . 252
Confidentiality . . . . . . . . . . 252
Risk Management . . . . . . . . 252
New Technology . . . . . . . . 252
Continuous Speech
Recognition (CSR) . . . . . . . 252
Integrating Digital Photographs
into Medical Transcription . . 253

**Unit 5:    Managing Facility
Finances            256**

**Chapter 17: Daily Financial
Practices            257**
Ⓐ **Patient Receipts**
Ⓐ **Purchase Orders**
Ⓐ **Payroll Procedures**
Ⓐ **Banking**
Determining Patient Fees . . 258
Usual, Customary, and
Reasonable Fees . . . . . . . . . . 259
Discussion of Fees . . . . . . . . 259
Adjustment of Fees . . . . . . . . 259
Credit Arrangements . . . . 260
Payment Planning . . . . . . . . 260
The Bookkeeping Function   260
Managing Patient Accounts . 260
The Importance of Good
Working Habits . . . . . . . . . . 261
The Pegboard System . . . . . . 261
Computerized Systems . . . . . 265
Banking Procedures . . . . . 266
Types of Accounts . . . . . . . . 266
Types of Checks . . . . . . . . . . 267
Deposits . . . . . . . . . . . . . . . . 267
Accepting Checks . . . . . . . . . 268
Lost or Stolen Checks . . . . . . 268
Writing and Recording
Checks . . . . . . . . . . . . . . . . . 268
Reconciling a Bank
Statement . . . . . . . . . . . . . . 269
Purchasing Supplies and
Equipment . . . . . . . . . . . . . 269
Preparing a Purchase Order . . 270
Verifying Goods Received . . . 271
Preparing the Invoice for
Payment . . . . . . . . . . . . . . . . 271
Petty Cash . . . . . . . . . . . . . 272
Establishing a Petty Cash
Fund . . . . . . . . . . . . . . . . . . . 272
Tracking, Balancing, and
Replenishing Petty Cash . . . . 272

**Chapter 18: Medical Insurance       281**
The Evolution of Medical
Insurance Coverage . . . . . . 283
Changes in Health Insurance
Today . . . . . . . . . . . . . . . . . . 283
Screening for Insurance . . . . . 283
Medical Insurance
Terminology . . . . . . . . . . . 284
Terminology Specific to
Insurance Policies . . . . . . . . 284
Terminology Specific to
Billing Insurance Carriers . . . 285
Types of Medical Insurance
Coverage . . . . . . . . . . . . . . 287
Traditional Insurance . . . . . . 287
Managed Care . . . . . . . . . . . 287
Medicare . . . . . . . . . . . . . . . 289
Other Types of Coverage . . . . 290
Prospective Payment
Systems and Diagnosis-
Related Groups . . . . . . . . 291
Legal and Ethical Issues . . . 291

**Chapter 19: Medical Insurance
Coding            295**
Ⓐ **Insurance Coding**
Insurance Coding Systems . 296
Procedure Coding . . . . . . . . 296
Diagnosis Coding . . . . . . . . 299
Coding the Claim Form . . . 301
Completing the HCFA-1500
(12-90) . . . . . . . . . . . . . . . 301
Overseeing the Claims
Process . . . . . . . . . . . . . . . 304
Point-of-Service Device . . . . 304
Maintaining Claim Register
or Diary . . . . . . . . . . . . . . . . 304
The Insurance Carrier's
Role . . . . . . . . . . . . . . . . . . . 305
Explanation of Benefits . . . . . 305
Following Up on Claims . . . . . 305
The Computerized Claims
Process . . . . . . . . . . . . . . . . . 305
Legal and Ethical Issues . . . 305
Healthcare Compliance . . . 306
Seven Basic Elements of a
Voluntary Compliance
Program . . . . . . . . . . . . . . . . 306

**Chapter 20: Billing and Collections   309**
Ⓐ **Pegboard Accounting**
Ⓐ **Superbill, Ledger Card,
Daily Log/Day Sheet**
Billing Procedures . . . . . . . 310
Credit and Collection
Policies . . . . . . . . . . . . . . . 311
Payment at Time of Service  311
Truth-in-Lending Act . . . . 311
Components of a Complete
Statement . . . . . . . . . . . . . . 311
Computerized Statements . . . 312
Monthly and Cycle Billing . 312
Monthly Billing . . . . . . . . . . 312
Cycle Billing . . . . . . . . . . . . 312
Past-Due Accounts . . . . . . 313
Collection Process . . . . . . . 313
Aging Accounts . . . . . . . . . 313
Computerized Aging . . . . . . . 313
Collection Techniques . . . . 314
Correspondence to
Insurance Carriers . . . . . . . . 314
Telephone Collections . . . . . 314
Collection Letters . . . . . . . . 315
Use of an Outside
Collection Agency . . . . . . . 315
Use of Small Claims Court . 317
Special Collection
Situations . . . . . . . . . . . . . 317
Bankruptcy . . . . . . . . . . . . . 317
Estates . . . . . . . . . . . . . . . . 317
Tracing "Skips" . . . . . . . . . . 317
Statute of Limitations . . . . 317

**Chapter 21: Accounting Practices     321**
Bookkeeping and
Accounting Systems . . . . . . 322
Single-Entry . . . . . . . . . . . . . 322
Pegboard . . . . . . . . . . . . . . . 322
Double-Entry . . . . . . . . . . . . 323
Computerized Systems . . . . . 323

Computer Service Bureaus . . 323
The Accounting Function . 323
Cost Analysis . . . . . . . . . . 324
Fixed Costs . . . . . . . . . . . . . 324
Variable Costs . . . . . . . . . . . 324
Financial Records . . . . . . 324
Income Statement . . . . . . . . 324
Balance Sheet . . . . . . . . . 324
Useful Financial Ratios . . . 326
Accounts Receivable Ratio . . 327
Collection Ratio . . . . . . . . . 327
Cost Ratio . . . . . . . . . . . . . 327
Expenses of the Ambulatory
Care Setting . . . . . . . . . . . 327
Accounts Payable . . . . . . . . 327
Payroll . . . . . . . . . . . . . . . . 327

# SECTION III: PROFESSIONAL PROCEDURES    331

**Unit 6:    Office and Human Resource Management    332**

**Chapter 22: The Medical Assistant as Office Manager    333**

The Medical Assistant as
Manager . . . . . . . . . . . . . 335
Qualities of a Manager . . . . 335
Management Styles . . . . . . 336
People-oriented Personality . 336
Things-oriented Personality . 336
Idea-oriented Personality . . . 336
Other Management Styles . . 336
Changing Styles for the
Twenty-first Century . . . . . . 337
The Importance of
Teamwork . . . . . . . . . . . . 337
Getting the Team Started . . . 338
Using a Team to Solve a
Problem . . . . . . . . . . . . . . 338
Planning and Implementing
a Solution . . . . . . . . . . . . . 338
Recognition . . . . . . . . . . . . 338
Supervising Personnel . . . . 338
Staff Meetings . . . . . . . . . . 339
Supporting Staff Members . . . 340
Travel Arrangements . . . . . 340
Itinerary . . . . . . . . . . . . . . . 340
Supervising Student
Practicums . . . . . . . . . . . . 341
Time Management . . . . . . . 342
Procedures Manual . . . . . . 342
Organization of the
Procedures Manual . . . . . . . 342
Updating and Reviewing
the Procedures Manual . . . . . 343
Marketing Functions . . . . . 343
Seminars . . . . . . . . . . . . . . 343
Brochures . . . . . . . . . . . . . 344
Newsletters . . . . . . . . . . . . 345

Press Releases . . . . . . . . . . . 345
Special Events . . . . . . . . . . . 345
Record and Financial
Management . . . . . . . . . . . 345
Payroll Processing . . . . . . . . 347
Facility and Equipment
Management . . . . . . . . . . . 348
Inventories . . . . . . . . . . . . . 348
Equipment and Supplies
Maintenance . . . . . . . . . . . 349
Risk Management . . . . . . . 349
Liability Coverage and
Bonding . . . . . . . . . . . . . . 349

**Chapter 23: The Medical Assistant as Human Resources Manager    357**

Tasks Performed by the
Human Resources
Manager . . . . . . . . . . . . . 358
The Office Policy Manual . 359
Recruiting and Hiring
Office Personnel . . . . . . . 359
Job Descriptions . . . . . . . . 359
Recruiting . . . . . . . . . . . . . 360
Preparing to Interview
Applicants . . . . . . . . . . . . . 360
The Interview . . . . . . . . . . . 361
Selecting the Finalists . . . . . . 362
Orienting and Training
New Personnel . . . . . . . . . 363
Evaluating Employees and
Planning Salary Review . . . 363
Performance Evaluation . . . . 363
Salary Review . . . . . . . . . . . 366
Dismissing Employees . . . . 366
Involuntary Dismissal . . . . . 367
Voluntary Dismissal . . . . . . . 367
Exit Interview . . . . . . . . . . . 367
Maintaining Personnel
Records . . . . . . . . . . . . . . 368
Complying with Personnel
Laws . . . . . . . . . . . . . . . . . 368
Special Policy
Considerations . . . . . . . . . . 368
Temporary Employees . . . . . 368
Smoking Policy . . . . . . . . . . 370
Discrimination . . . . . . . . . . . 370
Employees with Chemical
Dependencies or Emotional
Problems . . . . . . . . . . . . . . 370
Providing/Planning
Employee Training and
Education . . . . . . . . . . . . . 370
Conflict Resolution . . . . . . 371

**Unit 7:    Entry into the Profession    376**

**Chapter 24: Preparing for Medical Assisting Credentials    377**

Purpose of Certification . . . 378
Preparing for the
Examination . . . . . . . . . . 378

Registered Medical
Assistant (RMA) . . . . . . . . 379
Examination Format and
Content . . . . . . . . . . . . . . 379
Application Process . . . . . . . 380
Application Completion
and Test Administration
Scheduling . . . . . . . . . . . . 380
Certified Medical Assistant
(CMA) . . . . . . . . . . . . . . 380
Examination Format and
Content . . . . . . . . . . . . . . 380
Application Process . . . . . . . 381
Eligibility Categories and
Requirements . . . . . . . . . . . 381
Grounds for Denial of
Eligibillity . . . . . . . . . . . . . 381
How to Recertify . . . . . . . . 382

**Chapter 25: Employment Strategies    387**

Ⓐ **Resume Writing**
Developing a Strategy . . . . 388
Self-Assessment . . . . . . . . . . 388
Job Analysis and
Research . . . . . . . . . . . . . 388
Budgetary Needs
Analysis . . . . . . . . . . . . . . 390
Resume Preparation . . . . . . 391
Resume Specifications . . . . . . 391
Clear and Concise
Resumes . . . . . . . . . . . . . . 391
Accomplishments . . . . . . . . 391
References . . . . . . . . . . . . . 392
Accuracy . . . . . . . . . . . . . . 392
Resume Styles . . . . . . . . . . 392
Vital Resume Information . . . 396
Application/Cover
Letters . . . . . . . . . . . . . . . 396
Completing the Application
Form . . . . . . . . . . . . . . . . 396
The Look of Success . . . . . 398
Personal and Professional
Poise . . . . . . . . . . . . . . . . 398
The Interview Process . . . . . 399
Preparing for the Interview . . 399
The Actual Interview . . . . . . 399
Closing the Interview . . . . . . 400
Interview Follow-Up . . . . . 400
Follow-Up Letter . . . . . . . . 400
Follow Up by Telephone . . . . 401

**Appendix A    Common Medical Abbreviations and Symbols    405**

**Appendix B    Top 200 Drugs by Retail Sales in 2000    411**

**Appendix C    Medical Assistant Role Delineation Chart    415**

**Appendix D    Answers to Case Study Reviews    417**

**Glossary    424**

**Index    435**

# MANAGING AUTHORS

**Wilburta** (Billie) **Q. Lindh**, CMA, holds professor emeritus status at Highline Community College, Des Moines, Washington, and currently serves as program director and consultant to the Medical Assistant Program. She is a member of the SeaTac Chapter of the American Association of Medical Assistants (AAMA) and has lectured at AAMA seminars on the importance of communication. Lindh is co-author of *Therapeutic Communications for Allied Health Professions* published by Delmar. She has also co-authored *The Radiology Word Book* and *The Ophthalmology Word Book*, texts frequently used by transcriptionists. Lindh also authored the medical assistant chapter for *Guide to Careers in the Health Professions*.

**Marilyn S. Pooler**, RN, CMA-C, MEd, is a professor in the Medical Assisting Department at Springfield Technical Community College, Springfield, Massachusetts. Pooler has taught at Springfield for 24 years and previously served as chair of the Medical Assisting Department. She has served on the certifying board of the AAMA task force for test construction and is a member of the executive board of the New England Association of Allied Health Educators. She also is a site surveyor for AAMA, reviewing medical assisting programs at schools and colleges seeking accreditation.

**Carol D. Tamparo**, CMA-A, PhD, is Dean of Business and Allied Health at Lake Washington Technical College in Kirkland, Washington. Tamparo, who taught at Highline Community College in Des Moines, Washington, for 23 years, is a member of the SeaTac Chapter of the AAMA. Tamparo, a speaker at numerous AAMA seminars and educational conferences, is recognized as an expert on medical law, ethics, and bioethics. She is the co-author of *Diseases of the Human Body*; *Medical Law, Ethics, and Bioethics for Ambulatory Care*; and *Therapeutic Communications for Allied Health Professions*.

# ACKNOWLEDGMENTS

The managing authors personally acknowledge the following people:

To my husband, who continually supports and assists in so many ways, thank you. To my family for support and encouragement, and to Laura, who provided expertise for some chapters, thank you. To the students, graduates, and fellow colleagues who challenge me to stay current with skills and up-to-date with technology, thank you.

**Billie Q. Lindh**

Thanks to my friends who were very supportive of my efforts, and a special thanks to my husband, Jud, for his patience and understanding during this endeavor.

**Marilyn S. Pooler**

To all my students in health care programs who keep me current, to my school administrators and family members who have been supportive of this project, and to the health care providers who patiently and lovingly cared for my mother in an assisted living Alzheimer's unit until her death in April 2001, my thanks and deepest regard and respect.

**Carol D. Tamparo**

# REVIEWERS

Kaye Acton
Director of Medical Assisting Program
Alamance Community College
Graham, NC

Magdalena Andrasevits, NRCMA
Medical Assistant Program Director
Sanford-Brown College
North Kansas City, MO

Joseph DeSapio, RMA
Director of Facility and Library
    Resources
Medical Assisting Instructor
Ultrasound Diagnostic School
New York, NY

Eleanor K. Flores, RN, BSN, MEd
Briarwood College
Southington, CT

Tova Green
IVTC Fort Wayne
Fort Wayne, IN

Karen Jackson, NR-CMA
Medical Program Chair
Education America, Dallas Campus
Garland, TX

Barbara G. Kalfin, BS, AAS, CMA-C
Medical Assisting Extern Coordinator
Instructor, Medical Assisting Program
City College
Ft. Lauderdale, FL

Theresa Offenberger, PhD
Professor of Medical Assisting
Cuyahoga Community College
Cleveland, OH

Agnes Pucillo, LPN
Medical Assisting Program Director
Ultrasound Diagnostic School
Iselin, NJ

Patricia Schrull, RN, MBA, MEd,
    CMA
Program Director, Medical Assisting
    Program
Lorain County Community College
Elyria, OH

Janet Sesser, BS Ed. Admin., RMA,
    CMA
Corporate Director of Education,
    Allied Health
High-Tech Institute, Inc.
Phoenix, AZ

Kimberly A. Shinall, RN
President and CEO
KAS Enterprises
Virginia Beach, VA

Lois M. Smith, RN, CMA
Arapahoe Community College
Golden, CO

Susan Sniffin
Suffolk Community College
Great Neck, NY

Alisa M. Tetlow, RMA
Medical Assistant Program Director
Ultrasound Diagnostic School
Philadelphia, PA

Nina Thierer
Tidewater Technical Institute
Virginia Beach, VA

Fred Valdes, MD
Medical Department Chairman
City College
Ft. Lauderdale, FL

Sujana Wardell, RMA, RPT (AMT),
    AS
Program Director for Clinical and
    Administrative Medical Assisting
San Joaquin Valley College, Visalia
    Campus
Visalia, CA

Sally Wooten
Whitman Education Group
Miami, FL

Terri Wyman, CMA
Director of Health Information
    Specialties
Ultrasound Diagnostic School
Springfield, MA

# CONTRIBUTORS

**Sandra K. Anderson**, MS
Chapter 11: *Computers in the Ambulatory Care Setting*

**Bonnie Lou Deister**, MS, BSN, RN, CMA-C
Chapter 22: *The Medical Assistant as Office Manager* and Chapter 23: *The Medical Assistant as Human Resources Manager*

**Jeanette Girkin**, EdD, CMA
Chapter 15: *Written Communications*

**Mary K. Hickey**
Chapter 12: *Telephone Techniques* and Chapter 17: *Daily Financial Practices*

**Jan L. Johnson**, MEd, CMA
Chapter 13: *Patient Scheduling* and Chapter 14: *Medical Records Management*

**Benna Kisin**, CMT
Chapter 15: *Written Communications*

**Kathy A. McCall**, CMA-AC, BS, MA
Chapter 20: *Billing and Collections* and Chapter 21: *Accounting Practices*

**Sylvia Taylor**, BS, CMA
Chapter 2: *Health Care Settings and the Health Care Team*

**Virginia Lawless Thompson**
Chapter 9: *Emergency Procedures and First Aid*

**Ginny Torres**, CMA
Chapter 19: *Medical Insurance Coding*

# LIST OF PROCEDURES

9-1     Control of Bleeding
9-2     Applying an Arm Splint
9-3     Heimlich Maneuver for a Conscious Adult
9-4     Heimlich Maneuver for an Unconscious Adult or Child
9-5     Heimlich Maneuver for a Conscious Child
9-6     Back Blows and Chest Thrusts for a Conscious Infant Who Is Choking
9-7     Back Blows and Chest Thrusts for an Unconscious Infant
9-8     Rescue Breathing for Adults
9-9     Rescue Breathing for Children
9-10    Rescue Breathing for Infants
9-11    CPR for Adults
9-12    CPR for Children
9-13    CPR for Infants
12-1    Answering Incoming Calls
12-2    Handling Problem Calls
12-3    Placing Outgoing Calls
13-1    Checking in Patients
13-2    Cancellation Procedures
13-3    Establishing the Appointment Matrix
14-1    Steps for Manual Filing with a Numeric System
14-2    Steps for Manual Filing with a Subject Filing System
15-1    Preparing and Composing Business Correspondence Using All Components
15-2    Addressing Envelopes According to United States Postal Regulations
15-3    Folding Letters for Standard Envelopes
15-4    Preparing Outgoing Mail According to United States Postal Regulations
15-5    Preparing, Sending, and Receiving a Fax
17-1    Preparation for Posting a Day Sheet
17-2    Recording Charges and Payments Requiring a Charge Slip (Patient Visits)
17-3    Receiving a Payment on Account Requiring a Receipt
17-4    Recording Payments Received Through the Mail
17-5    Balancing Day Sheets
17-6    Preparing a Deposit
17-7    Reconciling a Bank Statement
17-8    Balancing Petty Cash
22-1    Preparing a Meeting Agenda
22-2    Making Travel Arrangements
22-3    Making Travel Arrangements Via Internet
22-4    Supervising a Student Practicum
22-5    Developing and Maintaining a Procedures Manual
23-1    Develop and Maintain a Policy Manual
23-2    Preparing a Job Description
23-3    Interviewing
23-4    Orient and Train Personnel

# PREFACE

The world of health care has changed rapidly over the past few years, and as we travel through the 21st century, health care professionals will encounter more challenges than ever before. As medical assistants you will be called on to do more and respond to an increasing number of administrative responsibilities, especially in this age of managed care. Now is the time to equip yourself with the skills you will need to excel in the field. Now is the time to maximize your potential, expand your base of knowledge, and dedicate yourself to becoming the best multifaceted, multiskilled medical assistant that you can be.

The new edition of *Delmar's Administrative Medical Assisting* will guide you on this journey. This text is part of a dynamic learning system that also includes an administrative skills CD-ROM and a workbook. Together, these learning tools conform to the standard and advanced areas of competence defined by AAMA's Role Delineation Study and AMT's Registered Medical Assistant Competency Inventory. They emphasize the importance of interpersonal communications in the medical environment. They explore changes in the health care setting including the development of standard precautions and the implications of managed care. This powerful learning system gives you an intimate look at the challenges you'll face and the opportunities you'll find as a medical assistant.

Unlike many texts, *Delmar's Administrative Medical Assisting*, 2nd edition, was written not just by one or two individuals but by many talented authors—experts who give you a sound and thorough understanding of the fundamentals. The text then moves beyond theory and develops all concepts in a real-life situation. What is it like to be working in the field? What are the problems you may encounter?

You'll discover common challenges faced by medical assistants through realistic scenarios woven into the chapter introductions. Case studies depict the ambulatory care setting where you, as a medical assistant, may very well be employed. Patient teaching tips provide practical advice. Proper documentation is emphasized.

## How the Text Is Organized

*Delmar's Administrative Medical Assisting*, 2nd edition, presents a logical, in-depth review of all administrative competencies required of today's multiskilled medical assistants—*in full color!*

- **Section I, General Procedures (Chapters 1 through 9)**, provides the groundwork for understanding the role and responsibilities of the medical assistant. Topics include the medical assisting profession, the health care team, history of medicine, therapeutic communications, coping skills for the medical assistant, legal and ethical issues, and emergency procedures and first aid.

- **Section II, Administrative Procedures (Chapters 10 through 21)**, provides up-to-date information on all administrative competencies required of medical assistants. Topics include creating the facility environment, computer use, telephone techniques, patient scheduling, medical records management, written communications, transcription, insurance and coding, managing facility finances, billing and collections, and accounting practices.

- **Section III, Professional Procedures (Chapters 22 through 25)**, examines the role of the medical assistant as office and human resources manager and provides tools and techniques to use when preparing for externship, medical assisting credentials, and employment.

- **Appendices** include (A) Common Medical Abbreviations and Symbols, (B) Top 200 Drugs, (C) the Medical Assistant Role Delineation Chart, and (D) Answers to the Case Study Reviews.

- **Glossary** includes definitions of all key terms, with related chapter numbers indicated.

- **The Medical Assisting Administrative Skills CD** is found on the inside back cover of this book. This interactive software challenges you to apply content, think critically, develop competency in skills, and improve your knowledge base.

## How Each Chapter Is Organized

All chapters include similar features and presentation and function as building blocks to a comprehensive medical assisting education. However, each chapter is also a self-contained module and can be studied in any order or independently of other chapters in the text.

Features include:

- A listing of *key terms*
- *Role delineation components*, both standard and advanced
- An *outline of chapter*
- *Objectives*
- An *introduction* with a real-life scenario

- *Graphic icons, tables, and figures*
- *Full-color illustrations and photographs*
- *Procedures* with step-by-step instructions
- *Patient teaching tips*
- *Spotlight on AAMA Essentials through CAAHEP* boxes
- *Case studies with review questions*
- *Summary*
- *Review questions*
- *Web Activities*
- *Bibliography* for further study

To receive the full value of *Delmar's Administrative Medical Assisting*, 2nd edition, it is important to understand the structure of the text and each chapter. Review the following information, plus "How to Use This Book" and "How to Use the Medical Assisting Administrative Skills CD-ROM." Together, these materials will make your medical assisting education comprehensive and meaningful, providing you with the skills and understanding to enable you to practice your profession with confidence and competence.

## EXTENSIVE TEACHING/LEARNING PACKAGE

The complete supplements package helps instructors efficiently manage time and resources and helps students develop the necessary skills and competencies required by the demanding profession of medical assisting.

### Instructor's Manual

Order #0-7668-2424-1
This compact resource is designed as a quick reference tool for classroom activity and instruction. Chapters include:

- Proficiency assessments
- Answers to text review questions
- Answers to text critical thinking questions
- Answers to workbook exercises
- Answers to workbook case studies

### Student Workbook

Order #0-7668-2425-X
The workbook helps you learn and reinforce the essential competencies needed to become a successful, multiskilled medical assistant. Each chapter includes:

- Vocabulary builder exercises
- Learning review
- Investigation activity
- Case study
- Skills assessment checklist

## *Instructor's Resource Kit (Comprehensive)*

Order #0-7668-2419-5
This dynamic resource is a must-have for all instructors. This comprehensive three-ring binder includes:

**Instructor's Guide.** Complete with teaching strategies and learning concepts, this print and electronic resource offers:

- Teaching/learning concepts
- Objectives and evaluation
- Instructional strategies
- Lesson plans
- Classroom activities

**Computerized and Printed Testbank.** Both electronic and printed testbanks are included, containing approximately 1,200 multiple choice questions.

**PowerPoint Slides.** The CD included in the *Instructor's Resource Kit* contains over 250 PowerPoint slides, making a backdrop with impact for your classroom presentations.

**Medical Assisting CD-ROM.** This is an innovative, comprehensive multimedia learning reference tool to enhance classroom presentations and increase student learning.

# HOW TO USE THIS BOOK

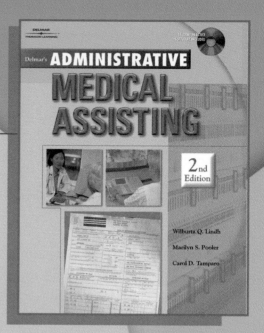

Delmar's *Administrative Medical Assisting, 2nd edition*, contains many features that make it an easy-to-use learning system. They include:

## 1 Key Terms

All key terms are listed at the beginning of each chapter. Within the text, the term is always boldfaced at its first occurrence for easy identification. Turn to the glossary for definitions of all key terms.

## 2 Chapter Outline

At the beginning of each chapter, you'll find an outline of all major headings. Review these headings of topic areas before you study the chapter. They are a road map to your understanding.

## 3 Objectives

Performance objectives test your knowledge of the key facts presented in the chapter. Use these objectives, together with review questions, to test your understanding of the chapter's content.

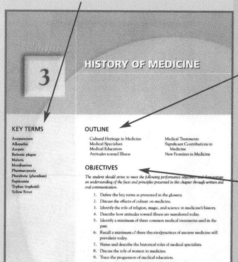

## 4 Role Delineation Components

This opening list in each chapter keeps the focus on the medical assistant's actual job functions as defined by the accrediting bodies.

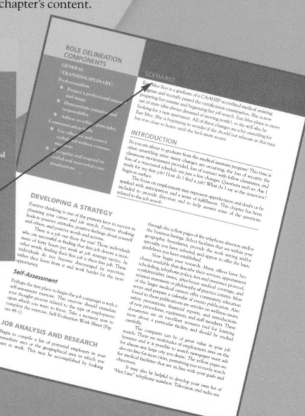

## 5 Real-Life Scenarios

The introductions to most chapters include an overview of the material *and* a real-life scenario based on two distinct ambulatory care settings and their physicians, medical assistants, and patients. Through these scenarios you'll come to understand some of the stimulating challenges faced by medical assistants and gain insight into how these challenges are overcome.

## 6 Patient Teaching Tips

This feature helps all current and future medical assistants anticipate patient concerns and provides sound suggestions for effective patient communication.

### Patient Teaching Tip

Encourage patients to think of themselves as members of the health care team for they can provide information about their medical history. Use good communication skills to encourage the patient to describe symptoms and provide other information that is useful in diagnosis and treatment.

*ied and Other Health Profession
*heir Roles*

## 7 Icons

Graphic icons pinpoint information that relates to legal, safety, computer, managed care, and global or cultural issues.

## 8 Procedures

Step-by-step procedures are now conveniently grouped together at the end of each chapter. They give detailed information on all important administrative, clinical, and general competencies as defined by AAMA and AMT.

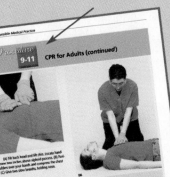

**Procedure 9-11**
**CPR for Adults (continued)**

Figure 9-27 (A) Tilt back head and lift chin. Locate hand on the breastbone two inches above xiphoid process. (B) Position your shoulders over your hands and compress the chest fifteen times. (C) Give two slow breaths, holding nose.

8. Do three more sets of fifteen compressions and two breaths.
9. Check the pulse and breathing for about 10-15 seconds.
10. If there is no pulse, continue sets of fifteen compressions and two breaths.
11. Dispose of waste in biohazard container.
12. Remove gloves, dispose of in biohazard container, and wash hands.
13. Document the procedure.

## 9 Spotlight on AAMA Essentials through CAAHEP

These psychology tips help you focus on the CAAHEP-mandated understandings required of medical assistants.

### SPOTLIGHT ON AAMA ESSENTIALS THROUGH CAAHEP

● Recognizing a patient's cultural background is part of caring for the patient as a whole person.
● Human kindness often eliminates fear of the unknown.
● A positive attitude helps to lessen a negative feeling.

*tines everyone who tests posi*
*ciency virus (HIV)*

## 10 Web Activities

This new feature at the end of each chapter gives you practice navigating the Internet by suggesting online activities to help you begin to use those sites.

## 11 Case Studies

The case studies with accompanying review questions encourage a problem/solution approach. Use the case studies to put your knowledge into practice and arrive at a deeper understanding of the profession. Answers to the case studies are included as an appendix of the text.

## 12 Review Questions

Test your comprehension of the chapter with structured multiple choice questions and open-ended critical thinking questions that require you to combine an understanding of chapter material with your personal insight and judgment.

## 13 Administrative Skills CD Quick Locator

This invaluable tool located in the table of contents tells you when to turn to your skills CD-ROM for practice activities that will strengthen your understanding of the chapter you are reading.

# HOW TO USE THE MEDICAL ASSISTING ADMINISTRATIVE SKILLS CD

The Administrative Skills CD is designed to accompany **Delmar's Administrative Medical Assisting, 2nd edition,** so you can review and reinforce the important concepts you are learning in the textbook. By using this CD, you'll challenge yourself and make your study of medical assisting concepts more effective and fun.

The Administrative Skills CD-ROM is designed with you, the user, in mind. Several medical assistants lead you on a verbal guided tour through the medical office.

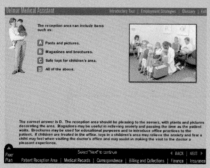

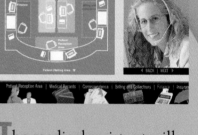

An introductory tour gives you an overview of the entire office. To navigate through the office, click on the area you wish to visit.

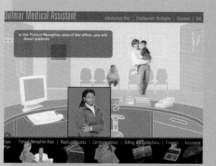

The medical assistant will give you an overview of the tasks and responsibilities associated with each area, and guide you through your many choices. In the patient reception area, for example, you may click on the active areas such as the computer, the phone, the answering machine, or the patient to branch into different content areas.

The medical assistant will give you instruction so you understand the various aspects of each area. Activities include multiple choice questions with correct and incorrect responses noted, scheduling appointments by dragging and dropping the information into the appointment book, filling out a message pad, and maintaining a telephone log.

In other areas such as billing and collections, you will be asked to complete a patient receipt by entering information into the correct area, fill out a daily log sheet, use the pegboard system, complete a super bill and ledger card by entering and highlighting information, complete a patient charge slip, write a check, and complete a deposit slip.

In the break room, you can test your knowledge of legal and ethical principles by completing a crossword puzzle.

A comprehensive glossary allows you to check your understanding of important key words and phrases.

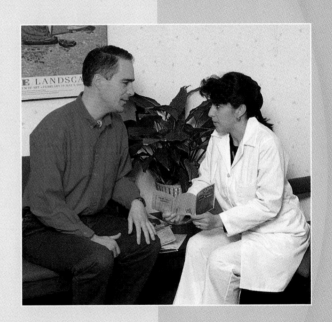

# GENERAL PROCEDURES

# INTRODUCTION TO MEDICAL ASSISTING AND HEALTH PROFESSIONS

# 1

# MEDICAL ASSISTING AS A PROFESSION

## KEY TERMS

Accreditation
Ambulatory Care Setting
Attribute
Baccalaureate
Certification
Certified Medical Assistant (CMA)
Competency
Compliance
Credentialed
Disposition
Empathy
Externship
Facilitate
Improvise
Integrate
Internship
License
Licensure
Litigious
Practicum
Proprietary
Registered Medical Assistant (RMA)

## OUTLINE

**Personal Attributes
of the Professional**
  Empathy
  Attitude
  Dependability
  Initiative
  Flexibility
  Desire to Learn
  Physical Attributes
  Ability to Communicate
  Ethical Behavior
**Historical Perspective
of Medical Assisting**

**American Association of
  Medical Assistants**
  Accreditation
  Certification
  Continuing Education
**Registered Medical Assistant**
**Education of the Professional
  Medical Assistant**
  Preparation for Externship
**Career Opportunities**
**Regulation of Health Care
  Providers**
  Scope of Practice

## OBJECTIVES

*The student should strive to meet the following performance objectives and demonstrate an understanding of the facts and principles presented in this chapter through written and oral communication.*

1. Define the key terms as presented in the glossary.
2. Identify and discuss nine personal attributes that are important for a professional medical assistant to possess.
3. Discuss the history of medical assisting.
4. Describe the American Association of Medical Assistants and list its three major functions.
5. Explain accreditation, certification, and continuing education as they pertain to the professional medical assistant.
6. Identify the importance of the accreditation process to an educational institution.
7. Recall two methods to obtain recertification.
8. List five means of obtaining continuing education units. *(continues)*

## OBJECTIVES (*continued*)

9. Describe the certifying agency that certifies medical assistants as registered medical assistants (RMA).
10. Describe the externship experience.
11. Recall two criteria for the selection of externship sites.
12. List three benefits of externship to student and site.
13. Describe the profession of medical assisting and analyze its career opportunities in relationship to your interests.
14. Differentiate among certification, licensure, and registration.
15. State the importance of understanding the scope of practice for the medical assistant.

## ROLE DELINEATION COMPONENTS

### GENERAL (TRANSDISCIPLINARY)

**Professionalism**

- Project a professional manner and image
- Adhere to ethical principles
- Demonstrate initiative and responsibility
- Work as a team member
- Adapt to change
- Promote the CMA credential
- Enhance skills through continuing education

**Legal Concepts**

- Maintain confidentiality
- Practice within the scope of education, training, and personal capabilities

## INTRODUCTION

Historically, medical science has been fascinating to most people. Perhaps you have been drawn to medical assisting because you too are intrigued by medicine and want to learn about advances in health care and want to become involved in providing care to patients. More than likely you have a desire to help others.

Medical assistants have always played an integral role in physicians' offices and ambulatory care settings such as clinics and urgent care facilities, where health care services are offered on an outpatient basis. And now more than ever, because of the explosion of knowledge and high technology in medicine, medical assistants are involved in an ever-widening scope of clinical and administrative duties. With the medical assistant's expanded role has come the responsibility to become a well-educated and highly competent professional dedicated to providing the highest quality of health care.

Consumers of health care have become increasingly aware, primarily through the media, of the availability of the latest advances, techniques, and discoveries in medicine. They realize that they have a right for health care to be provided to them by educated, skilled, and competent professionals.

As you study to become a medical assistant, it is important for you to understand what a professional is. According to *Merriam-Webster's Collegiate Dictionary*, 10th edition, it is "one who has acquired a specialized body of knowledge, skills, and attitudes."

You will learn to integrate, or unify, your desire and need to help others with the knowledge, skills, and attitudes you acquire through your studies. By blending all of these, you will be able to provide patients with the best health care possible and learn what it means to be a professional medical assistant.

## PERSONAL ATTRIBUTES OF THE PROFESSIONAL

There are certain characteristics or personal qualities that medical assistants should strive to cultivate. These are the attributes that identify a true professional; when caring for patients these qualities should come from the heart. They will enable the patient to trust you, the caregiver.

## Empathy

To have **empathy** means to consider the patient's welfare and to be kind. It means stepping into the patient's place, discovering what the patient is experiencing, and then recognizing and identifying with those feelings.

Medical assistants should treat patients as they themselves would want to be treated. A visit to the doctor is often a time of fear and anxiety. Apprehension can be allayed tremendously when patients realize that their caregiver understands their feelings and desires to make their lives more pleasant and comfortable. See Figure 1-1.

It is important to realize that patients' health problems can have a profound effect on the caregiver. By maintaining a balanced outlook, medical assistants can safeguard themselves from becoming too emotionally involved with patient problems. Empathy is extremely important in the health care profession; however, emotionalism can cloud one's judgment.

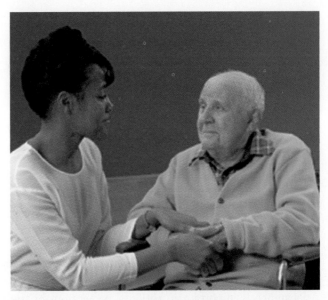

**Figure 1-1** The medical assistant should have a friendly disposition and communicate empathy for the patient.

## Attitude

A friendly, warm **disposition** and a sense of humor will help patients feel more at ease. A sincere affection for people can be conveyed by actions that **facilitate** open and honest communication. Your attitude should radiate genuine interest.

On occasion, difficult patients can test the tolerance level of the most experienced medical assistant because they seem never to be content with the care or services received. But no matter what the circumstances, patients should never be treated with disinterest or in an unfriendly manner. The medical assistant should always be pleasant and courteous.

When giving care to patients, do so unrestricted by your concerns about their attitudes, disease, race, religion, economic status, or sexual orientation.

As a member of the health care delivery team, the medical assistant needs to be cooperative and supportive of all other members, working with the team in an honest, open manner while keeping in mind the patient's right to privacy and confidentiality.

## Dependability

When providing for a patient's well-being, it is important to focus attention on activities in the office or clinic environment that will demonstrate being well-organized, accurate, and responsive to the patient's needs.

Being dependable means that employer and coworkers rely on the medical assistant to be respectful of them, of patients, and of equipment and materials. Other members of the health care team will expect duties and responsibilities to be carried out responsibly. A dependable person interacts with coworkers in a supportive manner, is punctual, and limits absences from work.

## Initiative

The willingness and ability to work independently shows initiative. A person with initiative is observant, notices work that needs to be done, and then takes action to complete those tasks without being told to do them. Employer and coworkers must be able to count on one another to anticipate patients' needs and be attentive to work that needs to be accomplished. The successful medical assistant will be ready to pitch in and recognize when others need assistance.

By asking appropriate questions and seeking information that will improve performance, medical assistants will demonstrate that they have the foresight and the "get up and go" needed to complete the numerous and varied tasks of the ambulatory care environment.

## Flexibility

The ability to be adaptable is a trait that serves all professionals well. When caring for ill people, unexpected situations arise daily and medical assistants must be able to respond to a variety of situations (many of them emergencies and unanticipated) without losing a sense of equilibrium. Finding solutions to problems and developing alternative action plans demonstrates flexibility. To **improvise,** or solve problems that arise either routinely or spontaneously, is a characteristic worth nurturing.

## Desire to Learn

A willingness to continually learn and grow is the mark of a true professional. With the growing technology in medicine, there is an ongoing necessity for constant learning. Medical assistants must be dedicated to high standards of performance, which can be accomplished by showing a desire to acquire information and by constantly updating their knowledge and skills. Keeping abreast of the latest diseases, treatments, procedures, and techniques can be achieved in a variety of ways, such as college courses, seminars, workshops, reading, and simply by being observant. The sharper the power of observation, the more the medical assistant will learn from physician, employer, and coworkers.

## Physical Attributes

Appearance is important in patients' perceptions of the delivery of their care. Imparting the look of a professional requires an appearance that is clean and fresh and wholesome; in general, an appearance that reflects good health habits (Figure 1-2). Good personal hygiene practices, weight control, healthy-looking skin, hair, teeth, and nails all contribute to a professional appearance. Rest, good nutrition, regular exercise, and recreation all promote good health.

Female medical assistants should wear appropriate light daytime makeup. For the safety of both the profes-sional and the patient, no necklaces or dangling earrings should be worn. The only jewelry worn should be single earposts or wedding rings. Hair should be neat and off the collar. Wear only clear, unchipped nail polish over short, manicured nails. Male medical assistants should be clean-shaven and have short hair. The only jewelry should be a wedding ring. Colognes, perfumes, and aftershave should not be worn at work. Tattoos should not be visible.

Patient care can place physical demands upon medical assistants. Lifting and moving patients is often required and the use of correct body mechanics will help minimize injuries to the back. While every reasonable accommodation is made for physically challenged medical assistants, to be mobile without assistance is important because medical assistants move about throughout the day while performing tasks and procedures. It is frequently necessary to bend, stoop, kneel, and crouch, especially when filing and retrieving patients' records, and for other tasks as well. Most procedures require that medical assistants have the ability to hear and see well for the accurate completion of tasks (Figure 1-3). Listening to blood pressures, taking a medical history, observing patients, performing phlebotomy, and identifying microorganisms under a microscope are some of the routine tasks and procedures performed daily in a medical facility.

Manual dexterity is also needed for manipulating certain instruments and for entering data using a computer.

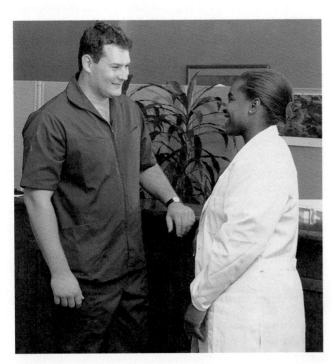

**Figure 1-2**  A professional, neat appearance makes patients feel at ease with their health care provider.

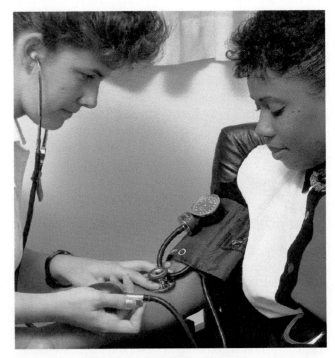

**Figure 1-3**  Measuring blood pressure is a task that requires the medical assistant to see and hear well.

## Ability to Communicate

It is important that medical assistants learn to develop the ability to communicate well verbally and nonverbally with patients, staff, and other professionals.

Compliance with the physician's treatment plan is important for a positive outcome of patients' illnesses (Figure 1-4). Also, patients will feel more comfortable and less threatened in a medical office or ambulatory center that encourages staff to keep them informed.

## Ethical Behavior

No discussion about personal attributes is complete without the mention of ethics. Ethics is a system of values each individual has that determines perceptions of right and wrong. Our life experiences mold this set of values, which is considered a personal code of ethics.

Medical ethics govern medical conduct or that behavior practiced as health care providers. These ethics involve relationships with patients, their families, fellow professionals, and society in general. Good ethical behavior will have a positive impact on the profession of medical assisting and on the medical community as well. By adhering to the medical assistants' Code of Ethics, we endeavor to elevate the profession to a position of dignity and respect. (A more in-depth discussion of this Code of Ethics can be found in Chapter 8.)

The personal qualities of empathy, healthy attitude, dependability, initiative, flexibility, the desire to learn, a wholesome physical presence, the ability to communicate well, and ethical behavior are some of the characteristics that any professional possesses and that medical assistants should strive to develop. When entering into the profession of medical assisting, it is important to learn more about these and other qualities and to begin to cultivate and refine them.

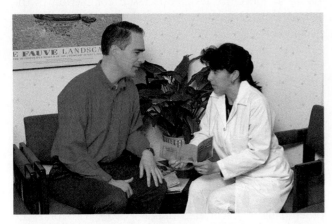

**Figure 1-4**  Patient education requires skill in communicating instructions to patients in language appropriate to their needs.

### SPOTLIGHT ON AAMA ESSENTIALS THROUGH CAAHEP

- It is your attributes that enable others to trust you as their caregiver.
- A true professional behaves in an ethical manner.
- Continuing education should be an ongoing and life-enhancing experience.

## HISTORICAL PERSPECTIVE OF MEDICAL ASSISTING

Historically, when physicians began their practices, it was common for them to hire individuals and train them on the job. Physicians originally hired nurses, but eventually they came to realize that nurses could not perform the variety of duties that are required in medical offices and ambulatory care centers. The nurse's role was limited to assisting the physician with clinical procedures, whereas the medical assistant's role was and is much broader and includes a large number of activities, procedures, and responsibilities, both administrative and clinical.

Today, with a much more informed patient comes the need for educated and credentialed medical assistants. Additionally, in today's litigious atmosphere, which makes health care providers vulnerable to malpractice suits, most employers recognize the importance of employing medical assistants who are professionally prepared through formal education. Employers want knowledgeable and dependable medical assistants so that physicians can focus their time and attention on the medical decisions, treatments, and techniques for which they have been educated and licensed. This leaves in the hands of the medical assistant, assisting the physician and the operation and management of the practice.

It was in 1978 that the profession of medical assisting was formally recognized by the United States Department of Education. Twenty-four years prior to this official recognition of the profession, a group of medical assistants gathered to establish a professional organization. With support, encouragement, and guidance from the American Medical Association (AMA), the American Association of Medical Assistants (AAMA) was founded in 1956 (Figure 1-5). The first president of the organization was Maxine Williams.

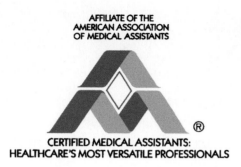

AFFILIATE OF THE
AMERICAN ASSOCIATION
OF MEDICAL ASSISTANTS

CERTIFIED MEDICAL ASSISTANTS:
HEALTHCARE'S MOST VERSATILE PROFESSIONALS

**Figure 1-5**　Logo of the American Association of Medical Assistants, a professional organization founded in 1956. (Courtesy of the AAMA)

In 1991, the AAMA's board of trustees approved the present definition of medical assisting:

> Medical Assisting is an allied health profession whose practitioners function as members of the health care delivery team and perform administrative and clinical procedures.

## AMERICAN ASSOCIATION OF MEDICAL ASSISTANTS

The American Association of Medical Assistants has three major purposes:

1. Accreditation
2. Certification
3. Continuing education

Accreditation and certification standards were developed by the AMA and the AAMA through the Commission on Accreditation of Allied Health Education Programs (CAAHEP) for schools wishing assurance that their medical assistant programs are of the highest quality and satisfy CAAHEP criteria.

### Accreditation

The AAMA works jointly with the AMA to define the essential components and appropriate standards of quality that educational institutions offer in their medical assistant curriculum. The United States Department of Education has approved the AAMA and AMA as an accreditation, or approving, body for educational programs for medical assistants. A medical assisting program that is accredited meets the standards as outlined in the *Standards and Guidelines for an Accredited Education Program for the Medical Assistant. Standards* are the minimum standards of quality used in accrediting programs that prepare individuals to enter the medical assisting profession. On-site review teams evaluate the program's compliance

with, or adherence to, the standards. All aspects of programs seeking accreditation status undergo scrutiny to ascertain the program's quality and to ensure continued compliance with the standards.

### Certification

As the profession grew and developed, some states came to require special licensure or certification to perform certain tasks, and in other states health professionals were challenged by the skill and broad spectrum of the medical assistant's ability. To defend medical assistants whose right to practice clinical procedures was being challenged, the AAMA responded at their 1995 convention with the following policy, which became effective February 1, 1998:

> that any candidate for the AAMA Certification Examination be a graduate of a CAAHEP-accredited medical assisting program. This requirement would become effective February 1, 1998. Anticipated benefits of the recommendation are to: (1) safeguard the quality of care to the consumer; (2) ensure the CMA's role in the rapidly evolving health care delivery system; and (3) continue to promote the identity and stature of the profession.

For a three-year trial period beginning in March 1998, graduates of medical assisting programs accredited by the Accrediting Bureau of Health Education Schools (ABHES) with 12 months of full-time health work experience or 24 months of part-time health work experience were eligible to take the AAMA certification examination.

Certification is voluntary, not mandatory, for medical assistants to practice, although the AAMA strongly urges those eligible to take the national certification examination. The exam measures professional competency at job entry level. Successful completion of the examination earns the individual the status of being certified and of being known as a certified medical assistant (CMA). The initials follow the individual's name. Conferring of the CMA status is referred to as being credentialed (Figure 1-6). It signifies recognition of competency by having attained a certain level of knowledge and skill.

In some areas of the United States, employers hire only certified medical assistants. The examination is offered twice yearly simultaneously at more than 200 test sites across the United States.

Recertification of the credential must be undertaken within five years from the date of certification in order to maintain current status as a CMA. Two routes are available to recertify. One is by accumulating approved continuing education hours, the other is by taking the certification examination again.

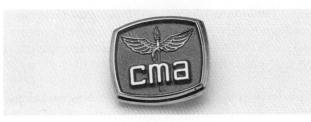

**Figure 1-6** CMA pin awarded by the American Association of Medical Assistants upon successful completion of the national certification examination.

The status of a medical assistant's credentials (whether current or not current) is a public record available at the AAMA executive office, 20 N. Wacker Dr., Suite 1575, Chicago, IL 60606-2963. The AAMA Board of Trustees approved a policy change at the association's 1999 annual convention in Nashville. Effective January 1, 2003, all certified medical assistants who are employed or seeking employment *must* have current status as a CMA in order to use the credential. The mandatory current status for use of the CMA designation protects patients, employers, and the medical assistant's right to practice. Certification and recertification attest to the medical assistant's desire for professional development.

At one time, the credentials CMA-A (Certified Medical Assistant, Administrative); CMA-C (Certified Medical Assistant, Clinical); CMA-AC (Certified Medical Assistant, Administrative and Clinical); and CMA-Ped (Certified Medical Assistant, Pediatrics) were awarded to candidates who successfully passed specialty examinations in addition to the basic CMA examination.

While these specialty examinations have been phased out for newly graduated medical assistants, current medical assistants who have already earned these specialty credentials can maintain them and continue to be recertified through the Continuing Education Unit method.

## *Continuing Education*

The AAMA vigorously encourages continuing education for all medical assistants. This can be accomplished through various means such as educational meetings, seminars, workshops, conventions, and the "Quest for Excellence," AAMA's series of home study courses for continuing education credit.

Membership in the AAMA is tri-level: local, state, and national. Educational meetings are held regularly at local and state meetings and conventions. The annual AAMA national convention provides an excellent forum for attaining knowledge through its educational offerings and for networking with other medical assistants.

Continuing an education is a lifelong process and serves as testimony to a commitment to professionalism.

## REGISTERED MEDICAL ASSISTANT

The American Medical Technologists (AMT) is a national agency that certifies several different health professionals including medical assistants. In 1972, the AMT began offering and administering a national certification examination to medical assistants. The AMT offers a computerized examination year-round to qualified candidates. Upon successful completion of the examination, medical assistants receive a certificate designating them as **registered medical assistants (RMA)**.

The association is similar to the AAMA. It has its own committees, conventions, bylaws, state chapters, officers, registrations, and revalidation examinations.

RMAs have been active in legislation to protect medical assistants, assuring improvement in medical assistant education, and providing for continuing education opportunities.

The RMA certification examination is given yearly in June and November at schools that have been accredited by the Accrediting Bureau of Health Education Schools (ABHES). To sit for the examination, applicants must have graduated from a medical assisting program accredited by ABHES or must meet certain experience requirements. AMT continuing education programs for renewal of the RMA credential also are available. The credential is awarded through the AMT (Figure 1-7). For more information, call 1-800-275-1268 or write to AMT, 710 Higgins Rd., Park Ridge, IL 60068.

## EDUCATION OF THE PROFESSIONAL MEDICAL ASSISTANT

Formal education of medical assistants takes place in community and junior colleges as well as in **proprietary** schools. The AAMA has established educational requirements for program directors to follow for their programs to be considered accredited. These requirements were previously known as the DACUM Competencies. In 1997, in coordination with the National Board of Medical Examiners, educators, and practicing CMAs, the AAMA developed the Medical Assistant Role Delineation Chart, which is the occupational analysis of the medical assisting profession, and is included as an appendix of this

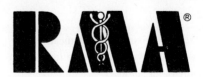

**Figure 1-7** Logo of Registered Medical Assistant, representing a credential awarded by the American Medical Technologists Association.

text. In addition, the entry-level competencies that must be mastered by students in academic programs and the *Standards* (formerly *"Essentials"*) *and Guidelines for an Accredited Education Program for Medical Assistants* will be revised to reflect the findings of the Role Delineation Study.

Educational institutions seeking accreditation for a medical assisting program must develop the curricula to these *Standards and Guidelines* to ensure the highest quality medical assistant education and employment preparedness.

While not a complete list, some of the administrative, general (transdisciplinary), and clinical courses include those shown in Table 1-1.

Another aspect of an educational medical assisting program is the externship, a period of time when students participate in a practicum. This provides an excellent opportunity to apply theory to practice.

## Preparation for Externship

Externship, practicum, and internship are all terms used to define the transition period between the classroom and actual employment. An externship is planned and supervised by a coordinator from the medical assisting program and the health care facility that agrees to become a partner in the education and employability of the student.

**Externship Sites.** Sites for externship are chosen carefully to ensure that a variety of experiences is available for the student. The sites should provide the student with adequate administrative, clinical, and general experiences. The staff at the various sites must be willing to make a commitment to the medical assistant's education by spending appropriate time observing and instructing the student.

**Benefits of Externship.** The externship experience is mutually beneficial to the student and staff at the health care facility that is providing the educational experiences.

Some of the benefits to the student are the opportunity to:

- Apply classroom knowledge and skill in a real-world medical setting

- Recognize improvement in performance and knowledge

- Understand that there may be more than one acceptable method of performance

- Begin to establish a network of support through colleagues

Some of the benefits to the externship site are:

- Greater alertness of staff because of their educational responsibilities to the student

- Opportunity for staff to observe students who will soon be seeking employment

- Possibility that staff will learn more about the profession of medical assisting

Educational institutions that confer associate or baccalaureate degrees require general education courses for graduation in addition to the administration and clinical courses.

There are four-year institutions of higher learning that offer a baccalaureate degree to medical assistants who have graduated with an associate's degree from a community or junior college. The graduate is accepted as a third-year student and can obtain a baccalaureate degree in such areas as health care management or health care facility administrator.

Because there is a demand for medical assistant educators, some medical assistants take education courses to become allied health educators.

| TABLE 1-1 | TYPICAL ADMINISTRATIVE, GENERAL, AND CLINICAL COURSES IN AN ACCREDITED MEDICAL ASSISTING PROGRAM |
|---|---|

**Administrative Courses**

Computer Applications
Manual Recording of Patients' Data
Scheduling Appointments
Maintaining Medical Records
Word Processing/Typewriting/Keyboarding
Billing/Collections/Managing Patients' Accounts
Coding/Insurance Claims
Telephone Triage
Personnel Management

**General Courses**

Anatomy and Physiology
Medical Terminology
Diseases
Patient Education
Medical Law and Ethics

**Clinical Courses**

Pharmacology/Administration of Medications
Assisting Techniques/Physical Examination
Assisting with Minor Surgery
Basic Laboratory Procedures/Routine Blood and Urine Testing
Cardiopulmonary Resuscitation

## CAREER OPPORTUNITIES

Medical assistants have been described as health care's most versatile, multifaceted professionals. The fact that medical assistants possess a broad scope of knowledge and skills makes them ideal professionals for any ambulatory care setting. Indeed, owing to such versatility, medical assistants find employment in a variety of settings: offices, clinics, hospitals, medical laboratories, insurance companies, government agencies, pharmaceutical companies, and educational institutions. Although the range of employment opportunities continues to grow, in the past decade, about four out of five medical assistants were employed in physicians' offices and clinics. About one in five worked in offices of other health care practitioners, such as chiropractors, optometrists, and podiatrists. The outlook for employment for medical assistants is very promising. According to the AAMA, there are presently 1.3 million medical assistants in the work force. The United States Department of Labor Bureau of Statistics listed medical assisting as one of the fastest growing allied health professions for the years 1998–2008.

Increased employment opportunities for medical assistants result from the increased medical needs of an aging population, growth in the number of health care practitioners and their desire to hire the most qualified person for the task, increased diagnostic testing, greater volume and complexity of paperwork and computer information, managed care's emphasis on ambulatory care, and the insurance-mandated shorter stay of patients in hospitals.

## REGULATION OF HEALTH CARE PROVIDERS

One way health care providers can be regulated is through the process of credentialing. Credentialing recognizes health care providers who are professionally and technically competent. Recognition comes from professional associations, certifying agencies, and the state or federal government. Regulation ensures:

- Competence of health care providers
- A minimum standard of knowledge, training, and skill
- The limiting of the performance of certain procedures to a specific occupation

Licensure, certification, and registration are three kinds of regulations/credentialing. See Table 1-2.

### Scope of Practice

Medical assisting is not licensed as a profession; however, some states require that medical assistants be graduates of an accredited medical assisting program in order to work as medical assistants.

Two examples of licensed professions are medicine and nursing. A license regulates the activities of these professions by enacting laws that specify educational requirements and by defining the scope of practice. A license is conferred upon an individual who successfully completes specialized educational requirements and successfully passes an examination administered by the state in which the individual resides. The state grants a license to that individual to practice medicine or nursing. Licensure forbids anyone who is not licensed from performing activities that are designated by that particular license. For example, the law states that the physician's license allows diagnosing and prescribing treatment. If someone were to diagnose or prescribe without a license, that individual would be committing an illegal act and would be practicing medicine without a license, which is considered a felony.

There are state laws that govern the practice of medicine and nursing (medical practice acts, nursing practice acts), and many states have acts that give physicians the right to delegate certain clinical procedures to

| TABLE 1-2 | COMPARISON OF REQUIREMENTS FOR CERTIFICATION, LICENSURE, AND REGISTRATION | | |
|---|---|---|---|
| | **Certification** | **Licensure** | **Registration** |
| Practice Requirement | Voluntary | Mandatory | Voluntary |
| Conferred by | Nongovernmental agency or professional association | Legislated by each state | Professional association |
| | If qualified and meets requirements | If qualified and meets requirements | Listed on an official roster |
| | Must pass examination | Must pass state examination | Passing examination not always required |
| How restrictive | Used by most professional associations | Most restrictive | Least restrictive |

qualified allied health professionals. Because medical assistants are not required to be licensed, they are allowed to perform clinical procedures only under the supervision of the physician or other licensed health care professional who is granted the right and who delegates the specific clinical procedures to them.

In some states, including California, Washington, and others, unlicensed health care providers are required to have authorization from the state to perform allergy testing, venipuncture, and to give injections. A registration fee and mandatory training are required. In such circumstances, medical assistants or other health care providers would be breaking the law if they performed these procedures without registration and training.

In some states, authorization is required for unlicensed health care providers to expose patients to X rays.

Medical assistants do not perform procedures for which they have not been educated and trained. The AAMA's Role Delineation Chart in the appendices is an excellent reference source that identifies which clinical, administrative, and general (transdisciplinary) procedures medical assistants are educated to perform. However, due to the variability of state statutes, the medical assistant would be wise to check with the executive director of the AAMA if there is doubt regarding the legality of performing certain clinical procedures.

## SUMMARY

Progress has been made in the advancement of the profession of medical assisting since the first group of medical assistants gathered to become organized and formed the American Association of Medical Assistants. For example, the number of certified medical assistants has exceeded 70,000 and continues to grow since certification began in 1963. The total number of medical assistants in the work force is 1.3 million and employment opportunities continue to grow. Educational requirements have become increasingly important. The AAMA continues to promote standards of excellence for its members, encouraging continuing education and awarding continuing education credits to members of AAMA via various means.

All of these factors are evidence of a strong professional perspective and should offer encouragement and support to any student or graduate of medical assisting.

Becoming a professional is a gradual process and cannot be learned in its entirety from a textbook. The challenge of becoming a professional medical assistant will require open-mindedness and a desire for continued learning and education, certification, and recertification of the CMA credential, and professional involvement through organizational participation.

As the scope of work done by medical assistants broadens and medical assistants seek and require formal education, the professional medical assistant will gain additional respect and be in even greater demand. Medical assistants must continuously pursue excellence, which is the hallmark of all professional behavior.

## REVIEW QUESTIONS

### Multiple Choice

1. Medical assisting has been recognized by the United States Department of Education as a profession since what year?
   a. 1956
   b. 1964
   c. 1978
   d. 1995
2. The AAMA was established as a professional organization in what year?
   a. 1945
   b. 1956
   c. 1962
   d. 1967
3. The "Quest for Excellence" is:
   a. a professional publication for medical assistants
   b. a code of professional behavior for medical assistants
   c. otherwise known as ethical behavior
   d. the AAMA's series of home study courses
4. The designation Registered Medical Assistant is awarded by:
   a. American Association of Medical Assistants (AAMA)
   b. Accrediting Bureau of Health Education Schools (ABHES)
   c. American Medical Association (AMA)
   d. American Medical Technologists (AMT)

5. Increased employment opportunities for medical assistants result from:
   a. decreases in diagnostic testing
   b. computers decreasing volume of paperwork
   c. managed care's emphasis on ambulatory care
   d. longer hospital stays for patients

## Critical Thinking

1. For each personal attribute used in your textbook to describe a professional, identify individuals from your family, friends, church, or community who possess one or more of these traits.
2. Patients and physicians desire professional medical assistants who have had the benefit of a formal education to care and work for them. Discuss the impact of this education on patients and employers. Why is it important to both groups?
3. Discuss the importance of certification and recertification.
4. Differentiate among certification, licensure, and registration.
5. Describe externship and its benefits.

## WEB ACTIVITIES

1. Visit the National Accrediting Agency for Clinical Laboratory Sciences (NAACLS) web site at http://www.naacls.org
   - What allied health professions other than medical technologist and clinical laboratory scientist are accredited by NAACLS?
   - Does NAACLS have a code of ethics for the medical assistant?
2. Visit the American Association of Medical Assistants web site at http://www.amaa-ntl.org
   - What allied health profession does the AAMA accredit?
   - What resources are available on the web for medical assistants interested in continuing education?
3. Visit the American Medical Technologists web site at http://www.amtl.com

## REFERENCES/BIBLIOGRAPHY

Balasa, D. (2000). Securing the future for medical assistants to practice. *Professional medical assistant*, January/February 2000, 6–7.

Keir, L., Wise, B. A., & Krebs, C. (1998). *Medical assisting: Administrative and clinical competencies* (4th ed.). Albany, NY: Delmar.

Kinn, M. E., & Woods, M. A. (1999). *The medical assistant: Administrative and clinical* (8th ed.). Philadelphia: W. B. Saunders.

Merriam-Webster (1998). *Merriam-Webster's collegiate dictionary* (10th ed.). Springfield, MA: Author.

Prickett-Ramutkowski, B., Barrie, A., Keller, C., Dazarow, L., & Abe, C. (1999). *Medical assistant: A patient-centered approach to administrative and clinical competencies* (1st ed.). Princeton, NJ: Glencoe/McGraw Hill.

# 2

# HEALTH CARE SETTINGS AND THE HEALTH CARE TEAM

## KEY TERMS

Acupuncture
Allied Health Professionals
Ambulatory Care Setting
Fringe Benefit
Health Maintenance Organization (HMO)
Holistic
Independent Physician Association (IPA)
Integrative Medicine
Managed Care
Managed Care Operation
Managed Competition
Partnership
Preferred Provider Organization (PPO)
Sole Proprietorship
Triage

## OUTLINE

**Ambulatory Health Care Settings**
  Individual and Group Medical Practices
  Urgent Care Centers
  Managed Care Operations
**The Impact of Managed Care in the Health Care Setting**

**The Health Care Team**
  The Role of the Medical Assistant
  Health Care Professionals and Their Roles
  Allied and Other Health Professionals and Their Roles
  The Role of Integrative or Alternative Health Care Therapies
  The Value of the Medical Assistant to the Health Care Team

## OBJECTIVES

*The student should strive to meet the following performance objectives and demonstrate an understanding of the facts and principles presented in this chapter through written and oral communication.*

1. Define the key terms as presented in the glossary.
2. Analyze the benefits and limitations of working in the different health care settings.
3. Assess the role and impact of managed care in the health care environment.
4. Identify and describe the three primary medical management models.
5. Describe the function of the health care team.
6. Discuss the role of the medical assistant in the health care team.
7. List and describe a minimum of twelve physician specialists.
8. List and describe a minimum of five nonphysician health care specialists.
9. List and describe a minimum of twelve allied health professionals.
10. Compare and contrast the types of nurses.
11. Critique alternative therapies and discuss their role in today's health care setting.

**GENERAL
(TRANSDISCIPLINARY)**

**Professionalism**

- **Project a professional manner and image**
- **Adhere to ethical principles**
- **Demonstrate initiative and responsibility**
- **Work as a team member**
- **Promote the CMA credential**

**Communication Skills**

- **Serve as liaison**

**Legal Concepts**

- **Practice within the scope of education, training, and personal capabilities**

## INTRODUCTION

There are few professions in our society as rich and complex as the health care profession. In recent years, especially, the health care environment has been very much in flux as the profession seeks ways to provide quality care while containing costs. This effort to curtail costs has resulted in the rise of what is known as managed care, which, in turn, has spawned a number of medical models such as health maintenance organizations (HMOs) and preferred provider organizations (PPOs), two well-known managed care entities.

Many other types of physician networks and alliances are also being established as providers merge in order to give patients the best of care while controlling their costs. Ambulatory care settings, where services are provided on an outpatient basis, have become increasingly pivotal to consumer health care as insurers direct dollars away from hospitals and toward outpatient care.

Just as the medical setting continues to evolve to meet new societal needs, health care technology is ever-changing. Health care is a dynamic, stimulating industry that requires the medical assistant and other professionals to constantly develop new skills if they are to contribute to the team effort. The range of skills within the health care team is astonishing, and includes physicians, or medical doctors, in more than 25 specialties, more than 20 kinds of allied health professionals, and an increasing number of nontraditional alternative practitioners.

## AMBULATORY HEALTH CARE SETTINGS

While medical assistants may work in a number of different environments, including laboratories or hospitals, most are employed in an **ambulatory care setting** such as a medical office (either a solo-physician or group practice), an urgent or primary care center, or a managed care organization such as an HMO.

Often, the medical assistant will choose to work in one setting rather than another based on interests, personality, and work preferences. For instance, the individual practice may provide medical assistants with the opportunity to use their full array of skills, while in urgent care centers, the work of the medical assistant may be more specialized in nature.

Medical assistants should also be aware of the three major forms of medical practice management and how they affect salary, benefits, and liability issues (Figure 2-1).

### Individual and Group Medical Practices

For years, the most common form of medical office was the individual physician or group practice. Although this model now competes with a variety of other models such as urgent care centers and HMOs, many medical assistants will still find the individual or group practice a challenging place of employment.

**Individual Practices.** In the individual practice, also called the solo practice, one primary physician sees and treats all patients. While this type of arrangement is limited in the number of people it can serve, many patients feel secure in this kind of health care setting for they come to know and trust their doctor. Because they always see the same doctor, they feel their health care is being managed in a personal way. The solo-physician practice, however, can be an expensive arrangement, because one doctor must undertake the costs of office space, equipment, and personnel.

**Group Practices.** In today's managed care environment, group practices are attractive arrangements where two or more physicians can share the high costs of space, equipment, and personnel. The advantages of a group practice are not solely economic, however; physicians learn from and consult one another, while patients receive the benefit of this exchange of information and knowledge. Often, a group practice may have more than one office and some employees may be asked to travel between sites to cut overhead. Group practices may also be formed to offer specialized care, such as oncology or women's health care.

In most smaller group practices, patients may

## FORMS OF MEDICAL PRACTICE MANAGEMENT

Medical assistants employed in ambulatory care settings or medical offices and clinics are likely to see three major forms of medical practice management. They are sole proprietorships, partnerships, and corporations.

Whatever form of management is chosen by physicians, they are responsible for the employees that serve with them. (Refer to the discussion of *respondeat superior* in Chapter 7.) Physician-employers and their medical assistants must have the kind of healthy working relationship where mutual trust and respect are apparent. The physician must understand the skill level of the medical assistant, and the medical assistant must feel secure enough to ask any questions necessary or admit any errors. Critical errors are often made when this trust does not exist between employer and employee. This causes a breakdown in the delivery of the best health care for patients.

### Sole Proprietorships

In the past, many physicians preferred a solo practice. A solo practice entitles the physician or sole proprietor to hold exclusive right to all aspects of the medical practice or sole proprietorship, including profits and debts. If the business fails, the sole proprietor's personal property may also be attached.

A sole proprietorship may employ other physicians to participate in the practice. The employed physician(s) would be entitled to any employee fringe benefits such as health insurance and paid vacation, but the solo practitioner is not so entitled.

It is predicted that the business of practicing medicine may become more generalized and government regulated. Trends indicate more group practices and managed care facilities may gain dominance over the sole proprietorship form of management for physicians. The accelerating cost of maintaining an office has become more prohibitive for a physician in a sole proprietorship, especially the new-graduate physician.

### Partnerships

When two or more physicians join together under a legal agreement to share in the total business operations of the practice, a partnership is formed. Several physicians who share a facility and practice medicine are often referred to as a group. Partners share expenses, income, debt, equipment, records, and personnel according to a predetermined agreement. Partners are liable for only their own actions, but may be liable for the whole amount of the partnership debts.

### Corporations

Physicians may form a corporation, usually referred to as a professional service corporation. The physician shareholders are considered employees of the corporation. A corporation allows income and tax advantages to all employees. A variety of fringe benefits can be offered to the employees, which may include pension, profit-sharing plans, medical expense reimbursement, and life, health, and disability insurance. These benefits are separate from salary. Another advantage is that professional employees of a corporation are liable only for their own acts, and personal property cannot be attached in litigation. A sole proprietor may incorporate if the practice is large enough.

The health maintenance organization (HMO) is one type of corporation in which physicians often practice. Basically, physicians are employees of the HMO and are paid by various methods; physicians in the HMO usually serve as the primary care physician (PCP). In this situation, a referral from the PCP may be necessary before a patient can see a specialist or allied health professional.

**Figure 2-1** Different forms of medical practice models and how they may affect the medical assistant.

request that they see the same physician for all appointments, although sometimes patients are assigned to the next available doctor. For emergencies, group practices have the staff and flexibility to ensure that there is always a doctor on call.

## Urgent Care Centers

Urgent care centers are usually private, for-profit centers that provide services for primary care, routine injuries and illnesses, and minor surgery. Sometimes lab services and a radiology department are located on the premises. Physicians and other health care professionals in the center are often salaried employees, not owners who share in the profits, and often are associated with other medical facilities.

The pace in most urgent care centers is brisk and typically a number of doctors are working at one time. Patients may be requested to make appointments, but in some centers drop-ins are accepted, especially for emergencies.

Because these centers can see a higher volume of patients, usually for a lower cost than the traditional solo-physician or small group practice, some experts predict that ambulatory care settings will continue to grow as private practices decrease in number.

## Managed Care Operations

 Health maintenance organizations, or HMOs, are probably the most familiar managed care operation. Originally, HMOs were designed to provide a full range of health care services under one roof. More recently, the HMO without walls has become established, which is typically a network of participating physicians within a defined geographic area.

Originally, the HMO with walls was conceived to provide patients with comprehensive health care services at one facility. Today, as managed care and managed competition sweep the health care industry, other arrangements include the **preferred provider organization (PPO)**, where physicians network to offer discounts to employers and other purchasers of health insurance, and the **independent physician association (IPA)**, whose members agree to treat patients for an agreed-upon fee.

## THE IMPACT OF MANAGED CARE IN THE HEALTH CARE SETTING

The emergence of **managed care** in today's society provides new administrative and clinical challenges to members of the health care team as they struggle to provide the best health care while working within limitations often imposed by insurance carriers. Virtually all health care settings, whether they are individual practices or urgent care centers, are experiencing the impact of managed care and **managed competition,** where physicians network and compete to serve patients better and more cost-efficiently.

Under managed care, critics charge, health care dollars have grown scarce, physicians must strive to provide the same quality for reduced reimbursement, preapprovals must be obtained for many services, and some services may be denied because they are not considered cost-effective.

Clinically, managed care may set limits on services or length of services. Second opinions are encouraged and sometimes required. In some systems, the patient selects a primary care physician, who is considered the gatekeeper and who must provide a referral for specialist care. Critics of managed care point out that restricting or denying services may lead to an increase in professional liability.

Administratively, paperwork and documentation have become increasingly important to assure proper reimbursement. While it is the patient's responsibility to understand the conditions of the insurance policy, these are often difficult to understand or interpret. The medical office or center must be fully aware of when a preapproval or treatment plan is required, when a second opinion is necessary for reimbursement, and of other clauses and restrictions that affect care and reimbursement for care.

At the same time, while managed care is challenging even the most resilient of providers, the very real need to keep costs down has also generated considerable creativity and energy among the health care profession as

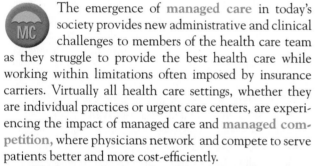

## SPOTLIGHT ON AAMA ESSENTIALS THROUGH CAAHEP

- Working as a team member and adapting to change makes a professional medical assistant stand out from others.
- Communication makes the difference between competency and negligence.
- Compassion and a caring attitude provide a positive experience for patients even when they are too ill to express their feelings.

physicians seek to use technology more efficiently, as they collaborate on new, cost-effective delivery methods, and as everyone involved in health care—insurers, providers, and patients—works together to contain costs by emphasizing prevention and lifestyle changes.

## THE HEALTH CARE TEAM

In every kind of health care setting, the team concept is critical to the quality of patient care. A primary care physician is most likely the main source of health care for patients. From time to time, however, a specialist will be sought or recommended. A number of different allied health professionals, including the medical assistant, will supply additional health care as ordered by the physician. Increasingly, patients are looking outside traditional medicine for portions of their health care. While alternative care may not be covered by medical insurance, traditional and nontraditional health care practices are nonetheless blending in many areas. For example, **acupuncture** is becoming recognized as effective in the treatment of chronic pain. In whatever manner health care is sought, all members of this health care team must communicate, sometimes in person and sometimes just through the medical history and record, with one another to assure quality patient care.

### The Role of the Medical Assistant

In the ambulatory care setting, a critical **allied health professional** is the medical assistant. The medical assistant, performing both administrative and clinical tasks under the direction of the physician, is an important link between patient and physician. The medical assistant serves in many capacities—receptionist, secretary, transcriptionist, bookkeeper, insurance coder and biller, patient educator, and clinical assistant. The latter requires the medical assistant to be able to administer injections and perform venipuncture, prepare patients for examinations, assist the physician with examinations and special procedures, and perform electrocardiography and various laboratory tests. Medical assistants triage and assess patient needs when scheduling appointments and tests. However, while medical assistants have a broad range of responsibilities, it is critical that they perform only within the scope of their training and personal capabilities and always function within ethical and legal boundaries and state statutes.

Because medical assistants are often the patient's first contact with the facility and its physicians, a positive attitude is important. They must be excellent communicators, both verbally and nonverbally, and project a professional image of themselves and their physician-employer. Medical assistants who believe in their work, who are proud of their career, and who convey compassion and caring provide a positive experience for patients who may be ill or in a great deal of discomfort.

## Health Care Professionals and Their Roles

The public is often confused by the title *doctor*. The term implies an earned academic degree of the highest level in a particular area of study. Physicians have earned the MD or Doctor of Medicine degree. A doctorate in medicine and/or a license to practice allows a person to diagnose and treat medical conditions. The doctor of medicine candidate will attend four years of medical school after receiving a baccalaureate degree. An internship of one to two years follows in a hospital or major medical center. If a physician chooses to specialize, as many do, a residency

### Patient Teaching Tip

Encourage patients to think of themselves as members of the health care team for they can provide invaluable information about their medical history. Use good communication skills to encourage patients to describe symptoms, identify their medications, and provide other information that is useful in diagnosis and treatment.

of two to five years in that specialty is required. In the medical field, the abbreviation *Dr.* is used and the title *doctor* is addressed to the person qualified by education, training, and licensure to practice medicine.

Other medical degrees include the Doctor of Osteopathy (DO), Doctor of Dentistry (DDS), Doctor of Optometry (OD), Doctor of Podiatric Medicine (DPM), Doctor of Chiropracty (DC), and Doctor of Naturopathy (ND). This group of doctors completes a different training regimen than that required for the Doctor of Medicine. The training is highly specialized and very specific but still grants the title of doctor upon completion, and when licensed, allows these health care professionals to diagnose and treat medical conditions.

In other nonmedical disciplines, the persons who have achieved a doctorate conferred by a college or university include the Doctor of Education (EdD) and the Doctor of Philosophy (PhD). Both the EdD and PhD have several areas of specialty.

Table 2-1 gives a selected listing of medical and surgical specialties, while Table 2-2 lists other health care specialists.

### TABLE 2-1 SELECTED MEDICAL AND SURGICAL SPECIALTIES

| American Board of Medical Specialties | General Certificates | Subspecialty Certificates | |
|---|---|---|---|
| Allergy & Immunology | Allergy & Immunology | Clinical & Laboratory Immunology | |
| Anesthesiology | Anesthesiology | Critical Care Medicine | Pain Management |
| Colon & Rectal Surgery | Colon & Rectal Surgery | | |
| Dermatology | Dermatology | Clinical & Laboratory Dermatological Immunology | Dermatopathology Pediatric Dermatology |
| Emergency Medicine | Emergency Medicine | Medical Toxicology Pediatric Emergency Medicine | Sports Medicine Undersea & Hyperbaric Medicine |
| Family Practice | Family Practice | Geriatric Medicine | Sports Medicine |

*(continues)*

**TABLE 2-1** (*continued*)

| American Board of Medical Specialties | General Certificates | Subspecialty Certificates | |
|---|---|---|---|
| Internal Medicine | Internal Medicine | Adolescent Medicine<br>Cardiovascular Disease<br>Clinical Cardiac Electrophysiology<br>Clinical & Laboratory Immunology<br>Critical Care Medicine<br>Endocrinology, Diabetes & Metabolism<br>Gastroenterology | Geriatric Medicine<br>Hematology<br>Infectious Disease<br>Interventional Cardiology<br>Medical Oncology<br>Nephrology<br>Pulmonary Disease<br>Rheumatology<br>Sports Medicine |
| Medical Genetics | Clinical Biochemical Genetics<br>Clinical Cytogenetics<br>Clinical Genetics (MD)<br>Clinical Molecular Genetics<br>Ph.D. Medical Genetics | Molecular Genetic Pathology | |
| Neurological Surgery | Neurological Surgery | | |
| Nuclear Medicine | Nuclear Medicine | | |
| Obstetrics & Gynecology | Obstetrics & Gynecology | Critical Care Medicine<br>Gynecologic Oncology | Maternal & Fetal Medicine<br>Reproductive Endocrinology |
| Ophthalmology | Ophthalmology | | |
| Orthopaedic Surgery | Orthopaedic Surgery | Hand Surgery | |
| Otolaryngology | Otolaryngology | Otology/Neurotology<br>Pediatric Otolaryngology | Plastic Surgery within the<br>Head and Neck |
| Pathology | Anatomic Pathology &<br>Clinical Pathology<br>Anatomic Pathology<br>Clinical Pathology | Blood Banking/Transfusion Medicine<br>Chemical Pathology<br>Cytopathology<br>Dermatopathology<br>Forensic Pathology | Hematology<br>Immunopathology<br>Medical Microbiology<br>Molecular Genetic Pathology<br>Neuropathology<br>Pediatric Pathology |
| Pediatrics | Pediatrics | Adolescent Medicine<br>Clinical & Laboratory Immunology<br>Development-Behavioral Peds<br>Medical Toxicology<br>Neonatal-Perinatal Medicine<br>Neurodevelopmental Disabilities<br>Pediatric Cardiology<br>Pediatric Critical Care Medicine<br>Pediatric Emergency Medicine<br>Pediatric Endocrinology | Pediatric Gastroenterology<br>Pediatric Hematology-<br>Oncology<br>Pediatric Infectious Diseases<br>Pediatric Nephrology<br>Pediatric Pulmonology<br>Pediatric Rheumatology<br>Sports Medicine |
| Physical Medicine<br>& Rehabilitation | Physical Medicine<br>& Rehabilitation | Pain Management<br>Spinal Cord Injury Medicine | Pediatric Rehabilitation<br>Medicine |
| Plastic Surgery | Plastic Surgery | Surgery of the Hand<br>Plastic Surgery within the Head and Neck | |
| Preventive Medicine | Aerospace Medicine<br>Occupational Medicine<br>Public Health & General<br>Preventive Medicine | Medical Toxicology<br>Undersea & Hyperbaric Medicine<br>Undersea Medicine | |
| Psychiatry & Neurology | Psychiatry<br>Neurology<br>Neurology with Special<br>Qualifications in Child<br>Neurology | Addiction Psychiatry<br>Child & Adolescent Psychiatry<br>Clinical Neurophysiology | Forensic Psychiatry<br>Geriatric Psychiatry<br>Neurodevelopmental<br>Disabilities<br>Pain Management |
| Radiology | Diagnostic Radiology<br>Radiation Oncology<br>Radiological Physics | Neuroradiology<br>Nuclear Radiology<br>Pediatric Radiology | Vascular & Interventional<br>Radiology |
| Surgery | Surgery | Pediatric Surgery<br>Surgery of the Hand | Surgical Critical Care<br>Vascular Surgery |
| Thoracic Surgery | Thoracic Surgery | | |
| Urology | Urology | | |

Copyright 2000 American Board of Medical Specialties

**TABLE 2-2   OTHER HEALTH CARE SPECIALISTS**

| Title | Degree | Function |
|---|---|---|
| Chiropractic Medicine | Chiropractors are licensed in their field of practice. They hold a degree of DC, or Doctor of Chiropractic. | Manipulative treatment of disorders originating from misalignment of the spinal vertebrae |
| Dentistry | Dentists are licensed in their field of practice, which can range from general to highly specialized. They hold the degree of DDS, or Doctor of Dental Surgery. | Diagnosing and treating diseases and disorders of the teeth and gums |
| Optometry | Optometrists are licensed in their field of practice. They hold the degree of OD, or Doctor of Optometry. | Measuring the accuracy of vision to determine if corrective lenses are needed |
| Osteopathy | Osteopaths are physicians who hold the title DO or Doctor of Osteopathy. | A therapeutic system that restores or preserves health through manipulation of the skeleton and muscles. Osteopaths also rely upon physical, medicinal, and surgical methods |
| Podiatry | Podiatrists are licensed in their field of practice. They hold the degree of DPM, or Doctor of Podiatric Medicine. | Diagnosing and treating diseases and disorders of the feet |
| Psychology | Psychologists are licensed in their field of practice. They hold the degree of PhD, or Doctor of Philosophy. (Some hold only a master's degree, or MA, and are not permitted to use the title *doctor.*) | Evaluating and treating emotional problems. These professionals give counseling to individuals, families, and groups |

## Allied and Other Health Professionals and Their Roles

In the health care team, allied health professionals bring specific educational backgrounds and a broad array of skills to the medical environment. Medical assistants are considered allied health professionals. Table 2-3 lists some of the allied health professionals recognized by the Commission on Accreditation of Allied Health Education Programs (CAAHEP) and other national accrediting bodies.

**TABLE 2-3   ALLIED HEALTH PROFESSIONS**

| Occupation | Abbreviations | Job Description |
|---|---|---|
| Anesthesiologist Assistant | AA | Performs preoperative tasks, performs airway management and drug administration for induction and maintenance of anesthesia during surgery under direction of a licensed and qualified anesthesiologist |
| Athletic Trainer | AT | Provides a variety of services including injury prevention, recognition, immediate care, treatment, and rehabilitation after athletic trauma |
| Cardiovascular Technologist | CVT | Performs diagnostic exams under the direction of a physician in (1) invasive cardiology, (2) noninvasive cardiology, and (3) noninvasive peripheral vascular study |
| Clinical Laboratory Scientist | CLS | Develops data on the blood, tissues, and fluids of the human body by using a variety of precision instruments |
| Clinical Laboratory Technician *Associate Degree* | CLT | Performs all routine tests in a medical lab and is able to discriminate and recognize factors that directly affect procedures and results. Works under direction of pathologist, physician, medical technologist, or scientist |
| Clinical Laboratory Technician *Certificate* | CLT | Performs many routine uncomplicated procedures in medical lab where discrimination is clear and errors are few and easily corrected. Works under direction of pathologist, physician, medical technologist, or scientist |
| Cytotechnologist | CT | Works with pathologists to detect changes in body cells that may be important in early diagnosis of cancer or other diseases primarily through microscopic analysis |

*(continues)*

**TABLE 2-3**   *(continued)*

| Occupation | Abbreviations | Job Description |
|---|---|---|
| Diagnostic Medical Sonographer | DMS | Provides patient services using medical ultrasound under the supervision of a physician |
| Electroneurodiagnostic Technologist | EEG-T | Possesses the knowledge, attributes, and skills to obtain interpretable recordings of a patient's nervous system functions |
| Emergency Medical Technician—Paramedic | EMT-P | Recognizes, assesses, and manages medical emergencies of acutely ill or injured patients in prehospital care settings, working under the direction of a physician (often through radio communication) |
| Health Information Administrator | RRA | Manages health information systems consistent with the medical, administrative, ethical, and legal requirements of the health care delivery system |
| Health Information Technician | ART | Possesses the technical knowledge and skills necessary to process, maintain, compile, and report patient data |
| Medical Assistant | MA, CMA, RMA | Functions under the supervision of licensed medical professionals and is competent in both administrative/office and clinical/lab procedures |
| Medical Illustrator | MI | Creates visual material designed to facilitate the recording and dissemination of medical, biological, and related knowledge through communication media |
| Nuclear Medicine Technologist | NMT | Assists the nuclear medicine physician to make diagnostic evaluations of the anatomic or physiologic conditions of the body and to provide therapy with unsealed radioactive sources |
| Occupational Therapist | OT | Educates and trains individuals in the application of purposeful, goal-oriented activity in the evaluation, diagnosis, and/or treatment of loss of the ability to cope with the tasks of living and impairment due to physical injury, illness, or emotional disorder, congenital or developmental disability, or the aging process |
| Occupational Therapy Assistant | OTA | Directs an individual's participation in selected tasks to restore, reinforce, and enhance performance; facilitates learning of those skills and functions essential for adaptation and productivity; diminishes or corrects pathology; and promotes and maintains health (under the direction of an occupational therapist) |
| Ophthalmic Medical Technician or Technologist | OMT | Assists ophthalmologists to carry out diagnostic and therapeutic procedures |
| Orthotist/Prosthetist | OP | Orthotists design and fit devices to provide care to patients who have disabling conditions of the limbs and spine; prosthetists design and fit devices for patients who have partial or total absence of a limb |
| Perfusionist | PERF | Operates extracorporeal circulation equipment during any medical situation where it is necessary to support or temporarily replace the patient's circulation or respiratory functions |
| Physician Assistant (includes Surgeon's Assistant) | PA | Practices medicine under the direction and responsible supervision of a doctor of medicine or osteopathy; performs diagnostic, therapeutic, preventive, and health maintenance services in any setting in which the physician renders care |
| Radiation Therapist | RADT | Administers radiation therapy services to patients under the supervision of radiation oncologists |
| Radiographer | RT(R) | Provides patient services using imaging modalities, as directed by physicians qualified to order and/or perform radiologic procedures |
| Respiratory Therapist | RRT | Applies scientific knowledge and theory to practical clinical problems of respiratory care |
| Respiratory Therapy Technician | CRTT | Administers general respiratory care |
| Surgical Technologist | ST | Works as integral member of the surgical team, which includes surgeons, anesthesiologists, registered nurses, and other surgical personnel delivering patient care and assuming appropriate responsibilities before, during, and after surgery |

Adapted from Health Professions Directory, 2000–2001, 28th ed. © American Medical Association, Chicago, IL

As a medical assistant, you may not work directly with all the identified allied health care professionals, but you are likely to have contact with many of them by telephone and written or electronic communication. Knowledge of the roles these health professionals play enables you to interact more intelligently with all members of the health care team.

In addition to the professionals listed in Table 2-3, you may encounter some or all of the following health care professionals in daily patient care.

## Health Unit Coordinator (HUC).
Health unit coordinators (HUC) perform nonclinical patient care tasks for the nursing unit of a hospital. This profession requires a self-motivated, mature individual who can handle the stress and hectic pace of coordinating personnel and their duties at the nurses' station. Also called unit secretary, administrative specialist, ward clerk, or ward secretary, a health unit coordinator receives on-the-job training with an emphasis on administrative office skills.

## Medical Laboratory Technologist (MLT).
Medical laboratory technologists physically and chemically analyze, as well as culture, urine, blood, and other body fluids and tissues. They work closely with physician specialists such as oncologists, pathologists, and hematologists. Knowledge of specimen collection, anatomy and physiology, biochemistry, laboratory equipment, asepsis, and quality control is essential. The American Society of Clinical Pathology (ASCP) is a professional organization that oversees credentialing and education in the medical laboratory professions. See Figure 2-2.

## Nurses.
The nursing profession is not listed in Table 2-3 because CAAHEP is not responsible for nurses' training

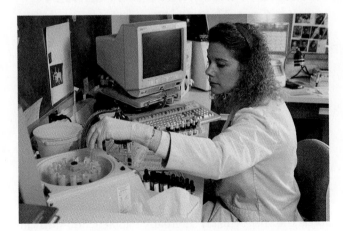

**Figure 2-2**  Medical technologists perform blood analyses and analyze and culture other body fluids as well. (Photo by Marcia Butterfield, courtesy of W. A. Foote Memorial Hospital, Jackson, MI)

and accreditation. Nurses are licensed by the state in which they practice. Although nurses' education and training are oriented to bedside care, some are employed in medical offices as clinical assistants, especially in offices where surgery is performed. Nurses play a number of roles on the health care team.

*Registered Nurse (RN).*  In the United States, RNs are professionals who have completed at a minimum, a two-year course of study at a state-approved school of nursing and passed the National Council Licensure Examination (NCLEX-RN). They are licensed only by the state to practice. Employment settings most often include hospitals, convalescent homes, clinics, and home health care.

*Licensed Practical Nurse (LPN).*  An LPN is a professional trained in basic nursing techniques and direct patient care. LPNs practice under the direct supervision of a registered nurse or physician and are employed in similar settings to RNs. Training includes completion of a state-approved program in practical nursing and successful completion of a national licensure examination.

*Nurse Practitioner (NP).*  A nurse practitioner is a registered nurse who, by advanced education (usually a master's degree) and clinical experience in a branch of nursing, has acquired expert knowledge in a specific medical specialty. Nurse practitioners are employed by physicians in private practice or in clinics, and sometimes practice independently, especially in rural areas.

## Registered Dietitian (RD).
Registered dietitians have specialized training in the nutritional care of groups and individuals and have successfully completed an examination of the Commission on Dietetic Registration. Dietitians assist patients in regulating their diets. Although they are typically employed in hospitals and clinics, they can also be found working with the public in personal nutritional counseling. Education includes a baccalaureate degree with a major in dietetics, food and nutrition, or food service systems management plus completion of an approved internship.

## Pharmacist (RPh).
Pharmacists are licensed by each state to prepare and dispense all types of medications as well as medical supplies related to medication administration. They may practice in hospitals, medical centers, and pharmacies. The minimum training for a pharmacist is a five-year baccalaureate degree; some pharmacists pursue a Doctor of Pharmacy degree (Pharm D), offered by major universities in the United States. Pharmacy technicians assist the pharmacist with preparation and administration

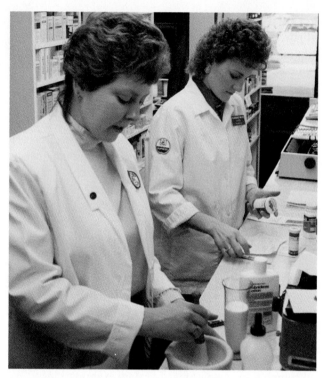

**Figure 2-3** Pharmacy technicians prepare medications to be dispensed. (Courtesy of the Michigan Pharmacists Association and the Michigan Society of Pharmacy Technicians)

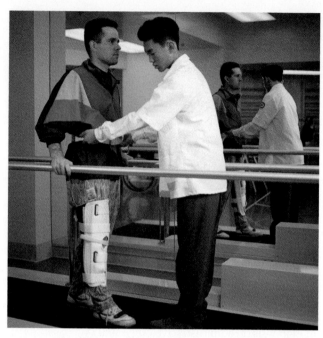

**Figure 2-4** Physical therapists work with disabled and physically challenged individuals and with patients who require physical rehabilitation.

of medications, as well as perform receptionist and billing duties. Professional certification of pharmacy technicians varies from state to state and is administered by state pharmacy associations. See Figure 2-3.

**Phlebotomist (LPT).** Phlebotomists are trained in the art of drawing blood for diagnostic laboratory testing. Phlebotomists are also referred to as lab liaison technicians. Phlebotomists may be nationally certified and are employed in medical clinics, hospitals, and laboratories. Training consists of one to two semesters in a community college program or on-the-job training.

**Physical Therapist (PT).** Physical therapists are licensed professionals who assist in the examination, testing, and treatment of physically disabled or challenged people. They also assist in physical rehabilitation of patients following an accident, injury, or serious illness using special exercises, application of heat or cold, *ultrasound* therapy and other techniques. Educational requirements for a physical therapist are a minimum of a four-year baccalaureate degree (bachelor of science) or a special certificate course after obtaining the bachelor of science in a related field. Physical therapists must also successfully complete a state licensure examination. See Figure 2-4.

**Physical Therapy Assistant (PTA).** Physical therapy assistants are trained to use and apply physical therapy procedures such as exercise and physical agents under the supervision of a physical therapist. The physical therapy assistant is a graduate of an accredited associate of science degree program and must pass a licensure or registry examination in selected states.

## The Role of Integrative or Alternative Health Care Therapies

Increasingly, integrative medicine or alternative forms of health care are being perceived as complements to traditional health care. As mentioned earlier, some nontraditional approaches, such as acupuncture, have been very successful in pain management or in reducing stress-related illnesses. For example, a patient being treated with medication for high blood pressure may also try to manage the hypertension with diet, exercise, and relaxation techniques. Sometimes this is considered a holistic approach to patient care, which takes into account the whole person.

While there is often controversy and confusion about the role of many alternative approaches, medical assistants should nonetheless be aware of the philosophy and intent of nontraditional therapies. Table 2-4 reviews some of the more common approaches.

| **TABLE 2-4** | **SELECTED EXAMPLES OF ALTERNATIVE APPROACHES TO HEALTH CARE** |
|---|---|
| **Type of Approach** | **Description of Approach** |
| Acupuncture | A piercing of the skin by long needles into any of 365 points along twelve meridians that transverse the body. Each point is related to a particular organ. Acupuncture is often successful in managing pain and has been successfully used to treat drug dependency. |
| Biofeedback | A relaxation technique that uses monitoring devices to gain information about certain automatic body responses such as heart rate or blood pressure in order to help the patient gain some voluntary control over that function. Biofeedback is often used to treat hypertension and migraine headaches. |
| Holism | An approach that treats the whole body, mind, and spirit. A holistic practitioner considers the needs of the patient in all areas, including physical, emotional, social, spiritual, and economic. |
| Homeopathy | A method of treating disease by administering very dilute doses of remedies that are typically made from natural substances. In more massive doses, these remedies would produce symptoms of the disease being treated. This is in contrast to traditional allopathic medicine, which typically treats disease with remedies that produce effects different from those caused by the disease itself. |
| Hypnotherapy | An approach that encourages patients to enter a trance-like state in which they are more open to suggestion. The hypnotherapist makes verbal suggestions in the attempt to bring some desired behavior change. |
| Naturopathy | Naturopaths are licensed in their field of practice and hold the degree of ND, Doctor of Naturopathy. Naturopaths diagnose and treat patients using the relationship between mind/body/spirit and nature. |
| Therapeutic Touch | Therapeutic touch uses the hands to facilitate healing and to restore wholeness, harmony, and well-being to the patient. Often practiced by nurses, therapeutic touch is considered a modern interpretation of ancient healing practices. It is thought to be effective for producing relaxation, reducing pain, and promoting wound healing. |

## *The Value of the Medical Assistant to the Health Care Team*

With their broad range of competencies in both administrative and clinical areas, medical assistants are increasingly valued as health care team members. Medical assistants are the great communicators, serving as liaison between physician and hospital staff and between physician and any number of allied and other health professionals. Because they are the first providers to see or speak with patients, they undertake responsibility for directing, informing, and guiding patient care while establishing a professional and caring tone for the entire health care team. The value of a competent, professional, caring medical assistant is immeasurable in today's fast-paced and challenging health care environment.

**CASE STUDY**

**2-1**

The number of sole proprietors is declining in this country.

### CASE STUDY REVIEW

1. Identify at least five reasons for this decline.
2. Describe the impact, if any, this decline has on quality health care.

## SUMMARY

The health care environment is a dynamic profession and one that changes rapidly in response to new technology and societal needs. In an effort to reduce the cost of health care, managed care has had and will continue to have a profound impact on all health care settings. A strong health care team is critical in the health care setting, as primary care physicians, specialists of all disciplines, and allied and other health professionals collaborate on the best way to provide patient care. Increasingly, selected alternative treatments may begin to complement traditional health care solutions. In almost any health care environment, but especially the ambulatory care setting, the medical assistant is a vital link in the team and is responsible for a range of responsibilities, both clinical and administrative.

## REVIEW QUESTIONS

### Multiple Choice

1. Medical assistants are employed for the most part in:
   a. hospitals
   b. nursing facilities
   c. ambulatory care settings
   d. insurance companies
2. A health maintenance organization is one kind of:
   a. managed care operation
   b. individual practice
   c. sole proprietorship
   d. hospital
3. With its emphasis on controlling costs, managed care is likely to affect:
   a. only hospitals
   b. all health care settings
   c. only physicians in private practice
   d. only patients
4. The health care team:
   a. should exclude the patient from being part of the team
   b. is only important in the hospital setting
   c. is made up of physicians and nurses
   d. is made up of physicians, nurses, allied and other health care professionals, patients, and sometimes a practitioner of nontraditional medicine
5. Integrative or alternative health care approaches:
   a. are increasingly accepted as complementary to traditional health care
   b. are always covered by insurance
   c. are not safe to practice
   d. are not important to understand
6. A medical assistant permitted by law to draw blood for diagnostic laboratory testing performs a procedure similar to those performed by a:
   a. health unit coordinator
   b. radiation therapist
   c. phlebotomist
   d. cytotechnologist
7. The distinct difference between the PA and the MA is that the PA:
   a. draws blood and gives injections
   b. practices medicine
   c. performs diagnostic services
   d. both b and c
8. Physicians just establishing their practice often seek to work with another physician in the same field. When expenses and profits are shared, this form of management is called a/an:
   a. HMO
   b. corporation
   c. sole proprietorship
   d. group or partnership
9. Managed care may be identified as care that:
   a. offers unlimited services
   b. forbids second opinions
   c. establishes a primary care physician as gate-keeper
   d. offers protection to physicians against liability
10. An alternative approach to medicine that treats patients using the relationship between mind/body/spirit/and nature is:
    a. homeopathy
    b. holism
    c. acupuncture
    d. naturopathy

### Critical Thinking

1. Evaluate the different health care settings and discuss the pros and cons of working in each setting.
2. From a patient point of view, which health care setting do you think offers more benefits? Why?
3. Review the three forms of medical management models. Which is probably the most advantageous from the physician's point of view? From the medical assistant's point of view?
4. Discuss the purpose of managed care. What impact is it having on health care?
5. What kinds of professionals make up the health care team?
6. Discuss the role of the medical assistant in the health care team. What qualities does the medical assistant need to possess?
7. If you were attending a family reunion and overheard a discussion about the title *doctor*, how would you clarify the situation? What are some examples of individuals who might be referred to as a doctor?
8. What organization recognizes allied health professionals?
9. Recall a few types of allied health professionals and, working in small groups, have each student create a scenario in which the medical assistant needs to coordinate with two or three allied professionals.
10. What role might alternative therapies play in the health care setting? Describe a few different alternative approaches and their philosophies.

## WEB ACTIVITIES

Visit http://www.abms.org for the most current list of the American Board of Specialties. What does board certified mean? Who credentials a specialist? How is this different from the certification or registration of medical assistants?

## REFERENCES/BIBLIOGRAPHY

American Board of Medical Specialties (1997). *The official ABMS directory of board certified medical specialists* (26th ed.). Evanston, IL: author.

Burton Goldberg Group (1995). *Alternative medicine*. Fife, WA: Future Medicine Publishing.

*Health professions directory* (27th ed.). (1999–2000). Chicago: American Medical Association.

Humphrey, D. D. (1996). *Contemporary medical office procedures* (2nd ed.). Albany, NY: Delmar.

*Mosby's medical, nursing and allied health dictionary* (5th ed.). (1998). St. Louis: Mosby-Year Book, Inc.

Smith, G. L., Davis, P. E., & Dennerll, J. T. (1999). *Medical terminology: A programmed systems approach* (8th ed.). Albany, NY: Delmar.

Stanfield, P. S. (1995). *Introduction to the health professions* (2nd ed.). Sudbury, MA: Jones & Bartlett Publishers.

*Taber's cyclopedic medical dictionary* (18th ed.) (1997). Philadelphia: F. A. Davis.

Warden, C. D. (1986). *Health care in the 1980s from a consumer's perspective*. Unpublished doctoral dissertation, Union Graduate School, Seattle, WA.

Weil, A. (1995). *Spontaneous healing*. New York: Alfred A. Knopf.

# Chapter 3

# HISTORY OF MEDICINE

## KEY TERMS

Acupuncture
Allopathic
Asepsis
Bubonic Plague
Malaria
Moxibustion
Pharmacopoeia
Pluralistic (Pluralism)
Septicemia
Typhus (Typhoid)
Yellow Fever

## OUTLINE

Cultural Heritage in Medicine
Medical Specialists
Medical Education
Attitudes toward Illness

Medical Treatments
Significant Contributions to
  Medicine
New Frontiers in Medicine

## OBJECTIVES

*The student should strive to meet the following performance objectives and demonstrate an understanding of the facts and principles presented in this chapter through written and oral communication.*

1. Define the key terms as presented in the glossary.
2. Discuss the effects of culture on medicine.
3. Identify the role of religion, magic, and science in medicine's history.
4. Describe how attitudes toward illness are manifested today.
5. Identify a minimum of three common medical treatments used in the past.
6. Recall a minimum of three theories/practices of ancient medicine still prevalent today.
7. Name and describe the historical roles of medical specialists.
8. Discuss the role of women in medicine.
9. Trace the progression of medical education.
10. Name at least five significant contributions to medicine.
11. Identify a minimum of three recent developments in medicine.

## INTRODUCTION

A historical overview of medicine must do more than identify a series of contributions by physicians. It must remind us that more than one discipline and more than one philosophy have contributed to medicine. This is perhaps more true now than ever as our world becomes smaller and our society becomes increasingly pluralistic, ethnically, culturally, and religiously.

## CULTURAL HERITAGE IN MEDICINE

Today's health professional will give care to individuals of varied cultures who hold differing philosophical beliefs toward medicine. The informed and caring health professional will recognize that a person's culture and ethnic heritage play an enormous role in any kind of health care. For example, if the cultural experience leans toward a more natural, nonmedical form of health care, treating the patient with prescription drugs will necessitate an explanation and rationale for the use of medications. Otherwise, the patient may refuse to take all or part of the medications, thus hindering recovery. It would be better to seek a treatment for the patient that embraces both the health care professional's desire to heal and the individual's wish to respect cultural tradition.

In every society, medicine has been an important element for its people. From the earliest time, culture was an important influence on medicine, and modern day medicine is in many ways a reflection of this diverse and rich heritage.

It is certain that religion, magic, and science all played a vital part in the history of medicine. Religion was important because it was perceived that certain gods were to be called upon for a cure through ceremonies, prayers, and sacrifices. Magic was practiced because it was such an important part of many societies and was seen as an essential ingredient to chase away evil spirits. The importance of science was demonstrated in the use of plants and minerals for medicinal purposes. The use of plants and minerals is found throughout medicine's history. Unearthed clay tablets reveal hundreds of plants, minerals, and animal substances used for medicinal purposes in ancient Mesopotamia and Babylon. The Chinese pharmacopoeia was rich in the use of herbs.

Skeletal remains of prehistoric cultures show advanced stages of arthritis, a nearly toothless jaw and only a 20- to 40-year lifespan for humans. Skull bones reveal round holes (trephination) believed to be necessary to release the evil spirits thought to be causing a person's illness. Mesopotamian cultures believed that illness was a punishment by the gods for violation of a moral code. Ancient Egyptians believed the body was a system of channels for air, tears, blood, urine, sperm, and feces. All the channels were thought to come together in the rectum, and were believed to become easily clogged. Thus, emetics, enemas, and purges of the anus were common treatments. In ancient India, plastic surgery was practiced. Punishment for adultery was cutting off the nose, therefore allowing physicians many opportunities to practice and refine the art of nose reconstruction.

The ancient Chinese examined and carefully monitored the pulse in each wrist. It was believed that the pulse had hundreds of characteristics important in medical treatment. There were five methods of treatment to bring a person back to the right track. They were:

1. Cure the spirit.
2. Nourish the body.
3. Give medications.
4. Treat the whole body.
5. Use acupuncture and moxibustion.

Acupuncture is the piercing of the skin by long needles into any of 365 points along twelve meridians that transverse the body and transmit an active life force called "ch'i" (pronounced chee). Each of these spots is related to a particular organ. Moxibustion requires the use of a powdered plant substance that is made into a small mound on the person's skin and then burned, usually raising a blister.

Even today's allopathic, or traditional, physicians would agree that the first four methods of treatment from Chinese culture are excellent guidelines for health care. There is an increasing awareness, also, that acupuncture has a valid place in allopathic medicine, especially for the control of pain.

## MEDICAL SPECIALISTS

Medicine's history gives early evidence of many "specialists" in the healing arts. They were known by various names—witch doctors, medicine men and women, shamans or healing priests, and physicians. These healers were more than ancestors of the modern physician, however, for they performed many functions that involved the welfare of the entire community or village. By today's standards, they were considered to be equivalent to spiritual advisers, social workers, counselors, and teachers.

While women were accepted as healers in primitive societies, later cultures reduced their status to that of being allowed to care only for women and to assist in childbirth. In any culture that granted women only secondary status, women are also considered unqualified to become physicians. In Chinese culture, the first reference to a female physician mentioned by name is in documents from the Han dynasty (206 B.C.–A.D. 220). In Muslim society, the reluctance of Arabic physicians to violate social taboo and touch the genitals of female strangers further encouraged relegating the practice of obstetrics and gynecology to midwives.

Women were not accepted as medical doctors in Western culture until the nineteenth and twentieth centuries. Italy granted women the status earlier than other cultures. In America, the first female physician was Elizabeth Blackwell, who was awarded her degree in 1849. While she was snubbed by the public, she soon earned the respect of her colleagues. When she refused to be absent from class when the male reproductive system was discussed, her fellow male students supported her actions.

From the earliest times, it appears that some payment was expected for medical services rendered. In many instances, the payment was dependent upon the status of the physician as well as the patient. At the same time, some cultures punished a physician who was not successful in treatment by forcing that physician to treat only those too poor to pay.

## MEDICAL EDUCATION

During the rise of Christianity, emphasis was placed on the soul rather than the body; therefore, early Christian monks held great control over medicine. This is evidenced by St. Benedict of Nursia (480–554) who forbade the study of medicine. The care of the sick was encouraged, but only through prayer and divine intervention. Thus, Christ's healing mission was institutionalized in a fashion that was to control medical care almost completely for the next 500 years, until the seventh century.

At that time, however, the religion of Islam moved to preserve the classical learning that had been achieved in medicine, and practitioners were not only able to return to the same methods as those practiced by earlier Greeks and Romans, but medical study was now encouraged.

Medical education in established universities began in the ninth century. These universities included Salerno in southern Italy, the University of Montpelier in southern France, and the University of Paris. By the time the Renaissance was at its height in the midfifteenth century, the physician had become licensed, was receiving great status, and was attending the ill in a velvet bonnet and fur-trimmed cloak.

Art and science were more closely related during the Renaissance than at any other period of time. Michelangelo (1475–1564) spent years on careful human dissection and this anatomical detail is evident in his paintings in the Sistine Chapel in the Vatican in Rome. Leonardo da Vinci (1452–1519) made anatomical preparations from which he produced drawings representing the skeletal, muscular, nervous, and vascular systems. His accurate sketch of the spinal vertebrae went undiscovered for more than 100 years.

## ATTITUDES TOWARD ILLNESS

Various attitudes prevailed toward the ill person. A sick person might be excused from daily activity, but was likely to be shunned if the disease was believed to be a punishment by the gods for mortal sin. This forced isolation may well have been beneficial to the community. In contrast, touching by Jesus was an important component of healing, as was the faith of the individual involved. The New Testament parable of the Good Samaritan helped establish a nexus between the early church and a concern for the sick. It was felt that though the body might be wasted and foul with disease, the purity of the soul guaranteed life everlasting. This was unlike the pagan religions that tended to abandon individuals thought to be ill because they were in disfavor with the gods.

 Native Americans had various feelings about illness. The ill were treated with kindness among the Navaho and Cherokee, and some who recovered from serious illness were considered to have extraordinary powers. However, if a tribe was faced with famine, suicide by the aged and infirm was considered a highest form of bravery. The Eskimos put their elderly unprotected onto ice floes. Neither the Romans nor the Greeks treated the hopelessly ill or deformed, and unwanted infants were disposed of quickly or left to die.

 Some of these attitudes are seen even today. The Western medical community and the consumers it serves are heatedly debating the right to choose life or death and the ethics and legality of physician-assisted suicide, which is acceptable in many other cultures. Even with our vast knowledge of medicine and the disease process, many individuals are still very fearful of any illness they do not understand or that they perceive as threatening their health—AIDS is a good example. This fear is often accompanied by public ill treatment of the individuals suffering from certain diseases. For example,

**SPOTLIGHT ON AAMA ESSENTIALS THROUGH CAAHEP**

- Recognizing a patient's cultural background is part of caring for the patient as a whole person.
- Human kindness often eliminates fear of the unknown.
- A positive attitude helps to lessen a negative feeling.

Cuba quarantines everyone who tests positive for the human immunodeficiency virus (HIV), even if they show no signs of illness.

## MEDICAL TREATMENTS

The writings of ancient Egypt reveal that when a woman suspected she was pregnant, she urinated over a mixture of wheat and barley seeds combined with dates and sand. If any of the grains sprouted, she was surely pregnant. If the wheat grew, she would have a boy. If the barley grew, it would be a girl. Urine is still used in modern tests to determine pregnancy.

Early medical treatments were often crude. For a sore throat, a physician might mix barley water, vinegar, and mulberry syrup for a gargle. Someone suffering with rheumatism might be given a prescription of chopped mice, lynx claws, and elk hooves. Rhubarb, senna, bitter apple, turpentine, camphor, and mercury were among the physicians' staples. Some physicians washed the instruments used in treating the ill; others scoffed at such a practice. **Malaria,** diphtheria, tuberculosis, **typhoid,** and dysentery were commonplace. Leprosy was prevalent and venereal diseases were rife. Smallpox was frequent in villages; sometimes the sufferer would be placed in a meat pickling vat and fumigated. The death toll from such diseases was particularly high among children. Finally in the eighteenth century, Edward Jenner made a great contribution to the prevention of disease by discovering a method of vaccination against smallpox.

Medicine progressed rapidly during the nineteenth century. Two very important discoveries occurred: anesthesia to alleviate pain during surgery and the realization that some bacteria cause disease. Once it had been proven that certain bacteria were causes of diseases and were transmissible agents responsible for contagion, greater care was taken to prevent that transmission. **Asepsis** became important to reduce the risk of infection. The Hungarian physician and obstetrician Ignaz Phillipp Semmeweis (1818–1865) was able to prove that physicians who came from an autopsy directly to the care of postpartum women, without scrubbing their hands and washing instruments, carried infection with them that often caused puerperal fever (**septicemia** following childbirth) and death to the new mothers.

The names of Louis Pasteur (1822–1895), Joseph Lister (1827–1912), and Robert Koch (1843–1910) are familiar to all bacteriologists. Louis Pasteur has sometimes been referred to as the father of preventive medicine as the result of his work in recognizing the relationship between bacteria and infectious disease (Figure 3-1). Joseph Lister revolutionized surgery because of his belief in Pasteur's theory of using carbolic acid as an antiseptic spray. He insisted that all instruments and physicians' hands be washed with the solution (Figure 3-2). Robert Koch used the culture-plate method for isolating bacteria

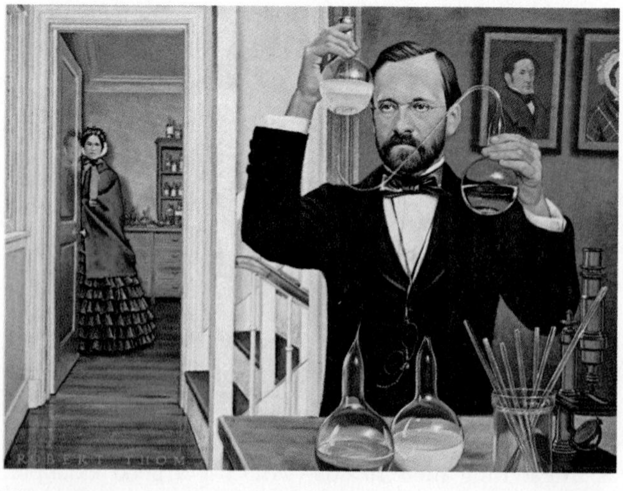

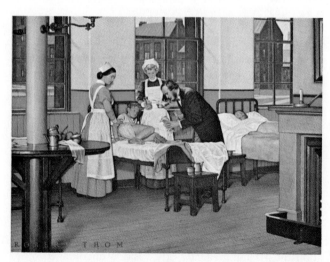

**Figure 3-1** Louis Pasteur, the father of preventive medicine. (Courtesy Parke-Davis & Company, © 1957).

**Figure 3-2** Joseph Lister revolutionized surgery by introducing antisepsis. (Courtesy Parke-Davis & Company, © 1957)

and demonstrated how cholera was transmitted by food and water. His discovery changed the way health departments cared for persons with infectious disease.

Fortunately, early in the twentieth century, society was finally liberated from many of the infectious and epidemic diseases that had scourged the human race for millennia. Smallpox vaccinations became common and causes of **yellow fever, typhus,** and **bubonic plague** were determined. Life expectancy increased. Tuberculosis became less frequent. In 1922, Frederick G. Banting and a medical student, Charles Best, were able to isolate and inject insulin into a fourteen-year-old boy who was dying of diabetes. Two weeks later, the boy was alive and alert. By 1923, insulin was available for general sale in pharmacies throughout the world. Antibiotics were discovered and the Salk and Sabin vaccines were found for poliomyelitis.

Yet, as we enter the twenty-first century, we are quite aware of the limitations of modern medicine. The rise of AIDS is a reminder that plagues are still possible. In developing countries torn with war and strife, cholera causes the deaths of thousands simply because there is no proper sanitation. In the microbial world, there are new, drug-resistant strains of malaria, tuberculosis, and other diseases that are not responding to known treatments. The challenge of medicine is as strong today as it was 100 years ago.

## SIGNIFICANT CONTRIBUTIONS TO MEDICINE

Hippocrates (c. 460–c. 377 B.C.) is the physician most recall from the Greek culture (Figure 3-3). It is not known

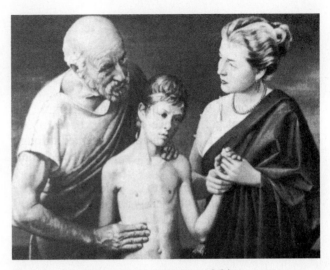

**Figure 3-3**   Hippocrates examining a child.

why his name surfaces above all other Greek physicians, for some were surely just as prominent. His writings, however, have contributed much to today's medical culture. Hippocrates is remembered by many for his well-known Hippocratic Oath, which established guidelines for a physician's practice of medicine. While few physicians swear to this oath today when they embark on their medical career, it is still recognized for its validity and wisdom. There are various translations of the Hippocratic Oath, although all communicate the same fundamental message.

It would be impossible to identify all the other individuals who made significant contributions to medicine in this text. There are several of note, however, who are mentioned in Table 3-1.

| TABLE 3-1   INDIVIDUALS OF NOTE IN THE HISTORY OF MEDICINE | |
| --- | --- |
| Moses c. 1205 B.C. | Advocate of health rules in Hebrew religion |
| Hippocrates c. 460–c. 377 B.C. | Greek physician; "father of medicine" |
| Andreas Vesalius A.D. 1514–1564 | Brussels physician; wrote first anatomical studies |
| Anton van Leeuwenhoek 1632–1723 | Dutch lens grinder; discovered lens magnification |
| John Hunter 1728–1793 | Founder of scientific surgery |
| Edward Jenner 1749–1823 | Developed smallpox vaccine |
| Rene Laennec 1781–1826 | Invented the stethoscope |
| W. T. G. Morton 1819–1868 | Massachusetts physician; introduced ether as anesthetic |
| Florence Nightingale 1820–1910 | Founder of modern nursing |
| Elizabeth Blackwell 1821–1910 | First female physician in America |
| Clara Barton 1821–1912 | Started American Red Cross in 1881 |
| Louis Pasteur 1822–1895 | "Father of bacteriology" |
| Joseph Lister 1827–1912 | Laid the groundwork on asepsis |
| Elizabeth G. Anderson 1836–1917 | First female physician in Britain |
| Robert Koch 1843–1910 | Bacteriologist; developed culture-plate method |
| Wilhelm Roentgen 1845–1923 | Discovered X rays (roentgenograms) |
| Sir Alexander Fleming 1881–1955 | Discovered penicillin in 1928 |

## THE OATH OF HIPPOCRATES

I swear by Apollo Physician and Aesculapius and Hygeia and Panacea and all the gods and goddesses, making them my witnesses, that I will fulfill according to my ability and judgment this oath and this covenant:

To hold him who has taught me this art as equal to my parents and to live my life in partnership with him, and if he is in need of money to give him a share of mine, and to regard his offspring as equal to my brothers in male lineage and to teach them this art—if they desire to learn it—without fee and covenant; to give a share of precepts and oral instruction and all the other learning to my sons and to the sons of him who has instructed me and to pupils who have signed the covenant and have taken an oath according to the medical law, but to no one else.

I will apply dietetic measures for the benefit of the sick according to my ability and judgment; I will keep them from harm and injustice.

I will neither give a deadly drug to anybody if asked for it nor will I make a suggestion to this effect. Similarly, I will not give to a woman an abortive remedy. In purity and holiness I will guard my life and my art.

I will not use the knife, not even on sufferers from stone, but will withdraw in favor of such men as are engaged in this work.

Whatever houses I may visit, I will come for the benefit of the sick, remaining free of all intentional injustice, of all mischief, and in particular of sexual relations with both female and male persons, be they free or slaves.

## NEW FRONTIERS IN MEDICINE

There has been phenomenal growth in medicine in the past two decades. Only a few advances are mentioned here. Much better imaging leading to much better diagnosis is now available. Where exploratory surgery might have been performed in the past to determine a diagnosis, noninvasive ultrasound, CT scans, and MRIs assist in diagnosis now. People who have worn glasses or contact lenses for many years are turning to eye laser surgery and implantable lenses.

Recently surgeons performed the first successful human larynx transplant. Consider the implications of an AIDS saliva test that creates a needle-free way to test for HIV. Needleless injections are now possible. There is a flu prevention inhaler and an osteoporosis pill.

Experimentation with aromatherapy reveals that some aromas actually improve brain function. Research has shown that individuals suffering from dementia often respond favorably to the odor of freshly roasted coffee and bread baking. Inhaling the scents of green apple, banana, and peppermint stimulates positive feelings. It is thought that with aromatherapy we will soon accelerate learning and speed up rehabilitation for people who have had a stroke.

Who can possibly predict what the future will bring in medicine?

## SUMMARY

Medicine's history leaves us with a rich heritage and a sound basis for the future of health care. Medical history continues to be in the making today. For example, research in gene manipulation has the potential benefit of being able to reverse the progression of many debilitating diseases. One day we will look upon medical discoveries of this decade and be impressed by how much further medicine has advanced.

## REVIEW QUESTIONS

### Multiple Choice

1. A pharmacopoeia is:
   a. a book describing drugs and their preparation
   b. an ancient religious rite used in medicine
   c. a source of magic
   d. used only by twentieth-century physicians

2. In later cultures, women were typically allowed to use their health care skills to:
   a. cure everyone in society
   b. care only for women and to assist in childbirth
   c. become physicians
   d. care only for the elderly

3. An accurate sketch of the spinal vertebrae was created during the Renaissance by:
   a. Leonardo da Vinci
   b. Michelangelo
   c. early Christian monks
   d. Louis Pasteur
4. Hippocrates is considered by many to be:
   a. the founder of scientific surgery
   b. the inventor of the smallpox vaccine
   c. the father of medicine
   d. the father of preventive medicine
5. The first woman physician in the United States was:
   a. Florence Nightingale
   b. Clara Barton
   c. Elizabeth Anderson
   d. Elizabeth Blackwell

## Critical Thinking

1. With a group of peers, identify the effects of culture on today's medicine.
2. How does the role of a medical specialist today compare to the role of a medical specialist in the past? Consider both similarities and dissimilarities.
3. You are a male physician on call in your hospital's emergency room when a woman, five months pregnant, is brought in. She is hemorrhaging. Her husband shuns you and demands a female physician. You quickly realize this couple is Muslim. Role play this scenario with a classmate. How can you solve the dilemma? Consider the possibility that your only female physician is out of the country on vacation.
4. You are the medical assistant. Your physician has just prescribed analgesics for a young Oriental woman suffering from migraine headaches. You overhear the young woman arguing with her mother who thinks that she should see a Chinese acupuncturist. What, if anything, would you do?
5. Discuss with a peer the role of women in medicine today. What difficulties, if any, might a female physician face today? Compare today's difficulties to those of female health care practitioners 100 years ago.
6. Write a one-page report on one significant person who contributed greatly to medicine.

## WEB ACTIVITIES

The World Wide Web is an ideal place to seek evidence of new and emerging technologies in medicine. One such avenue is "Medical Breakthroughs" reported by Ivanhoe Broadcast News, Inc. Identify at least two or three recent discoveries you find particularly interesting from your research on the Web.

## REFERENCES/BIBLIOGRAPHY

Keir, L., Wise, B. A., & Krebs, C. (1998). *Medical assisting: Administrative and clinical competencies* (4th ed.). Albany, NY: Delmar.

Kinn, M. E., & Woods, M. A. (1999). *The medical assistant: Administrative and clinical* (8th ed.). Philadelphia: W. B. Saunders.

Lewis, M. A., & Tamparo, C. D. (1998). *Medical law, ethics, and bioethics for ambulatory care* (4th ed.). Philadelphia: F. A. Davis.

Lyons, A. S., & Petrucelli, J. R., II (1978). *Medicine: An illustrated history*. New York: Harry N. Abrams, Inc.

*Taber's cyclopedic medical dictionary* (18th ed.) (1997). Philadelphia: F. A. Davis.

Warden, C. D. (1986). *Health care in the 1980s from a consumer's perspective*. Unpublished doctoral dissertation, Union Graduate School, Seattle, WA.

# *Unit*

## 2

# THE THERAPEUTIC APPROACH

# Chapter

## 4

# THERAPEUTIC COMMUNICATION SKILLS

## KEY TERMS

Active Listening
Bias
Body Language
Buffer Words
Closed Questions
Clustering
Communication Cycle
Compensation
Congruency
Decode
Defense Mechanism
Denial
Displacement
Encoding
Facial Expressions
Feedback
Gestures/Mannerisms
Hierarchy of Needs
Indirect Statements
Interview Techniques
Introjection
Kinesics
Masking
Modes of Communication
Open-Ended Questions
Perception
Position
Posture
Prejudice
Projection
Rationalization
Regression
Repression

*(continues)*

## OUTLINE

**Importance of Communication**
**Cultural Influence on Therapeutic Communication**
**Biases and Prejudices**
**The Communication Cycle**
  The Sender
  The Message
  The Receiver
  Feedback
**Listening Skills**
**Verbal Communication**
  The Five Cs of Communication
**Nonverbal Communication**
  Facial Expression
  Territoriality
  Posture
  Position
  Gestures and Mannerisms
  Touch

**Congruency in Communication**
  Perception
  Maslow's Hierarchy of Needs
**Technology and Communication**
**Roadblocks to Therapeutic Communication**
**Defense Mechanisms**
  Introjection
  Denial
  Compensation
  Regression
  Repression
  Sublimation
  Projection
  Displacement
  Rationalization
**Interview Techniques**
**Telephone Techniques**

## OBJECTIVES

*The student should strive to meet the following performance objectives and demonstrate an understanding of the facts and principles presented in this chapter through written and oral communication.*

1. Define the key terms as presented in the glossary.
2. Identify the importance of communication.
3. Recall at least four influences on therapeutic communication related to culture, and describe four common biases/prejudices in today's society.
4. List and define the four basic elements of the communication cycle.
5. Identify the four modes or channels of communication most pertinent in our everyday exchange.

*(continues)*

Roadblocks
Sublimation
Territoriality
The Message
The Receiver
The Sender
Therapeutic Communication
Touch

# OBJECTIVES (*continued*)

6. Discuss the importance of active listening in therapeutic communication.
7. Differentiate the terms verbal and nonverbal communication.
8. Analyze the five Cs of communication, and describe their effectiveness in the communication cycle.
9. Demonstrate the following body language or nonverbal communication behaviors: facial expressions, territoriality, position, posture, gestures/mannerisms, touch.
10. Identify and explain congruency in communication.
11. Discuss the use of Maslow's hierarchy of needs in therapeutic communication.
12. Discuss communication modification for electronically transmitted messages.
13. Recall eight significant roadblocks to therapeutic communication.
14. List and describe seven common defense mechanisms.
15. Discuss the possible impact on therapeutic communication that the unequal relationship between physician and patient might have.
16. Compare/contrast closed questions, open-ended questions, and indirect statements.
17. List four tools or considerations when communicating on the telephone.
18. Demonstrate the correct way to speak into the mouthpiece of a telephone by answering an incoming call and closing a telephone conversation.

# ROLE DELINEATION COMPONENTS

## GENERAL (TRANSDISCIPLINARY)

### Communication Skills

- Treat all patients with compassion and empathy
- Recognize and respect cultural diversity
- Adapt communications to individual's ability to understand
- Use effective and correct verbal and written communications
- Use medical terminology appropriately
- Use professional telephone technique

*(continues)*

# SCENARIO

In the two-doctor office of Doctors Lewis and King, four medical assistants constantly interact with patients, allaying their concerns, scheduling their appointments, instructing them on medications, and helping them understand their insurance coverage. On any given day, office manager Marilyn Johnson, CMA, is greeting patients warmly as they arrive for their appointments. Some patients, like Anna and Joseph Ortiz, are new to the practice. Marilyn's warm manner puts them at ease. Other patients, like Martin Gordon, who has prostate cancer, may be depressed and anxious. Marilyn tries to create an environment where they feel free to share their concerns and anxieties.

While Marilyn is busy with patients, administrative medical assistant Ellen Armstrong is on the telephone, scheduling appointments, answering patient questions, and making decisions about what calls need priority attention. Ellen projects a warm, courteous presence over the telephone; she maintains her composure, even when faced with difficult calls and tries always to ask the right questions of callers in a nonthreatening manner.

- Recognize and respond to verbal and nonverbal communications
- Receive, organize, prioritize, and transmit information
- Serve as a liaison
- Promote the practice through positive public relations

## INTRODUCTION

Of all the tasks and skills required of the medical assistant in the ambulatory care setting, none is quite so important as communication. Communication is the very foundation for every action taken by health care professionals in the care of their patients. Because medical assistants are often the liaison between patient and physician, it is critical to be aware of all the complexities of the communication process.

Every day, Marilyn and Ellen and the two clinical medical assistants at the offices of Doctors Lewis and King face many communication challenges. This chapter will describe effective communication principles, apply those principles to face-to-face communication as well as telephone communication, and describe the basic roadblocks to communication. The key word to all communication in the medical setting is *therapeutic*. In all conversation with patients, the more therapeutic the conversation, the more satisfied the patient will be with the care provided.

## IMPORTANCE OF COMMUNICATION

Communication in the health setting is the foundation for all patient care and is of the utmost importance. The majority of this communication in the ambulatory care setting will be therapeutic—it will utilize specific and well-defined professional skills. Patients' satisfaction with their medical care is as much related to the effectiveness of the communication between themselves and their chosen health care provider as it is to the actual care itself.

A patient choosing a physician wants a clear understanding of the physician's professional and technical skills as well as the physician's ability to communicate. The patient may question family members and friends regarding their personal physician's professional manner and communication skills. Questions often asked include: "Will your doctor talk with me so that I understand what is being said?" "Will your doctor listen to what I have to say?" "Can I talk to your doctor honestly and openly?"

When communication is therapeutic, patients feel validated and respected. **Therapeutic communication** skills create a feeling of comfort for patients even when difficult or unpleasant information must be exchanged.

## CULTURAL INFLUENCE ON THERAPEUTIC COMMUNICATION

 For true therapeutic communication to take place, the influence of culture must be considered. Cultural influences include one's ethnic heritage, geographic location and background, genetics, *No* (age,) gender, economics, educational experiences, life experiences, and value systems.

Any or all of these influences may exhibit themselves when health care is sought by patients. A patient's ethnic heritage may indicate a slant toward the Eastern influence in medicine as opposed to the traditional Western style more commonly taught and practiced in the United States today. Geographic location and background may reveal that a person is more comfortable with a family physician in a very small clinic than one in a large metropolitan multispecialty practice.

Age and gender are factors with a strong influence on communication. How and when do you communicate with a young child? What do you communicate to that child? How do you impress upon an elderly gentleman who has taken little medications throughout his lifetime that he now must take his pill every day? In a culture where the husband is the authority, how does the doctor discuss with the female patient the inadvisability of another pregnancy at this time?

Language barriers will prevent therapeutic communication if great care is not taken. If an interpreter is necessary, it is important to remember to speak directly to the patient, not the interpreter. If English is the second language or a heavy accent is involved, speaking clearly and slowly (not loudly) can greatly enhance communication. It must always be emphasized, however, that the lack of clear and understandable language does *not* imply lack of intelligence.

The influence of economics may reveal a discomfort if the office staff and patients have a different perception about how billing is managed and when and how payment is expected. A discussion of billing and payment procedures at the first office visit or before a major procedure will be beneficial to all concerned parties.

Educational and life experiences will, in part, determine how patients react to their care. Patients with family members being treated for a chronic illness will have more knowledge and understanding of that illness in their own lives. Individuals who have already suffered a great deal of loss and grief in their lives may handle the information of a life-threatening illness more easily than someone who has experienced little grief.

## BIASES AND PREJUDICES

Personal preferences, biases, and prejudices will enter into many physician-patient relationships. Such biases affect the types of communication possible. When individuals are not aware of their biases or prejudices, hostile attitudes may prevail.

For therapeutic communication to take place, biases must be examined, a person's comfort level with each bias determined, and measures taken to ensure that a hostile attitude is not present. Bias is defined as a slant toward a particular belief. Prejudice is defined as an opinion or judgment that is formed before all the facts are known; prejudice is a preconceived and unfavorable concept. Common biases and prejudices in today's society include:

1. A preference for Western style medicine
2. Choosing physicians according to gender
3. Prejudice related to a person's sexual preference
4. Discrimination based on race or religion
5. Hostile attitudes toward people with different value systems than one's own
6. A belief that people who cannot afford health care should receive less care than someone who can pay for full services

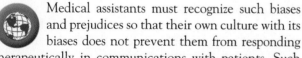 Medical assistants must recognize such biases and prejudices so that their own culture with its biases does not prevent them from responding therapeutically in communications with patients. Such recognition requires being aware of the differences among human beings and willingly accepting the uniqueness of each person.

## THE COMMUNICATION CYCLE

All communication, whether social or therapeutic, involves two or more individuals participating in an exchange of information. The communication cycle involves sending and receiving messages even when unconsciously aware of them.

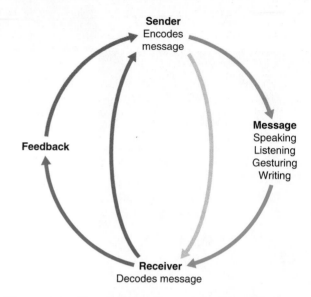

**Figure 4-1** The communication cycle and channels of communication.

Four basic elements are included in the communication cycle. They are (1) the sender, (2) the message and a channel or mode of communication, (3) the receiver, and (4) feedback (Figure 4-1).

### The Sender

The sender begins the communication cycle by encoding or creating the message to be sent. This is an important step, and much care should be taken in formulating the message. Before creating the message, the sender must observe the receiver to determine the complexity of the words to be used within the message, the receiver's ability to interpret the message, and the best channel by which to send the message.

### The Message

The message is the content being communicated. The message must be understood clearly by the receiver. Various levels of complexity in communication are used depending upon the ability of the receiver to recognize and understand the words contained within the message. Children do not have the vocabulary base nor the cognitive skills to communicate and understand the same as adults. The health of the receiver also must be considered. A patient who is stressed or in pain may find it difficult to concentrate on the message. If the patient is of a different nationality and/or culture from the sender, verbal communication may require special skill. When visual or hearing acuity is impaired, another challenge must be surmounted.

The four modes of communication, also called channels of communication, most pertinent in our everyday exchange include (1) speaking, (2) listening, (3) gestures or body language, and (4) writing. These modes or channels are affected by our physical and mental development, our culture, education and life experiences, our impressions from models and mentors, and in general by how we feel and accept ourselves as individuals. Each mode or channel of communication has its appropriateness and must be considered when formulating the message.

## The Receiver

The receiver is the recipient of the sender's message. The receiver must decode, or interpret, the meaning of the message. The primary sensory skill used in verbal communication is listening. It is hard work to concentrate and listen. When decoding the message, the receiver must be aware that not only the spoken words, but the tone and pitch of the voice and the speed at which the words are spoken carry meaning and must be evaluated.

## Feedback

Feedback takes place after the receiver has decoded the message sent by the sender. Feedback is the receiver's way of ensuring that the message that is understood is the same as the message that was sent. Feedback also provides an opportunity for the receiver to clarify any misunderstanding regarding the original message and to ask for additional information.

## LISTENING SKILLS

A vital part of feedback in the communication cycle is listening. A good listener is alert to all aspects of the communication cycle—the verbal and nonverbal message as well as verification of the message through appropriate feedback.

Active listening is one method used in therapeutic communication. In this technique, the received message is sent back to the sender, worded a little differently, for verification from the sender.

Sender:    "How can I possibly pay this fee when I have no insurance?"

Receiver:  "You're worried about paying your bill?"

The preceding example illustrates how the receiver is able to validate the sender's concerns at the same time the message is checked for accuracy. The door is then left open for a therapeutic response such as:

Sender:    "Our bookkeeper will be glad to work out a payment plan with you that will fit your resources."

## VERBAL COMMUNICATION

Verbal communication takes place when the message is spoken. However, one must keep in mind the fact that unless the words have meaning, and unless the sender and the receiver apply the same meaning to the spoken words, verbal communication may be misunderstood. If, for example, you overhear a conversation in a language foreign to you, you are indeed a witness to verbal communication, but you may not understand the message. To have any meaning, the spoken word must be understood by all parties of the communication (Tamparo & Lindh, 2000).

### The Five Cs of Communication

In their book *Professional Development*, Mary Wilkes and C. Bruce Crosswait (1991) identified the five Cs of Communication in business. They are (1) complete, (2) clear, (3) concise, (4) courteous, and (5) cohesive. These five Cs apply equally well in health care professions.

**Complete.** The message must be complete, with all the necessary information given. The medical assistant cannot expect the patient to be compliant if all the instructions are not given and understood.

**Clear.** The information given in the message must also be clear. The use of eye contact enhances clarity. Health care professionals must be able to articulate by using good diction and by enunciating each word distinctly. The patient must be allowed time to process the message and verify its meaning. The message must also be heard to promote understanding.

**Concise.** A concise message is one that does not include any unnecessary information. It should be brief and to the point (Figure 4-2). Patients must not be overloaded with technical terms that may not be understood or that tend to distract them by diverting their attention away from the balance of the message.

### Patient Teaching Tip

When patients speak a different language or when English is their second language, you may need to urge them to communicate nonverbally; you can encourage them to do so by using appropriate, nonthreatening gestures. Sometimes, it may be important to communicate verbally with a family member to gain specific information. Be sure not to violate any confidentiality of the patient, however.

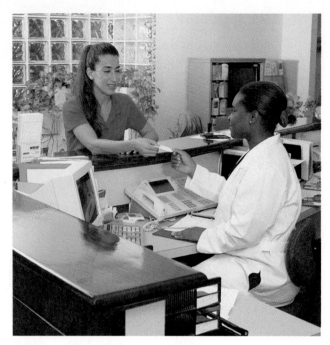

**Figure 4-2**   To say to the patient after greeting her by name, "I've completed an appointment card to remind you of your next appointment, Tuesday at 2:00 P.M." is an example of a concise message, brief and to the point.

**Courteous.** Courtesy is important in all aspects of communication. It only takes a moment to acknowledge a patient with a smile or by name. Knocking on the exam room door before entering validates the patient's right to privacy and builds self-esteem.

When a patient must be placed on hold on the telephone, thank the patient for waiting. Try not to keep the patient waiting too long if you must find information.

Remember to be courteous to colleagues in the office. Good working relationships and professionalism are always enhanced by simple courtesy.

**Cohesive.** A cohesive message is organized and logical in its progression. The cohesive message does not ramble and does not jump from one subject to another. The

## Patient Teaching Tip

Sensitive medical assistants will encourage patients to verbalize their concerns. The ability to ask questions in a nonprobing way and to elicit patient response is an important function in any ambulatory care setting, for it is critical to know a patient's history, current medications, and other relevant data.

patient should be able to follow the message easily. The medical assistant should always allow time to summarize detailed messages and utilize responding skills to verify that the patient fully understands the message.

When communicating within the health professions, keep in mind the following:

1. Good communication skills are necessary in establishing rapport with patients.
2. Patients feel respected and validated when called by their full name, such as Mary O'Keefe or Mrs. O'Keefe.
3. Patients should be encouraged to verbalize their feelings.
4. Give technical information to patients in a manner that they can understand.
5. Allow patients to make practical application to their personal health needs.

## NONVERBAL COMMUNICATION

Verbal communication alone is not always adequate in conveying the message being sent. In most instances, more than one mode or channel of communication is employed. Nonverbal communication, often referred to as **body language,** includes the unconscious body movements, gestures, and facial expressions that accompany speech. The study of body language is known as **kinesics** (Figure 4-3).

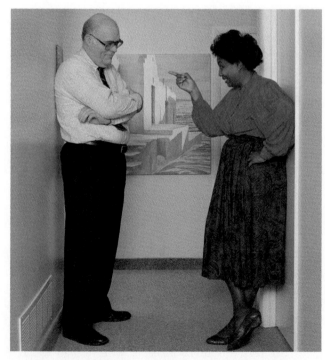

**Figure 4-3**   Body language can communicate more than spoken words.

Nonverbal communication is the language we learn first. It is learned seemingly automatically when infants learn to return a smile or respond to touches on the cheek. Much of our body language is a learned behavior and is greatly influenced by the primary caregivers and the culture in which we are raised.

Feelings and emotions are communicated most often through nonverbal means. The body expresses its true repressed feelings using body language. Most of the negative messages we communicate are also expressed nonverbally and usually are unintentional. Experts tell us that 70 percent of communication is nonverbal. The tone of voice communicates 23 percent of the message—only 7 percent of the message is actually communicated by the spoken word (Wilkes & Crosswait, 1991).

## Facial Expression

Facial expression is considered one of the most important and observed nonverbal communicators. Each facet or aspect of the anatomy of the face sends a nonverbal message.

Often expressions of joy and happiness or sorrow and grief are reflected through the eyes. The anatomy of the eyes does not change, but the movements of the structures surrounding the eyes enhance or magnify the message being communicated.

Children are told it is not polite to stare at people. It is acceptable to stare at animals in the zoo or art objects in the museum, but not at humans. Staring is dehumanizing and is often interpreted as an invasion of privacy.

The medical assistant must learn not to stare when patients present with ailments that make them "look" different. Patients such as these are individuals who have needs and who perhaps feel pain, discomfort, and have decreased self-esteem and value. These feelings will only be amplified if the medical assistant and other health professionals are unable to "see" them as humans. A lack of eye contact may also be viewed as avoidance or disinterest in being involved.

The movements of the eyebrow indicate many nonverbal cues as well. Surprise, puzzlement, worry, amusement, and questioning are often nonverbal messages reflected by the position of the eyebrow. Wrinkling of the forehead sends similar messages.

Cultural influences affect customs and different forms of facial expressions. In many Latin and Asian countries, it is unacceptable to look adults in the eye so people from these cultures often stare at the floor. This expression may be misinterpreted and misunderstood. Many persons of Eastern cultures communicate nonverbally differently from persons of Western cultures. These differences also may lead to confusion and misunderstanding.

## Territoriality

Territoriality is the distance at which we feel comfortable with others while communicating. In the classroom, for example, students claim their territory the first day of class. The area is well-defined by using books and papers or by placing the arm, hand, or chair on boundary lines. When another invades the territory, a shift in body position or the use of eye contact sends the message "This is my area." Individuals may feel threatened when others invade their personal space without permission. Some examples of comfortable personal space follow:

- Intimate
  touching to 6 inches
- Personal
  1½ to 4 feet
- Social
  4 to 12 feet
- Public
  12 to 15 feet

As with facial expressions, territoriality or personal space will be handled differently by various cultures. For example, there is no word for privacy in the Japanese language. Population numbers require crowding together publicly as well as privately. Public crowding is often viewed as a sign of warmth and pleasant intimacy in Japan. In the private home, several generations may live together; however, each considers this space to be his own and resents intrusion into it.

 Arabs like to touch their companions, to feel and to smell them. To deny a friend your breath is to be ashamed. When two Arabs talk to each other, they look each other in the eyes with great intensity.

The medical assistant may perform many invasive tasks during the course of an office visit. Examples include taking vital signs or giving injections, both of which require touching the patient. It is beneficial to explain procedures that invade another's space before beginning the procedure so that it will not be perceived as threatening. This helps to empower the patient by involving the patient in the decision-making process and builds a sense of trust in the medical assistant.

## Posture

Like territoriality, posture is important to allied health care professionals. Posture relates to the position of the body or parts of the body. It is the manner in which we carry ourselves, or pose in situations. We tend to tighten up in threatening or unknown situations and relax in nonthreatening environments. Those who study kinesics feel a posture involves at least half the body and that the position can last for nearly five minutes.

When the patient is seated with the arms and legs crossed, the message of closure or being opinionated may be relayed. On the other hand, sitting in a chair relaxed with the hands clasped behind the head indicates an attitude of being open to suggestions. Slumped shoulders may signal depression, discouragement, or in some cases even pain.

## Position

Position, the physical stance of two individuals while communicating, is a key factor to consider while communicating with the patient. Most physician-patient relationships utilize the face-to-face communication arrangement. When speaking with a patient, the physician or medical assistant will want to maintain a close but comfortable position enabling observation of all cues being sent, both verbal and nonverbal (Figure 4-4).

Standing over a patient can convey a message of superiority, and too much distance between the two parties may be interpreted as avoidance or being exclusive. Generally, leaning toward the patient expresses warmth, caring, interest, acceptance, and trust. Moving away from the patient may be interpreted as dislike, disinterest, boredom, indifference, suspicion, or impatience.

Whenever possible, it is best to have a chair in the examination room and to have the patient seated comfortably there to begin the communication cycle. The medical assistant or physician can sit on a stool that can easily be moved toward the patient. This arrangement aids the patient in feeling valued, listened to, and cared for as a fellow human being.

## Gestures and Mannerisms

Most of us use gestures and mannerisms when we "talk" with our hands. This form of body language may be useful in enhancing the spoken word by emphasizing ideas, thus creating and holding the attention of others.

## Touch

Touch is a powerful tool that communicates what cannot be expressed in words. Its appropriateness in the patient/health professional relationship has well-defined boundaries and requires the use of good judgment on the part of the professional. Infants who are not touched, cuddled, and loved do not grow and develop as those who receive these reassuring gestures. The touch that communicates caring, sincerity, understanding, and reassurance is usually welcomed and considered to be a therapeutic response. Most patients will understand and accept the touching behavior as it relates to the medical setting; however, we

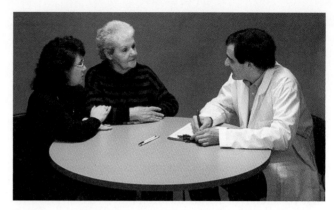

**Figure 4-4**    Positive posture and position encourage therapeutic communication.

must remember that not all patients are comfortable with touch. Whenever the patient is not comfortable with touch, ask permission and create as safe and reassuring an environment as possible.

## CONGRUENCY IN COMMUNICATION

There are some keys to successful communication to employ for communication to be effective. There must be congruency between the verbal and nonverbal communication. The two messages must agree; you cannot shake your head NO while saying YES verbally. This response sends a mixed message, and in most cases, the nonverbal messages will be accepted as the intended message.

It is also important to remember that most nonverbal messages are sent in groups of various forms of body language. The grouping of nonverbal messages into statements or conclusions is known as clustering. Masking involves an attempt to conceal or repress the true feeling

**SPOTLIGHT ON AAMA ESSENTIALS THROUGH CAAHEP**

- Respect your patient's cultural diversity, and adapt your skills to meeting the patient's needs.

- Remember that body language can often convey feelings not otherwise expressed through verbal communication.

- Consider that a patient may use defense mechanisms to mask true feelings.

or message. The perceptive professional will be aware of all these messages.

## Perception

Perception as it relates to communication is the conscious awareness of one's own feelings and the feelings of others (Fast, 1970). To be most useful and therapeutic as health professionals, we must first explore our own feelings and appreciate and accept ourselves.

Learning to use perception involves the ability to sense another's attitudes, moods, and feelings. It takes practice and experience to develop and use this skill effectively. Being attentive to other professionals and observing their use of perception will yield insight into its usefulness and provide an example to emulate. A word of caution—the use of perception may easily be misinterpreted, especially when going with your feeling or assessment of what is happening regarding the patient. Always follow perceived assessments with verbal validation before assuming your perception of the circumstance is correct.

Nonverbal communication is easily misinterpreted. Careful observation for congruency between verbal and nonverbal communication, and clustering nonverbal cues being sent into nonverbal statements will strengthen the ability to interpret the message accurately.

## Maslow's Hierarchy of Needs

Abraham Maslow is considered the founder of humanistic psychology and is most well known for his hierarchy of needs (Figure 4-5) (Miliken, 1998).

If you can understand this hierarchy, you can assess a patient's needs. If the most basic of needs are not met, it is highly unlikely that a patient can be successful with any

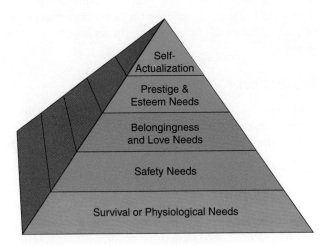

**Figure 4-5** Maslow's hierarchy of needs.

treatment protocol. Keeping this hierarchy in mind will help facilitate therapeutic communication.

## TECHNOLOGY AND COMMUNICATION

Face-to-face communication is the mode of choice in most physician offices today. However, technological devices are becoming more and more accepted as a means of communication. Technology-mediated communication and a greater reliance on cyberspace technology will greatly affect communication in the twenty-first century. Examples of new technologies in medical offices include fax machines, telecommunication conferences, e-mail, and laptop computers linked to a network of computers that communicate with satellite offices in another part of the community or even in another country.

Do these new communication methods change the communication cycle? There is still a message, a sender, a receiver, and feedback. What changes is the way in which the message is encoded and decoded. The content of the message will be examined for credibility rather than one's dress, eye contact, facial expression, vocal inflection, and posture. Technology does not convey emotions nearly as well as face-to-face or even telephone conversations. Another factor to consider is that your composed message may not look like what your reader sees. The software and hardware that you use for composing, sending, sorting, downloading, and reading may be completely different from what your recipient uses. Modifications to the format may change the intended emphasis or meaning of the message.

There are several advantages for the use of e-mail rather than postal mail (commonly referred to as "snail mail"). E-mail is less expensive and faster than mailing a letter. Because the turnaround time can be so fast, e-mail is more conversational than traditional paper-based media. An e-mail transmission is less intrusive than a telephone call and less bother than a fax. When one uses e-mail transmissions, differences in location and time zone are less of a problem. See Chapter 15 for additional information regarding e-mail.

## ROADBLOCKS TO THERAPEUTIC COMMUNICATION

Being sensitive to patients' unique personalities and needs will enable the health care professional to avoid roadblocks to communication (Table 4-1).

It must be the concern of each health care professional to facilitate communication by encouraging and enabling patients to express themselves honestly without

| TABLE 4-1 | ROADBLOCKS TO COMMUNICATION |
| --- | --- |
| **Roadblock** | **Example** |
| Reassuring clichés | "Don't worry, Mr. McKay, about not having a job; you'll find another one really soon." |
| Moralizing/lecturing | "If you were smart, Mrs. Johnson, you'd lose fifty pounds and you wouldn't have such a problem with your diabetes and hypertension." |
| Requiring explanations | "Why would you not want to have chemotherapy, Mr. Gordon? Seeing your wife die of cancer should surely make you want to seek treatment." |
| Ridiculing/shaming | "Ha, ha, Mr. Gordon! It's not *prostrate*—it's prostate cancer." |
| Defending/contradicting | "Mr. Marshal, I assure you the physician is *very busy.* He will not see you until he has finished with his other patients." |
| Shifting subjects | "Yes, Mrs. Jover, your work is very interesting, but I must ask you to sign this permission form to test for HIV." |
| Criticizing | "Mrs. O'Keefe, why in the world would you stay with an abusive husband?" |
| Threatening | "There is no way you will get rid of this cough if you do not stop smoking, Mr. Fowler." |

fear. Roadblocks close communication and prevent quality care of the total person.

## DEFENSE MECHANISMS

Defense mechanisms are used often by individuals and may further block the communication cycle. The use of defense mechanisms may be the result of individuals feeling threatened, ashamed, or guilty. In this situation, patients tend to respond defensively to protect themselves. Defense mechanisms are used unconsciously by all individuals at one time or another. They allow individuals to gain composure and/or control in a situation. They can become harmful when they prevent patients from seeing problems through to a satisfactory solution. Recognizing common defense mechanisms enables individuals to communicate effectively.

### Introjection

Introjection is the identification with another person or with some object. The patient assumes the supposed feelings and/or characteristics of the other personality or object.

### Denial

Denial (rejection of or refusal to acknowledge information) is often found in the health care setting. When patient Abigail Johnson does not comply with her diet, she is denying the consequences that might occur as a result.

### Compensation

Compensation is the overemphasizing of characteristics to make up for a real or imagined failure or handicap.

### Regression

Regression is moving back to a former stage to escape conflict or fear. When three-year-old Chris is faced with another baby in the family, he may feel left out, unwanted, and demand to be nursed or to have a bottle like the baby.

### Repression

Repression is temporary amnesia—being unable to cope with the overwhelming situation by temporarily forgetting. When Mary O'Keefe confronts her husband about his hostile attitude, he is likely to deny her allegation because he has repressed his frustration and anger at not having a satisfactory job.

### Sublimation

Sublimation is an example of redirecting a socially unacceptable impulse into one that is socially acceptable. If John O'Keefe could release his anger and frustration by playing handball, he would not be so hostile in other settings.

### Projection

Projection is the act of placing one's own feelings upon another. Juanita Hansen, who is suspected of child abuse, accuses the medical assistant of being unduly rough with her son.

### Displacement

Displacement occurs when individuals displace their negative feelings onto something or someone with no significance to the situation. Cele Little is agitated when Dr. Woo tells her that her hearing is seriously impaired and suggests going to an audiologist for a hearing aid. She yells at her sister, Dottie, about being so clumsy and falling and injuring her back.

## *Rationalization*

Rationalization is the act of justification, usually illogically, that one uses to keep from facing the truth of the situation. Leo McKay rationalizes that his stomach pains are the result of his lousy cooking and have nothing to do with the stress he may be feeling as the result of being laid off his job.

Recognizing defense mechanisms and understanding how best to communicate to get beyond the defense mechanisms to the truth is an art. It takes practice and patience. Medical assistants must be observant, always looking for the nonverbal cues while listening closely to the verbal message. Being present in the moment and giving each patient your full attention will enable you to communicate therapeutically.

## INTERVIEW TECHNIQUES

All health professionals must be adept at interview techniques—knowing how to encourage the best communication between themselves and the patient. It is important to remember that an unequal relationship exists between the health professional and the patient. The health professional, whether it be the physician or the medical assistant, is in the power position and has a great deal of control over the patient. Therefore, it is important to equalize the relationship as much as possible. That is the reason why some professionals use the term *client* rather than *patient*.

Early in the interview, the patient must feel comfortable enough to risk being honest with the health professional. The health professional must build an atmosphere of trust by showing concern for the patient. A gentle touch and a warm, caring facial expression may be all that is necessary. Always be honest and genuine in your responses to patients. Be sympathetic and empathic and create an environment that is free of hypocrisy.

When the medical assistant is interviewing the patient for the chief complaint, it is important to listen with a "third" ear. Listen to what the patient is not saying but is apt to exhibit through nonverbal communication.

You might choose to share your observation of the nonverbal message with the patient, thus encouraging the patient to verbalize more freely. When feelings are shared, validate and acknowledge those feelings through such statements as "I understand your distress." You can verify the communication by reflecting or paraphrasing what the patient has said.

You will be asking closed questions during the interview. Closed questions can be answered with a simple yes or no.

"Are you still taking your medication?"
"Are you in pain now?"

You will also use open-ended questions with the patient. These questions encourage therapeutic communication because the patient is required to verbalize more.

"What kind of help will you have at home during your recovery?"
"How are you coming along on this diet?"

Indirect statements will also prove helpful in facilitating therapeutic communication. An indirect statement will elicit a response from a patient without the patient feeling questioned.

"Tell me what you've been doing since you retired."
"I'd like to know more about your exercise program."

## TELEPHONE TECHNIQUES

It has often been said that the telephone is the lifeline of the physician's office. Communication over the telephone requires understanding on the part of each communicator (Figure 4-6).

Each medium uses the proper tools to get the job done. Speaking on the telephone is much like a conversation

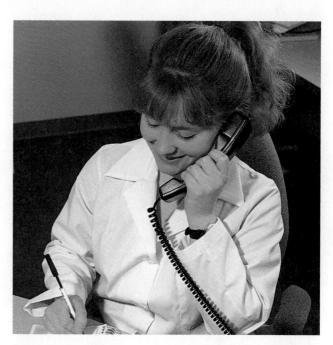

**Figure 4-6** When communicating over the telephone, listen with full attention to make certain the message sent and received is correct.

between two blindfolded individuals. The facial expressions cannot be seen, there is no eye contact, and there is no visual feedback. The listener will interpret mood by the tone and pacing of voice and the words spoken. When speaking on the telephone, quick conclusions are drawn. Often, we jump to conclusions, and the communication is misinterpreted.

The old, cold, aloof, formal business greeting comes across like frostbite in the medical office setting. It sounds curt, bored, and uncaring. Think of welcoming a new acquaintance into your home, then practice the same characteristics when speaking on the telephone. Speaking clearly, use words that will be easily understood, and ask questions to verify that the patient has understood the message being conveyed.

Concentrate on enunciating and being understood. If you hear, "What? I didn't understand you. I can't hear you," slow down and speak a little louder with distinct enunciation directly into the mouthpiece. The mouthpiece should be held one to two inches away from the mouth. Project your voice at the mouthpiece and then project another foot further. Your voice is the delivery system for your words and thoughts. Speak with confidence and conviction.

Have you ever called an office and had the firm name clipped off? The name of the office is important. To avoid clipping off the office name, practice using buffer words. **Buffer words** are expendable; if you clip them off, at least the office name remains intact. Use buffer words before the office name and before you identify yourself. "Good morning, this is Inner City Health Care. This is Walter, how may I help you?" *Good morning* and *this is* are buffer words.

All the techniques for effective face-to-face communication must be more intentionally observed when the communication is over the telephone because you cannot see the person with whom you are speaking. You must listen with full attention to make certain that the message sent and received is correct.

To close a telephone conversation to schedule an appointment, for example, consider the following:

1. Use the patient's name if it can be done without announcing the name to persons in the reception area.
2. Confirm the date and time of the appointment.
3. Identify the physician if there is more than one physician in the office.
4. Give any specific instructions that may be necessary.
5. Say goodbye.

For more information on telephone techniques, see Chapter 12.

## SUMMARY

Throughout this text you are reminded of the importance of effective communication techniques. Good communication takes practice. Use the techniques identified in this chapter with your family and with your peers. Watch for roadblocks, be aware of defense mechanisms, and remember the five Cs of communication.

**4-1**

It is a typically active day at the offices of Doctors Lewis and King. Despite the three emergencies in early afternoon and the full schedule of patients, everything is running smoothly with Dr. Lewis and the entire staff responding quickly but thoroughly to patient concerns.

At 4:00 P.M. another emergency patient arrives; at the same time Jim Marshal, an architect in a downtown firm, comes in early for a routine appointment and demands to be seen immediately. Jim, a regular patient, has a history of being difficult and impatient; being a bit arrogant, he tends to put his needs first. However, Dr. Lewis is occupied with another patient. It is critical to treat the patient with the emergency as soon as possible, and Jim is half an hour early.

Joe Guerrero, CMA, the office's administrative and clinical medical assistant, calmly asks Mr. Marshal to please wait until his scheduled appointment time. When he threatens to leave, Joe explains to Mr. Marshal that there are two patients ahead of him but that the doctor will see him at his scheduled appointment time.

*continues*

## CASE STUDY REVIEW

1. What communication roadblocks did medical assistant Joe Guerrero avoid in reacting to Jim Marshal's demands to see the doctor?

2. With another student, role-play the scenario, with one student taking the role of patient and one student the role of the medical assistant. Identify roadblocks to communication imposed by the patient. How is the medical assistant using the five Cs of communication to deal with the situation?

3. Do you think the medical assistant reacted appropriately? What else could he have done? What should he *not* do in this situation?

**CASE STUDY 4-2**

You have learned in this chapter that communication has not been successful until the cycle is complete. Consider the following scenario:

An 82-year-old woman with moderate dementia and a hearing impairment is brought to the surgeon's office for a follow-up appointment after hip replacement surgery. The woman's daughter accompanies her. The goal of the appointment is to make certain the hip is healing nicely and to discuss precautions before the patient returns to her assisted-living apartment. Almost immediately the conversation is directed toward the daughter because it is so much easier to explain to her what should be done.

## CASE STUDY REVIEW

1. What might the staff do to help the patient understand the following?
   - Use the walker consistently.
   - Shoes must be leather tennis shoe type or uniform style; consider Velcro closure as opposed to laces that have to be tied.
   - Do not wear pantyhose.
   - You will not be able to walk your dog on a leash.
2. Should the patient be left out of the conversation? Should the daughter be included?
3. In cases such as these, is something other than verbal communication indicated?

# REVIEW QUESTIONS

## Multiple Choice

1. Culture influences which of the following?
   a. biases and prejudices
   b. ethnic heritage, age, and gender
   c. educational and life experiences and value systems
   d. b and c only
2. In the cycle of communication, encoding means:
   a. deciphering a message
   b. creating the message to be sent
   c. sending the message
   d. receiving the message
3. Body language:
   a. is used to express feelings and emotions
   b. is not as important as verbal communication
   c. only makes up 7 percent of the message
   d. is only used in Eastern cultures

4. A comfortable social space is defined as:
   a. touching to 6 inches
   b. 1½ feet to 4 feet
   c. 12 to 15 feet
   d. 4 to 12 feet
5. A reassuring cliché is:
   a. a way of calming down a patient
   b. a means of rationalizing a decision
   c. a roadblock to communication
   d. always useful in daily communications
6. Redirecting a socially unacceptable impulse into one that is socially acceptable is an example of which of these defense mechanisms?
   a. sublimation
   b. rationalization
   c. projection
   d. displacement

7. When using an open-ended question with a patient, we expect:
   a. a yes or no answer
   b. them to tell us the truth
   c. a response that permits the patient to elaborate
   d. only the right answers
8. Buffer words:
   a. help us get through the day
   b. are meant to soothe a patient's feelings
   c. are expendable words used in answering a telephone call
   d. are important in face-to-face communication

## Critical Thinking

1. The 15-year-old girl awaiting a sports physical exam complains that she is overweight and has pimples. What is your therapeutic response?
2. Bill, who is 28 years old, comes for his annual checkup. When reviewing his social data sheet, you discover he is now living in an apartment and has a new phone number. He mumbles to you that his wife left him and won't let him see the kids. What is your verbal therapeutic response?
3. You try to be gentle and gracious with Edith. She is very fragile and difficult to please. While positioning her for an X-ray, she sneers and says, "You are about the roughest person who ever cared for me." What is your therapeutic response?
4. When you report to Herb that his cholesterol is quite high and that the doctor wants to discuss medication and diet, he responds, "That is impossible; you must have made some mistake." What is your therapeutic response?
5. Lenore uses a wheelchair for mobility. When you offer to help her, she says, "Buzz off! I can do this myself." What is your therapeutic response?
6. Leo, age 62, comments on his being laid off, "I simply don't know what I will do with all the extra time on my hands." What is your therapeutic response?
7. Martin says to you, "I wish it would just end," as you schedule him for another series of chemotherapy treatments. What is your therapeutic response?

8. Your physician/employer is leaving for hospital rounds. He must tell the Ward family that their father will never recover. If he does not die within the next thirty-six hours, the physician recommends disconnecting the ventilator. Your physician is close to this family; he has given them care for many years. What is your therapeutic response?

## WEB ACTIVITIES

Select three cultures of particular interest to you personally and search the World Wide Web for information regarding these cultures and communication traditions. How might this new information be applied to the physician whose clientele is primarily made up of these cultures? How might this new knowledge benefit a medical assistant employed in this type of setting?

## REFERENCES/BIBLIOGRAPHY

Blair, G. M. (January 23, 2000). *Conversation as communication* [On-line]. Available: http://www.ee.ed.ac.uk/~gerard/Management/art7.html

Fast, J. (1970). *Body language.* New York: M. Evans and Company.

Kinn, M. E., & Woods, M. A. (1998). *The medical assistant: Administrative and clinical* (8th ed.). Philadelphia: W. B. Saunders.

Miliken, M. E. (1998). *Understanding human behavior: A guide for health care providers.* Albany, NY: Delmar.

Purtillo, R. (1990). *Health professional/patient interaction.* Philadelphia: W. B. Saunders.

Sherwood, K. D. (January 25, 1999). *A beginner's guide to effective email* [On-line]. Available: http://www.webfoot.com/advice/email.top.html

*Taber's cyclopedic medical dictionary.* (18th ed.). (1997). Philadelphia: F. A. Davis.

Tamparo, C. D., & Lindh, W. Q. (2000). *Therapeutic communications for health professions.* Albany, NY: Delmar.

Wilkes, M., & Crosswait, C. B. (1991). *Professional development: The dynamics of success.* San Diego: Harcourt Brace Jovanovich.

# 5

# COPING SKILLS FOR THE MEDICAL ASSISTANT

## KEY TERMS

Burnout
Goal
Inner-Directed People
Long-Range Goals
Outer-Directed People
Parasympathetic Nervous System
Self-Actualization
Short-Range Goals
Stress
Stressors
Sympathetic Nervous System

## OUTLINE

**What Is Stress?**
    Adaptation to Stress
    Coping with Stress
**What Is Burnout?**
    Burnout in the Workplace
    What to Do If You Are Burned Out
    Preventing Burnout
**Goal Setting as a Stress Reliever**

## OBJECTIVES

*The student should strive to meet the following performance objectives and demonstrate an understanding of the facts and principles presented in this chapter through written and oral communication.*

1. Define the key terms as presented in the glossary.
2. Differentiate between stress and stressors.
3. Describe Hans Selye's GAS theory.
4. Identify seven approaches to coping with stressors in the ambulatory care setting.
5. Identify three characteristics associated with burnout in the workplace.
6. Identify seven signs or symptoms of burnout.
7. List five aspects of personality that promote burnout.
8. List a minimum of five ways to reduce the risk of burnout.
9. List five considerations when setting a goal.
10. Differentiate between long-range and short-range goals.

GENERAL
(TRANSDISCIPLINARY)

Professionalism

- **Project a professional manner and image**
- **Demonstrate initiative and responsibility**
- **Work as a team member**
- **Prioritize and perform multiple tasks**
- **Adapt to change**

At the office of Doctors Lewis and King, there are four full-time medical assistants who collaborate to make the office run smoothly, both administratively and clinically. One day a month, though, office manager Marilyn Johnson, CMA, is out of town, leaving Ellen Armstrong, the administrative medical assistant, in charge of a busy reception area and an ever-ringing telephone.

On these days, Ellen is particularly careful to organize her work so that things run as they should. She organizes some work the night before, she sets priorities so she is confident that the critical work will get done, and she tries to maintain her calm by taking a short break every couple of hours to review new needs that have come up during the day. While Ellen can't anticipate every emergency, she does try to influence the situation rather than let events control her.

## INTRODUCTION

Even in the most well-managed ambulatory care setting, medical assistants and other health providers are likely to feel the effects of stress from time to time. They may be overworked on certain days; they may face difficult patient situations; they may find that the administrative and paperwork load is getting ahead of them.

This chapter helps today's busy, multifaceted medical assistant pinpoint the symptoms of stress and provides ideas for coping with stress as it occurs. The better equipped the medical assistant is to confront and solve the sources of stress, the less likely stressors will become so overwhelming as to lead to burnout on the job. Goal setting, recognizing one's limitations and potentials, setting priorities, and keeping a balanced perspective can work together to reduce stress and enable the medical assistant to take pleasure in working with patients and colleagues.

## WHAT IS STRESS?

The body's response to change is termed **stress.** Stress is the "wear and tear" our bodies experience as we continually adjust to a changing environment. Stress has physical and emotional effects on the body, which create either eustress-positive feelings, or distress-negative feelings. Feeling positive leads to a sense of well being, increased motivation, and awareness of new opportunities and perspectives. Positive stress adds anticipation and excitement to life and is enhancing to our lives. Some stress is beneficial and helps us focus on details, achieve difficult goals, and perform at our best.

Negative feelings, or distress, may result in boredom, frustration, rejection, distrust, anger, and depression. Physical symptoms of distress may include cigarette smoking, obesity, and lack of exercise. It has been estimated that 50 percent of all diseases in the United States have a stress-related origin. Included in these diseases are hypertension, migraine headaches, ulcers, anxiety, allergies and asthma, and some types of cancer and cardiovascular disease (Tecco, 1999).

The demands to change that cause stress are called **stressors.** Stressors cause the body to go into arousal or alarm and may be anything from fear, worry, threat, or even challenging events. When we experience any type of stress that exceeds what our body can comfortably handle, we are more susceptible to depression and anxiousness. If we become very stressed, the ability to think clearly and objectively may be impaired.

### Adaptation to Stress

Hans Selye's General Adaptation Syndrome (GAS) theory proposes that adaptation to stress occurs in four stages, which he defines as alarm, fight-or-flight, exhaustion, and return-to-normal (Figure 5-1).

**Alarm.** Awareness of perceived stress is recognized by the body during the alarm stage. Pain is a part of this system as it tells us when body tissue is being damaged. A therapeutic response in the ambulatory care setting is to recognize the fact that pain does produce a stress response. The medical assistant who falls behind during the daily rush of scheduling may also experience a slight rise in blood pressure caused by the alarm stage of stress.

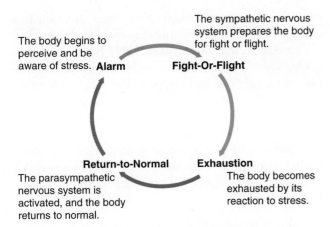

The body begins to perceive and be aware of stress. **Alarm**

The sympathetic nervous system prepares the body for fight or flight. **Fight-Or-Flight**

**Return-to-Normal** The parasympathetic nervous system is activated, and the body returns to normal.

**Exhaustion** The body becomes exhausted by its reaction to stress.

**Figure 5-1** Hans Selye's General Adaptation Syndrome (GAS) theory proposes that four stages are involved in adapting to stress.

**Fight-or-Flight.** The **sympathetic nervous system** prepares the body for fight-or-flight. The eyes dilate and the mouth becomes dry. The heart rate is increased, as is the pulse and respirations. Blood vessels in the skin constrict, and blood vessels in the heart and brain dilate. There is decreased motility in the gastrointestinal and genitourinary tracts. All these changes prepare the body for whatever action may need to be taken.

**Exhaustion.** The body can only stay in the fight-or-flight state for a limited time. If you have ever stretched a rubber band to the maximum and held it there for a period of time, eventually you tired of holding it and released the rubber band. If you were to examine the rubber band after its release, you would find that it has lost some of its elasticity, which can never be regained. The same principle applies to the blood vessels throughout the body. After repeated periods of dilation and relaxation, they become weakened. If you have ever overstretched a rubber band, you know it snaps in two. Blood vessels may burst when they are dilated to an extreme or have developed weakened areas.

**Return-to-Normal.** During the return-to-normal stage, the **parasympathetic nervous system** is activated, and the body returns to normal. The eyes constrict, salivary glands begin to function, and heart rate, pulse, and respirations decrease. Blood vessels dilate in the skin and constrict in the heart and brain. The gastrointestinal and genitourinary tracts begin to function again (Tamparo & Lindh, 2000).

Each stage in Selye's GAS theory is a mechanism to help protect the body and prepare it to escape from danger. When demands are placed on the body, stress occurs. The way a person reacts to those demands determines the

level of stress and whether health is threatened or harmed.

Stress is often considered harmful to health. In reality, stress is essential to one's well-being. The body continually goes through change in the course of a twenty-four-hour period. For example, a quick response while driving to work may be necessary to avoid a collision with another vehicle. During your working hours the telephone rings, the exam rooms are full, and the physician is called to the hospital on an emergency. Immediately the body's stress mode is activated. A moderate to high level of stress for short periods of time enables you to make quick judgments and decisions, to be organized and efficient, and to accomplish tasks within minimal time limits.

When too much stress is experienced or if the stress lasts for a long period of time, it begins to affect the body in a negative way. Often one of the first signs of stress may be a headache caused by an increase in blood pressure. Feeling tired even after plenty of rest may be another signal of stress. If these conditions continue, other vital organs, such as the heart and lungs, for example, may also be affected negatively. Cardiac or respiratory arrest, transient ischemic attack, or fainting may be experienced.

For the medical assistant, new technology, a demanding work load, responding to the needs of people who are ill or hurting, patient diversity, and the continuing need for creative problem solving are examples of the stressors encountered daily in ambulatory care settings.

## Coping with Stress

The following suggestions may be helpful in coping with stressors in the work environment.

1. Plan ahead
   - Review the schedule for the next day, and pull charts before leaving the office for the day.
   - Keep an accurate inventory of supplies; order before the last items are used.
   - Read journals and keep current with new technology.
   - Participate in continuing education activities.
2. Arrive early
   - Review the patient charts for the day; notice any special problems or needs.
   - Be sure that each exam room is well-equipped and ready for patients.
3. Personal assessment
   - Get plenty of rest.
   - Exercise and eat balanced meals.
   - Dress appropriately. Clothing or shoes that are too tight cause stress.

4. Laugh
   - Learn to laugh at life's little problems.
   - Laugh at yourself.
   - Establish an appropriate level of humor with other members of the staff.
5. Music, color, light
   - Soft background music has been proven to soothe and promote relaxation.
   - Use color and light to create a calm atmosphere.
6. Breaks
   - Build morning and afternoon breaks into the schedule, even if only five or ten minutes.
   - Close the office during the lunch hour, and if possible, leave the facility.
7. Work smarter, not harder
   - Employ time management techniques for reducing stress by completing one task before moving on to another.
   - Prioritize tasks; when possible do the most difficult task early in the day.
   - Do not procrastinate.
   - Be motivated.
   - Be a team member as well as working well independently.
   - Plan your work, then work your plan.

Incorporating these suggestions for coping with and relieving stress will help you operate efficiently and effectively in the ambulatory care setting. You may begin to experience what Abraham Maslow termed **self-actualization.** During self-actualization, you develop your full potential and experience fulfillment and job satisfaction. See Table 5-1 for some suggestions for relieving tension and stress during your daily work routine.

## WHAT IS BURNOUT?

According to New York psychologist Herbert J. Freudenberger, PhD, who coined the term, **burnout** is a state of fatigue or frustration brought about by a devotion to a cause, a way of life, or a relationship that failed to produce the expected reward (Gehmeyer, 2000). Burnout exhausts one's physical and mental resources, and leaves one feeling angry, helpless, and trapped. The military term for burnout is "battle fatigue." As a medical assistant you are a member of the health care team that battles disease and the ravages of disease on a daily basis.

Burnout does not occur suddenly as does stress. Rather, burnout is a gradual process that occurs slowly over a period of time. Typical signs and symptoms of burnout include:

- Emotional and physical exhaustion
- Anger
- Self-criticism
- Irritability
- Hair-trigger display of emotions
- Impatience
- Negativism
- A sense of being constantly under attack
- Inability to keep even daily frustrations in perspective

## *Burnout in the Workplace*

Burnout happens to people who previously were enthusiastic and bursting with energy and new ideas when first hired on the job or beginning a new experience. When individuals with a high need to achieve do not reach their goals, they are apt to feel angry and frustrated. Failing to recognize these signs as symptoms of burnout, they may throw themselves even more fully into work-related goals. Unless there is some type of revitalization outside of the workplace, burnout occurs.

Three characteristics associated with burnout in the workplace include:

- Role Conflict: When employees have conflicting responsibilities, they feel pulled in many directions. The perfectionist tries to do everything equally well without setting priorities. Fatigue and exhaustion associated with burnout begin to set in after a period of time.

- Role Ambiguity: The employee does not know what is expected and how to accomplish it because there may not be a role model to follow or ask, or established guidelines to follow.

- Role Overload: If the employee cannot say no and continues to accept more responsibility than they can handle, burnout is sure to set in (Gehmeyer, 2000).

| TABLE 5-1  TECHNIQUES FOR REDUCING STRESS AT WORK |
| --- |
| • Stretch or change positions. |
| • Slowly roll your head from side to side and forward and back. |
| • Slowly rotate your shoulders forward and backward several times. |
| • Turn away from the computer or close your eyes for several seconds. |
| • Walk around and deliver charts or lab specimens, and so on. |
| • Stand or sit tall and take a few deep breaths. |
| • Meditate for 30 seconds. |
| • Know your limits and be aware of your body's needs. |

## What to Do If You Are Burned Out

When you recognize the signs and symptoms of burnout, it is time to do some self-analysis by asking yourself some hard questions. Recall and analyze when you began feeling so tired and unable to relax and enjoy your work. Have you always been a perfectionist? Have you always had a higher need than most of your peers to do a job well? Are you irritable toward coworkers or patients? At what point did you lose your sense of humor? Do you always see work as a chore? Are you so intensely striving to achieve your goals that if you do not succeed you consider yourself a failure? Are you physically and emotionally exhausted?

The next step is to make some changes.

- Make a list of negative words or phrases that you most often use. Now replace the negatives with more neutral words or phrases.

- Create some job diversity for yourself. Drive to work via a different route; enter the building through a different door; change your work routine slightly; change your start time.

- Become creative. Redecorate your area.

- Establish some long- and short-term realistic goals and write them down.

- Take care of yourself; change your eating habits; exercise more; get more sleep.

- Renew friendships; go to lunch with coworkers; laugh with them.

- Implement time management techniques.

- Delegate responsibility to others who are capable.

Table 5-2 will help you assess your risk for burnout.

## Preventing Burnout

The best way to treat burnout on the job is to prevent it. This can be accomplished by leaving work-related issues at the office when leaving for the day. Other things you can do to reduce the risk of burnout include:

- Maintain a positive self-esteem and self-image

- Have regular physical examinations

- Take a vacation

- Give up unrealistic goals and expectations

- Develop interests outside of your profession

- Separate work from the rest of your life

- Develop time management techniques

- Develop clear and complete job descriptions for each position in the office

## GOAL SETTING AS A STRESS RELIEVER

Do you direct your life or do you allow others to influence and make decisions for you? **Outer-directed people** let events, other people, or environmental factors dictate their behavior. By contrast, **inner-directed people** decide for themselves what they want to do with their lives. Laurence Peter, author of *The Peter Principle*, stated, "If you don't know where you are going, you will end up somewhere else" (Wilkes & Crosswait, 1991).

Discoveries prove that goal-oriented employees are more effective and assertive than colleagues with no goals or future objectives. Recognizing the value of goal planning, many employers arrange planning sessions and/or

| TABLE 5-2 ASSESS YOUR RISK FOR BURNOUT | | |
|---|:---:|:---:|
| This simple test, developed by the Center for Professional Well-Being, can help you determine your predisposition to distress in your life. The more questions with a "yes" response, the greater your risk for burnout. | Yes | No |
| 1. Are you highly achievement-oriented? | ☐ | ☐ |
| 2. Do you tend to withdraw from offers of support? | ☐ | ☐ |
| 3. Do you have difficulty delegating responsibilities to others, including patients? | ☐ | ☐ |
| 4. Do you prefer to work alone? | ☐ | ☐ |
| 5. Do you avoid discussing problems with others? | ☐ | ☐ |
| 6. Do you externalize blame? | ☐ | ☐ |
| 7. Are your work relationships asymmetrical; that is, are you always giving? | ☐ | ☐ |
| 8. Is your personal identity bound up with your work role or professional identity? | ☐ | ☐ |
| 9. Do you often overload yourself and have a difficult time saying no? | ☐ | ☐ |
| 10. Is there a lack of opportunities for positive and timely feedback outside of your professional or work role? | ☐ | ☐ |
| 11. Do you abide by the laws "don't talk, don't trust, don't feel?" | ☐ | ☐ |

Musick, J. L. (1997). *How Close Are You to Burnout?* American Academy of Family Physicians. [On-line]. Available: http://www.aafp.org/fpm/970400fm/lead.html

seminars to encourage goal setting as a practical application for coping with stress and/or burnout and to develop career objectives. If this does not happen in your work environment, seek your own seminars for goal setting. Such an activity not only "centers" you in your current employment but helps you clearly picture your future plans and hopes.

What is a **goal**? The dictionary definition of a goal according to *Merriam-Webster's Collegiate Dictionary* is, "the result or achievement toward which effort is directed." To reach a desired goal, a person must implement planning along with a sincere desire to work hard. Skill in goal setting allows the medical assistant to clarify what must be accomplished and to develop a strategic plan to successfully achieve the goal.

A goal must be specific, challenging, realistic, attainable, and measurable. Specific goals are focused and have very precise boundaries. A goal that is challenging creates enthusiasm and interest in achievement. Realistic goals are practical or beneficial for the present and for future self-actualization. An attainable goal refers to the fact that the goal is possible to fulfill. Measurable goals achieve some form of progress or success. By reflecting on the process, one is encouraged to establish additional goals.

**Long-range goals** are achievements that may take three to five years to accomplish. Long-range goals give direction and definition to our lives and serve to keep us "on track" so to speak. Much discipline, perseverance, determination, and hard work will be expended in accomplishing long-range goals. Some adjustment and readjust-

ment to your goals may be necessary, however. The rewards of goal achievement include satisfaction, pride, a sense of accomplishment, and a job well done.

**Short-range goals** take apart long-range goals and reassembles the required activities into smaller, more manageable time segments. The time segments may be daily, weekly, monthly, quarterly, or yearly periods.

As a graduate and new employee, one of your long-range goals might be to become the office manager in the ambulatory care setting in which you are currently employed. You may wish to attain this goal within the next three to five years; by breaking it into three longer range goals and a series of short-range goals, you will be able to measure progress and feel a sense of accomplishment. Examples of long- and short-range goals might include:

*Long-range goal 1:*

To become proficient in all back-office clinical skills during the first year of employment.

*Short-range goals necessary to achieve this:*

- Practice accuracy and proficiency when performing tasks and skills.

- Practice efficiency by planning ahead for the equipment and supplies needed for each task performed.

- Evaluate your progress on a regular basis, and identify areas that need improvement.

*Long-range goal 2:*

To add front-office administrative tasks and skills to your routine during the second year of employment.

*Short-range goals necessary to achieve this:*

- Practice accuracy and proficiency when performing all front-office tasks and skills.

- Practice efficiency by planning ahead for the equipment and supplies needed for each task performed.

- Evaluate your progress on a regular basis, and identify areas that need improvement.

*Long-range goal 3:*

To begin to focus on office management during the third year of employment.

*Short-range goals necessary to achieve this:*

- Develop a procedures manual for all back- and front-office tasks and skills.

- Enroll in office management classes.

- Focus on team-building skills.

By year four, you will be ready to move into the office manager position.

Long-range and short-range goals work together to help make changes in our lives. Goals keep life interesting and give us something for which to strive. We can all reach goals successfully with some planning, hard work, discipline, and dedication.

## SUMMARY

Stress is very much a part of the medical profession. Each individual working in a medical career experiences consecutive days of demanding, emotionally and physically draining interactions with patients and staff members. This highly technical and ever-changing career requires its professionals to maintain a high level of skill and training and to be familiar with the newest technology.

Goal setting is one approach to reducing stress and burnout and promoting a sense of pride in the workplace, self-actualization, and possible employment promotion. Both long-range and short-range goal planning work together to help make changes in our lives.

**CASE STUDY 5-1**

Ellen Armstrong, CMA, is an administrative medical assistant with Doctors Lewis and King. This is her first job. She is just two years out of school, and she is trying to learn everything she can to achieve her long-range goal of becoming office manager at this or some other ambulatory care setting.

Ellen has a great deal in her favor, for she is good with patients, both face-to-face and over the telephone. She is not daunted by the complexity of administrative work her job requires. Ellen knows she has a great deal yet to learn and, although she is a bit intimidated by her, Ellen looks to Marilyn Johnson, CMA, the office manager, for guidance and advice.

### CASE STUDY REVIEW

1. How would you advise Ellen to go about achieving her long-term goal of office manager?
2. What are some of the short-term goals Ellen should set? Why are short-term goals important to her success?
3. Besides learning on the job, what else can Ellen do to achieve her goal?

**CASE STUDY 5-2**

Ellen Armstrong, CMA, has been employed for five years as an administrative medical assistant with Doctors Lewis and King. Ellen is a perfectionist and has pushed herself to achieve many of her short- and long-term goals. The office staff has become aware of the fact that Ellen does not have a sense of humor lately. She seems frustrated and irritable, and is becoming critical of herself and others. Ellen has felt physically and emotionally exhausted, yet she continues to focus on her high standard of job performance; however, work is becoming a chore. At the end of the day if everything has not been completed to her satisfaction, she feels like a failure.

### CASE STUDY REVIEW

1. Do you feel Ellen is stressed or experiencing burnout? What do you base your conclusions upon?
2. What might Ellen do to differentiate these two conditions?
3. What changes might Ellen implement to resolve this problem?

## REVIEW QUESTIONS

### Multiple Choice

1. Which answer is *not* true about stress?
   a. It does not occur suddenly.
   b. It has physical and emotional effects on the body.
   c. It may be positive or negative on its affects on the body.
   d. It is the body's response to change.
2. Hans Selye's GAS theory proposes that adaptation to stress occurs in how many stages?
   a. 2 stages
   b. 3 stages
   c. 4 stages
   d. 5 stages
3. Which is *not* a stage in the General Adaptation Syndrome?
   a. fight-or-flight
   b. exhaustion
   c. burnout
   d. alarm
4. Burnout occurs often if:
   a. a person is aged
   b. the individual works as a health care professional
   c. an individual has certain personality traits
   d. the individual isn't interested in the job
5. Signs and symptoms of burnout include all of the following *except*:
   a. emotional and physical exhaustion
   b. hair-trigger display of emotion
   c. feelings of accomplishment and pride in work
   d. irritability and impatience
6. Working smarter, not harder includes:
   a. taking a sick day now and then, even if you're not sick
   b. prioritizing your tasks and employing time-management techniques
   c. giving as much work to others as possible
   d. making sure others are not taking advantage of you
7. Self-actualization is a term used by:
   a. Laurence Peter
   b. Abraham Maslow
   c. Hans Selye
   d. Harry Levinson
8. Long-range goals are easy to achieve if:
   a. they are not too challenging
   b. they are divided into a series of short-range goals
   c. they don't involve too much hard work
   d. you never change or adjust them

### Critical Thinking

1. Discuss a minimum of five methods of dealing positively with stress.
2. Through self-analysis, determine whether you are an outer-directed person or an inner-directed person and what impact this trait may have upon your medical assisting career.
3. List two long-range goals you personally would like to attain within the next five years. Now determine the short-range goals necessary to achieve your long-range goals.
4. Discuss the causes and manifestations of burnout.
5. Discuss the causes of burnout in the workplace and ways in which it may be decreased.

## WEB ACTIVITIES

 Search the World Wide Web for additional information on burnout in the workplace. Compile your information into a report for your instructor. Be sure to include a bibliography identifying your web sources.

## REFERENCES/BIBLIOGRAPHY

Cooper, J. R. (1993). *The medical reporter: Beware of professional burnout* [On-line]. Available: http://none.coolware.com/health/medical_reporter/burnout.html

drkoop.com. (1998–2000). Wellness: Mental health, stress, ways stress affects individuals. [On-line]. Available: http://www.drkoop.com/wellness/mental_health/stress/page_337_765.asp

Gehmeyr, A. (June 14, 2000). *Burnout* [On-line]. Available: http://155.187.10.12/fun/burnout.html

Gehmeyr, A. (1993). *Prescription for burnout* [On-line]. Available: http://155.187.10.12/fun/burnout.html

Keir, L., Wise, B. A., & Krebs, C. (1998). *Medical assisting: Administrative and clinical competencies* (4th ed.). Albany, NY: Delmar.

*Merriam-Webster's collegiate dictionary* (10th ed.). (1994). Springfield, MA: Merriam-Webster.

Musick, J. L. (1997). *American Academy of Family Physicians: How close are you to burnout?* [On-line]. Available: http://www.aafp.org/fpm/970400fm/lead.html

*Stress management*. (2000). [On-line]. Available: http://www.ivf.com/stress.html

Tamparo, C. D., & Lindh, W. Q. (2000). *Therapeutic communications for allied health professions*. Albany, NY: Delmar.

Tecco, A. (1999). *Stress management* [On-line]. Available: http://www.drkoop.com/wellness/prevcenter/stress/stress.asp

Vikesland, G. (1999). *How to prevent burnout and ridding yourself of burnout* [On-line]. Available: http://www.employer-employee.com/Burnout.html

Wilkes, M., & Crosswait, C. B. (1991). *Professional development: The dynamics of success*. San Diego: Harcourt Brace Jovanovich.

# THE THERAPEUTIC APPROACH TO THE PATIENT WITH LIFE-THREATENING ILLNESS

*Chapter*

## 6

## KEY TERMS

Acquired Immunodeficiency Syndrome (AIDS)

Culture

Dementia

Durable Power of Attorney for Health Care

Human Immunodeficiency Virus (HIV)

Libido

Living Will

Physician Directive

Psychomotor Retardation

## OUTLINE

Life-Threatening Illness
  Cultural Perspective on Life-Threatening Illness
Choices in Life-Threatening Illness
The Range of Psychological Suffering

The Therapeutic Response to the Patient with AIDS
The Challenge for the Medical Assistant

## OBJECTIVES

*The student should strive to meet the following performance objectives and demonstrate an understanding of the facts and principles presented in this chapter through written and oral communication.*

1. Define the key terms as presented in the glossary.
2. Describe possible patient perspectives when facing a life-threatening illness.
3. Define "life-threatening" illness.
4. Discuss cultural manifestations of life-threatening illness.
5. Identify the strongest cultural influence in the life of a patient.
6. List at least four choices to be made when facing a life-threatening illness.
7. Briefly describe the use of living wills and physician directives.
8. Discuss the range of psychological suffering that accompanies life-threatening illnesses.
9. Discuss additional concerns/fears when the life-threatening illness is AIDS.
10. Recall a number of challenges faced by the medical assistant when caring for people with life-threatening illnesses.

## ROLE DELINEATION COMPONENTS

### GENERAL (TRANSDISCIPLINARY)

**Communication Skills**

- Treat all patients with compassion and empathy

**Legal Concepts**

- Maintain confidentiality

**Instruction**

- Instruct individuals according to their needs
- Teach methods of health promotion and disease prevention
- Locate community resources and disseminate information

## SCENARIO

You have seen the medical reports and have agonized with your physician who must tell Suzanne Markis when she comes in today that she has inoperable pancreatic cancer. When she arrives, you treat her as you normally would, making certain she suspects nothing from you. When she emerges from the physician's room, you make certain to meet her, take her arm, and ask if you can call someone for her. You do not present her with a bill or make another appointment at this time. You recognize that anything you say will probably not be remembered, so you focus entirely upon this patient and her immediate needs. In a day or two, as instructed by your physician employer, you will make a phone call to set an appointment for Suzanne and any family members she might want present to visit with your physician so any questions might be answered for them.

## INTRODUCTION

Everything learned in Chapter 4 regarding therapeutic communications is heightened and considered more difficult when the patient has a life-threatening illness. If you were told today that your life would probably be shortened because of a serious illness, your perspective would change completely. What was important yesterday may mean little or nothing now. Something that meant nothing to you yesterday suddenly takes on great importance to you now. It is essential for the medical assistant to remember this difference in perspective and what is likely to be important to patients with a life-threatening illness.

It also must be remembered that no two individuals respond to a life-threatening illness in the same way. Some respond with denial and act as if the information had never been shared with them. Others alter their lives radically and drastically change their priorities. Still others quietly continue their lives changing very little outwardly but recognize that their choices may now be limited (Figure 6-1).

## LIFE-THREATENING ILLNESS

A life-threatening illness is not easily defined. Some will use the word *terminal*; others refuse to use that word because they believe it removes any hope from the situation. Also, what is life-threatening for one individual may not be for another. For our purposes, life threatening is used to imply a life that in all probability will be shortened because of a serious or debilitating illness or disease. It may be defined as death that is imminent; it may be defined in terms of a serious illness that one will battle for many years but will ultimately shorten his/her life.

### Cultural Perspective on Life-Threatening Illness

Strong cultural manifestations will be seen in the treatment of a life-threatening illness and for anyone facing death. **Culture** is defined as how we live our lives, how we think, how we speak, and how we behave.

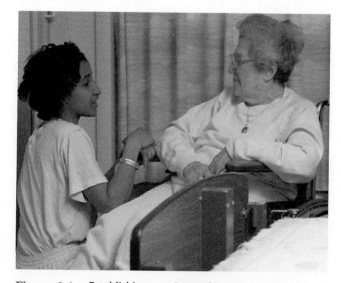

**Figure 6-1** Establishing a caring and trusting relationship will help the patient come to terms with a life-threatening illness.

## SPOTLIGHT ON AAMA ESSENTIALS THROUGH CAAHEP

- Taking care of a patient with a life-threatening illness should not constitute a fear of caring for that patient.

- Patients with life-threatening illnesses need not only skillful medical care but compassionate, sensitive treatment.

- Interacting with the seriously ill patient should include care that is appropriate to the patient's developmental age and cultural preferences.

Some cultures prefer that the life-threatening illness not be shared with the patient in the beginning, but with the family who helps to prepare the patient for the inevitable. A few cultures generally do not seek care for an illness until it is quite advanced; this practice can make pain management and treatment more difficult or impossible in some cases. Some cultures surround the person who is ill with great attention, never leaving the person alone. Other cultures view the illness as something that must be removed from the body, perhaps even believing that the individual has been visited upon with this illness due to some past sin or transgression.

In the same manner, pain is viewed. Some cultures believe it is to be endured quietly without complaint; others believe there is to be no pain and family members will go to great lengths to have health care providers relieve the pain. When questioning a patient about the pain level, it must be within a cultural perspective. For example, cultures with an Asian influence are more likely to describe pain in general terms related to the imbalance of the body than in terms of "piercing, intermittent, or throbbing" or on a scale of 1 to 10.

It must also be remembered that the strongest influence in managing any life-threatening illness in the life of the patient is *not* the health care team; it is the family and those closest to the patient. Therefore, great care must be taken to determine and understand the patient's cultural perspective as much as possible, and the patient must be given great respect. Many times the cultural influence may contradict the standard of care preferred by the health care provider. It is better to understand the culture and work within it than to deny it and continually work against the patient's belief system and influence of family.

## CHOICES IN LIFE-THREATENING ILLNESS

Many choices are available to a patient with a life-threatening illness, and many decisions are to be made. The urgency of the decisions will depend in part upon possible life expectancy. Sometimes these decisions may seem contrary to recommended medical intervention.

Patients have the right to choose or to refuse treatment in most cases. Some rush into a treatment protocol only to discover later that their choices have brought them pain, disability, and expense far beyond what originally was assumed. While it is the health care professional's goal to heal, if healing is not likely or possible, patients ought not to be "urged" into treatment protocols that are likely to be contrary to their personal wishes for the sake of treatment only.

While health care professionals are less comfortable with death than they are with saving life, there are some issues appropriate to discuss with patients especially when facing life-threatening illness. Those issues include the following:

1. **Living will** or **physician directive** documents may be used in making end-of-life decisions.
2. **Durable power of attorney for health care** allows another to make decisions for the patient when the patient is no longer able to do so.
3. Discussions of pain management and treatment may or may not be a part of a living will document but should be discussed at some point with the patient and/or patient's family.
4. Alternative methods of treatment should be discussed as well as the outcome if no treatment is sought.
5. Finances are to be considered. What will insurance cover (if there is insurance)? Who makes the decisions if managed care is an issue? What family resources can or will be used?
6. Emotional needs of the patient and family members are important. From where does the patient's primary support come? Friends, clergy, other?

It is not the responsibility of the health care professionals treating the individual with life-threatening illness to provide all these services, but a health care professional who raises these issues for patients and families to deal with is more closely in tune with a patient's power in the illness.

While some states were slow to recognize living wills, there is a piece of legislation that is available to all. The federal government passed the

Patient Self-Determination Act in 1991 giving all patients receiving care in institutions receiving payments from medicare and medicaid written information about their right to accept or refuse medical or surgical treatment. The act also requires that patients be given information about their options to create living wills and to appoint someone to act on their behalf in making health care decisions (durable power of attorney for health care). When facing a life-threatening illness, it can be very helpful to have some decisions made about what should be done and who can make decisions if the patient becomes unable to do so.

Any documents of this nature the patient has should be copied in the medical chart that goes with the patient when hospitalized. At any time the patient makes a change in such a document, the old document is to be replaced with the new one.

 The time when such documents are formulated can be the time for physicians to discuss with patients their right to decisions regarding pain management and treatment alternatives. Patients often fear pain and loss of independence more than anything when facing a life-threatening illness. It is better to have those discussions early in treatment than later when the patient may not be so clear on options. Sometimes treatment alternatives the patient may consider are not within the realm of recognized medical acceptability, but it is better to have that discussion than to ignore the possibility. Remember the earlier statement indicating that the family and friends bring more influence to bear than does the health care professional. If the physician and patient are seen as partners in the patient's care, then the patient may not be so fearful in discussing any nonmedically accepted protocol being considered.

Finances are no one's favorite subjects, especially physicians. However, such a discussion is important. Often patients fear not being able to meet their financial obligations as much as they fear the illness. What methods of payment are there? What does insurance cover? How far will insurance go? What restrictions does any managed care agency hold in a particular illness? Can the medical insurance be cancelled when the patient is no longer able to work or when a life-threatening illness is diagnosed?

Emotional support is vital when dealing with a life-threatening illness. Health care professionals will want to determine where that support comes from for the patient. Should a support group be suggested for the patient and family members? For some patients and families, an individual giving spiritual guidance is seen as a member of the family and a member of the health care team. For others, no spiritual influence is recognized or sought.

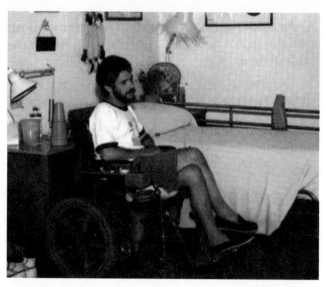

**Figure 6-2**   Patients living with a serious illness may experience a wide range of emotions.

## THE RANGE OF PSYCHOLOGICAL SUFFERING

The range of suffering associated with a life-threatening illness is extensive. Patients feel extreme distress. Anxiety and depression are common. At the time of diagnosis, patients' responses may include denial, numbness, and inability to face the facts. Sadness, hopelessness, helplessness, and withdrawal often are exhibited (Figure 6-2).

The range of psychological suffering leads to physical symptoms, such as tension, tachycardia, agitation, insomnia, anorexia, and panic attacks. The physician may be so intent on treating the physical ramifications of the illness that the psychological suffering is mostly ignored.

## THE THERAPEUTIC RESPONSE TO THE PATIENT WITH AIDS

It is not the intention of this chapter to specifically identify the many life-threatening illnesses and their particular needs. However, a few comments about patients testing positive for **human immunodeficiency virus (HIV)** and suffering from **aquired immunodeficiency syndrome (AIDS)** are important.

The discovery of infection with HIV is extremely stressful and is typically accompanied by the fear of developing AIDS. Patients are often preoccupied with illness and the fear of getting other life-threatening diseases. Patients are angry at the disease, at the discrimination that often accompanies it, at the prospect of a lonely, painful death, at the lack of effective treatment, at medical staff, and at themselves.

In many cases, guilt develops about past behavior and lifestyles, or about the possibility of having transmitted the disease to others. When the disease has been contracted through contaminated blood or blood products or by individuals who felt they were protected or safe from the disease, the anger may turn to rage.

Some patients contemplate suicide. Because social and physical assistance are needed, a strong network of friends and family is particularly important. In the case of homosexuals and those addicted to intravenous drugs, however, there are a large number who are estranged from their family's support system. People with AIDS may feel added strain if this is the first knowledge their families have of any high-risk behaviors associated with the transmission of the disease.

Patients with AIDS are apt to suffer central nervous system involvement. Forgetfulness and poor concentration may be followed by **psychomotor retardation** (the slowing of physical and mental responses), decreased alertness, apathy, withdrawal, diminished interest in work, and loss of **libido** (sexual drive). Some patients later experience confusion, progressive impairment, and profound **dementia** (progressive impairment of intellectual function).

## THE CHALLENGE FOR THE MEDICAL ASSISTANT

As a medical assistant, you face the challenge of caring for people with a life-threatening illness; you must comfort those who face great suffering and death. You will become a source of information for patients and their support members. You must be particularly sensitive and respectful toward individuals who may be viewed as social pariahs. You will have to examine your own beliefs, lifestyle, and biases. You must be comfortable treating all patients, no matter what the illness is or how it was contracted.

As well as assisting your physician or employer in providing the best possible medical care, many nonmedical forms of assistance may be required by patients suffering from a life-threatening illness. You may need to make referrals to community-based agencies or service groups. Health departments, social workers, trained hospice volunteers, and AIDS volunteers may also be helpful to you, your patients, and their families.

The best therapeutic response to the patient with a life-threatening illness will build upon the person's own coping abilities, capitalize on strengths, maintain hope, and show continued human care and concern. Patients may want up-to-date information on their disease, its causes, modes of transmission, treatments available, and sources of care and social support. Be prepared to recommend support groups where patients can discuss their feelings and express their concerns. Treat patients with concern and compassion and assure them everything will be done to provide continuity of care and relief from distress. Patients may be encouraged to call upon clergy for spiritual support.

> For example, at Inner City Health Care, Dr. Ray Reynolds is known for his compassion and great warmth toward people. On difficult days at the center, this attitude holds him in good stead. Sometimes, he tends to take on the more challenging cases: patients with life-threatening diseases, often young people with AIDS who should be in the prime of their lives.
>
> Clinical medical assistant Wanda Slawson always tries to learn from Dr. Reynolds' example. While she is quieter and not as outgoing as Dr. Reynolds, Wanda always tries to be both courteous and comforting to patients, especially those who are anxious. She makes it a point always to help patients discover a new way to cope with debilitating diseases.

**6-1** The extended family of Wong Lee is concerned about his illness and his care. Chronic obstructive pulmonary disease (COPD) has ravaged his body. He is on oxygen all the time now. He wants to remain at home to die; his family wants that, too. Yet you are uncertain of how much information to give to members of this expanded family when they call. You wish to protect Mr. Lee's confidentiality.

## CASE STUDY REVIEW

1. Are the questions the extended family members raise intended to harm or help Mr. Lee?

2. Is there a durable power of attorney for health care in place?

3. What, if any, of this concern is related to the culture?

4. What can you and your physician-employer suggest to be of help to everyone involved?

**6-2**

Inner City Health Care, a multi-doctor urgent care center in a large city, has a large roster of patients, some of whom have AIDS. While clinical medical assistant Bruce Goldman tries not to be, sometimes he is wary of patients who he thinks might be homosexual. When patient Bill Swartz was seen for a change in a mole on his calf, Bruce did his best to interact in a professional manner even though he suspected Bill was homosexual. After this patient exchange, medical assistant Bruce Goldman decided it was time to deal with his prejudices against homosexuals and his fear of AIDS and all AIDS patients.

## CASE STUDY REVIEW

1. While medical assistant Bruce Goldman may not admit it, he is threatened by AIDS. What should he know about AIDS transmission that may reduce his fears?

2. In the future, Bruce would like to be more open and supportive when he is dealing with an AIDS patient. What are some of the things he can do to help patients?

3. What are some things Bruce can do to reduce wariness regarding patients he feels might be homosexuals?

## SUMMARY

Medical assistants must be aware that when caring for people with a life-threatening illness, having even the slightest fear of death can undermine the ability to respond professionally, with empathy and support. If you feel yourself losing the ability to be helpful, it is time to briefly step aside. This does not mean withdrawal from your position or refusal to care for your patients. It means that you do whatever is necessary so that your perspective is not lost. It may mean taking a day off from work to "fill up your soul" and to give your psyche a rest. If the ambulatory care setting has an abundance of patients with life-threatening illnesses, it may require that you spend some time in a support group of your own so that you are better able to cope. Never be afraid to feel sad or weep with your patients. It is better to sense their pain and, at times, feel the pain with them, than it is to be so clinically objective you miss their true needs.

## REVIEW QUESTIONS

### Multiple Choice

1. When a practice treats patients with AIDS, it is important for medical assistants to:
   a. warn other patients about the dangers of transmission
   b. segregate AIDS patient reception areas from other patient areas
   c. be supportive and free of prejudice
   d. deny any information to patients regarding the seriousness of the illness

2. The Patient Self-Determination Act:
   a. allows a patient to have a choice of physicians
   b. ensures a patient's right to accept or refuse treatment
   c. gives patients the right to formulate advance directives

   d. all of the above
   e. only b and c

3. The strongest influence in a patient with a life-threatening illness is:
   a. the physician
   b. the hospital
   c. the family
   d. the patient

4. Life-threatening illness is defined as:
   a. a life shortened due to serious illness or disease
   b. death that is imminent
   c. serious illness to battle for many years but may shorten life
   d. all of the above

5. Culture may be defined as:
   a. how we live our lives
   b. how we think

c. how we speak and behave

d. all of the above

6. Therapeutic communication with a patient with a life-threatening illness:
   a. is no different than communicating with any patient
   b. is heightened and considered more difficult
   c. is left to nonmedical support staff
   d. comes naturally and requires no special skill

7. Cultural influence may in part determine:
   a. when/how to involve family members
   b. whether spiritual support is sought
   c. how the illness and pain associated with it is managed
   d. all of the above

8. Durable power of attorney for health care:
   a. enables someone other than the patient to make only health care decisions
   b. enables someone other than the patient to make any decisions for the patient
   c. makes certain that patients' financial responsibilities are met
   d. makes certain a patient's wishes are followed
   e. only a and d

9. Additional problems people with AIDS may encounter are:
   a. loss of family and friends for support
   b. being treated as social pariahs in some settings
   c. that living wills are not recognized
   d. only a and b

10. Effective pain management may depend upon:
    a. patient's needs
    b. family wishes
    c. cultural systems
    d. all of the above
    e. only a and c

## Critical Thinking

1. Research other sections in this text that discuss end-of-life legal documents. Describe additional information you find.

2. Discuss with a friend what cultural influences might affect each of you if you were facing a life-threatening illness. What choices would each of you make?

3. In a paragraph seen only by yourself, describe your greatest fears in caring for patients with AIDS.

4. List common psychological reactions people might have from learning they have a life-threatening illness.

5. Research other sections in this text that discuss AIDS. What additional information do you find beneficial?

6. What steps would you personally take to make certain you do not burn out from caring for persons with a life-threatening illness?

7. List the advantages/disadvantages of the physician directives available.

8. Discuss with a nurse or a nursing student in your school how health care professionals deal with the psychological suffering in persons with a life-threatening illness.

9. Discuss with a classmate your concerns in dealing with patients with a life-threatening illness. Would you choose to work where you seldom lost a patient to a life-threatening illness? If so, what are the reasons?

10. Research the agencies available in your community that can provide support for people and family members facing life-threatening illness.

## REFERENCES/BIBLIOGRAPHY

Lewis, M., & Tamparo, C. (1998). *Medical law, ethics, and bioethics for ambulatory care*. Philadelphia: F. A. Davis Company.

Purnell, L., & Paulanka, B. (1998). *Transcultural health care: A culturally competent approach*. Philadelphia: F. A. Davis Company.

Tamparo, C., & Lindh, W. (2000). *Therapeutic communications for health professionals*. Albany, NY: Delmar.

# 3

# RESPONSIBLE MEDICAL PRACTICE

# Chapter

## 7

# LEGAL CONSIDERATIONS

## KEY TERMS

Agent
Civil Law
Criminal Law
Defendant
Doctrine
Durable Power of Attorney
Emancipated Minor
Expert Witness
Expressed Contract
Implied Consent
Implied Contract
Incompetence
Informed Consent
Libel
Litigation
Malpractice
Mandate
Minor
Negligence
Noncompliant
Plaintiff
Risk Management
Slander
Statute
Subpoena
Tort

## OUTLINE

**Civil and Criminal Law**
**Medical Practice Acts and the**
**  Medical Assistant's Role**
  Patient Rights
**The Physician, the Medical**
**  Assistant, and the Law**
**Contracts**
  Termination of Contracts
**Standard of Care and the 4 Ds of**
**  Negligence**
**Torts**
  Battery
  Defamation of Character
  Invasion of Privacy

**Medical Records**
  Informed Consent
  Implied Consent
  Consent and Legal Incompetence
  Subpoenas
  Confidentiality
  Statute of Limitations
**Public Duties**
  Drug Screening
  AIDS
  Abuse
**Good Samaritan Law**
**Physician's Directives**
**Americans with Disabilities Act**
**  (ADA)**

## OBJECTIVES

*The student should strive to meet the following performance objectives and demonstrate*
*an understanding of the facts and principles presented in this chapter through written and*
*oral communication.*

1. Define the key terms as presented in the glossary.
2. Compare/contrast civil and criminal law.
3. Define the medical assistant's role in legal issues.
4. Describe the use of contracts in the ambulatory care setting.
5. Discuss the standard of care for health care professionals.
6. Explain the 4 Ds of negligence.
7. Define and give examples of torts.
8. Explain the necessity of informed consent.
9. Describe how to handle subpoenas.
10. Recall the special consideration for patients related to the issues of confidentiality, the statute of limitations, public duties, and AIDS.   *(continues)*

11. Describe procedures to follow in documenting and reporting abuse.
12. Discuss Good Samaritan Laws, physician's directives, and the Americans with Disabilities Act.

## ROLE DELINEATION COMPONENTS

### GENERAL (TRANSDISCIPLINARY)

**Legal Concepts**

- **Prepare and maintain medical records**
- **Document accurately**
- **Use appropriate guidelines when releasing information**
- **Follow employer's established policies dealing with the health care contract**
- **Follow federal, state and local legal guidelines**
- **Maintain awareness of federal and state health care legislation and regulations**
- **Comply with risk management and safety procedures**

## SCENARIO

At the ambulatory care center of Doctors Lewis and King, a two-doctor family physician office, Dr. Lewis and Dr. King are especially careful about establishing stringent risk management procedures to protect patients from harm and the practice from potential liability.

Dr. King has worked with office manager Marilyn Johnson, CMA, to assemble a policy and procedures manual outlining everything from how telephone calls are answered to how patient medical records are documented and stored. Marilyn, in turn, seeks the input of the other administrative and clinical medical assistants as she frequently updates the manual. To ensure that they are providing the best care for patients while protecting themselves, four times a year the entire staff meets to review office policies, changing them as necessary or incorporating new procedures to meet new situations or legal mandates.

## INTRODUCTION

The law as it relates to health care has grown increasingly complex in the past decade. The agendas of federal and state governments include an investigation of quality health care, a desire to control health care costs (while hoping to assure equitable access to health care), and an interest in protecting the patient. A full discussion of health law requires several volumes; therefore, only the laws designated to protect the patient will be identified in this chapter, and emphasis will be placed on the ambulatory care setting.

Being aware of the law and its implications and establishing sound practices and procedures will both safeguard patient rights and protect the health care professional.

## CIVIL AND CRIMINAL LAW

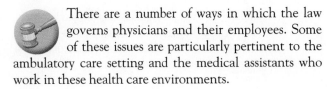

The most frequent law exercised in the ambulatory care setting is **civil law**, or law as it is related to individuals. Restitution awarded when a civil wrong is committed is usually monetary in nature. **Criminal law** addresses wrongs committed against the welfare and safety of society as a whole; punishment is usually imprisonment or a fine.

If a charge is brought against a physician as the **defendant** in a civil case, the goal is to reimburse the **plaintiff**, the person bringing charges (usually a patient), with a monetary amount for suffering, pain, and any loss of wages. For example, a physician who has caused harm to a patient in the course of treatment may be sued in a civil case by the patient for the recovery of time lost from work as well as the pain and suffering that was the result of treatment.

In a criminal case, charges are brought against the defendant by the state with the intent of preventing any further harm to society. For example, a physician practicing medicine without a proper license may be subject to disciplinary action from a professional association and criminal action by the courts.

## MEDICAL PRACTICE ACTS AND THE MEDICAL ASSISTANT'S ROLE

Each state has medical practice acts that regulate the practice of medicine with the intent of protecting its citizens from harm. These **statutes**, or laws, govern licensure, standards of care, professional liability and negligence, confidentiality, and torts. Some states also regulate personnel who may be employed in the ambulatory care setting. For example, some states require that medical assistants be licensed or certified to be able to perform any invasive procedures. Other states require additional training in radiology for the medical assistant to be able to take X rays. Further, some states are so strict in their regulations that medical assistants perform mostly clerical functions. Certainly, medical assistants desiring to utilize their skills must be aware of state regulations and always perform only within the scope of those regulations.

### *Patient Rights*

The Patient's Bill of Rights was developed by the American Hospital Association in 1973 and revised in 1992 to establish more effective patient care and greater satisfaction for patient, physician, and hospital (Figure 7-1). While this Bill of Rights was written with the hospital patient in mind, patients in ambulatory care settings should be accorded the same rights. Although no list of rights can guarantee the

kind of treatment patients have a right to expect, medical assistants should make every effort to conduct activities with the concern of the patient in mind.

## THE PHYSICIAN, THE MEDICAL ASSISTANT, AND THE LAW

There are a number of ways in which the law governs physicians and their employees. Some of these issues are particularly pertinent to the ambulatory care setting and the medical assistants who work in these health care environments.

## CONTRACTS

A contract is a binding agreement between two or more persons. A physician has a legal obligation, or duty, to care for a patient under the principles of contract law. The agreement must be between competent persons to do or not to do something lawful in exchange for a payment.

A contract exists when the patient arrives for treatment and the physician accepts the patient by providing treatment. An example of a valid contract occurs when a patient calls the office or clinic to make an appointment for an annual physical examination. Assuming both physician and patient are competent and that the physician performs the lawful act of the physical examination and the patient pays a fee, all aspects of the contract exist.

There are two types of contracts, expressed and implied. An **expressed contract** can be written or verbal and will specifically describe what each party in the contract will do. A written contract requires that all necessary aspects of the agreement be in writing. An **implied contract** is indicated by actions rather than by words. The majority of physician-patient contracts are implied contracts. It is not required that the contract be written to be enforceable as long as all points of the contract exist. An implied contract can exist either by the circumstances of the situation or by the law. When a patient complains of a sore throat and the physician does a throat culture to diagnose and treat the ailment, an implied contract exists by the circumstances. An implied contract by law exists when a patient goes into anaphylactic shock and the physician administers epinephrine to counteract shock symptoms. The law says that the physician did what the patient would have requested had there been an expressed contract.

For a contract to be valid and binding, the parties who enter into it must be competent; therefore, the mentally incompetent, the legally insane, persons under heavy drug or alcohol influences, infants, and some minors cannot enter into a binding contract.

# A PATIENT'S BILL OF RIGHTS

*First adopted by the American Hospital Association in 1973.*

*This revision approved by the AHA Board of Trustees on October 21, 1992.*

1. The patient has the right to considerate and respectful care.

2. The patient has the right to and is encouraged to obtain from physicians and other direct caregivers relevant, current, and understandable information concerning diagnosis, treatment, and prognosis.

    Except in emergencies when the patient lacks decision-making capacity and the need for treatment is urgent, the patient is entitled to the opportunity to discuss and request information related to the specific procedures and/or treatments, the risks involved, the possible length of recuperation, and the medically reasonable alternatives and their accompanying risks and benefits.

    Patients have the right to know the identity of physicians, nurses, and others involved in their care, as well as when those involved are students, residents, or other trainees. The patient also has the right to know the immediate and long-term financial implications of treatment choices, insofar as they are known.

3. The patient has the right to make decisions about the plan of care prior to and during the course of treatment and to refuse a recommended treatment or plan of care to the extent permitted by law and hospital policy and to be informed of the medical consequences of this action. In case of such refusal, the patient is entitled to other appropriate care and services that the hospital provides or transfer to another hospital. The hospital should notify patients of any policy that might affect patient choice within the institution.

4. The patient has the right to have an advance directive (such as a living will, health care proxy, or durable power of attorney for health care) concerning treatment or designating a surrogate decision maker with the expectation that the hospital will honor the intent of that directive to the extent permitted by law and hospital policy.

    Health care institutions must advise patients of their rights under state law and hospital policy to make informed medical choices, ask if the patient has an advance directive, and include that information in patient records. The patient has the right to timely information about hospital policy that may limit its ability to implement fully a legally valid advance directive.

5. The patient has the right to every consideration of privacy. Case discussion, consultation, examination, and treatment should be conducted so as to protect each patient's privacy.

6. The patient has the right to expect that all communications and records pertaining to his/her care will be treated as confidential by the hospital, except in cases such as suspected abuse and public health hazards when reporting is permitted or required by law. The patient has the right to expect that the hospital will emphasize the confidentiality of this information when it releases it to any other parties entitled to review information in these records.

7. The patient has the right to review the records pertaining to his/her medical care and to have the information explained or interpreted as necessary, except when restricted by law.

8. The patient has the right to expect that, within its capacity and policies, a hospital will make reasonable response to the request of a patient for appropriate and medically indicated care and services. The hospital must provide evaluation, service, and/or referral as indicated by the urgency of the case. When medically appropriate and legally permissible, or when a patient has so requested, a patient may be transferred to another facility. The institution to which the patient is to be transferred must first have accepted the patient for transfer. The patient must also have the benefit of complete information and explanation concerning the need for, risks, benefits, and alternatives to such a transfer.

9. The patient has the right to ask and be informed of the existence of business relationships among the hospital, educational institutions, other health care providers, or payers that may influence the patient's treatment and care.

10. The patient has the right to consent to or decline to participate in proposed research studies or human experimentation affecting care and treatment or requiring direct patient involvement, and to have those studies fully explained prior to consent. A patient who declines to participate in research or experimentation is entitled to the most effective care that the hospital can otherwise provide.

11. The patient has the right to expect reasonable continuity of care when appropriate and to be informed by physicians and other caregivers of available and realistic patient care options when hospital care is no longer appropriate.

12. The patient has the right to be informed of hospital policies and practices that relate to patient care, treatment, and responsibilities. The patient has the right to be informed of available resources for resolving disputes, grievances, and conflicts, such as ethics committees, patient representatives, or other mechanisms available in the institution. The patient has the right to be informed of the hospital's charges for services and available payment methods.

**Figure 7-1**   A Patient's Bill of Rights. (Reprinted with permission of the American Hospital Association)

Medical assistants are considered **agents** of the physicians they serve and as such must be cautious that their actions and words may become binding on their physicians. For example, to say that the doctor can cure the patient may cause serious legal problems when in fact a cure may not be possible.

## Termination of Contracts

A broken contract or breach of contract occurs when one of the parties does not meet contractual obligations. A physician is legally bound to treat a patient until:

- The patient discharges the physician
- The physician formally withdraws from patient care
- The patient no longer needs treatment and is formally discharged by the physician

**Patient Discharges Physician.** When the patient discharges the physician, the physician should send a letter to the patient to confirm and document the termination of the contract. The notice should be sent by certified mail with return receipt requested. Keep a copy of the letter in the patient's record (Figure 7-2).

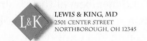

January 6, 20--

CERTIFIED MAIL

Jim Marshal
76 Georgia Avenue
Millerton, TX 43912

Dear Mr. Marshal:

This will confirm our telephone conversation today in which you discharged me as your attending physician in your present illness. In my opinion your condition requires continued medical supervision by a physician. If you have not already done so, I suggest that you employ another physician without delay.

You may be assured that after receiving a written request from you, I will furnish the physician of your choice with information regarding the diagnosis and treatment which you have received from me.

Very truly yours,

*Winston Lewis*

Winston Lewis, MD
WL:ea

**Figure 7-2**   Letter confirming physician's discharge by the patient.

**Physician Formally Withdraws from the Case.** To avoid any charges of abandonment, the physician should formally withdraw from the case as, for example, when the patient becomes **noncompliant** or the physician feels the patient can no longer be served. Again, notice should be sent to the patient by certified mail with return receipt requested and a copy of the notice should be filed in the patient's record (Figures 7-3 and 7-4).

Inner City Health Care
222 S. First Avenue
Carlton, MI 11666

May 9, 20--

CERTIFIED MAIL

Lenny Taylor
260 Second Street
Carlton, MI 11666

Dear Mr. Taylor:

You will recall that we discussed our physician-patient relationship in my office on May 6, 20--.

Your son, George Taylor, and Bruce Goldman, my medical assistant were also present. As you know, the primary difficulty has been your failure to cooperate with the medical plan for your care.

While it is unfortunate that our relationship has reached this stage, I will no longer be able to serve as your physician. I will be available to you on an emergency basis only until June 10, 20--. Meanwhile, you should immediately call or write the Medical Society, 123 Omega Drive, Carlton, MI 11666, Tel. 123-456-7899 and obtain a list of gerontologists. Any delay could jeopardize your health, so please act quickly.

Your physical (and/or mental) problems include: hypertensive heart disease, decreased kidney function, and arteriosclerosis. You could have additional medical problems that may also require professional care. Once you have found a new physician have him or her call my office. I will be happy to discuss your case with the physician assuming your care, and will transfer a written summary of your case to them upon the receipt of a written request from you to do so.

Thank you for your anticipated cooperation and courtesy.

Very truly yours,

*James Whitney*

James Whitney, MD
JW:kr

**Figure 7-3**   Letter reiterating "for the record" the physician's decision to withdraw from the case discussed during meeting with patient.

Inner City Health Care
222 S. First Avenue
Carlton, MI 11666

December 5, 20--

CERTIFIED MAIL

Rhoda Au
41 Academy Road
Carlton, MI 11666

Dear Ms. Au:

I find it necessary to inform you that I am withdrawing further professional medical service to you because of your persistent refusal to follow my medical advice and treatment.

Since your condition requires medical attention, I suggest that you place yourself under the care of another physician without delay. If you so desire, I shall be available to attend you for a reasonable time after you have received this letter, but in no event later than January 7, 20--. This should give you sufficient time to select a physician from the many competent practitioners in this area.

You may be assured that, upon receiving your written request, I will make available to the physician of your choice your case history and information regarding the diagnosis and treatment which you have received from me.

Very truly yours,

*Mark Woo*

Mark Woo, MD
MW:kr

**Figure 7-4** Letter notifying patient of physician's withdrawal as attending physician.

**The Patient No Longer Needs Treatment.** Unless a formal discharge or withdrawal has occurred, a physician is obligated to care for a patient until the patient's condition no longer requires treatment.

## STANDARD OF CARE AND THE 4 DS OF NEGLIGENCE

Physicians, medical assistants, and all health care providers have the responsibility and duty to perform within their scope of training and to always do what any reasonable and prudent health care professional in the same specialty or general field of practice would do. That is what is expected of every physician when a contact is made by a patient. Failure to do what any reasonable and prudent health care professional would do in the same set of circumstances can be seen as a breach of the standard of care.

**Negligence** is defined as the failure to exercise the standard of care that a reasonable person would exercise in similar circumstances. Negligence occurs when someone suffers injury because of another's failure to live up to a required duty of care. This is a primary cause of malpractice suits. **Malpractice** is professional negligence. The four elements of negligence, sometimes called the 4 Ds, are:

1. Duty: duty of care
2. Derelict: breach of the duty of care
3. Direct cause: a legally recognizable injury occurs as a result of the breach of duty of care
4. Damage: wrongful activity must have caused the injury or harm that occurred

If an individual has knowledge, skill, or intelligence superior to that of a layperson, that individual's conduct must be consistent with that status. Medical assistants are held to a high standard of care by virtue of their skills, knowledge, and intelligence. As professionals, medical assistants are required to have a standard minimum level of special knowledge and ability. This is what is known as duty of care.

Physicians and members of their staff may be called to testify in court to the standard of care. In such a case, they are usually considered **expert witnesses**. An expert witness is one who has knowledge and experience enough in a field to be able to testify to what is the reasonable and expected standard of care. Expert witnesses are expected to tell what they know to be fact and are best counseled to use lay terms rather than complicated medical language. The goal is for jurors and judges to understand the nature of any medical information shared. Visual aids, charts, and computer simulations are often used to illustrate or clarify testimony given by expert witnesses.

## TORTS

A **tort** is a wrongful act that results in injury to one person by another. Medical assistants may commit a tort that may result in **litigation**. If it can be proven that the injury resulted from the medical assistant (or other health care professional) not meeting the standard of care governing their respective professions, then litigation is a possibility. If, however, the medical assistant (or other health care professional) commits a wrongful act but the patient suffers no injury or harm, then no tort exists. If, for example, the medical assistant changes a wound dressing, breaks sterile technique, and the patient suffers a severely infected wound, the medical assistant has committed a tort and can be held liable, and legal action can be taken. On the other hand, if the medical assistant changes a wound dressing, breaks sterile technique, and the patient's wound does not become infected, no harm has been suffered, and a tort does not exist. If a medical assistant fails to report to the physician a negative result on a blood test that causes the physician to fail to make an early diagnosis of a disease, the assistant's omission of an act has caused a breach in the standard of care.

There are two major classifications of torts, intentional and negligent. Intentional torts are deliberate acts of violation of another's rights. Negligent torts are not deliberate and are the result of omission and commission of an act. Malpractice is the unintentional tort of professional negligence; that is, a professional either failed to act in a reasonable and prudent manner and caused harm to the patient or did what a reasonable and prudent person would not have done and caused harm to a patient.

There are two Latin terms that can be used to describe aspects of negligence. These are known as **doctrines**. *Res ipsa loquitur*, or "the thing speaks for itself," is the term used in cases that involve situations such as a nick made in the bladder when the surgeon is performing a hysterectomy. The negligence is obvious. The other doctrine, *respondeat superior*, "let the master answer," expresses that physicians are responsible for their employees' actions. If a medical assistant violates the standard of care, therein lies the basis for a suit of medical malpractice. For example, the medical assistant used the incorrect solution to clean the patient's wound and the patient sustained injuries to the wound. The physician-employer can be sued under the doctrine of *respondeat superior* because the physician-employer is responsible for the acts of employees committed in the scope of their employment. The medical assistant also can be sued because individuals are responsible for their own actions.

Some common areas of negligence may result in torts when the standard of care is not adhered to; practicing good **risk management** makes the medical assistant and the physician-employer less vulnerable to litigation.

- Protect patients from falling from an examination table, wheelchair, or stretcher.
- Check for faulty electrocautery. Have repair done by qualified technicians.
- Check patient identification by correctly identifying patient before performing a procedure or administering a medication.
- Never leave a patient unattended. If you must leave, pass the responsibility for the patient's care on to another individual.
- Be particularly watchful with patients who have special needs such as the elderly, pediatric patients, and those with physical and emotional disabilities.

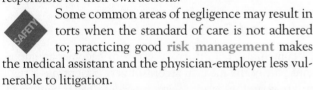

**SPOTLIGHT ON AAMA ESSENTIALS THROUGH CAAHEP**

- Looking at a neighbor's medical record out of curiosity, and not as part of your responsibility as a medical assistant, is not against the law, but it is unethical.
- Practicing good risk management, such as protecting patients from falling, checking identification, and never leaving a patient unattended, makes the medical assistant less vulnerable to litigation.
- A healthy relationship between the medical assistant and the patient, as well as respect for one another's rights, lowers the potential for the likelihood of a lawsuit.

- Properly label and identify all specimens. Handle specimens properly.
- Make certain the patient has signed a consent for surgery and other care.
- Follow all policies and procedures established by your employer.
- Do not misrepresent your qualifications.
- Document fully only facts and do not alter medical records.
- Admit any error that may have occurred.

Some specific examples of common torts that can occur in the office or clinic are battery, defamation of character, and invasion of privacy.

## Battery

The basis of the tort of battery is unprivileged touching of one person by another. A patient must consent to being touched. When a procedure is to be performed on a patient, the patient must give consent in full knowledge of all the facts. It does not matter whether the procedure that constitutes the battery improves the patient's health. Patients have the right to withdraw consent at any time.

One example of battery is when a medical assistant insists on giving the patient an injection the physician ordered for the patient even though the patient refuses the injection. Another example can be seen when a physician performs additional surgery beyond the original procedure (the surgeon performed a hysterectomy for which consent was given, but is liable for battery for removing an abdominal nevus from the patient's abdomen without consent). It does not matter that the physician does not charge for the additional procedure. It also does not matter if the patient would have given consent if asked in advance.

## Defamation of Character

The tort of defamation of character consists of injury to another person's reputation, name, or character through spoken or written words for which damages can be recovered. Two kinds of defamation are **libel** and **slander**. Libel is false and malicious writing about another such as in published materials, pictures, and media. An example can be seen when the medical assistant writes in the patient's record, "Mr. O'Keefe's wife appears to be the cause of his ulcer." A copy of Mr. O'Keefe's records were later sent to a new physician who reviewed the record and saw the remarks quoted by the medical assistant.

Slander is false and malicious spoken words. Slander can be seen in the following comment directed by a patient toward the physician, "Dr. Woo is incompetent. He should have his license revoked." The statement is overheard by the office receptionist and other patients waiting in the reception area.

In order for a tort of defamation of character (either libel or slander) to exist, a third party must see or hear the words and understand their meaning.

## Invasion of Privacy

Invasion of privacy is another kind of tort. It includes unauthorized publicity of patient information, medical records being released without the patient's knowledge and permission, and patients receiving unwanted publicity and exposure to public view. For example, if a minor unmarried girl has been examined for possible pregnancy, and the medical assistant telephones the laboratory report to the girl's home and inadvertently gives the results to someone other than the patient, her privacy has been invaded. A second situation exists when persons other than those providing care and performing examinations and procedures (essential or nonessential personnel) are allowed to be present without the patient's consent. Yet another example of the patient's right to privacy being violated is when the patient is asked to walk from the examination room across the hall to a treatment room while wearing only a patient gown in full view of other patients and personnel.

Medical assistants and other health care professionals should:

- Close a door, pull a curtain, or provide a screen when looking at, handling, or examining the patient's body

- Expose only body parts necessary for treatment (drape the patient's body, exposing only that part which is being treated)

- Discuss patients with no one except those individuals involved in the patient's care and then discuss only those aspects that relate to the needs of the patient for care

It is not an invasion of privacy to disclose information required by a court order (**subpoena**) or by statute to protect the public health and welfare, as in the reporting of violent crime.

## MEDICAL RECORDS

A major responsibility of the physician and the medical assistant is to maintain an accurate and up-to-date record of the patient's care. Whatever style of record is used, the credibility of the medical record will be a key factor in any litigation.

All matters related to a patient's care must be charted, and these charts must be an accurate reflection of actual care rendered and charges made. An act not recorded is generally considered an act not done. Charts that are incomplete or illegible are not easily defensible. Necessary corrections should be made by drawing one line through the error and placing the correction above it with the person's initials and date. All entries should be properly signed and dated, also. Consistency in the medical records becomes a powerful defense for the physician.

## Informed Consent

Documentation of **informed consent** becomes an important part of the medical records. Every patient has a right to know and understand any procedure to be performed. The patient is to be told in language easily understood:

1. The nature of any procedure and how it is to be performed
2. Any possible risks involved as well as expected outcomes of the procedure
3. Any other methods of treatment and those risks
4. Risks if no treatment is given

It is the responsibility of the health care provider to make certain the patient understands. If an interpreter is necessary, the physician must procure one.

Often, consent forms will be signed if there is to be a surgical or invasive procedure performed (Figure 7-5). The medical assistant may be asked to witness the patient's

```
CONSENT FOR TREATMENT

Date _____ Time _____

    I authorize the performance of the following
procedure(s) _____ on
_____ (name of patient) _____ to be performed by
_____ (name of physician) _____, MD.

    The following have been explained to _____
by Dr. _____ (name physician) _____.

    Nature of the procedure _____ (describe procedure)
_____.

    For the purpose of _____
_____.

    The possible alternative methods of treatment are
_____.

    The possible consequences of the procedure are
_____.

    The risks involve the possibility of _____
_____.

    The possible complications of this procedure are
_____.

    I have been advised of the serious nature of this pro-
cedure and have been further advised that if I desire a
more detailed explanation of any of the foregoing or
further information about the possible risks or compli-
cations, it will be given to me.

    I do not request a more detailed listing and explana-
tion of the above information.

                    Signed _____
                            (Patient/Parent/Guardian)
Witnessed by: _____
```

**Figure 7-5**    Model formal consent for treatment form.

signature and may be expected to follow through on any of the physician's instructions or explanations but is not expected to explain the procedure to the patient. The signed consent form is kept in the medical chart and a copy is also given to the patient.

## Implied Consent

Two circumstances related to consent are worth mentioning at this point. **Implied consent** occurs when there is a life-threatening emergency or the patient is unconscious or unable to respond. The physician, by law, is allowed to give treatment without a signed consent. Implied consent occurs in more subtle ways, also. The patient who rolls up a shirt sleeve for the medical assistant to take a blood pressure reading is implying consent to the procedure by the action taken.

## Consent and Legal Incompetence

Consent for treatment is not valid if the patient is legally incompetent to give consent. Legal **incompetence** means that a patient is found by a court to be insane, inadequate, or to not be an adult. In such instances, consent must be obtained from a parent, a legal guardian, or the court on behalf of the patient. Consent for treatment may be given only by the natural parent or legal guardian as determined by the court for a **minor** child, typically defined as one under eighteen years of age or the age of majority. An **emancipated minor** is one considered by the courts to be an adult. Emancipated minors may be defined as persons living on their own, who are self-supporting, who may be married, or who are in the military. They can legally give consent for treatment.

Consent problems may arise when providing care to minors. Consent for medical care such as treatment of sexually transmitted diseases, pregnancy, alcohol or drug abuse, abortion, or birth control pose special problems. Some states allow minors to give their consent in these special situations.

Questions of ability to give consent related to minors and emancipated minors often must be determined on a case-by-case basis because state statutes vary. Placing a telephone call to the state attorney general's office can help clarify issues, questions, and concerns that involve consent and treatment of minors.

## Subpoenas

The medical records may be subpoenaed and/or the physician and health care provider (*subpoena duces tecum*) may be subpoenaed to testify in court. The subpoena is a court order naming a specific date, time, and reason to appear. The staff in the ambulatory care setting usually will have ample time to make certain the record is current and complete prior to its inclusion in court. Out of courtesy, the physician will notify patients whose records have been subpoenaed. If, for any reason, the patient does not want the record released, the physician must call for legal advice on how to respond to the subpoena.

Certain records, because of their sensitive nature, may require more than a subpoena to be released. These include records related to sexually transmitted diseases, including AIDS and HIV testing, mental health records, substance abuse records, and sexual assault records. For the courts to have access to these records, a court order is required in some states.

## Confidentiality

The care taken with subpoenas and court orders for certain information is to assure patients of confidentiality. The information in the medical record, including the information a patient shared with the physician and medical assistant, is private.

No patient information can be given to another (another physician, patient's attorney, insurance company, federal or state agency) without the expressed written consent of the patient. Care must be exercised at all times to ensure that the patient's right to confidentiality is not breached. For example, information given to unauthorized personnel associated with the physician's or clinic's practice in regard to the patient's condition or financial status regarding payment of bills violates the patient's right to confidentiality. Likewise, when discussing issues over the telephone that can be overheard—such as the patient's account being turned over to a collection agency—the patient's right to confidentiality has been violated.

There are certain disclosures of information about a patient's conditions and suspected illnesses that are required by law. Legally required disclosures are necessary when the public needs to know certain information for its safety and welfare. The disclosures supersede the patient's right to privacy and confidentiality. See "Public Duties" in this chapter.

## Statute of Limitations

No discussion of medical records is complete without a brief statement regarding the statute of limitations which will, in part, determine how long medical records are kept. Generally speaking, all records should be retained until after the statute has run, usually three to six years. Statutes of limitations most commonly begin at the time a negligent act was committed, when the act was discovered, or when the care of the patient and the patient-physician relationship ended. It is easy to understand why many physicians choose to keep their records indefinitely.

State and federal statutes set maximum time periods during which certain actions can be brought or rights enforced; there is a time limit for individuals to initiate legal action. The statute of limitations varies from one jurisdiction to another and a lawsuit may not be brought after the statute of limitations has run. For example, in the Commonwealth of Massachusetts, the statute of limitations for an act of medical malpractice committed on an adult is three years. If harm to a patient resulted from a medical assistant administering the wrong dose of medication to a patient in Massachusetts, a lawsuit must be brought within three years from the time the medication error was made, with the three years commencing at the time the negligent act was committed.

## PUBLIC DUTIES

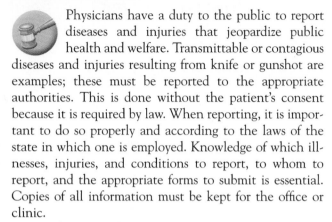 Physicians have a duty to the public to report diseases and injuries that jeopardize public health and welfare. Transmittable or contagious diseases and injuries resulting from knife or gunshot are examples; these must be reported to the appropriate authorities. This is done without the patient's consent because it is required by law. When reporting, it is important to do so properly and according to the laws of the state in which one is employed. Knowledge of which illnesses, injuries, and conditions to report, to whom to report, and the appropriate forms to submit is essential. Copies of all information must be kept for the office or clinic.

Other generally required reportables include: births, deaths, childhood immunizations, rape, and abuse toward a child, elder, or domestic partner.

Some states have laws specific to the release of information relative to mental or psychological treatment, human immunodeficiency virus testing, acquired immunodeficiency syndrome diagnosis and treatment, sexually transmitted diseases, and chemical substance abuse.

Local or state health departments can provide lists of diseases and injuries to report and will also provide the appropriate forms.

## Drug Screening

States vary in the laws they have regarding the abuse of alcohol and other drugs. In general, employers are allowed to screen an employee for chemical substances if they believe the employee's work performance is being affected by the abuse.

Great controversy surrounds preemployment and random screening for drugs in the workplace. Some states allow widespread random testing of employees. It is important that the worker's right to privacy not be violated. A tort of defamation of character could be claimed against an employer if the results of the testing become known to others.

Get the patient's written consent when asked to collect a specimen for drug screening. Be certain the laboratory that performs the screening is qualified to perform the test. The possibility of liability is great if the ambulatory care setting does not have specific policies and procedures to employ in regard to specimen collection and testing. It should be carefully documented on the patient's record which medical personnel are responsible for the specimen from the time it was collected until the results are known.

The release of patients' records that pertain to chemical substance abuse is protected by federal laws under the Federal Drug Abuse Prevention, Treatment, and Rehabilitation Act. The law prohibits disclosure of information that identifies the patient as a chemical substance abuser. Also, information about the patient's treatment cannot be divulged without the patient's written consent. The records can, however, be released by order of a subpoena to another health care professional during an emergency situation or if the records are to be used for research and program evaluation.

## AIDS

The Americans with Disabilities Act of 1990 (ADA) offers protection to persons with AIDS or diseases associated with AIDS. Controversy surrounds the mandatory testing for human immunodeficiency virus (HIV) in medical assistants and other health care professionals and the release of the results to patients who say they have the right to know the HIV status of their caregivers. Health care professionals insist on their right to privacy.

Patients also insist on their privacy. A written informed consent form specific to HIV testing is signed by the patient prior to testing. Laws regarding HIV and AIDS vary from state to state. The best approach regarding release of information regarding the HIV status of a patient is never to disclose this or any confidential patient information.

## Abuse

Child abuse, elder abuse, and domestic violence are becoming more common in our society and as a result, patients suffering such abuse may be seen in the ambulatory care setting. In all cases of abuse, medical records hold valuable information if a court procedure ensues. Careful documentation is critical. State laws are fairly specific in mandates to report child abuse, but laws related to elder abuse and domestic violence are not so detailed. In any case, the rights of the victim must be protected.

**Child Abuse.** The law mandates, or requires, that physicians and health care professionals, teachers, social workers, and certain others who suspect child abuse report the incident to the proper authorities. Confidentiality in the physician-patient relationship does not exist when parents abuse children. If a person has a reason to suspect abuse and reports the abuse to the police and in the case of child abuse to the child protective agency, this individual is protected against liability as a result of making the report. Failure to report could result in criminal or civil penalties. Usually, the Child Protective Unit of the State Department of Social Services is called in to investigate suspected cases of child abuse. Some injuries that are commonly seen in child abuse are bruises, welts, burns, fractures, and head injuries.

If a suspicion of abuse exists, the physician and health care professional should:

- Treat the child's injuries
- Send the child to the hospital for further treatment when necessary
- Inform parents of the diagnosis and that it will be reported to the police and social services agency
- Notify the child protective agency (keep phone number posted)
- Document all information
- Provide court testimony if requested

**Elder Abuse.** Elder abuse may consist of neglect, physical abuse, punishment, physical restraint, or abandonment. Examples are seen when elders are overmedicated or undermedicated, physically restrained, intimidated by shouting or profanity, sexually abused, neglected or abandoned, or in any other way have their rights and dignity violated. The person reporting the abuse is generally a health care professional, and the reporting agency is most likely one of a social service or welfare nature.

**Domestic Violence.** Incidents of spousal abuse have escalated since the 1970s. The battered women's syndrome is recognized as a significant problem. The violence of it is a criminal act and failure to report it may be considered a misdemeanor in some states. Victims of domestic violence should be treated as soon as possible after the assault so as to preserve evidence for legal purposes. Community agencies such as rape hot lines are available and the physician may refer the patient for additional services.

## GOOD SAMARITAN LAW

Most states have laws regarding the rendering of first aid by health care professionals at the scene of an accident or sudden injury. Good Samaritan laws, although not always clearly written, encourage physicians and health care professionals to provide medical care within the scope of their training without fear of being sued for negligence. In an emergency situation, medical assistants cannot be held liable should an injury result from some form of first aid rendered or from first aid they omitted to render as long as they acted in a reasonable way within the scope of their knowledge. Medical assistants and other health care professionals with skills in cardiopulmonary resuscitation (CPR) who are present when CPR is needed must perform the procedure on the victim or otherwise could be declared negligent. Emergencies that arise in the ambulatory care setting generally are not covered by Good Samaritan laws.

## PHYSICIAN'S DIRECTIVES

Medical assistants in the ambulatory care setting will be asked to attach physicians' directives or living wills to patients' charts (Figure 7-6). These directives are legal documents in which patients indicate their wishes in the case of a life-threatening illness or serious injury. Such documents should always accompany the patients to the hospital for any treatment or care. They may be updated from time to time, and the patient can ask to rescind such a document at any time. Medical assistants must remember that these documents reflect the choices of their patients and are to be respected as such.

Another document often seen in the ambulatory care setting is the **durable power of attorney** for health care or Designation of Health Care Surrogate (Figure 7-7). These documents allow a patient to name another person who is appointed as the official spokesperson for the patient should the patient be unable to speak for herself. The documents may allow another person to manage finances and personal matters or just to make medical decisions. These documents should be recognized and honored.

Every state has different versions of the Living Will and Designation of Health Care Surrogate forms as well as requirements for filling them out. To assure the correct language is used, these forms should be prepared either by an attorney familiar with your state requirements, or by contacting Partnership for Caring, 1035 30th Street NW, Washington, DC 20007, 800-989-9455.

## AMERICANS WITH DISABILITIES ACT (ADA)

The federal government established new laws in 1990 to protect physically challenged persons. Barrier-free accommodations are required in public and commercial facilities. The ADA law applies to businesses with at least fifteen employees, but some states have more stringent laws.

---

| INSTRUCTIONS | **FLORIDA DESIGNATION OF HEALTH CARE SURROGATE** |
|---|---|
| PRINT YOUR NAME | Name:_____<br>    *(Last)*         *(First)*         *(Middle Initial)*<br><br>In the event that I have been determined to be incapacitated to provide informed consent for medical treatment and surgical and diagnostic procedures, I wish to designate as my surrogate for health care decisions: |
| PRINT THE NAME, HOME ADDRESS AND TELEPHONE NUMBER OF YOUR SURROGATE | Name:_____<br>Address: _____<br>_____ Zip Code: _____<br>Phone: _____<br><br>If my surrogate is unwilling or unable to perform his or her duties, I wish to designate as my alternate surrogate: |
| PRINT THE NAME, HOME ADDRESS AND TELEPHONE NUMBER OF YOUR ALTERNATE SURROGATE | Name: _____<br>Address: _____<br>_____ Zip Code: _____<br>Phone: _____<br><br>I fully understand that this designation will permit my designee to make health care decisions and to provide, withhold, or withdraw consent on my behalf; to apply for public benefits to defray the cost of health care; and to authorize my admission to or transfer from a health care facility. |
| ADD PERSONAL INSTRUCTIONS (IF ANY) | Additional instructions (optional): |
| © 2000 PARTNERSHIP FOR CARING, INC. | |

| | FLORIDA DESIGNATION OF HEALTH CARE SURROGATE — PAGE 2 OF 2 |
|---|---|
| | I further affirm that this designation is not being made as a condition of treatment or admission to a health care facility. I will notify and send a copy of this document to the following persons other than my surrogate, so they may know who my surrogate is: |
| PRINT THE NAMES AND ADDRESSES OF THOSE WHO YOU WANT TO KEEP COPIES OF THIS DOCUMENT | Name: _____<br>Address: _____<br>Name: _____<br>Address: _____ |
| SIGN AND DATE THE DOCUMENT | Signed: _____<br>Date: _____ |
| WITNESSING PROCEDURE | Witness 1:<br>      Signed: _____ |
| TWO WITNESSES MUST SIGN AND PRINT THEIR ADDRESSES | Address: _____<br><br>Witness 2:<br>      Signed: _____<br>Address: _____ |
| © 2000 PARTNERSHIP FOR CARING, INC. | *Courtesy of Partnership for Caring, Inc.*     10/99<br>1035 30th Street, NW  Washington, DC 20007  800-989-9455 |

**Figure 7-6**    Living will declaration. Choice In Dying makes available legally recognized document forms to residents of states that have enacted right-to-die laws. For people in states that have not enacted right-to-die laws, Choice In Dying provides statutory advance directives for each state free of charge, as well as other materials and services relating to end-of-life medical care. (Reprinted by permission of Choice in Dying, 200 Varick Street, New York, NY 10014, 212-366-5540)

| | |
|---|---|
| **INSTRUCTIONS** | **FLORIDA LIVING WILL** |

**FLORIDA LIVING WILL**

**INSTRUCTIONS**

**PRINT THE DATE**

**PRINT YOUR NAME**

Declaration made this _____ day of _____, _____,
*(day)* *(month)* *(year)*

I, _____, willfully
and voluntarily make known my desire that my dying not be artificially
prolonged under the circumstances set forth below, and I do hereby
declare that:

**PLEASE INITIAL EACH THAT APPLIES**

If at any time I am incapacitated and
_____ I have a terminal condition, or
_____ I have an end-stage condition, or
_____ I am in a persistent vegetative state

and if my attending or treating physician and another consulting
physician have determined that there is no reasonable medical
probability of my recovery from such condition, I direct that life-
prolonging procedures be withheld or withdrawn when the application of
such procedures would serve only to prolong artificially the process of
dying, and that I be permitted to die naturally with only the
administration of medication or the performance of any medical
procedure deemed necessary to provide me with comfort care or to
alleviate pain.

It is my intention that this declaration be honored by my family and
physician as the final expression of my legal right to refuse medical or
surgical treatment and to accept the consequences for such refusal.

In the event that I have been determined to be unable to provide express
and informed consent regarding the withholding, withdrawal, or
continuation of life-prolonging procedures, I wish to designate, as my
surrogate to carry out the provisions of this declaration:

**PRINT THE NAME, HOME ADDRESS AND TELEPHONE NUMBER OF YOUR SURROGATE**

Name: _____

Address: _____

_____ Zip Code: _____

Phone: _____

© 2000 PARTNERSHIP FOR CARING, INC.

**FLORIDA LIVING WILL — PAGE 2 OF 2**

I wish to designate the following person as my alternate surrogate, to
carry out the provisions of this declaration should my surrogate be
unwilling or unable to act on my behalf:

**PRINT NAME, HOME ADDRESS AND TELEPHONE NUMBER OF YOUR ALTERNATE SURROGATE**

Name: _____

Address: _____

_____ Zip Code: _____

Phone: _____

**ADD PERSONAL INSTRUCTIONS (IF ANY)**

Additional instructions (optional):

I understand the full import of this declaration, and I am emotionally
and mentally competent to make this declaration.

**SIGN THE DOCUMENT**

Signed: _____

**WITNESSING PROCEDURE**

Witness 1:

Signed: _____

Address: _____

**TWO WITNESSES MUST SIGN AND PRINT THEIR ADDRESSES**

Witness 2:

Signed: _____

Address: _____

© 2000 PARTNERSHIP FOR CARING, INC.

*Courtesy of* **Partnership for Caring, Inc.** 6/00
1035 30th Street, NW Washington, DC 20007 800-989-9455

**Figure 7-7** Health care surrogate form. (Reprinted by permission of Choice in Dying, 200 Varick Street, New York, NY 10014, 212-366-5540)

The ADA allows preemployment physical examinations only after an individual has been offered employment. Medical records of these persons are kept
confidential and separate and accessible only to persons
who must know what restrictions the patient may bring to
a job. Job qualifications and the specific standards for
employment must be the same for all applicants. Disabled
persons cannot be screened using different standards for
employment.

Former drug users and those who are being rehabili-
tated also are covered by the ADA and cannot be denied
employment because of their past history of drug use.

Employers are required to post notices regarding
employee and applicant rights and obligations.

**CASE STUDY 7-1**

Three weeks ago, Dr. King treated a new patient, Boris Bolski, for lower back pain, which the patient felt
was the result of consistent heavy lifting at his job. Medical assistant Joe Guerrero assisted Dr. King during the examination and, today, both Joe and Dr. King were served with subpoenas by Mr. Bolski's attorney. Mr. Bolski is alleging that unsafe conditions at his workplace caused severe strain on his back and he
is suing his employer for damages. Dr. King and Joe Guerrero were called as expert witnesses to a civil
hearing; Joe, especially, is a bit nervous about this, as he has never been on the witness stand in court and
is not sure what is expected of him.

## CASE STUDY REVIEW

1. How will Mr. Bolski's medical record help Joe answer questions at the hearing?

2. What information should Joe gather in order to be prepared to testify?

3. As an expert witness, what is Joe expected to communicate to the judge in this case?

## SUMMARY

Changing societal values have contributed to an explosion of lawsuits in medical practice. Patients are more aware than ever of their rights, especially those of confidentiality and the right to privacy, consent, and records ownership. They readily seek redress when they perceive their rights to be violated.

A healthy relationship between physicians and patients and between medical assistants and patients, as well as respect for the patient's rights, lowers the likelihood of a lawsuit.

Knowledge of the laws that regulate medical and business practices in your state is necessary in order to be in compliance. Sources of information regarding state and federal laws can be obtained from the state medical society, the physician's liability insurance company, the state medical assistant society, the state attorney general's office, or the public library.

## REVIEW QUESTIONS

### Multiple Choice

1. The type of contract that most often exists between physician and patient is:
   a. expressed
   b. implied
   c. privileged
   d. civil
2. Which of the following claims of negligence would fit into the category of *res ipsa loquitur*?
   a. improper use of X-ray equipment
   b. failure to use X-ray equipment
   c. incorrect administration of anesthesia
   d. discovery of a surgical instrument inside the patient's body
3. Slander is defamation through:
   a. spoken statements that damage an individual's reputation
   b. written statements that damage a person's reputation
   c. written falsehoods about an individual
   d. a, b, and c
4. Occasionally, a physician will be sued for the negligence of a partner or employee, even though the physician is not guilty of any negligent act. This is done on the basis of the doctrine of:
   a. *res ipsa loquitur*
   b. *respondeat superior*
   c. proximate cause
   d. contract law
5. The standard of care expected of a physician is held by the courts to mean:
   a. on a par with all other physicians engaged in the same medical specialty anywhere
   b. reasonable, attentive, diligent care comparable to other physicians of the same specialty in the same or similar community

   c. the best possible under the circumstances
   d. the same as the national norm
6. Physician's directives:
   a. allow patients to direct how their billing is to be handled
   b. are designed to encourage physicians to render first aid in an emergency
   c. direct physicians based on a patient's wishes in life-threatening circumstances
   d. are not considered legal documents
7. A subpoena:
   a. is a court order requesting data and/or an appearance in court
   b. is sufficient to enforce a release of any type medical record or information
   c. may be ignored without consequences
   d. allows the person being served to select a specific date or time to appear
8. The 4 Ds of negligence are:
   a. duty, danger, damage, and disaster
   b. derelict, direct cause, damage, and danger
   c. danger, direct cause, damage, disaster
   d. duty, derelict, direct cause, damage
9. Emancipated minors:
   a. are considered adults and can consent to treatment
   b. live on their own and are self-supporting
   c. may be married or serve in the military
   d. all of the above
   e. only b and c
10. Torts:
    a. include battery, defamation of character, invasion of privacy
    b. are always intentional in nature
    c. do not require that harm has occurred
    d. do not include malpractice

## Critical Thinking

1. Chris is a six-year-old girl whom Dr. King has seen for a broken leg. Chris' parents fail to follow Dr. King's treatment plan for Chris. What, if any, action can Dr. King take? What is the legal term for this situation?

2. Audrey, the medical assistant at Lewis & King MD, has accidentally used an incorrect solution to irrigate a patient's eyes. The patient suffers injuries to both eyes. Can Audrey's error be considered malpractice? Explain your reason.

3. Explain the standard of care as it applies to medical assistants. Give an example.

4. Jaime arrived in the clinic having sustained a serious laceration at his construction site. Dr. Woo ordered Demerol R 100 mg. 1.m - stat which Wanda, the medical assistant, administers. Dr. Woo determines surgery is required. Should a consent form be prepared? If so, by whom, and what should be included?

5. Give two examples of routine office or clinic procedures that might constitute violation of the patient's right to privacy.

6. Discuss the federal law regarding HIV testing, AIDS, and drug screening.

7. What are public duties? Discuss the physician's and medical assistant's obligations in regard to public duties.

8. What is the Good Samaritan Law? What must a medical assistant and any other health care professional remember when giving first aid at the scene of an accident?

9. Describe three types of abuse. Tell what your role and responsibilities are as a medical assistant when Juanita brings her son Henry into the clinic. Henry appears to have bruises on his face and chest.

10. Lenore McDonnell, who uses a wheelchair, has applied for employment in a large bookstore in town. She has not yet been offered the job. She has an appointment today for a preemployment physical examination and tells Audrey, the medical assistant, that the bookstore wants a copy of the results of Dr. Lewis' findings. Discuss the situation in light of the Americans with Disabilities Act.

## WEB ACTIVITIES

Research the World Wide Web for the statute of limitations related to claims injuries. What is the time span in your state?

## REFERENCES/BIBLIOGRAPHY

Cowdrey, M., & Drew, M. (1995). *Basic law for the allied health professions* (2nd ed.). Sudbury, MA: Jones and Bartlett.

Flight, M. (1998). *Law, liability, and ethics for medical office professionals* (3rd ed.). Albany, NY: Delmar.

Lewis, M. A., & Tamparo, C. D. (1998). *Medical law, ethics, and bioethics for ambulatory care* (4th ed.). Philadelphia: F. A. Davis Company.

McWay, D. A. (1997). *Legal aspects of health information management*. Albany, NY: Delmar.

# 8

# ETHICAL CONSIDERATIONS

## KEY TERMS

Bioethics
Ethics
Genetic Engineering
Surrogate

## OUTLINE

**Ethics Defined**
**Bioethics Defined**
**Keys to the AAMA Code of Ethics**
**AMA Ethical Guidelines**
    Advertising
    Media Relations
    Confidentiality
    Medical Records
    Professional Fees and Charges
    Professional Rights and Responsi-
      bilities
    Abuse

**Bioethical Dilemmas**
    Allocation of Scarce Medical
      Resources
    Abortion and Fetal Tissue
      Research
    Genetic Engineering/Manipula-
      tion
    Artificial Insemination/Surrogacy
    Dying and Death
    HIV and AIDS

## OBJECTIVES

*The student should strive to meet the following performance objectives and demonstrate an understanding of the facts and principles presented in this chapter through written and oral communication.*

1. Define the key terms as presented in the glossary.

2. Identify the two prominent Codes of Ethics.

3. Compare/contrast the AAMA and the AMA Codes of Ethics.

4. Recall the five principles of the AAMA Code of Medical Ethics.

5. Relate the five principles of the AAMA code to patient care in the ambulatory care setting.

6. Recall the seven principles or standards of conduct adopted by the AMA.

7. Discuss the guidelines identified in at least six ethical issues presented by the *Current Opinions of the Council on Ethical and Judicial Affairs of the AMA*.

8. Restate the dilemmas encountered by the following bioethical issues: (a) allocation of scarce medical resources; (b) abortion and fetal tissue research; (c) genetic engineering/manipulation; (d) artificial insemination/surrogacy; (e) dying and death.

83

**GENERAL (TRANSDISCIPLINARY)**

**Professionalism**
- **Adhere to ethical principles**
- **Promote the CMA credential**

**Legal Concepts**
- **Maintain confidentiality**
- **Prepare and maintain medical records**
- **Use appropriate guidelines when releasing information**

On occasion, ethical dilemmas occur because patients are unsure of the role of the medical assistant. For example, the medical assistants of Inner City Health Care are truly multidisciplinary and have a range of administrative and clinical skills. However, patients sometimes think of them as nurses who have an entirely different set of skills. While most of the medical assistants gently correct patients and make it a point to practice only within their area of expertise, occasionally newer members of the medical assistant staff may feel more "important" when patients regard them as nurses or physicians' assistants.

A few weeks ago, medical assistant Liz Corbin, who is in her early twenties, was taken aback when Walter Seals, the office manager, spoke up about Liz's tendency to let patients assume she was a nurse. While Liz never deliberately intended to mislead patients, she never corrected them about their misconceptions. Walter pointed out that to present a good example of the medical assisting profession, Liz should gently but firmly help patients understand that she was a medical assistant with a specific range of skills that complemented, but did not substitute for, nursing skills.

## INTRODUCTION

It is impossible in today's world to function as a medical assistant without an awareness of the impact of ethics and bioethics on health care. Just as an understanding of the law and working within the law is vital information for the medical assistant, it is equally important to understand ethics and bioethics.

From the previous chapter, you have come to realize that there are many circumstances and situations that occur in health care that are guided and directed by state and federal laws. You, personally, are expected to be above reproach in all your actions in this regard. You must also work with your employer and other members of the health care team to assure that each member of the staff functions within the law—protecting both patients and providers.

Ethics plays a huge role in such an endeavor. To function ethically demands that you never function outside the law. Ethics, however, demands something more—ethics

calls for honesty, trustworthiness, integrity, confidentiality, and fairness. To function ethically, you must know yourself well and understand weaknesses and any vulnerabilities that might prevent you from acting ethically.

The scenario described above is just one situation in which medical assistants may need to reflect on their actions and be sure that they are acting ethically and within the range of their skills. Medical assistants also need to recognize the warning signs that they, or some other staff member, may be about to breach a code of ethics. Often, this kind of breach occurs when one has, or seeks to have, too much power; when one attempts to take too much authority; and when one has too little knowledge and experience. When a breach seems about to occur, the individuals involved should be encouraged to step back and review their actions and the likely consequences of those actions.

## ETHICS DEFINED

Traditionally, **ethics** has been defined in terms of what is right or wrong. For health care professionals, ethics is often defined by a code or creed as seen in the Code of Ethics from the American Association of Medical Assistants (AAMA) or the Principles of Medical Ethics from the American Medical Association (AMA). While these codes, and many others like them, are essential and very helpful, they lose their vitality unless they are understood

by individuals who possess a personal and sound moral code or set of values.

Unlike the law, which seldom changes unless challenged and examined in the courts, codes of ethics constantly change and evolve just as personal values and morals change and evolve. Every time values are challenged and examined, a medical assistant's personal ethical codes become stronger, the understanding of others' perceptions becomes clearer, and professionalism is enhanced.

## BIOETHICS DEFINED

Bioethics brings the entire focus of ethics into the field of health care and into those ethical issues dealing with life. Never before in the history of medical care has bioethics been such a topic of concern. In the past, most bioethical decisions were made by physicians and esteemed members of the medical and/or legal profession. However, advancing technology giving patients and consumers numerous choices regarding their health care causes each one of us to take an active role in bioethics.

Medical assistants will encounter ethical and bioethical issues across the lifespan. In Figure 8-1, a few issues are identified for contemplation and discussion. Issues of bioethics common to every medical office are the allocation of scarce medical resources, abortion and fetal tissue research, genetic engineering or manipulation, and the many choices surrounding life, dying, and death.

For medical assistants to fully comprehend a discussion of ethics and bioethics, they must be familiar with the Code of Ethics of AAMA (Figure 8-2) and the AMA's Principles of Medical Ethics (Figure 8-3).

## A FEW ISSUES FOR CONTEMPLATION AND DISCUSSION

### Infants

- In premature, deformed, or severely disabled infants, ethical issues include the decision to provide or withhold treatment. Health care professionals and parents are not always in agreement. Central to this issue, also, is the expense involved in certain treatments and deciding who pays the cost of treatment.
- Vulnerability of infants can lead to issues of negligence, abuse, or rejection. Parents are also vulnerable because they may be unable to cope with the needs of the entire family.

### Children

- Children who are ill-fed, housed, educated, and clothed exhibit great needs for preventive, curative, and rehabilitative health care.
- Minors with sexually transmitted diseases can seek treatment without the parents' knowledge. Treatment also must be offered without parental consent to pregnant, infected, or addicted minors.
- Child abuse presents an ethical dilemma, especially when a child confides physical, sexual, or emotional abuse to a health care worker but does not want the information divulged. Health care professionals, as mandated reporters, must report suspected child abuse. Will the child/patient view this as a violation of confidence or suffer dire consequences as a result of the reported abuse?

### Adolescents

- Adolescents as young as 13 to 18 years old may seek abortion without parental knowledge or consent. Is this a violation of parents' right to medical information regarding their children? Or should the adolescent, fearful of parental reaction, have the right to decide?
- The adolescent's growing autonomy, need for independence, changing values, and desire for peer acceptance lead to a number of ethical issues that may involve the health care environment. These include the adolescent's decision to be sexually active, to use birth control, to protect against sexually transmitted diseases, and to use drugs and/or alcohol.

### Adults

- Many low-income women do not have sufficient access to prenatal care, which has proven to be a cost-saving medical measure that is critical to the health of both mother and infant.
- As employers seek to reduce the cost of health insurance benefit programs, many individuals and families are finding themselves shifted from one insurance program to another, leaving them with little or no continuity of care. Also, in some managed care programs, adults may receive medical services from a number of health care professionals with whom they have no opportunity to establish an ongoing physician-patient relationship.
- Even with a physician's directive or a living will, a dying patient's wishes may not be followed. Technological advances in medicine have created a situation where patients may not be able to exercise a choice in the death issue.

### Senior Adults

- Dementia is a common problem that is physically and financially exhausting for the caregiver, who is usually a spouse or adult child. How do caregivers cope with their own needs and the needs of dependent adults? Often, the elderly may reject nursing home placement, and there may be limited funds for such long-term care.
- Elderly patients have the right to maintain dignity and privacy, but their dependency on others may deprive them of these basic rights.
- Physician-assisted suicide for terminally ill patients is a prominent issue in our society, especially when elderly patients sense a total loss of dignity.

**Figure 8-1**    **Ethical issues across the lifespan.** (Compiled by Carol Tamparo, CMA-A, PhD, and Marilyn Pooler, RN, CMA-C, MEd)

## AAMA CODE OF ETHICS

The Code of Ethics of AAMA shall set forth principles of ethical and moral conduct as they relate to the medical profession and the particular practice of medical assisting.

Members of AAMA dedicated to the conscientious pursuit of their profession, and thus desiring to merit the high regard of the entire medical profession and the respect of the general public which they serve, do pledge themselves to strive always to:

A. render service with full respect for the dignity of humanity;
B. respect confidential information obtained through employment unless legally authorized or required by responsible performance of duty to divulge such information;
C. uphold the honor and high principles of the profession and accept its disciplines;
D. seek to continually improve the knowledge and skills of medical assistants for the benefit of patients and professional colleagues;
E. participate in additional service activities aimed toward improving the health and well-being of the community.

## CREED

I believe in the principles and purposes of the Profession of Medical Assisting.
I endeavor to be more effective.
I aspire to render greater service.
I protect the confidence entrusted to me.
I am dedicated to the care and well-being of all people.
I am loyal to my employer.
I am true to the ethics of my profession.
I am strengthened by compassion, courage, and faith.

**Figure 8-2**   AAMA Code of Ethics and Creed. (Copyright by the American Association of Medical Assistants, Inc. Revised October, 1996)

## KEYS TO THE AAMA CODE OF ETHICS

Medical assistants should consider the more salient points in the AAMA code of ethics and ask themselves the following questions:

A. *Render service with full respect for the dignity of humanity.*
   - Will I respect every patient even if I do not approve of his or her morals or choices in health care?
   - Will I honor each patient's request for information and explain unfamiliar procedures?

## PRINCIPLES OF MEDICAL ETHICS: AMERICAN MEDICAL ASSOCIATION

### Preamble

The medical profession has long subscribed to a body of ethical statements developed primarily for the benefit of the patient. As a member of this profession, a physician must recognize responsibility not only to patients, but also to society, to other health professionals, and to self. The following Principles adopted by the American Medical Association are not laws, but standards of conduct which define the essentials of honorable behavior for the physician.

I. A physician shall be dedicated to providing competent medical service with compassion and respect for human dignity.
II. A physician shall deal honestly with patients and colleagues, and strive to expose those physicians deficient in character or competence, or who engage in fraud or deception.
III. A physician shall respect the law and also recognize a responsibility to seek changes in those requirements which are contrary to the best interests of the patient.
IV. A physician shall respect the rights of patients, of colleagues, and of other health professionals, and shall safeguard patient confidences within the constraints of the law.
V. A physician shall continue to study, apply, and advance scientific knowledge, make relevant information available to patients, colleagues, and the public, obtain consultation, and use the talents of other health professionals when indicated.
VI. A physician shall, in the provision of appropriate patient care, except in emergencies, be free to choose whom to serve, with whom to associate, and the environment in which to provide medical services.
VII. A physician shall recognize a responsibility to participate in activities contributing to an improved community.

**Figure 8-3**   American Medical Association Principles of Medical Ethics. (Source: Code of Medical Ethics Current Opinions with Annotations, 2000–2001 Edition, American Medical Association, Copyright 2000)

- Will I give my full attention to acknowledging the needs of every patient?
- Will I be able to accept the indigent, the physically and mentally challenged, the infirm, the physically disfigured, and the persons I simply do not like as equal and valid human beings with an equal right to service?

B. *Respect confidential information obtained through employment unless legally authorized or required by responsible performance of duty to divulge such information.*

- Will I refrain from needless comments to a colleague regarding a patient's problem?
- Will I refrain from discussing my day's encounters with patients with my family and friends?
- Will I always protect a patient's chart and everything in it from unnecessary observation?
- Will I keep patients' names and the circumstances that bring them to my place of employment confidential?

C. *Uphold the honor and high principles of the profession and accept its disciplines.*

- Am I proud of serving as a medical assistant?
- Will I always perform within the scope of my profession, never exceeding the responsibility entrusted to me?
- Will I encourage others to enter the profession and always speak honorably of medical assistants?

D. *Seek to continually improve the knowledge and skills of medical assistants for the benefit of patients and professional colleagues.*

- Will I always be willing to learn new skills, to update my skills, and seek improved methods for assisting the physician in the care of patients?
- Will I keep my certification current and valid?
- Can I always remember that I am a member of a group of broad-based health care professionals and that my goal is to complement rather than to compete with that team?

E. *Participate in additional service activities aimed toward improving the health and well-being of the community.*

- Will I be able to serve in the community where I reside and work to further quality health care?
- Will I promote preventive medicine?
- Will I practice good health care management for myself, being a model for others to follow?

## AMA ETHICAL GUIDELINES

The American Medical Association and its nine-member Judicial Council publish a guide for ethical behavior for physicians that is beneficial to medical assistants who act in concert with their physician/employer. The guidelines are based on the Code of Medical Ethics in the publication *Current Opinions of the Council on Ethical and Judicial Affairs of the American Medical Association, 2000.* Information shared here is not meant to be exhaustive; however, physicians and their employees will find it helpful to con-

sider information on the following topics, which was summarized from this publication. The complete guide can be purchased from the AMA in Chicago, IL.

## Advertising

Physicians and professional people have traditionally not advertised; however, it is not illegal or unethical to do so if claims made are truthful and not misleading. Advertisements may include credentials of physicians and a description of the practice, kinds of services rendered, and how fees are determined. Managed care agencies may advertise their services and the names of participating physicians. Testimonials from patients are best avoided. Indeed, most physicians discover that word-of-mouth advertisement from patients is the best source of advertisement for their practice.

## Media Relations

Physicians and all of their employees are not allowed to discuss a patient's medical condition with any member of the media without the patient's expressed approval. This does not apply to information that is considered "public domain," which includes births, deaths, accidents, and police records. While more hospitals than ambulatory care settings will be involved in media relations, the following is an example of information that is considered public domain and does not require the patient's consent.

"Jaime Carrera, a local construction worker, suffered a severe laceration to the head as a result of an accident at the construction site. He remains hospitalized in good condition."

## Confidentiality

 Physicians must not reveal confidential information about patients without their consent unless they are otherwise required to do so by law. Confidentiality must be protected so that patients will feel comfortable and safe in revealing information about themselves that may be important to their health care. The following list contains examples of the kinds of reports that allow or require health professionals to report a confidence.

- A patient threatens another person and there is reason to believe that the threat may be carried out.

- Certain injuries and illnesses *must* be reported. They include injuries such as knife and gunshot wounds, wounds that may be from suspected child abuse, and communicable diseases such as influenza, AIDS, and sexually transmitted diseases.

- Information that may have been subpoenaed for testimony in a court of law.

When in doubt, it is always recommended that a physician have the patient's permission to reveal any confidential information.

 Extra caution must be taken to protect the confidentiality of any patient's data that is kept on a computer database. As few people as possible should have access to the computer data, and only authorized individuals should be permitted to add or alter data. Adequate security precautions must be utilized to protect information stored on a computer.

## Medical Records

The medical chart and the information in it are the property of the physician and the patient. No information should be revealed without the patient's consent unless required by law. The record is confidential. Physicians should not refuse to provide a copy of the record to another physician treating the patient so long as proper authorization has been received from the patient. Also, physicians should provide a copy of the record or summary of its contents if a patient requests it. A record cannot be withheld because of an unpaid bill.

Upon a physician's retirement or death, or when a practice is sold, patients should be notified and given ample time to have their records transferred to another physician of their choice.

## Professional Fees and Charges

Illegal or excessive fees should not be charged. Fees should be based on those customary to the locale and should reflect the difficulty of services and the quality of performance rendered. Fee splitting (a physician splits the fee with another physician for services rendered with or without the patient's knowledge) in any form is unethical. Physicians may charge for missed appointments (if patients have first been notified of the practice) and may charge for multiple or very complex insurance forms. Physicians and their employees must be diligent to assure that only the services actually rendered are charged or indicated on the insurance claim. Only what is documented in the patient's chart is to be billed.

## Professional Rights and Responsibilities

 Physicians may choose whom to serve, but may not refuse a patient on the basis of race, color, religion, national origin, or any other illegal discrimination. It is unethical for physicians to deny treatment to HIV-infected individuals on that basis alone if they are qualified to treat the patient's condition. Once a physician takes a case, the patient cannot be neglected nor refused treatment unless official notice is given from the physician to withdraw from the case.

Patients have the right to know their diagnoses, the nature and purpose of their treatment, and to have enough information to be able to make an informed choice about their treatment protocol. Physicians should inform families of a patient's death and not delegate that responsibility to others.

Physicians should expose incompetent, corrupt, dishonest, and unethical conduct by other physicians to the disciplinary board. It is unethical for any physician to treat patients while under the influence of alcohol, controlled substances, or any other chemical that impairs the physician's ability.

Physicians who know they are HIV positive should refrain from any activity that would risk the transmission of the virus to others.

Any activity that might be regarded as a "conflict of interest" (for example, a physician holding stock in a pharmaceutical company and prescribing medications only from that company) should be avoided. Financial interests are not to influence physicians in prescribing medications, devices, or appliances.

## Abuse

 It is the responsibility of physicians and their employees to report all cases of suspected child abuse, to protect and care for the abused, and to treat the abuser (if known) as a victim also. This is not an

---

**SPOTLIGHT ON AAMA**
**ESSENTIALS THROUGH CAAHEP**

- Medical ethics involves providing patients of all socioeconomic backgrounds with quality care.

- Professional and empathetic medical assistants never judge patients whose belief systems differ from their own.

- If a medical assistant suspects that an HIV-seropositive patient is infecting an unsuspecting person, he or she should make every attempt to protect the individual at risk and to encourage the infected person to cease endangering other people.

easy task. Abuse is not easy to witness. While there are very specific laws regarding suspected child abuse, and in most states medical assistants are mandated to report abuse, the laws are vague or nonexistent in elderly and spousal abuse. However, whatever form the abuse takes, it is best to treat all forms of abuse in the same manner by providing a safe environment for those abused and seeking treatment for the abuser and the abused.

## BIOETHICAL DILEMMAS

Guidelines for bioethical issues are even harder to define than are guidelines for ethics, because each of the bioethical issues calls upon us to make decisions that directly affect a person's life. In some instances, the bioethical issue requires a choice about who lives and requires a definition of the quality of life. Such dilemmas are difficult, if not impossible, to approach from a neutral point of view even though medical assistants should strive not to impose their own moral values upon patients or coworkers.

### *Allocation of Scarce Medical Resources*

The issue faced daily by health care workers is the allocation of scarce medical resources. Even with the government's attempts at health care reform, medical resources still will not be available to everyone. When the receptionist determines who receives the only available appointment in a day, when patients are turned away because they have no insurance or financial resources to pay for services, when Medicare/Medicaid patients are denied services because of low return from state and federal insurance programs, scarce medical resources are being denied.

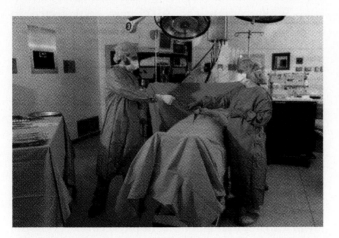

**Figure 8-4** Scarce medical resources may limit surgery options for patients whose conditions are not immediately life threatening; some patients may lack insurance and not be able to afford necessary surgical procedures. (Photo courtesy of the U.S. Army)

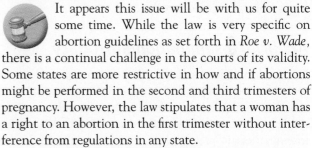

Weightier decisions might include who gets the surgery, a kidney transplant, or the experimental bone marrow transplant, Figure 8-4. These allocations are being made and will continue to require decisions on the part of the health care team. Rationing of health care may become more widespread as managed care operations try to achieve a balance between providing access to care while still curtailing costs.

Decisions made by Congress, health systems agencies, and insurance companies are termed macroallocation of scarce medical resources. Decisions made individually by physicians and members of the health care team at the local level are termed microallocation of scarce resources. No matter what the level, physicians and medical assistants will be involved.

### *Abortion and Fetal Tissue Research*

It appears this issue will be with us for quite some time. While the law is very specific on abortion guidelines as set forth in *Roe v. Wade,* there is a continual challenge in the courts of its validity. Some states are more restrictive in how and if abortions might be performed in the second and third trimesters of pregnancy. However, the law stipulates that a woman has a right to an abortion in the first trimester without interference from regulations in any state.

A physician must decide whether to perform abortions and under what circumstances (within the legal parameters). A physician cannot be forced to perform abortions, nor can any employee be forced to participate or assist the physician to perform an abortion. Employees not wishing to participate in abortions are advised to seek employment where they are not performed.

There are many unanswered ethical questions related to abortion that make it difficult for health care professionals. Should abortion be considered a form of birth control? If not, should birth control be readily available to all who seek it regardless of age? Is it ethical to deny a woman on welfare an abortion while providing one to the woman who either has money for the procedure or whose insurance pays for it? And, of course, the major unanswered question that must be determined by every physician is: when does life begin?

The abortion issue raises another bioethical issue—fetal tissue research and transplantation. Research has shown that transplanted tissue from aborted fetuses can be instrumental in benefiting individuals with serious, life-threatening diseases. This issue is political as well as bioethical, and it changes with each major political shift in our government. If fetal tissue research is allowed, the primary ethical concern is that that fact not be used to encourage women to have abortions; rather, the tissue would be available only after a decision had already been made regarding abortion.

## Genetic Engineering/Manipulation

So much is possible today in the area of genetic engineering and more is being discovered daily. Through genetic engineering, we have the potential of identifying genes that predispose individuals to certain illnesses and diseases and manipulating or altering those genes to prevent or lessen the disease or illness. Who among us would not want to be free of certain illnesses? But at what cost? How far do we go in genetic engineering? Would we prefer a society where everyone is healthy and beautiful? If it is determined that a fetus suffers from a serious defect, should abortion be encouraged? If we manipulate the genes prior to implantation, are we playing god? If fertilization takes place *in vitro,* is discarding defective embryos a reasonable and presumed choice?

## Artificial Insemination/Surrogacy

For many individuals, artificial insemination is the only means by which they can conceive. Physicians can be called upon to perform artificial insemination for couples, single women, or lesbians who want a child. If artificial insemination is practiced, the AMA recommends the signed consent of each party involved. It is also recommended that physicians practicing AID (Artificial Insemination by Donor), not continually use the same donors for semen, and that meticulous screening be performed prior to the insemination.

Surrogacy is another bioethical issue. Men have been used as surrogates, or substitutes, for decades with the practice of artificial insemination, but society has a more difficult time with surrogate mothers than artificial insemination with male donors. Under what circumstances should a surrogate mother be considered? How should the rights of each individual in the exchange be protected? For many of these issues, there is little or no protection or guidance under the law; therefore, physicians and their employees must make decisions on the basis of their own belief systems. The AMA is not supportive of surrogacy as a viable route to parenthood.

## Dying and Death

Patients are making more choices regarding their death. We all have the right to direct health care professionals regarding our death in the case of a life-threatening ill-

ness. Through a living will or a physician's directive, we can mandate that life support systems be removed. Sometimes, patients make these decisions before physicians are ready to remove the life support. Other times, physicians can determine when a case is hopeless far quicker than the patient or the patient's family. What should be done then? When a physician is committed to sustaining life, it is very difficult to make decisions to terminate life. In 1994, Oregon voters passed a physician-assisted suicide law. Other states are considering similar laws.

In 1990, Congress passed a bill called the Patient Self-Determination Act, which encourages patients to make living wills and advance directives before life-sustaining measures become necessary. Nearly all states have legislation regarding advance directives.

Choices available to patients who are dying always cause us to ask ourselves what is "quality of life"? While the answer to that question is different for everyone, it is a question often in conflict with today's medical technology that can, in many instances, keep a patient alive much longer than the patient might prefer. The benefits of advanced technology will continue to be weighed against what many consider the right to die with dignity and a minimum of medical intervention.

## HIV and AIDS

The general public's fear of AIDS has caused some serious bioethical issues. Patients who may suspect they have come into contact with HIV or AIDS should be tested for the virus. Their confidentiality must be protected as much as possible since persons with AIDS often face loss of employment, medical insurance, and even loss of family and friends. It is unethical to deny treatment to HIV-infected individuals because they test positive for HIV.

While persons with AIDS must be protected, so must the public. Therefore, if physicians suspect that an HIV-seropositive patient is infecting an unsuspecting individual, every attempt should be made to protect the individual at risk. Health professionals must first encourage the infected person to cease endangering any person. Second, if the patient refuses to notify the person at risk or wishes the physician to notify the person, the physician can contact authorities. Many states and cities have Partner Notification Programs that will anonymously notify the patient at risk, keeping the source confidential. The Program informs them that it has been brought to their attention that they are a "person at risk" and provides them with free testing. Third, the physician can notify the person at risk.

**8-1**

At the end of a busy afternoon, Juanita Hansen, a single mother in her twenties, brings in her son Henry after he fell down a flight of steps. He is badly bruised and crying and also seems to be somewhat fearful of his mother. Medical assistant Liz Corbin recognizes Henry, for his mother brought him in the week before when he fell off his bike. At that time, Liz had assisted Dr. Esposito in examining Henry and both were concerned about the possibility of child abuse, for Henry had been in before for various "accidents." Today, when Liz assists Dr. Esposito once again to examine Henry, it becomes clear that Henry is probably the victim of abuse.

## CASE STUDY REVIEW

1. Because Liz and Dr. Esposito strongly suspect that Henry is being repeatedly abused, what are they obligated to do?
2. How can Liz best help Henry to cope with his situation?
3. How can Liz attempt to help Henry's mother come to terms with the fact that she is physically abusing her son?

## SUMMARY

As medical technology continues to advance, a greater need for ethical guidelines will be necessary. Physicians and health care professionals at all levels must stay abreast of the issues and carefully consider all aspects prior to any decision making.

Medical assistants must, however, keep the following legal and ethical guidelines in mind: (1) always practice within the law; (2) preserve the patient's confidentiality; (3) maintain meticulous records; (4) obtain informed, written consent; (5) do not judge patients whose belief system differs from yours.

## REVIEW QUESTIONS

### Multiple Choice

1. Typically, ethics has been defined in terms of:
   a. what is right and wrong
   b. whether an action is legal
   c. the expedient thing to do
   d. professionalism in the workplace
2. Bioethics has to do with:
   a. biological reproduction
   b. the act of artificial insemination
   c. genetic engineering
   d. ethical issues that deal with life and health care
3. The Code of Ethics of AAMA:
   a. is concerned with principles of ethical and moral conduct
   b. defines the duties the medical assistant can perform
   c. is intended for physicians only
   d. applies only to patient rights

4. When a physician or medical assistant suspects child abuse, she should:
   a. give the parent a warning
   b. report it to the proper authorities
   c. not impose her values on the parents
   d. give the child some hints on how to protect against abuse
5. When a patient has HIV:
   a. it is ethical for the physician not to provide treatment
   b. it is unethical for the physician not to provide treatment
   c. other patients should be warned of the possibility of infection
   d. all friends and family members of the patient should be notified
6. A copy of a medical record may be granted to:
   a. a physician the patient is being referred to
   b. a physician's attorney when subpoenaed or released by patient

c. the patient
d. all of the above
e. only a and b

7. A patient's living will or physician's directive:
   a. is a legal document to be kept in the chart
   b. can be changed at any time by the patient
   c. should accompany the patient to the hospital
   d. all of the above
   e. only a and c

8. Your physician employer is considering changing the practice's announcement in the yellow pages of the phone book. Which of the following is not recommended?
   a. Name and specialty of practice
   b. Names and credentials/specialties of participating physicians
   c. Patient testimonials
   d. Managed care participation

9. Which of the following is true?
   a. A physician can choose whom to serve.
   b. A physician may charge for completing multiple and complex insurance claims.
   c. Physicians and their employees cannot be forced to perform abortions.
   d. All of the above
   e. None of the above

10. You are most likely to make ethical decisions correctly when:
    a. you have a clear picture of the situation
    b. you leave emotion out of the decision as much as possible
    c. you understand your weaknesses and vulnerabilities
    d. honesty and integrity are hallmarks of your entire life
    e. all of the above

## Critical Thinking

1. In your own words, define ethics and bioethics.
2. List the similarities of and the differences between the AAMA Code of Ethics and the AMA Principles of Medical Ethics.
3. The physician observes another physician put a patient at risk while under the influence of alcohol and does nothing about it. What would constitute ethical behavior?

4. A physician attends a medical seminar related to medical practice every month and charges the seminar fee to the business. Would you consider this ethical or unethical? Why?

5. A physician refuses to accept any more Medicaid patients for medical care. Is this the physician's right? Is it ethical?

6. A medical assistant whispers to the receptionist, "There goes the guy with AIDS." How should the receptionist view this behavior?

7. The services reported on the insurance claim are more complex than those actually rendered. Is this ethical or unethical? State your reasons.

8. The physician refuses to perform a legal abortion. Do you consider this an ethical issue? Why?

9. A physician performs artificial insemination for a lesbian couple; however, the medical assistant refuses to participate or assist the physician. What are the ramifications of the medical assistant's behavior? Do you believe the medical assistant has a right to refuse?

10. Referring to Figure 8-1, select an ethical issue with which you may have had some personal experience. Now, form a small group, with each student leading a discussion on a different issue.

## WEB ACTIVITIES

Using the World Wide Web, research particular guidelines to be used for artificial insemination either by donor or by husband. Look under the Current Opinions of the Council on Ethical and Judicial Affairs.

- What are the guidelines for medical records? Why?

- Why is frozen sperm recommended?

## REFERENCES/BIBLIOGRAPHY

American Medical Association. (2000). *Code of medical ethics. Current opinions of the council on ethical and judicial affairs, 2000.* Chicago: Author.

Flight, M. (1998). *Law, liability, and ethics for medical office personnel* (3rd ed.). Albany, NY: Delmar.

Lewis, M. A., & Tamparo, C. D., (1998). *Medical law, ethics, and bioethics for ambulatory care* (4th ed.). Philadelphia: F. A. Davis Co.

# EMERGENCY PROCEDURES AND FIRST AID

## KEY TERMS

Cardiopulmonary Resuscitation (CPR)
Crash Tray or Cart
Crepitation
Emergency Medical Services (EMS)
First Aid
Fracture
Heimlich Maneuver
Hypothermia
Lackluster
Occlusion
Rescue Breathing
Shock
Splint
Sprain
Standard Precautions
Strain
Syncope
Triage
Universal Emergency Medical
   Identification Symbol
Wound

## OUTLINE

**Recognizing an Emergency**
   Responding to an Emergency
   Primary Survey
   Using the 911 or Emergency
      Medical Services System
   Good Samaritan Laws
   Blood, Body Fluids, and Disease
      Transmission
**Preparing for an Emergency**
   The Medical Crash Tray or Cart
**Common Emergencies**
   Shock
   Wounds
   Burns

   Musculoskeletal Injuries
   Heat- and Cold-Related Illnesses
   Poisoning
   Sudden Illness
   Cerebral Vascular Accident
      (CVA)
   Heart Attack
**Procedures for Breathing Emer-
gencies and Cardiac Arrest**
   Heimlich Maneuver (Abdominal
      Thrust)
   Rescue Breathing
   Cardiopulmonary Resuscitation
      (CPR)

## OBJECTIVES

*The student should strive to meet the following performance objectives and demonstrate an understanding of the facts and principles presented in this chapter through written and oral communication.*

1. Define the key terms as presented in the glossary.
2. Learn to recognize, prepare for, and respond to emergencies in the ambulatory care setting.
3. Understand the legal and disease transmission considerations in emergency caregiving.
4. Perform the primary assessment in emergency situations.
5. Identify and care for different types of wounds.
6. Understand the basics of bandage application.
7. Discriminate among first-, second-, and third-degree burns.
8. Assess injuries to muscles, bones, and joints.
9. Describe heat- and cold-related illnesses.

*(continues)*

10. Describe how poisons may enter the body.
11. Recall the eight types of shock.
12. Define a cerebral vascular accident.
13. Describe the signs and symptoms of a heart attack.
14. Demonstrate proficiency in Heimlich maneuver, rescue breathing, and cardiopulmonary resuscitation (CPR).

## ROLE DELINEATION COMPONENTS

**CLINICAL**

**Patient Care**

- Adhere to established triage procedures
- Recognize and respond to emergencies
- Obtain patient history and vital signs
- Prepare and maintain examination and treatment areas
- Prepare patient for examination, procedures, and treatment

**GENERAL (Transdisciplinary)**

**Instruction**

- Instruct individuals according to their needs

## SCENARIO

Inner City Health Care, which is located in Carlton, Michigan, has its share of cold, snowy winters and when the temperature drops near freezing, that snow sometimes turns to ice. Last night, as Clinical Medical Assistant Wanda Slawson, CMA, was leaving for the evening, she noticed a woman from an adjacent office slip and fall in the parking lot. Wanda immediately went over to the woman to lend assistance and saw that, in falling, the woman had cut the palm of her hand. Apparently, she had tried to break her fall with her hand only to sustain a large wound that was now bleeding moderately. Fortunately, Wanda knew that one of the physicians was still in the office and she led the woman back to the building, reassuring her all the way. Once in the office, Wanda assisted Susan Rice, the physician, to examine the wound. After determining that sutures were not needed, Dr. Rice and Wanda cleansed the wound, applied a dry, sterile dressing, and covered it with an elastic bandage. The patient was instructed to call her physician first thing in the morning.

## INTRODUCTION

While the ambulatory care setting is primarily designed to see patients under nonemergency conditions, occasionally the physician will need to administer emergency care and the medical assistant will be called upon to assist the physician in this care. For the medical assistant who may need to triage or assess the patient's condition, the first and most critical step in responding to an emergency is developing the skill to recognize when emergency measures should be taken.

While some emergencies can be treated in the office, others cannot and the medical assistant must know when to call for outside help. If the emergency occurs in the ambulatory care setting, the physician usually provides immediate care. It is possible, however, that the medical assistant may be the first emergency caregiver should the physician be out of the office. The medical assistant also may be called upon to provide care in an emergency outside of the office environment.

This chapter will acquaint the medical assistant with types of emergency situations that may occur either inside or outside of the office. However, this chapter is merely an introduction to emergency topics and does not substitute for first aid and cardiopulmonary (CPR) instruction taught either through the college curriculum or through the American Red Cross or the American Heart Association. These hands-on classes are vital teaching tools and all medical assistants should take them on a regular basis in order to continually update their skills.

## RECOGNIZING AN EMERGENCY

An emergency is considered any instance in which an individual becomes suddenly ill and requires immediate attention. Some common signs that an individual has an emergency include unusual noises, such as yelling, moaning, or crying. A person may appear to be behaving strangely when choking or if having difficulty breathing. To recognize when an emergency exists, it is important to have sharp senses of hearing, sight, and smell and be acutely sensitive to any unusual behaviors.

In the ambulatory care setting, medical assistants will encounter a range of emergency situations requiring first aid techniques. **First aid** is designed to render immediate and temporary emergency care to persons injured or otherwise disabled prior to the arrival of a physician or transport to a hospital or other health care agency.

Emergency situations can include:

- Wounds
- Bleeding
- Burns
- Shock
- Fractures
- Poisoning
- Sudden illnesses such as fainting
- Illnesses related to heat and cold
- Heart attack
- Choking and breathing crises

Some of these will be life-threatening; all will require immediate care. In either case, it is critical to remain calm, to follow the emergency policies and procedures established by the ambulatory care setting, and to be well-versed in first-aid and cardiopulmonary resuscitation techniques.

### *Responding to an Emergency*

Once it has been determined that an emergency exists, it is essential to act quickly. Before making any decisions about how to proceed, it is necessary to assess the nature of the situation. Does it include respiratory or circulatory failure, severe bleeding, burns, poisoning, or severe allergic reaction?

Sometimes, it is possible that more than one type of care must be administered. In this case, it is necessary to **triage** the situation, which is a method of prioritizing treatment. When an individual suffers more than one illness or injury, care must be given according to the severity of the situation. When two or more patients present with emergencies simultaneously, triage also determines which patient is treated first. The main principle of triage states that absence of breath and severe bleeding are immediate life threats. See Table 9-1 for the common ordering of triage situations.

To identify the nature of the emergency and respond effectively, it is critical that the patient be assessed. If the patient is conscious, ask for personal identification and identification of next of kin. Try to obtain information about symptoms being experienced in order to identify the problem. Always check for a **universal emergency medical identification symbol** (Figure 9-1) and accompanying identification card, which will describe any serious or life-threatening health problems of the patient. Quickly observe the patient's general appearance, including skin color and size and dilation of pupils. Check pulse.

| TABLE 9-1 | EXAMPLES OF TRIAGE SITUATIONS | |
|---|---|---|
| **First Priority** | **Next Priority** | **Least Priority** |
| Airway and breathing problems | Second-degree burns not on the neck and face | Fractures |
| Cardiac arrest | Major or multiple fractures | Minor injuries |
| Severe bleeding that is uncontrolled | Back injuries | Sprains |
| Head injuries | Severe eye injuries | |
| Poisoning | | |
| Open chest or abdominal wounds | | |
| Shock | | |
| Second- and third-degree burns | | |

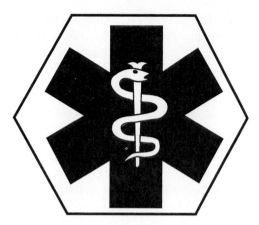

**Figure 9-1**    The universal emergency medical identification symbol.

## Primary Survey

If the patient is unresponsive, it is critical to assess the ABCs, which include:

- Airway (A)

- Breathing (B)

- Circulation (C)

To assess whether the unresponsive patient is breathing and to determine if there is an open airway, place your face close to the patient's face and look, listen, and feel.

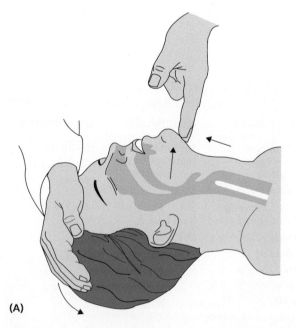

(A)

### Patient Teaching Tip

Alert patients to the importance of carrying the universal emergency medical identification symbol and its accompanying identification card if the patient suffers from severe heart disease, diabetes, or has other life-threatening illnesses or allergies.

Look at the patient's chest and notice whether the chest rises and falls with breathing. Listen for air entering and leaving the nose and mouth and feel for moving air.

If the individual is not breathing, first open the airway by either tilting the head and lifting the chin (Figure 9-2A); or by the jaw-thrust maneuver, which involves placing both thumbs on the patient's cheekbones and index and middle fingers on both sides of the lower jaw (Figure 9-2B). **CAUTION:** Do not attempt to tilt the head and lift the chin when the patient has a head, neck, or spinal cord injury.

If the patient still does not breathe after the airway has been opened, rescue breathing must be performed, which is covered later in this chapter.

To assess circulation, check for the presence of a pulse at the carotid artery on the side of the neck below the ear. If no pulse is present, the patient may be in cardiac arrest and must be given cardiopulmonary resuscitation. CPR techniques are covered in detail later in this chapter.

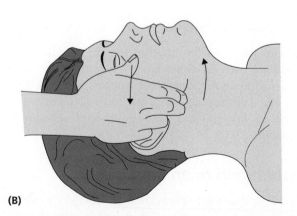

(B)

**Figure 9-2**    If the individual is not breathing, first open the airway: (A) By tilting the head and lifting the chin or (B) By the jaw-thrust maneuver, which involves placing both thumbs on the patient's cheekbones and index and middle fingers on both sides of the lower jaw.

## Using the 911 or Emergency Medical Services System

The **Emergency Medical Services (EMS)** system is a local network of police, fire, and medical personnel who are trained to respond to emergency situations. Other community experts and volunteers also act as resources in an EMS system. In many communities, the network is activated by calling 911. Even when preliminary emergency care is provided by the ambulatory care physician, the patient may still need to be transported or may require follow-up care. It is also possible that the physician may not be equipped to deliver the type of emergency care required, in which case one person should call for EMS help while another stays with the patient until help arrives. Never leave a seriously ill or unconscious patient unattended.

## Good Samaritan Laws

When delivering or assisting in delivering emergency care, the medical assistant may be concerned about professional liability. Most states have enacted Good Samaritan laws, which provide some degree of protection to the health care professional who offers first aid.

Most Good Samaritan laws provide some legal protection to those who provide emergency care to ill or injured persons. However, when medical assistants or any other individuals give care during an emergency, they must act as reasonable and prudent individuals and provide care only within the scope of their abilities. Remember that a primary principle of first aid is to prevent further injury.

While Good Samaritan laws give some measure of protection against being sued for giving emergency aid, they generally protect *off-duty* health care professionals. Also, conditions of the law vary from state to state. As part of establishing emergency care guidelines, every ambulatory care setting should understand the explicit and implicit intent of the Good Samaritan Law in its state. See Chapter 7 for more information on legal guidelines.

## Blood, Body Fluids, and Disease Transmission

 When providing emergency care, medical assistants should always protect themselves and the patient from infectious disease transmission. Serious infectious diseases, such as hepatitis B (HBV) and HIV, which causes AIDS, can be transmitted through blood and body fluids.

By establishing and following strict guidelines, the risk of contacting or transmitting an infectious disease while providing emergency care is greatly reduced.

- Always wash hands thoroughly before (if possible) and after every procedure.
- Use protective clothing and other protective equipment during the procedure.
- During the procedure, avoid contact with blood and body fluids, if possible.
- Do not touch nose, mouth, or eyes with gloved hands.
- Carefully handle and safely dispose of soiled gloves and other objects.

**Standard precautions** were issued by the Centers for Disease Control and Prevention (CDC) in 1996 and combine many of the basic principles of universal precautions with techniques known as body substance isolation. These augmented 1996 guidelines represent the standard in infection control and are intended to protect both patients and health care professionals.

## PREPARING FOR AN EMERGENCY

Emergencies are unexpected but can and should be anticipated and prepared for in the ambulatory care setting. Being properly prepared assures that the office has the materials and resources needed to respond to emergencies.

An in-office handbook of policies and procedures should be developed and should be familiar to all staff. Telephone numbers for the local emergency medical services (often this is 911) and the poison control center should be posted and kept in an established place so that there is no delay in calling for outside assistance. Materials and supplies should be maintained in proper inventory. All personnel should be trained in the basics of first aid and CPR, so that every staff member can respond to or

**SPOTLIGHT ON AAMA ESSENTIALS THROUGH CAAHEP**

- Treat all patients with compassion and empathy.
- Identifying a patient's cultural needs during an emergency may help to save his or her life.
- Listening to how a patient "feels" is just as important as how the patient appears.

assist the physician in providing care. Proper documentation should be completed after any emergency situation. The office environment itself should be a safe one and as accident-proof as possible. Wipe up spills to avoid falls on a slippery floor, keep corridors clutter-free, and keep medications out of sight. These basic risk management techniques will help medical personnel focus on giving emergency care and also protect the facility from any possible litigation.

## The Medical Crash Tray or Cart

Every health care facility should have a **crash tray or cart**, with a carefully controlled inventory of supplies and equipment (Figure 9-3). These first-aid supplies should be kept in an accessible place, and the inventory should be routinely monitored to assure that all supplies are replaced and that all medications are up to date and have not reached their expiration date.

A smaller practice may require only a portable tray for emergency and first-aid supplies; larger urgent care centers may respond more frequently to emergencies and thus may need a cart that can hold a large inventory and variety of supplies. Whether a tray or cart is used, supplies should be customized to the facility and the type of emergencies frequently encountered. Remember that only physicians can order medications or treatment.

Following is a brief list of some common supplies found on most trays and/or carts.

**General supplies:**

- Adhesive and hypoallergenic tape
- Alcohol wipes
- Bandage scissors
- Bandage material
- Blood pressure cuff (standard, pediatric, large)
- Constriction band
- Defibrillator
- Gloves
- Hot/cold packs
- IV tubing
- Needles and syringes for injection
- Orange juice for diabetics (refrigerated)
- Penlight (with extra batteries)
- Personal protective equipment
- Spirits of ammonia

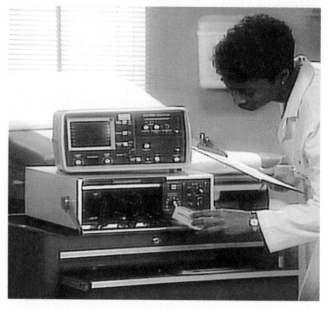

**Figure 9-3**   Medical crash cart.

- Sterile dressings
- Stethoscope

**Emergency medications:**

- Activated charcoal
- Aramine
- Aspirin
- Atropine
- Dextrose
- Diphenhydramine
- Epinephrine
- Glucagon
- Insulin
- Lidocaine
- Nitroglycerin tablets
- Phenobarbital and diazepam (controlled substances; must be kept in a locked cabinet)
- Sodium bicarbonate
- Spirits of ammonia
- Sterile water
- Syrup of ipecac
- Verapamil
- Xylocaine and marcaine

**Respiratory supplies:**

- Airways of all sizes for nasal and oral use
- Ambu bag™
- Bulb syringe for suction
- Oxygen mask
- Oxygen tank

This list represents just some of the supplies to be found on a well-stocked crash cart or tray. The type and list of supplies should always be overseen by facility physicians and tailored to the emergency demands of the practice. The medical assistant should be familiar with the equipment and medication on the crash cart or tray. Practice "drills" simulating various emergency situations are helpful for preparing staff members for actual emergencies.

# COMMON EMERGENCIES

Included in this discussion are shock, wounds, burns, musculoskeletal injuries, heat- and cold-related illnesses, poisoning, sudden illness, cerebral vascular accident, and heart attack.

## Shock

When a severe injury occurs, shock is likely to develop. **Shock** is basically a condition in which the circulatory system is not providing enough blood to all parts of the body, causing the body's organs to fail to function properly.

Shock is always life threatening, and EMS should be activated. The body's attempt to compensate for a massive injury or illness, especially those involving severe bleed-ing, often leads to other problems. During shock several things occur.

- The heart becomes unable to pump blood properly.
- Consequently, the body does not get enough oxygen, which is carried by the blood.
- The body tries to compensate by sending blood to critical organs and reducing the flow of blood to arms, legs, and skin.

**Signs and Symptoms of Shock.** Learn to recognize the signs and symptoms of shock.

- Patient may be restless or feel irritable.
- Weakness, dizziness, thirst, or nausea may occur.
- Breathing may be shallow and rapid.
- Skin is cool, clammy, and pale.
- Pulse is weak and rapid.
- Blood pressure is low.
- Area around the lips, eyes, and fingernails may turn blue from lack of oxygen.
- The patient may be confused and/or become suddenly unconscious.
- Dilated pupils and **lackluster** eyes are notable.

**Types of Shock.** There are eight major types of shock, including respiratory, neurogenic, cardiogenic, hemorrhagic, anaphylactic, metabolic, psychogenic, and septic. See Table 9-2 for a description of each.

| TABLE 9-2 | EIGHT TYPES OF SHOCK WITH DESCRIPTIONS |
|---|---|
| **Type of Shock** | **Description** |
| Respiratory | Trauma to the respiratory tract (trachea, lungs) which causes a reduction of oxygen and carbon dioxide exchange. Body cells cannot receive enough oxygen. |
| Neurogenic | Injury or trauma to the nervous system (spinal cord, brain). Nerve impulse to blood vessels impaired. Blood vessels remain dilated and blood pressure drops. |
| Cardiogenic | Myocardial infarction with damage to heart muscle; heart unable to pump effectively. Inadequate cardiac output. Body cells not receiving enough oxygen. |
| Hemorrhagic | Severe bleeding or loss of body fluid from trauma, surgery, or dehydration from severe nausea and vomiting. Blood pressure drops, thus blood flow is reduced to cells, tissues, and organs. |
| Anaphylactic | Results from reaction to substance to which patient is hypersensitive or allergic (allergen extracts, bee sting, medication, food). Outpouring of histamine results in dilation of blood vessels throughout the body, blood pressure drops and blood flow is reduced to cells, tissue, and organs. |
| Metabolic | Body's homeostasis impaired; acid-base balance disturbed (diabetic coma or insulin shock); body fluids unbalanced. |
| Psychogenic | Due to overwhelming emotional factors; i.e., fear, anger, grief. Sudden dilation of blood vessels, results in fainting because of lack of blood supply to the brain. In most cases, may not be life-threatening unless it leads to physical trauma as a result of a fall. |
| Septic | An acute infection, usually systemic, that overwhelms the body (toxic shock syndrome). Poisonous substances accumulate in bloodstream and blood pressure drops impairing blood flow to cells, tissues, and organs. |

**Treatment for Shock.** A person suffering from shock needs immediate medical attention. Call for outside emergency help first, then care for the patient until help arrives. **CAUTION:** Shock requires immediate medical help. Shock is progressive and if not treated immediately, most types are life threatening. Once shock reaches a certain point, it is irreversible.

To care for a patient in shock, follow these procedures.

- Lie the patient down. This minimizes pain and decreases stress on the body.

- Loosen clothing.

- Check for an open airway.

- Control any external bleeding.

- Help the patient maintain normal body temperature. A blanket over and under the patient can help avoid chilling. Do not overheat.

- Reassure the patient.

- Elevate the legs about 12 inches, unless you suspect spinal injuries or broken bones involving the hips or legs.

- Do not give the patient anything to eat or drink.

- Ascertain that outside help has been called and stay with the patient until help arrives.

## Wounds

Typically, **wounds** are classified as open wounds or closed wounds. In the closed wound, there is no break in the skin; a bruise, contusion, and hematoma are common closed wounds. An open wound represents a break in the skin and can be classified as an abrasion, avulsion, incision, laceration, or puncture wound.

**Closed Wounds.** Most closed wounds do not present an emergency situation. If there is pain and swelling, the application of a cold compress can be effective. Protect the patient's skin by placing a cloth beneath the source of cold; apply the compress for 20 minutes, then remove for 20 minutes; continue for 24 hours. Then apply heat 20 minutes on and 20 minutes off for the next 24 hours. A common procedure for treating closed wounds is to RICE it:

- Rest

- Ice

- Compression

- Elevation

Some closed wounds, such as hematomas, can be very dangerous and may cause internal bleeding. If the patient is in severe pain and was subject to an injury caused by high impact, call for help and keep the patient comfortable until the help arrives. Watch for symptoms of shock and monitor vital signs.

**Open Wounds.** Open wounds can be minor tears in the skin or more serious breaks, but all open wounds represent an opportunity for microorganisms to gain entry and cause an infection. Some major open wounds may involve heavy bleeding, which will need to be controlled, probably by suturing. A tetanus injection is indicated for an open wound if the patient has not had a booster in the past seven to ten years.

There are five common types of open wounds.

1. *Abrasions* are a superficial scraping of the epidermis. Because nerve endings are involved, they can be painful. However, they are not usually serious, unless they cover a large area of the body. Administer first aid by cleaning the area carefully with soap and water, apply an antiseptic ointment if prescribed by a physician, and cover with a dressing.

2. In an *avulsion*, the skin is torn off and bleeding is profuse. Avulsion wounds often occur at exposed parts: fingers, toes, ear. First, control bleeding (Procedure 9-1) if necessary. Then clean the wound. If there is a skin flap, reposition it. Apply a dressing, then bandage as necessary. Note that pieces of the body may be torn away. If possible, save the body part, keep moist, and transport with the patient.

3. *Incisions* are wounds that result from a sharp object, such as a knife or piece of glass. Incisions may need sutures. The wound must be cleaned with soap and water and a dressing applied.

4. *Lacerations* tear the body tissue and can be difficult to clean, so care must be taken to avoid infection. If there is not severe bleeding, which in itself is a cleansing mechanism, these wounds may need to be soaked to remove debris. If there is severe bleeding, it must be controlled immediately (Procedure 9-1). Lacerations with severe bleeding are likely to need suturing.

5. *Punctures* pierce and penetrate the skin and may be deep wounds while appearing insignificant. Usually, external bleeding is minimal, but the patient should be assessed for internal bleeding. Because a puncture wound is deep, the risk of infection is great and the patient should be advised to watch for signals of infection, such as pain, swelling, redness, throbbing, and warmth.

**Use of Tourniquets in Emergency Care.** In the past, tourniquets were regularly used in the field to control hemorrhaging from an extremity when all other attempts to control bleeding were unsuccessful. However, because tourniquet application was meant to completely stop blood flow, many times this complete lack of blood flow resulted in the death of the arm or leg. Often, the affected extremity needed to be amputated.

To remedy this situation, a "constriction band" was substituted for the tourniquet and is now widely used. The constriction band is made of a material similar to that used in the tourniquet. When the band is applied to an extremity to control bleeding, it is applied tightly enough to stem the rapid loss of blood but loosely enough to allow a small amount of blood to continue to flow. A pulse should be felt distally to the constriction band. The use of the constriction band applied in this manner allows a blood supply to the remainder of the extremity unlike the tourniquet, which cuts off all blood flow.

### Dressings and Bandages.
When a patient presents with an open wound, after treatment it is critical to dress and bandage it properly to curtail infection. This covering of the wound is accomplished by a series of dressings and bandages.

Typically, dressings are sterile pads placed directly on the wound; they often have nonstick, sterile surfaces, but they are absorbent and will soak up blood and protect the wound from microorganisms. They are often made of a gauze-type material.

Bandages, which are nonsterile, are placed over the dressing. They hold the dressing in place and are made to conform to the area to be covered. Sometimes, as in a Band-Aid, the dressing and bandage are combined. Roller bandages, such as those made of elastic, can be placed over a dressing and used to control bleeding or swelling.

Kling gauze, a type of gauze that stretches and clings as it is applied, and roller bandages, long strips of soft material wound on itself, are other types of bandage materials.

Bandages and their applications can take many shapes and forms, depending on the type of injury and the injury site. In all cases, a bandage must be secure, but not constricting. Avoid too tight or too loose a wrap.

- Spiral bandages are useful for injuries to the arms or legs (Figure 9-4).
- A figure-eight bandage will hold the dressing in place on a wound on the hand or wrist, knee, or ankle (Figure 9-5).
- Fingers, toes, arms, and legs can also be bandaged using a tubular gauze bandage (Figures 9-6, 9-7, and 9-8). Using a cylindrical applicator, a quantity of gauze is stretched over the wound site.
- Commercial arm slings are used to support injured or fractured arms (Figure 9-9). To apply, support the injured arm above and below the injury site while applying the sling.

## Burns

Most burns are commonly caused by heat, chemicals, explosions, and electricity. Critical burns can be life threatening, requiring immediate medical care. According to the American Red Cross, critical burns:

- Involve breathing difficulty
- Cover more than one body part
- Involve the head, neck, hands, feet, or genitals

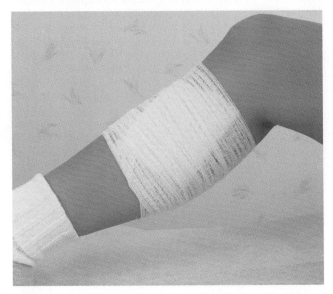

**Figure 9-4**  The spiral bandage is an option for arm and leg injuries.

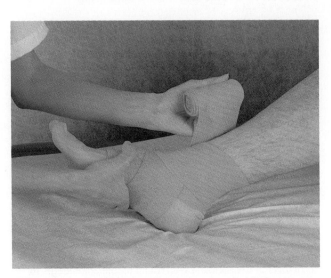

**Figure 9-5**  An elastic figure-eight bandage holds dressings in place or can be used for immobilization as with an ankle sprain.

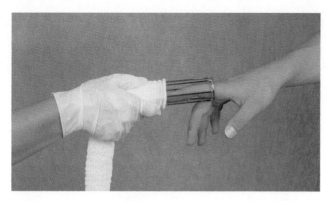

**Figure 9-6**    There are several types and sizes of tubular gauze applicators, including plastic, solid metal, and metal cage applicators; the metal cage is shown here. All applicators use a seamless elastic gauze bandage (also available in various sizes) that slides over the applicator. The applicator with the gauze then fits over the appendage to be wrapped.

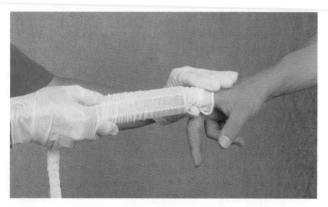

**Figure 9-7**    The gauze bandage is stretched over the appendage by pulling the applicator away from the base of the appendage. At the same time, the bandage should be held in place at the appendage base with the other hand.

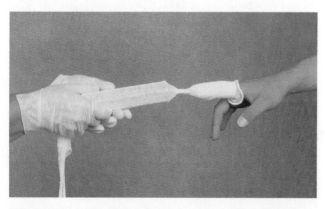

**Figure 9-8**    Once the applicator has been pulled off the finger, a layer of the bandage will remain on the appendage. To apply another layer, the applicator is again fitted over the finger and a new layer is applied in the same manner as before.

● are any burns to a child or elderly person (other than minor burns)

To distinguish critical from minor burns, it is important to understand the degrees of burns and what they mean.

**First-, Second-, and Third-Degree Burns.** First-degree burns are superficial burns that involve only the top layer of skin. The skin appears red, feels dry, is warm to the touch, and is painful. First-degree burns usually heal in a week or so with no permanent scarring (Figure 9-10).

In a second-degree burn, the skin is red and blisters are present. The healing process is slower—usually a month—and some scarring may occur. Second-degree burns affect the top layers of the skin, are very painful, and

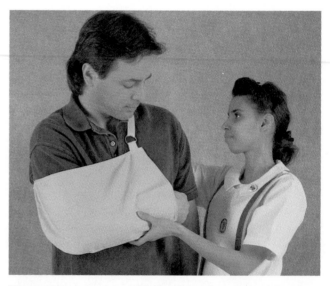

**Figure 9-9**    A commercial sling is used to support injured or fractured arms.

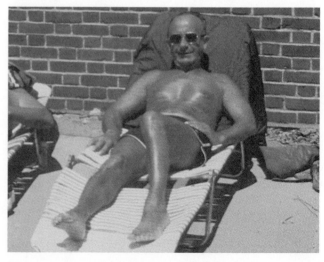

**Figure 9-10**    First-degree burns involve the top layer of skin. (Courtesy of the Phoenix Society of Burn Survivors, Inc.)

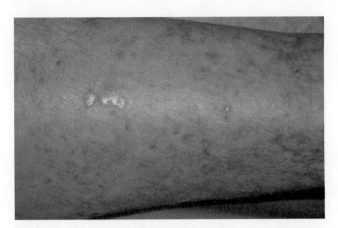

**Figure 9-11** Second-degree burns affect the top layers of skin. The healing process is slower and scarring may occur. (Courtesy of the Phoenix Society of Burn Survivors, Inc.)

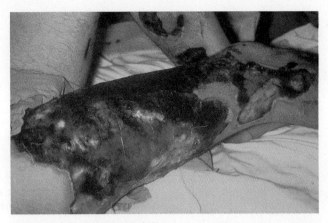

**Figure 9-12** Third-degree burns are the most serious, affecting or destroying all layers of skin plus the fat, muscle, bones, and nerves. (Courtesy of the Phoenix Society of Burn Survivors, Inc.)

may take three to four weeks to heal. Some scarring may occur (Figure 9-11).

Third-degree burns are the most serious, affecting or destroying all layers of skin, plus the fat, muscles, bones, and nerves under the skin. These burns look charred or brown. There may be great pain or, if nerve endings are destroyed, the burn may be painless. Victims of third-degree burns must receive immediate medical attention both for the burn and for shock. Of serious concern with a third-degree burn, is the likelihood of infection and the amount of scarring that can result in loss of body function. Skin grafts may be necessary (Figure 9-12).

Figure 9-13 shows the relative penetration level of each degree of burn into the skin and underlying structures.

**General Guidelines for Caring for Burns.** Treatment for burns depends on the type of agent causing the burn. General treatment strategies for any degree of burn include the following:

- Cool the burn with large amounts of cool normal saline.
- Cover the burn with a sterile dressing if one is available and burn is minor. Otherwise, cover the burn with a sheet or other smooth textured cloth for a burn over a large area of the body.
- Be sure the patient is protected from being either chilled or overheated.

However, it is important to follow these guidelines:

- Do not apply ice or ice water to a burn.
- Do not touch a burn, except with a clean sterile dressing.
- Do not clean a severe burn, break blisters, or use any kind of ointment.
- Do not remove pieces of clothing that may be sticking to the burn.

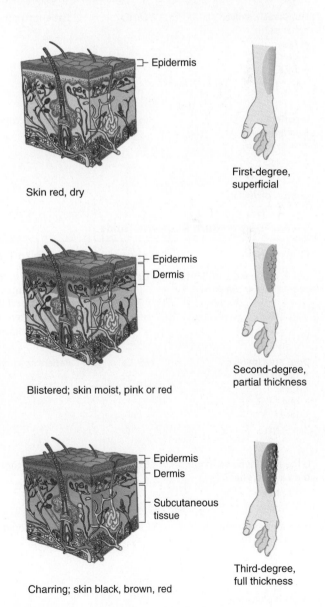

**Figure 9-13** Classification of burn injuries.

**First Aid for Burns.** First aid for burns is outlined in Table 9-3.

**Types of Burns.** Most burns are caused by heat; however, burns can also be caused by chemicals, electricity, and solar radiation.

*Chemical Burns.* These can occur in the workplace or even in the home with "ordinary" household chemicals. In order to stop the burning process, the chemical must be removed from the skin. Have someone call an ambulance while you flush the skin or eyes with cool water. Remove any clothing contaminated by the chemicals unless they

## TABLE 9-3    FIRST AID FOR BURNS

### First-Degree Burn Response Guide

| Questions | Responses | Action to Take | Rationale |
|---|---|---|---|
| Is skin reddened without blisters? | YES ⇨ | Submerge in cool normal saline 2–5 minutes. | Stops burning process. |
| NO ⇩ | | | |
| Does area involve:<br>• hands?<br>• feet?<br>• genitals?<br>• face? | YES ⇨ | Patient to come to office. | These are potential danger areas and require evaluation by the physician. |
| NO ⇩ | | | |
| Is patient:<br>• elderly?<br>• very young? | YES ⇨ | Patient to come to office. | These groups are very susceptible to burn complications. |
| NO ⇩ | | | |
| Consult physician. | | | Physician has final decision whether patient is seen. |

### Second-Degree Burn Response Guide

| Questions | Responses | Action to Take | Rationale |
|---|---|---|---|
| Is skin reddened with blisters or splitting of the skin? | YES ⇨ | Submerge in cool normal saline 10–15 minutes if skin is intact. Use compresses if skin is broken. Do not break blisters. Do not use anesthetic creams or sprays. | Stops burning process. If blisters are broken, can allow infection in burn. Creams or spray may slow healing process and increase severity of a burn. |
| NO ⇩ | | | |
| Does area involve:<br>• hands?<br>• feet?<br>• genitals?<br>• face? | YES ⇨ | Patient to come to office. | These are potentially dangerous areas and require medical attention. |
| NO ⇩ | | | |
| Is the area involved larger than a child's hand? | YES ⇨ | Patient to come to office. | Burns of this size are very susceptible to complications. |
| NO ⇩ | | | |
| Is patient experiencing trouble breathing? | YES ⇨ | Patient should go to emergency room. | There may be swelling of the airways because of heat. |
| NO ⇩ | | | |
| Consult physician. | | | Physician has final decision whether patient is seen. *(continues)* |

**TABLE 9-3** *(continued)*

**Third-Degree Burn Response Guide**

| Questions | Responses | Action to Take | Rationale |
|---|---|---|---|
| Is skin gray, black, or charred appearing? Can muscle, fat, or bone be seen in wound? | YES ⇨ | Call EMS immediately. Do not ⇨ apply cold; do not remove burnt clothing from burn area. | Life-threatening emergency that requires prompt attention. |
| NO ⇩ | | | |
| Is patient experiencing:<br>• pallor?<br>• loss of consciousness?<br>• shivering? | YES ⇨ | Patient in shock: ⇨<br>• maintain body temp.<br>• elevate feet if appropriate.<br>• monitor breathing.<br>• call EMS. | Need to control shock due to loss of fluid. |
| NO ⇩ | | | |
| Consult physician. | | | Physician has final decision whether patient is seen. |

adhere to the skin. If clothing clings to the skin, it can be cut with scissors. Do not attempt to pull clothing away from burned area.

*Electrical Burns.* Electrical burns can be caused by power lines, lightning, or faulty electrical equipment in the home or workplace. **It is important to remember never to go near a patient injured by electricity until you are sure the power has been shut off because you could be injured.** If there is a downed line, call the power company and emergency medical services (EMS).

A victim of an electricity burn may be suffering from two burns: one where the power entered the body, and one where it exited. Often, the burns themselves may be minor. Of more serious consequence are the possibilities of shock, breathing difficulties, and other injuries. CPR is often needed here.

*Solar Radiation.* Most "sunburns," while not advisable nor good for the skin, present minor burns. If the patient has a severe burn, however, he should see a physician who will cover the burn area to reduce infection and protect the patient against chill.

## Musculoskeletal Injuries

Most injuries to muscles, bones, and joints are not life threatening, but they are painful and, if not properly treated, can be disabling. Some injuries, such as those to the spinal cord, can be quite serious and can result in paralysis. These injuries are not typically seen in the ambulatory care setting.

**Types of Injuries.** A sprain is an injury to a joint, often an ankle, knee, or wrist, that involves a tearing of the ligaments. Most sprains are minor and heal quickly; others are more severe, include swelling, and may not heal properly if the patient continues to put stress on the sprained joint. Signs of a sprain are rapid swelling, discoloration at the site, and limited function. Many times it is difficult to determine whether the patient has sustained a sprain or a fracture because the degree of pain may not be a true indicator of the patient's injury. As with most closed wounds, treating the injury with the RICE method is beneficial.

A strain results from the overuse or stretching of a muscle or group of muscles, as with improper lifting or

**Patient Teaching Tip**

Some burns can be prevented. Advise patients who insist on sunbathing to protect themselves against harmful rays by using a sunscreen and avoiding the sun between 10 A.M. and 2 P.M.

**Patient Teaching Tip**

Advise patients not to run should their clothing catch on fire. They should fall to the ground or wrap themselves in a blanket or rug and roll on the ground to extinguish the flames.

moving heavy objects. Applications of ice and heat (as described for treatment of sprains), as well as rest, are indicated for treatment of strains.

Dislocations are painful and involve the separation of a bone from its normal position. These usually occur from the kind of wrenching motion that might result from a fall, automobile accident, or sports injury.

**Fractures** involve a break in a bone and can be caused by a fall, by a blow, from bone disease, or from sports injuries. There are several types of fractures, but all are classified as either open fractures or closed fractures. An open fracture involves an open wound and is characterized by a protruding bone. In a closed fracture, the skin is not broken. Signs and symptoms that occur with a fracture may include swelling, discoloration, pain, deformity, and immobility of the body part. It is not unusual for patients to tell you that they heard the bone break or that they sensed a grating feeling. **Crepitation** is the term that describes the grating sensation experienced when bone fragments rub together. Fractures are further defined as follows:

- Incomplete or greenstick: fracture in which the bone has cracked but the break is not all the way through. Frequently seen in children.

- Simple: complete bone break in which there is no involvement with the skin surface.

- Compound: fracture in which the bone protrudes though the skin surface, creating the possibility of infection.

- Impacted: fracture in which the broken ends are jammed into each other.

- Comminuted: more than one fracture line and several bone fragments are present.

- Spiral: fracture that occurs with a severe twisting action, causing the break to wind around the bone.

- Depressed: fracture that occurs with severe head injuries in which a broken piece of skull is driven inward.

- Colles: fracture often caused by falling on an outstretched hand. Involves the distal end of the radius and results in displacement, causing a bulge at the wrist.

See Figure 9-14 for examples of these fractures.

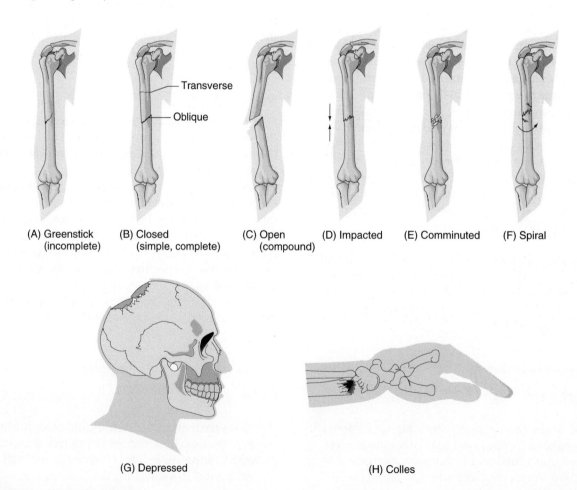

(A) Greenstick (incomplete)   (B) Closed (simple, complete)   (C) Open (compound)   (D) Impacted   (E) Comminuted   (F) Spiral

Transverse
Oblique

(G) Depressed

(H) Colles

**Figure 9-14**   Types of fractures.

**Assessing Injuries to Muscles, Bones, and Joints.** Sometimes it is difficult to determine the extent of an injury, especially in closed fractures. There are some assessment techniques to call upon, however, to gauge the seriousness of an injury.

- Note the extent of bruising and swelling.

- Pain is a signal of injury.

- There may be noticeable deformity to the bone or joint.

- Use of the injured area is limited.

- Talk to the patient: what was the cause of the injury? What was the sound or sensation at the time of injury?

**Caring for Muscle, Bone, and Joint Injuries.** Most injuries to muscles, bones, and joints are treated in a similar way; all require rest, elevation of the injured part, immobilization, and the application of ice to the injury.

After calling for outside care (always check for life-threatening symptoms, such as breathing difficulties, bleeding, or head, neck, or back injuries), it is important to immobilize the injured area if the patient must be moved. EMS personnel employ a variety of splints to immobilize bones and joints. See Procedure 9-2 for splinting an arm in the ambulatory care setting.

## Heat- and Cold-Related Illnesses

The condition of patients who have been subject to extreme heat and cold can deteriorate very rapidly and either a heat- or cold-related illness can result in death. Individuals especially vulnerable to extreme exposures include the very young and very old; individuals who must work out of doors; and people who may suffer from poor circulation.

**Heat-Related Illnesses.** Illnesses related to heat, in increasing degree of severity, include heat cramps, heat exhaustion, and heat stroke. Heat cramps, the least serious, involve cramping in the legs and abdomen due to excessive body exposure or exercise in hot weather. Heat cramps should be considered a signal to stop, slow down, rest in a cool place, and drink plenty of water. Salt tablets should not be taken. The individual should lightly stretch the muscles. Heat cramps can progress to heat exhaustion or heat stroke, both more serious conditions.

Heat exhaustion, often experienced by people who work or exercise in extreme heat, is a more serious reaction and is signaled by exhaustion, cold and clammy skin, profuse sweating, headache, and general weakness. The individual should come out of the heat immediately, apply cool, wet towels, and slowly drink cool water. The physician will advise the patient not to resume activity in the heat.

Heat stroke is the least common, but the most dangerous of heat-related illnesses and requires immediate medical attention. Heat stroke is characterized by red, dry, hot skin, an abnormal, weak pulse, and breathing that is shallow and fast. In heat stroke, the body systems are extremely taxed. EMS should be alerted; until they arrive, stay with the patient, watch for breathing problems, and attempt to lower body temperature by applying cool, wet towels or sheets.

**Cold-Related Illnesses.** Exposure to extreme cold for prolonged periods can lead to frostbite or hypothermia.

Frostbite, which typically affects the extremities such as fingers, toes, ears, and nose, involves the freezing of exposed body parts. Symptoms include skin that becomes off-color, that is cold, or that takes on a waxy appearance. Severity can range from the superficial (frostnip) to more penetrating stages, which may require amputation.

Individuals with frostbite need immediate medical attention. To care for frostbitten extremities, warm the area of injury by wrapping clothing or blankets around the affected body part. Be careful in handling the frozen part. It is best to have the patient transported as soon as possible to emergency care. This type of facility is better able to properly rewarm the frozen part, preventing further tissue damage.

Hypothermia is a serious illness in which the body temperature falls to a perilously low level. It can result in death if the individual does not receive care and if the progression of hypothermia is not reversed. Hypothermia occurs when a person falls through the ice or is exposed to cold temperatures, for example, after getting lost in the woods while hiking. Symptoms include shivering, cold skin, and confusion.

After checking for breathing problems and alerting EMS, care for the patient. Make the individual comfortable, provide a source of warmth, such as a blanket, and *gradually* warm the body. If clothing is wet or cold, remove and put on dry clothing. In extreme cases, it may be necessary to provide rescue breathing, which is covered later in this chapter.

## Poisoning

Poisons can enter the body in four ways:

- *Ingestion.* Ingested poisons enter the body by swallowing. Swallowed poisons may include medications, plant material, household chemicals, contaminated foods, and drugs.

- *Inhalation.* Poisons are inhaled into the body in poorly ventilated areas where cleaning fluids, paints and chemical cleaners, or carbon monoxide may be present.

- *Absorption*. Poisons absorbed through the skin include plant materials such as poison oak or ivy, lawn care products such as chemical pesticides, and other chemical powders or liquids.

- *Injection*. Drug abuse is the most common cause of injected poisons. The stingers of insects inject poisons into the body and can be extremely dangerous and lead to anaphylactic shock in allergic individuals.

Whenever a patient calls regarding poisoning or there is a suspicion of poisoning, call the local poison control center or the local emergency number and ask for advice. Telephone numbers of the poison control center should be posted in a familiar and accessible place.

The treatment for poisoning will vary according to the source of the poisoning and must be tailored to the specific incident. The physician will have advised staff regarding specific poisoning antidotes. Generally, do not give the patient anything to eat or drink; try to determine what poison the patient was exposed to and, if ingested, how much was taken; if the patient vomits, save some of the vomitus for analysis.

If prescribed by a physician, two medications used to treat poisoning include syrup of ipecac, which can induce vomiting, and activated charcoal, which is used to absorb certain swallowed poisons.

**Insect Stings.** The medical assistant in the ambulatory care setting is likely to receive a number of calls every summer from patients who have been stung by insects, typically yellow jackets, hornets, honeybees, or wasps. In the nonallergic patient, the sting is likely to result in localized swelling and tenderness and slight redness. The physician will recommend that these localized symptoms be managed with a topical cream and oral antihistamines. Swelling can be significant and cause for serious concern if the sting occurred in a vulnerable area of the body such as the mouth or tongue. Swelling in these locations can be

## Patient Teaching Tip

Remind patients who are parents of young children to remove any potential sources of poisoning from their homes or to keep them in locked cabinets. Also advise them to include the nearby poison control center in their list of emergency phone numbers. They should also keep syrup of ipecac and activated charcoal on hand.

## Patient Teaching Tip

Advise all patients with known allergic reactions to be particularly careful when working or playing outdoors. Insects are not usually aggressive until their nests are approached; however, often these nests are not easy to detect and an individual may approach one without being aware of its presence. Patients with allergies to insects should always wear shoes out-of-doors, wear light-colored clothing, preferably with long sleeves and pant legs, look before taking a sip from a beverage when outdoors, and inspect lawn areas, shrubbery, and building walls periodically for evidence of stinging insect nests.

frightening and dangerous because it can impair breathing. An antihistamine, administered as soon as possible after the sting, may help to curtail symptoms somewhat. Treatment for insect stings in nonallergic individuals consists of removing the stinger by scraping it off with the edge of something rigid such as a credit card or your fingernail. Tweezers can cause more venom to be dispersed into the patient's body tissues so should not be used. Wash the area with soap and water, apply a cold pack to the site, and watch for an anaphylactic reaction.

The individual who experiences an allergic reaction or hypersensitivity to a sting needs to be seen immediately, for in severe cases a sting may induce an anaphylactic reaction which can lead to death. If allergic, individuals who have been stung are likely to experience symptoms within a half-hour after the incident. Symptoms are generalized throughout the body and may include hives, itching, lightheadedness, and may progress to difficulty breathing, faintness, and eventual loss of consciousness.

For individuals with known allergic reactions, the physician will prescribe epinephrine, which patients should carry with them and self-inject should they not be able to get immediate emergency care. The patient should then seek immediate emergency treatment. For individuals who present at the ambulatory care setting with an apparent allergic reaction to a sting, the physician will prescribe epinephrine. Attempt to allay patient apprehension and monitor vital signs while waiting for EMS personnel to arrive.

### Sudden Illness

Sudden illness is, by definition, an unexpected occurrence. While the cause of the illness may be inexplicable, it is important to respond sensibly and responsibly within the parameters of knowledge and resources.

Sudden illnesses include, but are not limited to, fainting, seizures, diabetic reaction, and hemorrhage.

**Fainting.** Also known as **syncope**, fainting involves a loss of consciousness, caused by an insufficient supply of blood to the brain. Loss of consciousness may simply be the result of a fainting episode or it may indicate a more serious medical problem such as diabetic coma or shock. A fall during a fainting incident may result in bodily harm.

If a patient in the office or clinic "feels faint," indicated by lightheadedness, weakness, nausea, or unsteadiness, have the individual lie down or sit down with head level with the knees. This may prevent a fainting spell. As a part of office policy, aromatic spirits of ammonia may be administered to revive the patient who faints. **CAUTION:** Hold the crushed ampule of ammonia at least six inches away from the patient's nose and eyes. Move it back and forth since the fumes are very irritating to eyes and mucous membranes.

If a patient faints, gradually lower the patient to a flat surface, loosen any tight clothing, and check breathing and for any life-threatening emergencies. Elevate the legs if there is no back or head injury. If vomiting occurs, place the patient on the side. While fainting is typically not serious in itself, 911 or EMS may need to be called since the problem may be indicative of a more complex medical condition.

**Seizures.** Seizures or convulsions occur when normal brain functioning is disrupted, which can occur for a variety of reasons including fever, disease such as diabetes, infection, or injury to the brain. Epilepsy is a common cause of convulsions. Involuntary spasms or contractions of muscles characterize seizures.

To the onlooker, seizures look frightening and painful, which may lead inexperienced individuals to try to stop the seizure when they see it occurring in another individual. A patient suffering from a seizure should never be restrained; simply care for the victim of a seizure with compassion and medical understanding. The goal is to protect the patient from self-injury during the episode. Also, do not force anything between the patient's clenched teeth—individuals experiencing seizures cannot "swallow" their tongues.

Most patients will recover from a seizure in a few minutes. During the seizure, protect the patient from injury, cushion the patient's head, and roll the patient to the side if any fluid is in the mouth. After the seizure subsides, calm and comfort the patient.

If a patient is known to regularly have seizures, and the patient's seizure subsides in a matter of minutes, EMS personnel do not need to be summoned. Repeated seizures during the same time frame, however, dictate a call to emergency services, as does any seizure if the patient is diabetic, pregnant, injured, or does not regain consciousness after the incident.

**Diabetes.** Diabetes is defined by the American Diabetes Society as the "inability of the body to properly convert sugar from food into energy."

Under normal functioning, the body produces a hormone called insulin, which transports sugars into body cells. In some cases, the body does not produce insulin or does not produce enough insulin; this results in diabetes.

Diabetes occurs in two major types:

- Type I, or insulin-dependent diabetes.

- Type II, or noninsulin-dependent diabetes, which usually occurs in adults. In Type II, the body produces insulin in insufficient quantities.

Complications from diabetes, which you may encounter in a medical office or clinic setting, include diabetic coma (acidosis) and insulin shock or reaction. The physician will prescribe either insulin or glucose prior to the patient being transported to the hospital. Both are serious emergencies that require immediate EMS assistance. See Table 9-4 for common causes and symptoms of diabetic coma or insulin shock.

**Hemorrhage.** The different sources of bleeding determine the seriousness of hemorrhage, or bleeding.

*External Bleeding.* External bleeding includes capillary, venous, and arterial bleeding. Capillary bleeding, often from cuts and scratches, usually clots without first-aid measures. Bleeding from a vein, which is characterized by dark red blood that flows steadily, needs to be controlled quickly (see Procedure 9-1) to avoid excessive blood loss. Bleeding from an artery produces bright red bleeding that spurts from the wound; this is the most serious type of bleeding and occurs when an artery is punctured or severed. Like venous bleeding, arterial bleeding requires immediate emergency care, for serious loss of blood and profound irreversible shock can quickly ensue.

Epistaxis, or nosebleed, may be the result of breathing dry air for a long period of time; may result from injury or blowing the nose too hard; may be caused by high altitudes; may be caused by hypertension (high blood pressure); or may result from overuse of medications such as aspirin and anticoagulants.

To control nosebleeds, seat the patient, elevate the patient's head, and pinch the nostrils for at least ten minutes. Assist the patient to sit with head tilted forward so blood running down the back of the throat will not be aspirated. If bleeding cannot be controlled, the physician may request that you activate EMS.

**TABLE 9-4   CAUSES AND SYMPTOMS OF DIABETIC COMA AND INSULIN SHOCK**

| Diabetic Coma or Acidosis | | Insulin Shock or Reaction | |
| --- | --- | --- | --- |
| Causes | Too little insulin, too much to eat, infections, fever, emotional stress | Causes | Too much insulin or oral hypoglycemic drug, too little to eat, an unusual amount of exercise |
| Symptoms | Skin: Dry and flushed | Symptoms | Skin: Moist and pale |
| | Behavior: Drowsy | | Behavior: Often excited |
| | Mouth: Dry | | Mouth: Drooling |
| | Thirst: Intense | | Thirst: Absent |
| | Hunger: Absent | | Hunger: Present |
| | Vomiting: Common | | Vomiting: Usually absent |
| | Respiration: Exaggerated, air hungry | | Respiration: Normal or shallow |
| | Breath: Fruity odor of acetone | | Breath: Usually normal |
| | Pulse: Weak and rapid | | Pulse: Full and pounding (gives patient feeling of heart pounding) |
| | Vision: Dim | | Vision: Diplopia (double) |
| | Blood glucose over 200 mg/100 ml | | Blood glucose low (40–70 mg/100 ml) |
| First aid | Keep patient warm | First aid | If conscious, give patient sugar or any food containing sugar (fruit juice, candy, crackers, etc.) |
| | Obtain medical help immediately | | Obtain medical help immediately |

*Internal Bleeding.* Internal bleeding may be minor or serious depending on the cause of the injury. A contusion, or bruise, will result in minor internal bleeding. A sharp blow may induce severe internal bleeding.

Because there is no visible blood flow, it is important to recognize other symptoms of internal bleeding. Symptoms are similar to those of shock and include a rapid, weak pulse, shallow breathing, cold, clammy skin, dilated pupils, dizziness, faintness, thirst, restlessness, and a feeling of anxiety. There may be pain, tenderness, or swelling at the injury site. The abdomen may be board-like.

If internal bleeding is suspected, ask another staff member to call EMS; until they arrive, stay with the patient and take measures to prevent shock. Monitor vital signs.

## Cerebral Vascular Accident (CVA)

The common term for a cerebral vascular accident (CVA) is stroke. A stroke is the result of a ruptured blood vessel in the brain; it can also be caused by the **occlusion** of a blood vessel or by a clot. Both these situations can result in blood spilling over brain cells and depriving them of oxygen, causing them to die. Symptoms of a stroke

## Patient Teaching Tip

Advise the patient not to blow the nose for several hours following an epistaxis.

include numbness in face, arm, leg on one side of the body, loss of vision, severe headache, mental confusion, slurred speech, nausea, vomiting, and difficulty in breathing and swallowing. Paralysis may be present. If a patient is suspected of having a stroke, call EMS, loosen tight clothing, lie the patient down and keep her comfortable. Position the patient's head to facilitate flow of secretion from the mouth to avoid choking and maintain an open airway. Do not give anything by mouth and monitor vital signs. Immediate emergency care is critical for all individuals experiencing strokes. If the stroke is caused by a clot that blocks blood flow, a recently released drug may be able to protect the individual from permanent injury. Rapid transport to the hospital is important for treatment to be instituted as soon as possible. Treatment with the clot-dissolving drug must be given within three hours of onset of symptoms.

## Heart Attack

Heart attack, also known as myocardial infarction, is usually caused by blockage of one or more of the coronary arteries. Symptoms include tightness of the chest, pain radiating down one or both arms, or pain radiating into the left shoulder and jaw. Other signs include rapid and weak pulse, excessive perspiration, agitation, nausea, and cold, clammy skin.

If you suspect the patient is experiencing a heart attack, contact EMS immediately, loosen tight clothing, and keep the patient comfortable. Prepare to give oxygen and other medications such as aspirin as directed by the physician. Monitor vital signs. If the patient suffers an episode of cardiac fibrillation, cardioversion or defibrillation may be necessary.

## PROCEDURES FOR BREATHING EMERGENCIES AND CARDIAC ARREST

Breathing or respiratory emergencies occur for a variety of reasons, including choking, shock, allergies, and other illnesses or injuries such as drowning and electrical shock. When an individual stops breathing, artificial breathing must be given quickly, for without a constant supply of oxygen, brain damage or death will occur.

When the breathing problem is accompanied by cardiac arrest, the rescue breathing must be accompanied by chest compressions. This is known as **cardiopulmonary resuscitation (CPR)**. Cardiac emergencies may occur in the medical office due to the large number of patients who have heart disease.

The procedures that follow will help you respond to breathing emergencies in your clinic or office until EMS arrives. The techniques vary for conscious and unconscious individuals, and for adults, children, and infants. These procedures are for review purposes only; it is essential that every medical assistant take first aid and CPR courses and frequent refresher courses.

### Heimlich Maneuver (Abdominal Thrust)

A common cause of breathing difficulty results from choking. If an individual signals distress from choking, assist the patient in coughing up the object (Figures 9-15 and 9-16). If the patient cannot cough up the object, and the breathing airway is becoming completely blocked, act immediately. It is apparent that the airway is becoming blocked when the patient cannot cough or speak and the patient uses the universal sign for choking.

Have someone call an ambulance while you perform abdominal thrusts, known as the **Heimlich maneuver**. Patients can be taught to give themselves abdominal thrusts if they are alone and choking (Figure 9-17).

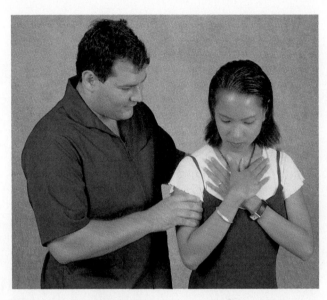

**Figure 9-16**    Assist the patient in coughing up an object by encouraging continuous coughing.

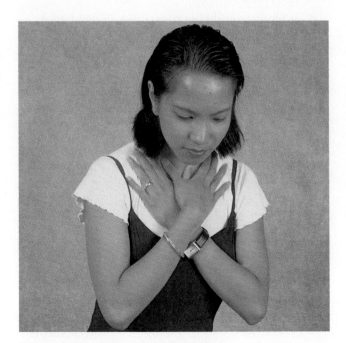

**Figure 9-15**    Universal sign for choking.

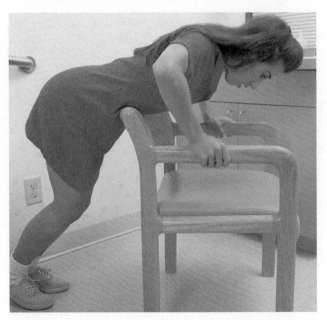

**Figure 9-17**    If alone, individuals can self-administer the Heimlich maneuver by using the back of a chair or similar hard object.

## Patient Teaching Tip

Teach patients to perform the abdominal thrust when they are alone and choking. To perform the Heimlich maneuver when alone, use the fist or thrust against a chair back or any other hard object of adequate height that reaches just below the navel. See Figure 9-17.

Procedures 9-3, 9-4, 9-5, 9-6, and 9-7 describe how to perform the Heimlich maneuver for adults, children, and infants; these reflect the American Red Cross updates effective July 2001.

### Rescue Breathing

Individuals in respiratory arrest require immediate emergency care. **Rescue breathing**, previously called mouth-to-mouth resuscitation, provides oxygen to the patient until emergency personnel arrive.

When performing rescue breathing procedures in the ambulatory care setting, it is recommended that resuscitation mouthpieces be used and that direct mouth-to-mouth (i.e., with no personal protective equipment) resuscitation never be used.

Procedures for rescue breathing differ for adults, children, and infants. See Procedures 9-8, 9-9, and 9-10.

### Cardiopulmonary Resuscitation (CPR)

The combination of rescue breathing and chest compressions is known as CPR, which stands for cardiopulmonary resuscitation. Alone, CPR cannot save an individual from cardiac arrest—it represents preliminary care until advanced medical help is available to the heart attack victim. See Procedures 9-11, 9-12, and 9-13.

When performing CPR, the rule is that you do not stop until

- another trained person can take over
- EMS arrives and takes over care of the patient
- you are physically exhausted and not able to continue
- the environment becomes unsafe for any reason

## *Procedure*

### 9-1    Control of Bleeding

**STANDARD PRECAUTIONS:**

   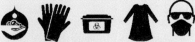 

**PURPOSE:**
To control bleeding caused by an open wound.

**EQUIPMENT/SUPPLIES:**
Sterile dressings
Sterile gloves
Mask and eye protection
Gown
Biohazard waste container

**PROCEDURE STEPS:**
1. Wash hands.
2. Put on gloves.
3. Apply eye and mask protection and gown if splashing is likely to occur.
4. Assemble equipment and supplies.
5. Apply dressing and press firmly (Figure 9-18A).
6. Apply pressure bandage over the dressing.

7. If bleeding continues, elevate arm above heart level (Figure 9-18B).
8. If bleeding still continues, press adjacent artery against bone (Figure 9-18C). Notify the physician if bleeding cannot be controlled.

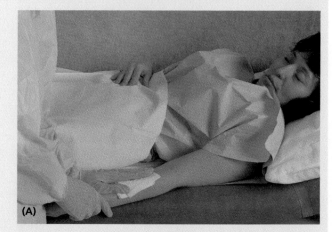

(A)

**Figure 9-18**    (A) Apply dressing and press firmly.

*(continues)*

## Procedure

### 9-1 (*continued*)

9. Dispose of waste in biohazard container.
10. Remove gloves, dispose of in biohazard container.
11. Wash hands.
12. Document procedure.

**CAUTION:** If bleeding is not controlled, the patient may go into hemorrhagic shock. Be prepared to call EMS immediately.

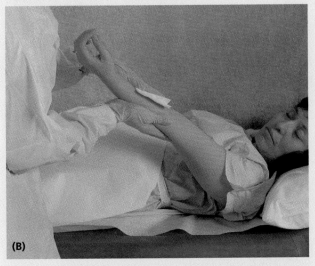
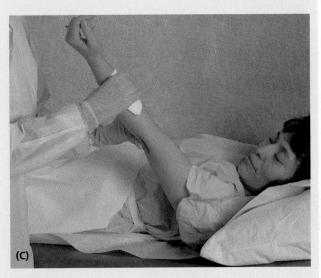

**Figure 9-18** (B) Elevate arm above heart level. (C) Press artery against bone.

## Procedure

### 9-2 Applying an Arm Splint

**STANDARD PRECAUTIONS:**

**PURPOSE:**
To immobilize the area above and below the injured part of the arm in order to reduce pain and prevent further injury.

**EQUIPMENT/SUPPLIES:**
Thin piece of rigid board; cardboard can be used if necessary
Gauze roller bandage

**PROCEDURE STEPS:**
1. Place the padded splint under the injured area.
2. Hold the splint in place with gauze roller bandage.
3. After splinting, check circulation (note color and temperature of skin, check pulse) to ascertain that the splint is not too tightly applied.
4. A sling can now be applied to keep the arm elevated, which increases comfort and reduces swelling.
5. Wash hands.
6. Document the procedure.

## *Procedure* 9-3  Heimlich Maneuver for a Conscious Adult

**STANDARD PRECAUTIONS:**

**PURPOSE:**
To open up a blocked airway.

**EQUIPMENT/SUPPLIES:**
None needed

**PROCEDURE STEPS:**
1. Place the thumb side of your fist against the middle of the abdomen, just above the umbilicus and below the xiphoid process.
2. Grasp your fist with your other hand and give quick upward thrusts (Figure 9-19).
3. Repeat the procedure until the patient coughs up the object. If the person becomes unconscious, perform abdominal thrusts for an unconscious individual (Procedure 9-4).
4. Wash hands.
5. Document the procedure.

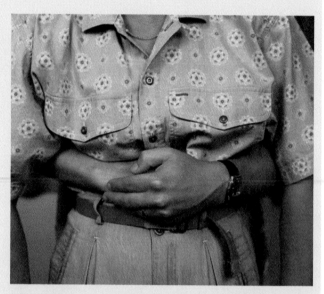

**Figure 9-19**    Grasp your fist with your other hand and give quick thrusts.

## *Procedure* 9-4  Heimlich Maneuver for an Unconscious Adult or Child

**STANDARD PRECAUTIONS:**

   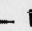 

**PURPOSE:**
To open up a blocked airway.

**EQUIPMENT/SUPPLIES:**
Gloves
Resuscitation mouthpiece
Biohazard waste container

**PROCEDURE STEPS:**
1. Have someone call emergency services.
2. Put on gloves if available.
3. Lie person on back. Open victim's mouth and look

for foreign object. Position resuscitation mouthpiece. Tilt back person's head (Figure 9-20A).
4. Give two breaths (Figure 9-20B).
5. If air will not go in, retilt head to try to give two breaths again. If air will not go in, give 15 chest compressions.
6. Find hand position on breastbone 2 inches above xiphoid and compress 2 inches deep. (For child, give five compressions, 1½ inches deep.)
7. Lift the jaw, look for object, and sweep it out of the mouth with finger, if seen (Figure 9-20E).
8. Tilt back the head, lift the chin, and give breaths again slowly. Continue giving breaths and compressions, looking for object and sweeping it out

*(continues)*

# Procedure
## 9-4 *(continued)*

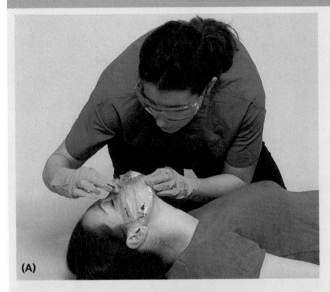

(A)

if seen. Continue breathing until breaths go in. If the airway is cleared and victim does not begin to breathe on his own, prepare to perform CPR (Procedure 9-11).

9. Dispose of waste in biohazard container.
10. Remove gloves, dispose of in biohazard container, and wash hands.
11. Monitor vital signs.
12. Document the procedure.

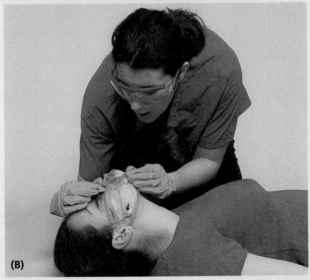

(B)

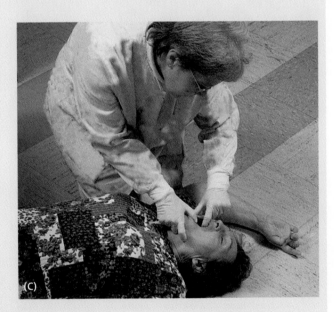

(C)

**Figure 9-20** (A) Tilt back head. (B) Give breaths. (C) Lift jaw and sweep out mouth.

## Procedure
### 9-5
# Heimlich Maneuver for a Conscious Child

**STANDARD PRECAUTIONS:**

**PURPOSE:**
To open up a blocked airway.

**EQUIPMENT/SUPPLIES:**
None needed

**PROCEDURE STEPS:**

1. Place the thumb side of your fist against the middle of the child's abdomen, just above the umbilicus and below the xiphoid process (Figure 9-21A).

2. Grasp your fist with your other hand. Give quick upward thrusts (Figure 9-21B). Repeat the procedure until the object is expelled or until the patient loses consciousness (see Heimlich maneuver for unconscious child, Procedure 9-4).

3. Wash hands.

4. Document the procedure.

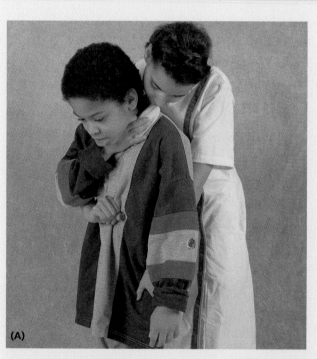

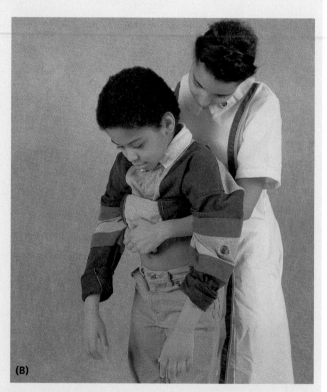

**Figure 9-21** (A) Place the thumb side of your fist against the middle of the abdomen, just above the umbilicus and below the xiphoid process. (B) Grasp your fist with your other hand and give quick upward thrusts.

## Procedure 9-6

# Back Blows and Chest Thrusts for a Conscious Infant Who Is Choking

**STANDARD PRECAUTIONS:**

**PURPOSE:**
To open up a blocked airway and assist an infant unable to cough, cry, or breathe.

**EQUIPMENT/SUPPLIES:**
None needed

**PROCEDURE STEPS:**
1. With the infant face down on your forearm, give five back blows between the infant's shoulder blades with the heel of your hand (Figure 9-22A).

2. Position the infant face up on your forearm.
3. Give five chest compressions ½ to 1 inch deep, on about the center of the breastbone (Figure 9-22B).
4. Look in the infant's mouth for the object. Repeat the back blows and chest compressions and look for object until the infant begins to breathe on own. If the infant becomes unconscious, use back blow and chest compression techniques for unconscious infants (Procedure 9-7).
5. Wash hands.
6. Document the procedure.

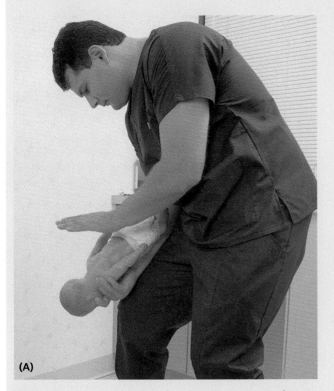
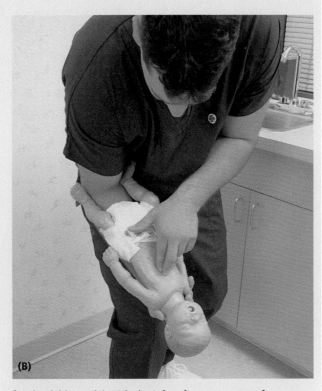

**(A)**   **(B)**

**Figure 9-22** (A) With the infant face down on your forearm, give five back blows. (B) With the infant face up on your forearm, give five chest thrusts.

## Procedure 9-7

# Back Blows and Chest Thrusts for an Unconscious Infant

**STANDARD PRECAUTIONS:**

**PURPOSE:**
To open up a blocked airway.

**EQUIPMENT/SUPPLIES:**
Gloves
Resuscitation mouthpiece

**PROCEDURE STEPS:**
1. Have someone call emergency services.
2. Don gloves. Tap the infant gently to check for consciousness.
3. Gently tilt back the infant's head. Do not hyper-extend (Figure 9-23A).
4. Listen and watch for breathing.
5. Apply resuscitation mouthpiece. Give two breaths, covering infant's nose and mouth with your mouth (Figure 9-23B).

6. If air will not go in, retilt head, attempt to give breaths again.
7. If breaths still will not go in, give chest compressions ½ to 1 inch deep.
8. Lift jaw and tongue and check for object. If you see the object, sweep it out (Figure 9-23C).
9. Tilt back head and give one breath again.
10. Repeat breaths and chest compressions, and check for object until breaths go in. If the infant does not begin to breathe on his own, prepare to perform CPR.
11. Remove gloves. Wash hands.
12. Document the procedure.

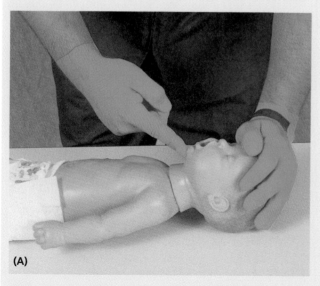

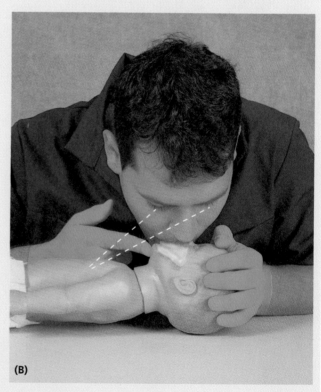

**Figure 9-23**    (A) Gently tilt back head. (B) Give two breaths, covering the infant's nose and mouth.    (*continues*)

*Procedure*
**9-7** **(continued)**

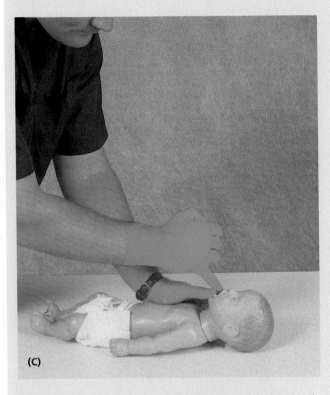

(C)

**Figure 9-23** (C) Lift jaw and tongue. Check for object and, if seen, sweep out.

## Procedure

### 9-8    Rescue Breathing for Adults

**STANDARD PRECAUTIONS:**

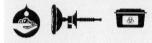

**PURPOSE:**
To respond to a breathing emergency.

**EQUIPMENT/SUPPLIES:**
Biohazard waste container
Resuscitation mouthpiece

**PROCEDURE STEPS:**
1. Have someone call emergency services.
2. Tilt back the head, lift the chin, position resuscitation mouthpiece, and pinch the nose closed (Figure 9-24A).
3. Give two slow breaths. Breathe into patient until the chest gently rises. Turn your face to the side and listen and watch for air to return.
4. Check for pulse on the carotid artery (Figure 9-24B).
5. If pulse is present, but the person is not breathing, give one slow breath every five seconds. Do this for one minute.
6. Recheck pulse and breathing every minute.
7. Continue rescue breathing as long as pulse is present and the person is not breathing. Continue until breathing is restored or another person takes over.
8. Dispose of waste in biohazard container.
9. Wash hands.
10. Document procedure.

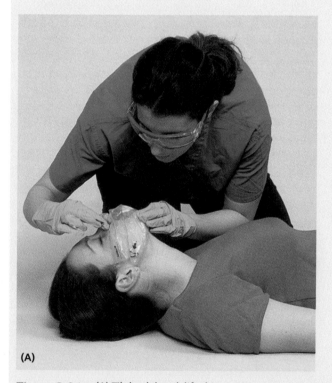

(A)

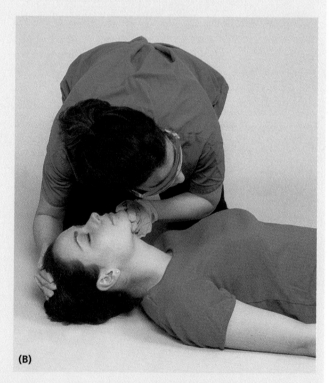

(B)

**Figure 9-24**    (A) Tilt back head, lift chin, position resuscitation mouthpiece, pinch nose closed, and give two short breaths. (B) Check for pulse at the carotid artery.

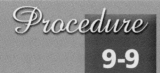

## Procedure
## 9-9    Rescue Breathing for Children

**STANDARD PRECAUTIONS:**

**PURPOSE:**
To respond to a breathing emergency.

**EQUIPMENT/SUPPLIES:**
Gloves
Resuscitation mouthpiece

**PROCEDURE STEPS:**
1. Have someone call emergency services.
2. Don gloves.

3. Tilt back the head, lift the chin, position the resuscitation mouthpiece, pinch the nose closed, and give two short breaths (Figure 9-25A). If air does not go in, retilt head and breathe again.
4. Check for a pulse at the carotid artery (Figure 9-25B).
5. If pulse is present, but the child is not breathing, give one slow breath every three seconds. Do this for one minute.
6. Recheck pulse and breathing every minute.
7. Continue rescue breathing as long as pulse is present but the child is not breathing.
8. Remove gloves. Wash hands.
9. Document the procedure.

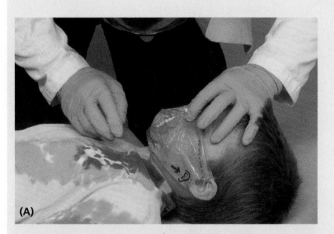
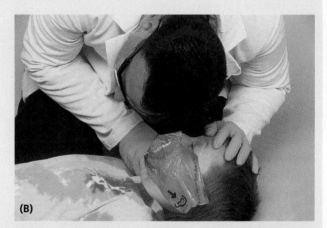

**Figure 9-25**    (A) Tilt back head, lift chin, position resuscitation mouthpiece, pinch nose closed, and give two short breaths. (B) Check for pulse at the carotid artery.

# *Procedure* 9-10     Rescue Breathing for Infants

## STANDARD PRECAUTIONS:

## PURPOSE:
To respond to a breathing emergency.

## EQUIPMENT/SUPPLIES:
Gloves
Resuscitation mouthpiece

## PROCEDURE STEPS:
1. Have someone call emergency services.
2. Don gloves.
3. Tilt back the head (Figure 9-26A).
4. Position resuscitation mouthpiece. Seal your lips tightly around the infant's nose and mouth (Figure 9-26B).
5. Give two slow breaths. Breathe into the infant until the chest rises.
6. Check for a pulse at the brachial artery (Figure 9-26C).
7. If pulse is present, but infant is not breathing, give one slow breath every three seconds. Do this for one minute.
8. Recheck pulse and breathing every minute (Figure 9-26D).
9. Continue rescue breathing as long as pulse is present but the infant is not breathing.
10. Remove gloves. Wash hands.
11. Document the procedure.

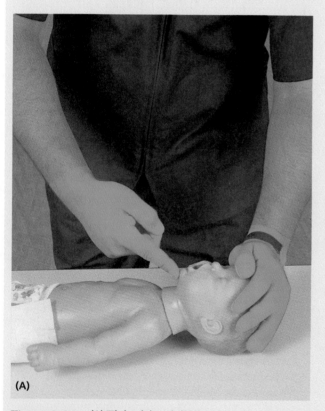

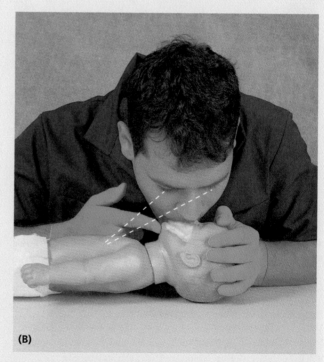

**Figure 9-26** (A) Tilt back head. (B) Position resuscitation mouthpiece. Seal lips around nose and mouth, and give two slow breaths.

*(continues)*

## *Procedure*
### 9-10 *(continued)*

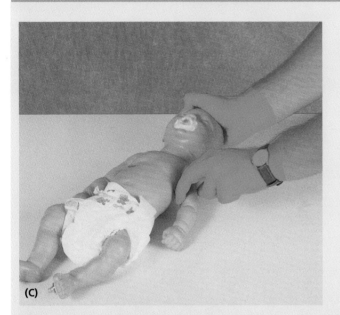
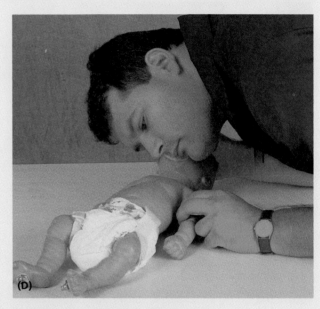

**Figure 9-26** (C) Check for pulse at the brachial artery. (D) Recheck pulse and breathing every minute.

## *Procedure*
### 9-11 CPR for Adults

**STANDARD PRECAUTIONS:**

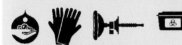

**PURPOSE:**
To respond to a breathing and cardiac arrest emergency.

**EQUIPMENT/SUPPLIES:**
Biohazard waste container
Resuscitation mouthpiece
Gloves

**PROCEDURE STEPS:**
*Ask, "Are you OK?" If no response:*
1. Have someone call emergency services.
2. Put on gloves if available.
3. Tilt back head and lift chin.

4. Look, listen, and feel for breathing for 10–15 seconds. If the patient is not breathing, keep the airway open, pinch the nose, position the mouthpiece, seal your mouth over the device, and give two breaths through the mouthpiece into the patient's lungs.
5. Check the pulse at the carotid artery for 10 to 15 seconds. If the patient has a pulse, continue rescue breathing. If the patient does not have a pulse, start chest compressions.
6. After locating the area on the abdomen 2 inches above the xiphoid (Figure 9-27A), position your shoulders over your hands and compress the chest about 2 inches fifteen times (Figure 9-27B).
7. Give two slow breaths, holding the nose (Figure 9-27C).

*(continues)*

*Procedure*

**9-11** **(continued)**

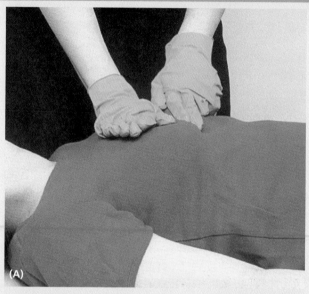

(A)

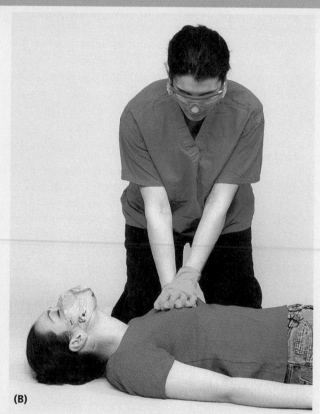

(B)

**Figure 9-27** (A) Tilt back head and lift chin. Locate hand on the breastbone two inches above xiphoid process. (B) Position your shoulders over your hands and compress the chest fifteen times. (C) Give two slow breaths, holding nose.

8. Do three more sets of fifteen compressions and two breaths.
9. Check the pulse and breathing for about 10–15 seconds.
10. If there is no pulse, continue sets of fifteen compressions and two breaths.
11. Dispose of waste in biohazard container.
12. Remove gloves, dispose of in biohazard container, and wash hands.
13. Document the procedure.

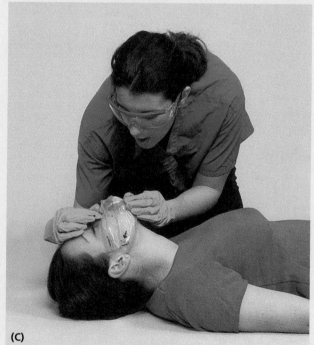

(C)

# *Procedure*

## 9-12 CPR for Children

**STANDARD PRECAUTIONS:**

**PURPOSE:**
To respond to a cardiac arrest emergency.

**EQUIPMENT/SUPPLIES:**
Gloves
Resuscitation mouthpiece

**PROCEDURE STEPS:**
1. Put on gloves.
2. Tap child to check consciousness level. Activate EMS.
3. Tilt head, look, listen, and feel for breathing. If there is no breathing, give two slow breaths. Check carotid artery for pulse.
4. Locate one hand on the breastbone and one hand on the forehead to maintain an open airway. Use heel of hand only. Position your shoulders over the child's chest and compress the chest five times (Figure 9-28A).

5. Position resuscitation mouthpiece. Give one slow breath, while pinching the nose (Figure 9-28B).
6. Repeat cycles of five compressions and one breath for about 1 minute.
7. Check the pulse and breathing for about 5–10 seconds (Figure 9-28C).
8. If there is no pulse, continue sets of five compressions and one breath.
9. Recheck the pulse and breathing every few minutes.
10. Remove gloves. Wash hands.
11. Document the procedure.

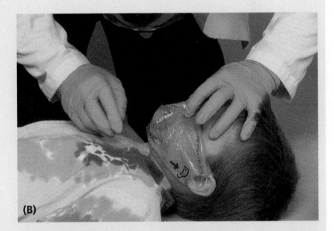

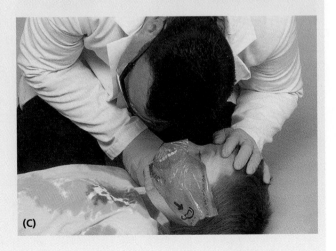

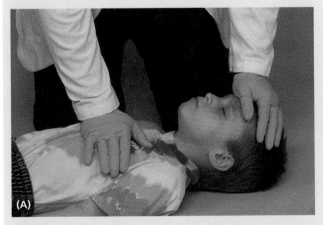

**Figure 9-28** (A) Position your shoulders over the child's chest and compress the chest five times. (B) Give one slow breath, holding the nose. (C) Check pulse and breathing for 5 seconds.

*Procedure*

## 9-13    CPR for Infants

**STANDARD PRECAUTIONS:**

**PURPOSE:**
To respond to a cardiac arrest emergency.

**EQUIPMENT/SUPPLIES:**
Gloves
Resuscitation mouthpiece

**PROCEDURE STEPS:**
1. Don gloves.
2. Gently tap the infant to determine consciousness level. Activate EMS.
3. Tilt head. Look, listen, and feel for breathing. If there is no breathing, position resuscitation mouthpiece and give two slow breaths, covering mouth and nose. Check brachial artery for pulse for 5–10 seconds.
4. Find your finger position on the center of the sternum.
5. Compress the infant's chest five times about ½ inch to ¾ inch.
6. Give one slow breath (Figure 9-29A).
7. Repeat cycles of five compressions and one breath for 1 minute.
8. Recheck brachial pulse and breathing for about 5–10 seconds (Figure 9-29B).
9. If there is no pulse, continue cycles of five compressions and one breath.
10. Recheck the pulse and breathing every few minutes.
11. Remove gloves. Wash hands.
12. Document the procedure.

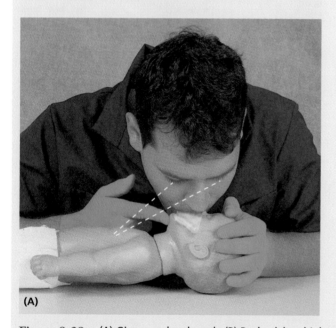

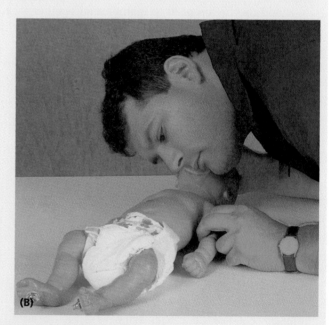

**Figure 9-29**    (A) Give one slow breath. (B) Recheck brachial pulse and breathing for 5–10 seconds.

**9-1**

Annette Samuels, a regular patient at Inner City Health Care, is walking her dog one morning, stops to rest on a grassy knoll, and notices a yellow jacket on her arm. She brushes it away, unthinkingly, and then realizes it is stinging her. She receives two more stings and suddenly notices she is at a nest site. Annette is now a half-hour walk from home but not really concerned because she has never had an allergic reaction to a bee sting. However, a few minutes into her walk, her palms become itchy, her ears start to burn, and she feels lightheaded. She is not having difficulty breathing. She is determined to get home and she does, at which point she notices she is covered with hives. She calls Inner City Health Care to ask: should she come in?

### CASE STUDY REVIEW

1. Wanda Slawson, CMA, is triaging calls the morning Annette is stung. What questions should she ask Annette?
2. Because Annette obviously is having a hypersensitive or an allergic reaction, she is advised to seek emergency care immediately. What first-aid measures might be taken?
3. What advice about precautions should Wanda give Annette?

**9-2**

Abigail Johnson has arrived at Inner City Health Care for her scheduled nine o'clock appointment. As she checks in with Bruce Goldman, the medical assistant, she complains of feeling nauseated, having some pressure in her chest, and being short of breath.

### CASE STUDY REVIEW

1. What immediate actions should Bruce take to respond to Mrs. Johnson's complaints?
2. What equipment/supplies/medications should be ready and available for Dr. Lewis?
3. Because of the possibility of myocardial infarction, what action would Dr. Lewis direct Bruce to take after Mrs. Johnson has been stabilized?
4. What patient education can Bruce employ in this situation?

## SUMMARY

While many of the emergencies covered in this chapter may never be seen by the medical assistant in the ambulatory care setting, it is nonetheless important to develop a broad base of information about the various types of potential emergency situations. This knowledge gives the medical assistant the confidence and the preparation to manage the emergencies that do occur with speed, accuracy, and understanding until outside emergency help arrives. Staff will need to assess their response to emergencies on a continual basis. Was protocol followed? Were there difficulties in the delivery of care? Were staff and equipment pre-

pared and ready to deal with these potentially life-threatening situations? Staff meetings should be held to discuss these and other questions that may have arisen and to allow staff the opportunity to talk about any fears or concerns they might have. It must be stressed that this chapter is at best an introduction to the topic of emergency procedures and first aid; it is highly recommended that all medical assistants in all ambulatory care settings, whether large or small, enroll in either a Red Cross or American Heart Association first aid and CPR program and take refresher courses at least every two years to update skills.

## REVIEW QUESTIONS

### Multiple Choice

1. Good Samaritan laws:
   a. are designed to protect the public
   b. only protect non-health-care professionals
   c. require that all individuals providing assistance act within the scope of their knowledge and training
   d. only protect health care professionals on the job
2. First-degree burns:
   a. are the most serious and penetrate all layers of skin
   b. affect only the top layer of skin
   c. often leave scar tissue
   d. usually take more than a month to heal
3. A fracture in which the bone protrudes through the skin is called:
   a. greenstick fracture
   b. compound fracture
   c. depressed fracture
   d. comminuted fracture
4. To control a nosebleed, it is important to:
   a. have the patient lie down
   b. tilt the patient's head back
   c. tilt the patient's head forward
   d. call 911 immediately
5. Another name for a heart attack is:
   a. cerebral vascular accident
   b. cardiac arrest
   c. angina pectoris
   d. myocardial infarction

### Critical Thinking

1. Discuss the Good Samaritan law and define its purpose and the extent of its protection.
2. Recall what ABC stands for and describe actions that may need to be taken when doing a primary survey of a patient in distress.
3. Define the purpose of a crash cart or tray and compile a list of the major supplies and medications it should contain.
4. Describe shock and tell how and why it is important to prevent a patient from going into shock.
5. Recall three types of bandages and give examples of their use.
6. Describe the difference between first-, second-, and third-degree burns.
7. Recall and describe the four ways that poisons may enter the body.

8. What is hemorrhaging and what kinds of bleeding may the medical assistant encounter? What are the symptoms of each?
9. Explain when and why Heimlich maneuver, rescue breathing, and CPR techniques are performed.
10. What courses should every medical assistant take at least every two years and why?

## WEB ACTIVITIES

1. Search the web for sites and resources on the Emergency Medical Services (EMS) System. Are there any cities or towns within 100 miles of your place of residence that do not use the EMS System?
2. What sites can you recommend to patients and their families who are looking for first aid information about diabetes and heart attack?
3. What organizations could you use to search for information that deal with first aid for convulsions?
4. Search the web for information regarding first aid for insect stings.
5. What sites are available for information about poisonings?

## REFERENCES/BIBLIOGRAPHY

American Red Cross. (1993). *Community first aid & safety*. St. Louis, MO: Mosby-Year Book, Inc.

Bonewit-West, K. (2000). *Clinical procedures for medical assistants* (5th ed.). Philadelphia: W. B. Saunders.

Frew, M. A., Frew, D., & Lane, K. (1995). *Comprehensive medical assisting, competencies for administrative and clinical practice* (3rd ed.). Philadelphia: F. A. Davis.

Keir, L., Wise, B. A., & Krebs, C. (1998). *Medical assisting: Administrative and clinical competencies* (4th ed.). Albany, NY: Delmar.

Kinn, M. E., & Woods, M. A. (1999). *The medical assistant: Administrative and clinical competencies* (8th ed.). Philadelphia: W. B. Saunders.

Prickett-Ramutkowski, B., Barrie A., Keller, C., Dazarow, L., Abel, C. (1999). *Medical assisting: A patient-centered approach to administrative and clinical competencies* (1st ed.). Princeton: Glencoe/McGraw Hill.

*Taber's cyclopedic medical dictionary* (18th ed.). (1997). Philadelphia: F. A. Davis.

Tuttle-Yoder, J., & Fraser-Nobbe, S. (1996). *STAT! Medical office emergency manual*. Albany, NY: Delmar.

# II

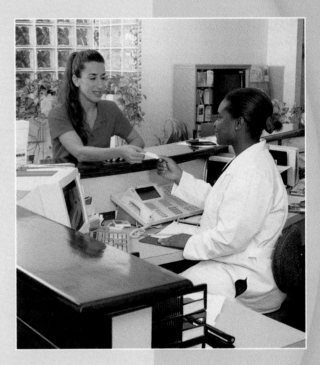

# ADMINISTRATIVE
# PROCEDURES

# INTEGRATED ADMINISTRATIVE PROCEDURES

# Chapter 10

# CREATING THE FACILITY ENVIRONMENT

## KEY TERMS

Accessibility
Americans with Disabilities Act
(ADA)

## OUTLINE

The Reception Area
Office Design and Environment
    Americans with Disabilities Act

The Receptionist's Role
Opening the Facility
Closing the Facility

## OBJECTIVES

*The student should strive to meet the following performance objectives and demonstrate an understanding of the facts and principles presented in this chapter through written and oral communication.*

1. Define the key terms as presented in the glossary.
2. Describe a comfortable and pleasing reception area.
3. List at least six physical characteristics that may leave patients with an inaccurate impression of the medical facility.
4. Discuss how to ensure a patient's privacy.
5. Describe the role of color in the office environment.
6. Review the purpose of the Americans with Disabilities Act.
7. Discuss the importance of the physical office environment to the patient's care.
8. Identify the important personality characteristics the medical receptionist should possess.
9. Describe the procedure to use when an unexpected delay causes patients to wait for the physician.
10. List at least three tasks to perform upon opening and closing the facility.

### GENERAL (TRANSDISCIPLINARY)

**Professionalism**

- **Project a professional manner and image**

**Legal Concepts**

- **Maintain and dispose of regulated substances in compliance with government guidelines**
- **Comply with established risk management and safety procedures**

**Operational Functions**

- **Evaluate and recommend equipment and supplies**

The design of any ambulatory setting often evolves as the needs of the office and patients change. In the office of Doctors Lewis and King, which is a two-doctor family practice, the environment has always been warm and welcoming, which is particularly important because the physicians see many children. However, the office was initially designed in the early 1980s, before the Americans with Disabilities Act was passed by the United States Congress.

Once this Act was passed in 1990, the office manager, Marilyn Johnson, CMA, was very aware of the need to comply with its mandates. In addition, Doctors Lewis and King wanted to make all their patients—including those with disabilities—as comfortable as possible. Working with a local architect, Marilyn was able to incorporate changes into the practice's existing space: a ramp was added outside, doorways were widened to provide wheelchair access, and new Braille signage was installed outside for the visually impaired patients. While the changes were not without expense, the staff of Doctors Lewis and King willingly complied with the ADA not only because it is law but because it gave more access to more patients.

## INTRODUCTION

The environment of the medical office or clinic contributes almost as much to a patient's well-being as does the medical attention given by the physician and medical assistants. The physical environment can foster a feeling that embraces and welcomes patients or causes them to feel alienated and intimidated.

Interior designers and experts in space planning are advising all individuals involved in designing clinics, medical offices, and hospitals that patient comfort must be considered as important as the facility's functional utility and ease of maintenance. The Americans with Disabilities Act (ADA) also must be taken into account when creating any medical office environment, and provisions must be made to accommodate patients who are physically challenged.

The creation of a health care facility involves many variables. Some are concrete elements, such as lighting, color choice, and furniture arrangement. Yet others are intangible and are expressed in a receptionist's greeting and attitude toward patients. Together, these elements make an ambulatory setting the kind of environment where patients will feel comfortable and secure.

## THE RECEPTION AREA

A reception area is just that—a place of reception; it should never be thought of as the waiting room. This is the area that can make the patient feel welcome, secure, and comfortable. Adequate and comfortable seating affords patients room to have their own space.

 Proper seating placement also respects cultural biases. For example, some Americans do not like to be touched by strangers. Middle Eastern and Latin cultures, by contrast, encourage closeness and touching, and individuals from these cultures may cluster themselves close together in the reception area (Figure 10-1).

Current magazines that are appropriate to the clinic clientele, plants, and other features such as a professionally maintained built-in aquarium will help set a welcoming tone. The fabric and texture of draperies, upholstery, and carpet should be pleasing, comfortable, and easy to maintain. It is helpful if there is a place for patients to hang heavy coats or wet umbrellas.

Many physicians provide educational materials for patients in the reception area. For example, new parents always appreciate pamphlets related to raising children. It is also appropriate to have available in the reception area a patient information brochure that describes the services of the office, the function of medical staff members, measures to take in case of an emergency, and other issues that patients may need to consider. See Chapter 22 for more information on developing brochures for patient use.

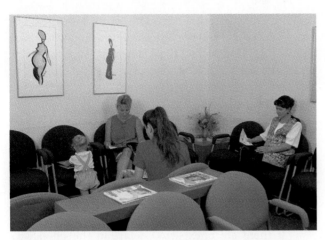

**Figure 10-1** An inviting and pleasant reception area has seating arranged so that patients are comfortable sitting together or away from other patients.

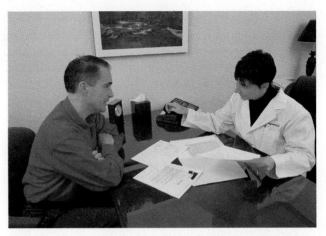

**Figure 10-2** Patients should be afforded as much dignity and empowerment as possible. Many patients may feel more comfortable discussing conditions, procedures, or treatments in the physician's office rather than in the examination room.

## OFFICE DESIGN AND ENVIRONMENT

Even when the office or clinic is housed in an older building not originally constructed as a medical facility, there is much that can be done to create an environment that enhances patient comfort. Remember to see things from the patient's point of view. If the facility is a labyrinth of corridors where patients can easily get turned around, make certain that directions are clear. Be sure that examination rooms are not made more frightening by an assortment of exposed medical equipment and strange-looking dials, hoses, and nozzles. Be alert to odors that are often distasteful to patients even if the odors are from necessary antiseptics.

A reception window or desk should not make the patient feel closed off from the receptionist; it should provide privacy for the receptionist while allowing a full view of the reception area. A poorly illuminated room may suggest that the physician is trying to hide something—poor housekeeping, dust-encrusted baseboards, soiled carpets, or faded draperies. Lighting can be soft and inviting while providing proper illumination.

Some rooms in the facility, by their very nature, cause patients to feel intimidated. Consider the patient who is naked on an examination table except for a paper or cloth gown interacting with the physician who is fully clothed and wearing a white lab coat and comfortably seated at a counter desk. Consider also the patient who is about to have a sigmoidoscopy and must be placed on a special examination table tilted into the knee-chest position. Both these situations place the patient at an unequal level with the physician for discussion and negotiation. The goal in medical care should be to empower the patient with as much control as possible (Figure 10-2).

Privacy is always important to patients. Provide space for them to hang their clothes and undergarments out of view. A mirror is especially helpful when dressing. Always ask if a patient needs help in disrobing, and always knock before entering a room. Remember, too, that privacy implies that the patient's conversation cannot be overheard in any other part of the facility.

Color can do much to establish an inviting environment. Greens and blues are good in areas that require quiet and extended concentration. Cool colors cause individuals to underestimate time and make heavier items seem lighter, objects smaller, and rooms larger. Warm colors with high illumination cause increased alertness and an outward orientation. The aged will have difficulty distinguishing pastels because of failing eyesight. Strongly contrasting patterns and extremely bright colors can be overwhelming, and even intimidating or threatening in their effect.

Accessories and artwork can easily add a special touch to a facility. While fresh flowers might be a nice touch, fresh flowers harbor microorganisms, and some patients may be allergic to them. There is the tendency to use living plants in the medical facility, but some silk plants and flowers also may be appropriate. It would be worth the investment to have a professional designer look through the facility to make suggestions regarding color, artwork, and the general environment of the office.

### *Americans with Disabilities Act*

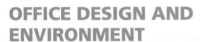**Accessibility,** or making facilities and equipment available to all users, is a major consideration when creating the health care environment. The **Americans with Disabilities Act (ADA)** was passed by the United States Congress

in 1990. The purpose of this act is to provide a clear and comprehensive national mandate to end discrimination against individuals with disabilities and to bring them into the economic and social mainstream of life. In addition to accessibility regulations, this act also provides employment protection for persons with disabilities. ADA applies to businesses with fifteen or more employees; however, some states may have stricter legislation. Even before ADA became legislation, most health care facilities attempted to make their premises barrier-free and accessible to patients with special needs. While many ambulatory care settings will have less than fifteen employees, accessibility for all patients in all settings is very important.

A professional designer can provide advice on how the facility must be accessible to persons who are physically challenged. For example, all doors and hallways must accommodate a wheelchair. There must be a bathroom facility available for handicapped individuals. Signage in Braille accommodates patients with visual disabilities. Elevators must be provided if the facility is on more than one level. Be alert also, to patients whose impairment is not obvious—individuals with impaired hearing or vision and individuals whose infirmity (temporary or permanent) may prevent them from doing certain physical activities.

## THE RECEPTIONIST'S ROLE

The receptionist is the person on the health care team who must always keep a positive "We can help you" attitude, have a smile for each patient, and a genuine "I care about you" personality. This individual, who often is a medical assistant with other duties as well, must be able to perform telephone triage, retrieve records, greet patients, present a bill, make appointments, and log data into the computer all the while remembering that the patient's

comfort is of primary concern. The receptionist must genuinely like people and not be upset when they are grumpy, irritable, or depressed and worried about an illness. The receptionist is the person who sets the social climate for the interchange between the patient and the physician and the rest of the staff, Figure 10-3.

Patients who are very ill should not have to wait in the reception area but should be shown to an examination room away from other patients. The receptionist or medical assistant may also have to entertain children who may be intent on disrupting patients. This is especially necessary if the parent seems unconcerned about keeping youngsters under control, Figure 10-4.

If there are unexpected delays in the physician's schedule, be certain to notify patients of the delay tactfully and graciously and offer them the alternative of making other arrangements. Keep in mind that the patient's time is as valuable as the physician's.

## OPENING THE FACILITY

When the facility is opened in the morning, everything should be in readiness. The receptionist or administrative medical assistant, who arrives at least twenty minutes before the first patient, will make a visual check of each room to be certain it is prepared and ready for the day.

Rooms should be of a comfortable temperature, well-organized, pleasantly illuminated, and spotless. All necessary supplies and equipment should be checked for readiness. At all times, patient comfort and safety should be paramount. Patient charts for the day should be retrieved if not done so the prior evening. The receptionist will also check the answering service or machine for any telephone messages.

An effective way to check a room's readiness is to place yourself in the room as a patient. Ask yourself how

**Figure 10-3**    A friendly greeting from the medical assistant who is serving as receptionist is reassuring to most patients.

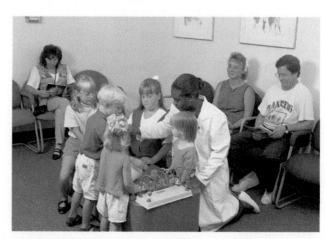

**Figure 10-4**    The receptionist or medical assistant may need to entertain children while parents are in the examination room or physician's office.

you feel about being there, what mood the surroundings create for you, and whether you would feel welcome and comfortable as a patient.

## CLOSING THE FACILITY

At the close of the day, each room should be checked to make certain all equipment is shut down and doors and windows are secured. Be sure that all materials of a sensitive nature are under lock and key. (This is not easily accomplished in facilities that use open-shelf filing, however.) Any drugs identified in the Controlled Substances Act list of narcotics and non-narcotics must be in a locked and secure cabinet and should also be checked when leaving the office. Any petty cash kept on the premises must be locked in a safe container.

It is best, also, to put each room and area in readiness for the next day.

 Local law enforcement officers can advise you on appropriate indoor and outdoor lighting as well as any other security measures to make both during and after office hours.

Always contact the answering service to notify them that the office is closed and where and how the medical staff can be reached in an emergency.

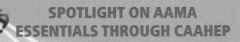

**SPOTLIGHT ON AAMA ESSENTIALS THROUGH CAAHEP**

- A friendly greeting, a pleasant smile, and a professional attitude, always help to reassure most patients coming into the office.

- Creating an environment that is inviting, pleasant, and arranged in a comfortable manner helps patients feel at ease when coming into the office either for the first time or as a returning patient.

- Affording patients as much dignity and empowerment as possible helps them to feel more comfortable when discussing their medical condition.

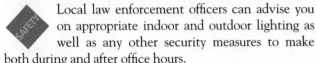

**CASE STUDY 10-1**

Even though she appears collected on the outside, Abigail Johnson, age somewhere in the seventies, is really quite nervous about having her annual physical. Clinical medical assistant Audrey Jones senses her patient's underlying tension and wants to do what she can to get Abigail to relax. She knows that the patient suffers from hypertension and may be feeling guilty about going off the strict diet that was designed to manage both her high-blood pressure and her diabetes. At this moment, Audrey is helping Abigail get ready to see Dr. King, her physician. She does not want to intrude on her patient's privacy but does want her to relax a bit.

### CASE STUDY REVIEW

1. What are some of the actions Audrey can take to ensure her patient's privacy?

2. In what ways can the physical environment itself become a calming influence for the patient, Abigail?

3. How will Audrey's sympathetic attitude affect her patient?

## SUMMARY

Keep in mind that the environment in which patient care is given must promote health rather than aggravate illness and feed anxiety. The environment must be clean, fresh, cheerful, and nonthreatening with contemporary furnishings, appropriate colors, proper lighting, and soothing textures.

Even if patients are not consciously aware of the message they are getting from the office design and environment, they are subconsciously receiving it. The office environment reveals things that might subconsciously undermine a patient's confidence in the physician and the health care team.

## REVIEW QUESTIONS

### Multiple Choice

1. Which of the following is appropriate for the reception area of an ambulatory care setting?
   a. heavily scented flowers
   b. medical journals with colored pictures
   c. dim lighting
   d. live or silk plants
2. One of the goals in treating patients is:
   a. to give them as much control as possible
   b. to see them as quickly as possible
   c. to disregard their desire for privacy
   d. to be sure they arrive on time for their appointment
3. One design element to avoid in a medical office is:
   a. a mirror for dressing
   b. the colors green and blue
   c. strongly contrasting patterns
   d. accessories and artwork
4. The Americans with Disabilities Act is mostly concerned with:
   a. segregating individuals according to type of disability
   b. providing access and opportunity for physically challenged individuals
   c. only the work environment
   d. getting economic benefits for physically challenged people
5. In any medical office, the receptionist's key responsibility is to:
   a. not keep the physician waiting
   b. make sure all plants are watered
   c. greet patients in a friendly, warm manner
   d. be efficient, even if it means ignoring patient requests
6. Making a visual check of each examination room is a function of:
   a. only the physician
   b. opening the office
   c. closing the office
   d. b and c above
7. The American with Disabilities Act applies to businesses with ___ employees:
   a. 10
   b. 5
   c. 15
   d. one or more
8. Children in the reception area:
   a. should sit still and be quiet
   b. may need to be entertained by the receptionist
   c. are not the responsibility of the office staff
   d. should be able to go into the examination room with a parent

### Critical Thinking

1. What would an interior designer or space planner do to create a pleasant atmosphere for patients in a medical office? If there is an interior design program in your school, consult with their students on planning a medical office environment.
2. Describe the most pleasant office you have seen. What made it stand out? In what ways was it special? What were your first impressions?
3. Recall your physician's office. Is it accessible to all patients? If not, what would you do to make it accessible to all patients?
4. As the administrative medical assistant employed in a busy ambulatory setting, how will you keep your personality pleasant, warm, and genuinely friendly and caring even on days when you are having your own personal difficulties?
5. With a fellow student, role-play a situation in which a very frustrated and angry patient must be calmed by the medical receptionist. Assume the patient is angry because of a long wait in the reception area.
6. Discuss what you might do to entertain children aged 4 and 6 while their mother is in the examination room.
7. If you felt the facility in which you are employed could benefit from the services of an interior designer either for minor adjustments or a major remodel, what suggestions would you make to your physician employer to convince him/her of the benefits of such a suggestion?

## WEB ACTIVITIES

 Using the World Wide Web, search for sites identifying companies whose specialty it is to create pleasant interior environments for medical office clinics. Start with the words "interior design and medical facilities." Identify what you are able to locate. What about the pictures displayed is pleasing to you? Why?

## REFERENCES/BIBLIOGRAPHY

Keir, L., Wise, B. A., & Krebs, C. (1998). *Medical assisting: Administrative and clinical competencies* (4th ed.). Albany, NY: Delmar.
Kinn, M. E., & Woods, M. A. (1999). *The medical assistant: Administrative and clinical* (8th ed.). Philadelphia: W. B. Saunders.

# Chapter 111

# COMPUTERS IN THE AMBULATORY CARE SETTING

## KEY TERMS

Algorithm
Antivirus Program
Application Software
Benchmark
Bit
Byte
Central Processing Unit (CPU)
Data Input Device
Data Output Device
Data Storage Device
Data Storage Memory
Database Management Software
Documentation
Ergonomics
Field
Firewall
Floppy Disk
Footer
Gigabyte
Graphics Software
Hacker
Hard Disk
Hardware
Header
Information Retrieval System
Internet
Jaz® Drive
Macro
Mainframe Computer
Megabyte
Merge Operation
Microcomputer
Minicomputer
Motherboard                  *(continues)*

## OUTLINE

Types of Computers
Components of a Computer
   System
   Hardware
   Power Outage, Electrical Surge,
      and Static Discharge Protection
      Devices
   Software
   Documentation

Common Software Applications
   in the Medical Office
   Word Processing
   Graphics
   Spreadsheets
   Databases
   Virus Protection
Patient Confidentiality in the
   Computerized Medical Office
Computerizing the Medical Office
The Safe Use of Computers

## OBJECTIVES

*The student should strive to meet the following performance objectives and demonstrate an understanding of the facts and principles presented in this chapter through written and oral communication.*

1. Define the key terms as presented in the glossary.

2. Recall ten examples of what computers can do to improve efficiency in the ambulatory care setting.

3. Describe the six points that must be considered when moving from a manual to a computerized system.

4. Identify the four main types of computers.

5. Define a computer system and identify its components.

6. Explain the difference between system and application software.

7. Differentiate between the five major categories of application software.

8. Explain how database management concepts might be used in an ambulatory care setting.

9. Discuss patient confidentiality and guidelines for maintaining confidentiality.

10. Explain why ergonomics is important, and recall at least six guidelines for setting up a computer workstation.

Network Interface
Optical Disk
Orphan
Password
Patch
Personal Computer (PC)

Random Access Memory (RAM)
Read-only memory (ROM)
Record
Server
Software
Sort

Spreadsheet Software
Supercomputer
System Software
Widow
Word Processing Software
Zip® Drive

## ROLE DELINEATION COMPONENTS

### GENERAL (TRANSDISCIPLINARY)

**Legal Concepts**

- Maintain confidentiality
- Prepare and maintain medical records
- Use appropriate guidelines when releasing information
- Comply with established risk management and safety procedures
- Develop and maintain personnel, policy, and procedure manuals (advanced)

**Operational Functions**

- Evaluate and recommend equipment and supplies
- Apply computer techniques to support office operations

## SCENARIO

Inner City Health Care, an urgent care center in a large urban area, recently made the transition from a manual to a computerized system. It was a change long overdue, and it required a great deal of fact-finding and research before office manager Walter Seals could convince the center's physicians to purchase a network of computers for the five-physician center.

Once he persuaded his employers of the computer's potential value to the center, Walter, an administrative medical assistant, proceeded very carefully. He spoke with other ambulatory care settings that were already computerized, to establish **benchmarks**, or comparisons. He selected a computer vendor who was familiar with the software needs of a medical office. He made sure all staff would receive training in the use of the computer. Finally, he selected a two-week period when the office was routinely closed for summer vacation to have the computer system installed and operational.

## INTRODUCTION

In a little more than a decade, computers have revolutionized the world of health care. Computers assist in performing sensitive surgeries, diagnosing illnesses, and developing patient treatment strategies. In addition to these dramatic clinical applications, computers have changed the nature of the ambulatory care setting from an administrative point of view, streamlining critical tasks such as patient data collection, correspondence, reports, and insurance claim filing.

Yet, by itself, the computer cannot make a medical practice function more smoothly. Talented medical assistants, who understand the uses and potential of the computer, are the key behind an effective computerized office.

Computers are no longer a luxury in the ambulatory care setting; they have become an essential way of doing business. The medical assistant in most ambulatory care settings must be computer literate. In addition, the medical assistant also must be aware of procedures to prevent compromise of confidential medical records.

## TYPES OF COMPUTERS

Although the medical assistant will be primarily concerned with the uses of the minicomputer and the microcomputer, commonly known as the personal computer, it is helpful to understand the capabilities of the four major types of computers.

**Supercomputers**, the fastest and the most powerful computers, are used in medical research to combat cancer and to trace the genetic components for birth defects. They are the most expensive and complex of computers. Relatively few of these systems are up and running. Supercomputer technology is still under development but holds great promise for the advancement of sophisticated medical interventions.

**Mainframe computers**, the next largest in size and processing ability, are used for large volumes of repetitive calculations. With their high processing speeds, mainframes are invaluable for large governmental provider service programs like Medicaid and Medicare.

**Minicomputers**, grouped between mainframes and microcomputers in terms of size, speed, and capacity, process data in health care facilities in a variety of ways, including patient account processing, insurance claim processing, and statistical analysis of research data. Minicomputers handle large amounts of processing and challenge the capabilities of older mainframe systems (Figure 11-1).

**Microcomputers** are the most widely used type of computer in today's health care facility. The smallest of the four types of computers, microcomputers range in size

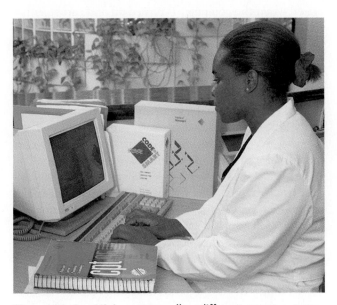

**Figure 11-1** Minicomputers allow different operators to use the same application at the same time. There is no data storage unit (disk or drive) at the operator's station, only a keyboard and monitor.

from easily transportable systems such as handheld, laptop, or notebook systems, to the more common desktop or **personal computer (PC)** (Figure 11-2).

The medical assistant will work with the computer on a daily basis in many different ways. Microcomputers may be used in a medical practice to schedule appointments, maintain patient accounts, and process insurance claims. Handheld micros may be used to input patient information during examination.

## COMPONENTS OF A COMPUTER SYSTEM

A system is an assembly of parts that function together to perform a particular task. A computer system consists of hardware, software, and documentation of the installation.

### *Hardware*

The components of a computer system you can see and touch are referred to as **hardware**. Hardware consists of the central processing unit (CPU), data input devices, and data output devices. Each of these items is made up of many subcomponents. However, we will only concern ourselves with the primary function and unique technology employed to perform that function.

**Central Processing Unit.** The **central processing unit (CPU)** of a computer is the brain of the system. It carries out instructions defined by the program software on the data input and sends the result to the selected output device. The actual heart of the CPU is a silicon microchip approximately 3 inches square with sometimes hundreds of connections to other electronic components. The circuitry printed on the microchip contains logic **algorithms** for performing functions such as addition, subtraction, and multiplication. (Word processing example: The operator presses the letter *a* on the keyboard or data input device. The input device sends the numeric symbol for *a* to the CPU. The CPU then combines this input and whether the shift or caps key was pushed with data previously input when the word processing program was set up and sends the output to memory and to the monitor for you to view the letter A.)

**Data Input Devices.** **Data input devices** convert hard copy, motion, temperature, position, and other analog signals into digital input for use by a computer. The most common data input devices are the keyboard and mouse. Other input devices are electronic tablets with pointers, pens, airbrush tools, scanners, touch screens, and a host of electronic clinical instruments that can directly

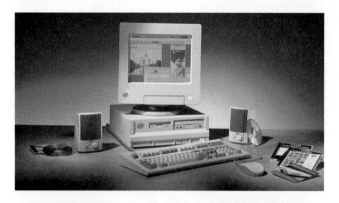

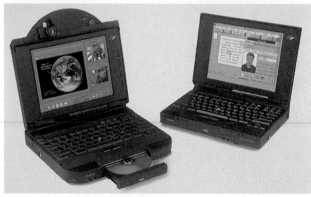

**Figure 11-2**    Microcomputers come in a variety of sizes and types: (Top) Traditional desktop personal computer. (Bottom) Versatile laptop and Thinkpad models. (Courtesy of International Business Machines Corporation)

record patient laboratory data into a patient's file as either a printed or an electronic record.

**Data Output Devices.** Data output devices are the user's eyes, showing how the program has manipulated the input data. The most common data output device is the monitor or screen, which provides real-time feedback of what is taking place with input data. It is used interactively by most operators to make in-process changes to format of data output and to correct input errors. Printers, plotters, and facsimile (fax) machines are output devices that provide hard copy for filing, mailing, or transmission to remote locations. Use of a fax machine or connection to the Internet requires a modem to interface between the computer and a telephone line or cable. Modems can be internal to the computer case or external in the form of an add-on device connected by a cable or plug-in slot on the computer case. Modems operate at different speeds of data transfer, and the fastest device compatible with the telephone, cable system, or Internet provider should be utilized. **CAUTION:** Fax transmission of sensitive data requires special protocols to ensure that unauthorized persons do not receive it. Data storage devices also function

as output devices to electronically store output for future manipulation or transmission. The same caution should apply when transmitting output electronically as with electronic fax machine transmission of output or data. See the section on Patient Confidentiality in the Computerized Medical Office.

**Data Storage Devices.** Data storage devices are devices capable of permanently or temporarily storing digital data. Data storage device capacity is often referred to as memory. Along with computer speed, this area of the computer has seen the greatest improvement, with capability doubling every few years or less. Computers used by most of us today have no functional limitation for memory, with portable memory cartridges providing unlimited memory expansion.

Data storage devices consist of **read-only memory (ROM)**, **random access memory (RAM)**, and **data storage memory**. The computer manufacturer permanently writes data or instructions into the memory on ROM chips, which are installed directly onto the **motherboard**. They contain instructions for operations such as booting the computer when the power is turned on. RAM memory is also in the form of chips and is part of the motherboard. It provides the computer with registers in which to store in-process data. RAM memory is erased or "lost" when the computer is turned off or experiences a power failure. RAM memory is important to the user, in that too small a RAM capacity will cause the computer to run slowly and sometimes not run some software programs. Data storage memory is permanent in that it is not erased when the computer is turned off and can be either read-only or random access. Read-only data storage memory is used to store application programs for loading onto the computer. The following paragraphs describe several devices for providing data storage.

**Hard disks** are nonportable storage devices, usually installed directly into the computer cabinet that contains the CPU. A hard disk is a read-write device, and the memory is permanent except if the device experiences mechanical failure. Because of the failure potential of these devices, it is considered good practice to back up frequently the stored data by making a copy of files on a portable data storage device. The frequency for data backup is dependent on rate at which data is entered into your system, and upon how long original records are maintained. Original records should never be destroyed until the stored data is backed up.

**Floppy disks** are portable memory storage devices that can be readily removed and transported. The most common floppies are 3.5 inches square and hold about 1.4 **megabytes** of data, although minicomputers use larger disks that hold correspondingly more data.

Zip® drives and Jaz® drives are found on many new computers. They are slightly thicker than a floppy disk but hold between 100 and 2,000 megabytes of data. They are portable and interchangeable from one computer to another.

**Optical disks** are portable memory storage devices that can be of the read-only or read-write type. The read-only devices are basically a compact disk commonly used to record digital music and are used to store computer programs for loading onto your computer or to store catalogs, maps, and charts or similar data-intensive applications. The storage capacities of optical disks run into the **gigabyte** range.

**Servers** are not true data storage devices. They usually contain or are connected to massive hard drives, but in many networked systems they become the storage devices for the user workstations. Servers may be located remote from workstations or even on the Internet. When servers are used, special protocols must be employed to protect confidentiality of records. See the section on Patient Confidentiality in the Computerized Medical Office.

## Power Outage, Electrical Surge, and Static Discharge Protection Devices

Protection devices must be an integral part of a medical office computer system. Computer systems should have an uninterruptible power supply, usually a battery backup, to prevent power outages from shutting down the system or destroying data. The power supply should also have a surge protection capability to prevent voltage surges on the utility line from damaging computer components. Static electricity can also be highly damaging to computers by transferring thousands of volts of electrical charge to components that are damaged by only a few hundred volts. This is the type of charge we all experience during dry weather when we get a shock from touching a grounded object and draw a spark. Nylon stockings, synthetic clothing, and walking on a synthetic fiber carpet all create static charges. To prevent damage from static discharges, grounding mats are required at all workstations.

## Software

**Software**, frequently referred to as a computer program, can be thought of as a set of instructions that a computer follows to control computer hardware and to process data. System software and application software are both required by a computer to accomplish its tasks.

**System software**, frequently just called the operating system, tells the computer hardware what to do and when to do it. Some of the modern systems operate with a graphic interface that utilizes graphic symbols for input to the system and is much more user friendly than systems requiring alphanumeric inputs. Microsoft Windows® and Macintosh systems are probably the best known of the graphic interface operating systems.

**Application software** performs a specific data processing function. Word processing, accounting, scheduling, and insurance coding are examples of application software functions. Application software must be compatible with the operating system and the computer system hardware. The label on the application package usually defines the minimum system properties for the program to function as designed and in a fashion acceptable to the user. It is usually better to have a system, which has a slightly faster speed, greater RAM capacity, and more memory than required by the program.

## Documentation

Computer system **documentation** consists of the manuals and documents that define how programs operate. Documentation tells how to execute specific functions and gives the specifications for specific hardware, such as the frequency of the internal clock, RAM, and hard disk available memory. Although it is more likely provided on an optical disk that originally provided the specific program, documentation can be in printed format.

Updates to program documentation are increasingly made available on the web site of the company providing the program, along with **patches** for glitches discovered in the basic program. Third party documents defining how to use application software are becoming increasingly popular and are frequently more user-friendly than documentation from the software supplier. All documentation, including licenses, recovery software, and program disks that come with the computer system, add-on hardware, and software should be maintained in a safe location for the life of the equipment and software and then disposed of when the system or software is phased out of use.

## COMMON SOFTWARE APPLICATIONS IN THE MEDICAL OFFICE

In a medical environment, application software can be used either for general or specialized purposes (Figure 11-3). When applications are needed to fulfill specific purposes, customized software might be used. Custom software can be purchased as a prewritten application designed for a specific industry (such as The Medical Manager® software for the medical field, Figure 11-4), or it can be written to meet the needs of a single organization.

**Scheduling**

Appointment scheduling
Follow-up scheduling
Patient recall lists
Patient reminders

**Word processing**

Articles
Consultation reports
Correspondence
Labels and addressing
Medical transcription
Memos
Thank you letters
Welcome-to-practice letters

**Clinical**

Access to national data banks
CME (continuing medical education) programs
Drug interaction and allergy checks
Medical records
Patient education brochures
Prescription writing
Protocols, diagnosis, and treatment
Research
Retrieving medical research from on-line sites
Treatment plans

**Accounting**

Accounts payable
Cash report
Cash register

Charge slips
Check writing
Cross-posting in multiphysician practices
Daily log
Deposit slip
General ledger
Income and expense statement
Monthly statements to patients
Payroll
Profit and loss statements
Retirement plan accounting
W-2 forms

**Billing, collecting, and insurance**

Accounts receivable
Aging accounts receivable
Billing forms
Collection letters
Electronic transmission of claims
Insurance claim processing
Patient billing

**Practice management**

Employee vacation and sick-time records
Hospital lists and charges
Inventories and drug supplies
Ordering drugs and supplies
Patient profiles by age, diagnosis, and so on
Practice profiles by diagnosis, procedure, service
Production reports by physicians
Referrals

**Figure 11-3**    The computer has great value for the ambulatory care setting.

While custom software can be very expensive, it is valuable because it has many special features developed especially for medical offices (Figure 11-5).

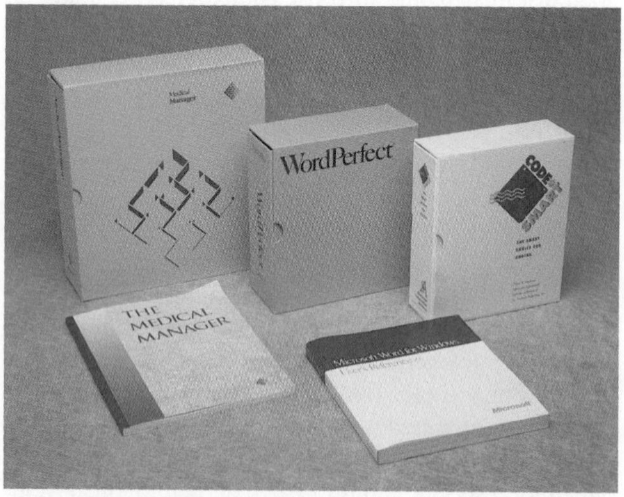

**Figure 11-4**    Examples of popular application software and documentation packages common to many medical offices.

General-purpose software useful in the ambulatory care setting includes word processing, graphics, spreadsheet, database, and on-line communications programs.

## Word Processing

Word processing is largely concerned with the production of textual material. Documents created using **word processing software** may include standard reports, medical transcription, memos, business letters, and articles.

Word processing software allows the medical assistant to produce a document needed quickly and easily; the advantages of word processing over typewriting are considerable, for corrections are easily made and material can be cut or copied and pasted from one file to another.

### Common Word Processing Features

● Block operations allow the user to highlight and move "blocks" of text to another position within the document. Text can be copied, appended, deleted, moved, and added to another document. It can be changed

- Provides immediate access to patient records, insurance information and eligibility, office notes, and reports
- Procedure entry routines capture information necessary for any type of claim or HMO report
- Electronic communications include ability to request, receive, and transfer information electronically. An example of this is electronic insurance claim filing
- Advanced billing features may include:
  - Capability for maintaining enrollment lists, automatically calculating co-pay amounts, and monitoring benefit limits for managed care
  - Capability for government reporting such as Worker's Compensation documents
  - Collection tracking system for patient bills and insurance claims
- Automates the scheduling of patient appointments, cancellations, and recalls
- Electronic medical records can store, organize, and present data on various aspects of a patient's medical history on demand
- Automated reporting allows practice to predefine reports and billing jobs to be printed automatically and even unattended

**Figure 11-5**   Some medical management software capabilities.

from lowercase to all caps, the font or typestyle can be altered, and it can be made italic or boldface.

- Page formatting can create a variety of looks for the printed page. Text can be right and left justified, centered, or aligned on the left with a ragged right. Other page format features include pagination, the placement of numbers on the page, **widow** and **orphan** control (where paragraphs end or begin on the page), and the use of **headers** and **footers** that mark each page of the document in some consistent way.

- Spell check is a feature of most word processing programs. Medical spell checkers can be added to most word processing programs and can be used to check medical terminology in word processed documents or transcribed medical reports. See also the transcription section in Chapter 16. While spell checkers are useful tools, they are not a replacement for proofreading.

- **Macros** are keystrokes that have been saved separately so that the saved keystrokes may be inserted into any document. Macros are useful for increasing productivity when working with repetitive types of

## SIX OPERATIONS FUNDAMENTAL TO OPERATING SOFTWARE

### 1. File creation.
When alphanumeric or numeric data are entered, the information is stored in primary memory (RAM) and made available to the user for viewing on a monitor.

### 2. Formatting.
Formatting a file, depending on the software, usually refers to the arrangement of information so that its appearance is concise and easy to read. For word processing files, this process entails setting margins, line spacing, tab settings, and other variations. For a spreadsheet file, the process may involve choices about the size of the columns, the placement of headings over columns, and the placement of headings.

### 3. Editing.
Once a file has been created and formatted, modifications may be made to the original file. Spelling corrections can be made and formatting changes can be implemented. Sections of the document may be cut and pasted.

### 4. Saving.
If the file is to be retained permanently, it must be saved to a secondary storage medium. When working on any document, it is advisable to use the save command frequently; power interruptions and other events may cause the file to be deleted.

### 5. Printing.
A hard copy (printed page) is created when the file is complete and all changes have been made. Text viewed on the monitor is called a soft copy.

### 6. Retrieval.
Saved files may be retrieved from storage at any time. Accessing them is a process known as retrieval.

materials. For example, a letterhead used on every business letter could easily be saved in a macro format and used repeatedly.

- **Merge operations** are also time savers when working with repetitive material. Merges are often used on the individualized form letter. Ambulatory care settings may use merge operations in mailing patient education memos.

- **Sorting** refers to rearrangements of information. Sorts can be performed on alphanumeric (letters and numerals) or numeric (numerals) data. Frequently, sorts are used to arrange labels for mailings by zip code.

- Importing and exporting data allow users to carry a text file into another applications program. Moving data from one program to another can be cumbersome, time consuming, and frustrating without the ability to import (bring in) and export (send out) easily and efficiently.

- Multicolumn output is the arrangement of text on a page in two or more columns for documents such as newsletters and patient education brochures. See Chapter 22 for techniques on developing patient information brochures.

- Desktop publishing refers to the ability to combine text and graphics into documents and produce them in a high-quality format, usually with the use of an inkjet or laser printer. Word processing packages vary greatly in their ability to provide all the options necessary for effective desktop publishing environments.

## Graphics

Pictorial representations help to summarize and highlight important ideas and assist professionals in communicating material effectively. **Graphics software** transforms numeric information into line graphs, pie charts, or bar graphs (Figure 11-6). These graphic representations summarize trends in an easy-to-read format.

Graphics programs often allow the medical assistant to import files from spreadsheet or database applications, so that data from these files can be summarized graphically and displayed on screen. Drawing applications also provide a means of creating and developing custom artwork for patient brochures and newsletters.

When more than one application is grouped together and made available in a single prewritten, prepackaged format, the application is said to be integrated. Popular integrated packages include Microsoft Works and Lotus Works.

## Spreadsheets

**Spreadsheet software** "crunches" or calculates numbers. These programs act as electronic calculators, performing mathematical calculations and recalculations. These calculations occur so quickly and accurately that financial and other types of numeric data can be summarized and analyzed in ways that used to be difficult and time consuming. In fact, the introduction of spreadsheets began what we know now as the computer revolution.

Spreadsheets take the form of a worksheet, much like an accountant's columnar pad. The worksheet consists of empty rows and columns. Each row and each column is labeled, either numerically or alphabetically, to give

entries a title. The intersection of row and column has a unique location, identified by the coordinates of the row and column, for example, D5 or AA7760. This intersection is called the cell location or cell address.

Common features found in most spreadsheet packages include the ability to format numbers. Values can be displayed in decimal format, in a currency format with a dollar sign, or as a percent sign (%). Labels can be formatted to be left justified over a column of cells, right justified over a column of cells, or centered over the column.

Spreadsheets are useful for expense sheets, tax reporting, and other financial reporting. Medical billing packages are usually based on spreadsheet software.

## Databases

Databases serve to organize large quantities of related data into useful forms. **Database management software** is frequently used to handle employee information, manage inventory systems, record number of patient visits, and manage other patient information. Databases also are used in information retrieval services, which provide access to on-line sites.

**Database Management Systems.** Databases or database management systems (DBMS) are built from the concept of data organization. Data is organized from its most simple component, the bit, to the most complex data structure, the database. **Bits** are the smallest unit of data that the computer can process. **Bytes**, the equivalent of characters (a, b, 1, 2, @, #, and so on), are made up of codes of bits. Each byte that can be input from a keyboard can be translated into a unique code. These codes make up what is referred to as machine language, the language the computer works with in order to process data.

Bytes are combined together to make fields. **Fields** are pieces of information or data elements. Examples of fields include first names, last names, and disease categories like hypertension or obesity. Fields are pieces of information that we collect about individual entities. These entities are known as **records**, and most of the time entities represent individuals.

Databases can be quite complex, based on sophisticated mathematical models. One of the most flexible models for the database is the relational model. Because of its flexibility, it has been used with microcomputer systems and is becoming more popular with the use of minicomputers and mainframes.

**Structuring or Defining the Database.** The first step in working with a database is the creation of the database structure itself.

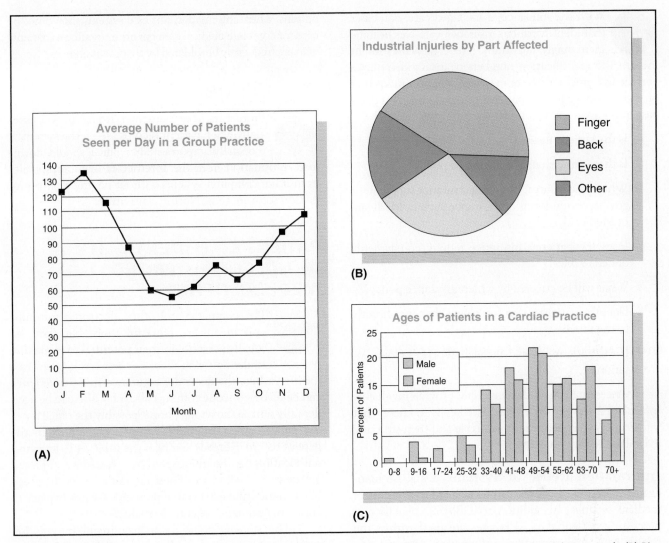

**Figure 11-6** Graphs and charts are excellent for presenting information that can be interpreted at a glance: (A) Line graph. (B) Pie chart. (C) Bar graph.

Creating an imaginary patient database for a medical practice will be helpful for illustrative purposes. Consider a two-physician practice with 1,000 patients. The office maintains information on all its patients, including general identifying information, accounting information, and medical records.

A database is needed that will maintain the general identifying information. Minimally, the fields necessary for the database would need:

- Patient name
- Patient address
- Work phone
- Home phone
- Patient insurance

Other fields might also be included such as:

- Gender
- Social Security number
- Date of birth
- Occupation
- Place of employment

These headings provide the basic structure for the database.

The variables involved in health care databases are numerous and might include identification of the patient, identification of the insurance carrier or carriers, type of insurance, limits in plan benefits, diagnosis and procedure codes, and information concerning the primary care physician.

With the influence of managed care, databases that identify patient insurance variables become increasingly important. These databases might include the identification numbers of insurance policies and the insurance carriers or managed care operations that provide coverage for the patient. In developing this database, it is important to consider the following questions:

- Is the patient insured?

- Is there more than one insurance policy?

- Who is the insurer? Does this insurance supplement governmental forms of insurance such as Medicare or Medicaid?

- Does the patient's insurance require co-payments or deductibles?

- What will be covered by which insurance policy?

- Does the patient assign (turn over) benefits directly to the provider?

- Is the patient covered through Worker's Compensation?

Once established, databases can provide invaluable information in very little time. The key is to know what information you need readily available and then structure a database to that objective.

**Information Retrieval Systems.** Database management software (DBMS) can be adapted to a variety of medical settings. In addition to DBMS's capability of processing patient data, databases are used within the health care environment as information retrieval systems. Through the Internet, it is possible to connect electronically with information retrieval systems to reference topics in health sciences literature. Most medical libraries and many hospitals have the capacity to use the MEDLARS (Medical Literature Analysis and Retrieval Systems) literature database. This database, through the National Library of Medicine, allows researchers to conduct literature reviews on any of their twenty on-line bibliographies.

Information systems that complete biomedical journal searches are also becoming available on a subscription service basis to individual purchasers for use on their microcomputers. One on-line service is Medline; it contains more than six million references on journal articles relevant to health care professionals.

Information retrieval systems are also available for patient use. Cancer treatment protocols, descriptions of treatment regimens, and prognosis information by diagnostic category are now available to individuals who wish to gather information on cancer diagnoses and treatment

options. These information retrieval systems should not be used for complete medical care but are a resource to patients who are frequently bewildered by treatment choices.

## Virus Protection

 Protecting your computer from viruses, especially when patient records are on the system, is especially important. No office should download information from the Internet or even accept files from other computer systems without having a virus protection software (e.g., Norton Antivirus).

## PATIENT CONFIDENTIALITY IN THE COMPUTERIZED MEDICAL OFFICE

The computer and other electronic transmission media are powerful tools, but they are equally powerful in their potential to jeopardize patient confidentiality. A record or test result faxed to a location where the fax is not contained in a secured area can be read by anyone coming past. A fax also can be accidentally sent to the wrong phone, possibly the office fax of the patient since this information is commonly in the patient record. Records sent over the Internet to an external location can be intercepted by a hacker and posted on the web for all to see. These are just a few of the possible scenarios that can occur if protocols are not in place to ensure maintenance of confidentiality.

The starting point for a meaningful information security system is a comprehensive security policy that is understood and supported by staff and employees. All staff and vendors having access to the computer system should be educated on the security policy and should be asked to sign a contract affirming that they will adhere to the policy before they are given access to confidential data.

The next essential step is to ensure that computer literate personnel are employed to set up and structure databases. Protocols should be established defining who can access and modify databases, providing identification, dating, and authentication mechanisms for those changes and additions. Procedures should be in place to ensure that people other than the intended recipient cannot accidentally read misdirected files, and that sufficient firewalls or precautions are taken to prevent people from hacking into the system through Internet or network interfaces. Antivirus programs should be part of the system to prevent loss of the database and/or the unintentional dissemination of files.

Passwords incorporating employee personal identification numbers (PIN) or passwords that are employee-specific are quite successful in controlling access to files and providing an authentication mechanism. Locating fax machines in restricted access areas under the supervision of people with access to all sensitive data can control faxes. Both the sender and the recipient can make sending files on the Internet secure by the use of encryption programs. Development of a firewall to allow outside computers to access your computer while restricting access to your databases is essentially impossible. The U.S. government, with unlimited facilities, hasn't been able to develop a foolproof system, so other approaches are required for an office of limited resources. Probably the best approach is not to allow outside computers access to your database computers, and to communicate to an outside network or Internet using a dedicated computer. Files to be transferred would be loaded into the dedicated computer using one of the portable data storage devices. This would also limit damage in the event a virus invaded your system.

The American Medical Association (AMA) supports the adoption of standards to protect individual confidential information. Figure 11-7 summarizes AMA Policy E5-07, "Confidentiality—Computers," issued prior to April 1977 and updated in 1994 and 1998. Sample security policy guidelines, employee and vendor training, and confidentiality statements have been developed by the Computer-Based Patient Records Institute (CPRI). Their web site is www.cpri-host.org. They are located at 4915 St. Elmo Avenue, Suite 401, Bethesda, MD 20814.

## COMPUTERIZING THE MEDICAL OFFICE

While the computerization of an ambulatory care setting may seem like a daunting process, the task is made more manageable if problems are anticipated beforehand. While computerization can simplify cumbersome tasks, and ultimately lead to greater productivity, initially staff members may experience some frustration until they become proficient in the use and language of computers.

When computerizing a medical office, it is important to know what to expect, to understand the uses and limits of computers, and to organize the transition thoroughly, with proper attention to these details:

1. *Know what the office needs in a computer system.* To be useful, a computer system must serve the needs of the facility. Make a list of why you want the computer: it might include word processing, insurance claim filing, and managing a database. You also might want on-line and e-mail capabilities.

2. *Network by talking to other people in the medical industry.* It is advisable to ask questions of other ambulatory care centers that have been through the

**SPOTLIGHT ON AAMA ESSENTIALS THROUGH CAAHEP**

● When computerizing the medical office, asking for input from members of the staff will ultimately make implementation of the system a much more positive experience for all involved.

● Being willing to help others to learn new skills and tackle new office tools, such as the computer, helps to promote adaptability and eventually helps you get ahead in your career.

● A medical assistant who is familiar with computers and how they can be used in the ambulatory care setting can help others understand their usefulness, and thus, help lessen the stress caused by learning something new.

manual-to-computerization process. Ask them what computer hardware they prefer, what software applications they advise for different functions, and what problems they encountered during their transition.

3. *Work with a trusted, knowledgeable vendor.* It is important to establish a relationship with a computer vendor who understands not only computers but the needs of a medical office. Reliable vendors should be able to advise you of the best system and software and help you anticipate and allow for future needs as the medical practice grows.

4. *Involve all staff members.* If staff members are not familiar with the use of computers, they may feel threatened and, initially, think that using a computer is more time consuming than doing a task manually. The transition takes time and training. Organize staff training sessions, either on- or off-site, so that all employees are familiar with the basics of computer operation.

5. *Install the operation during a down period.* The installation of a computer network can be very disruptive to patients and the office environment. If possible, schedule the installation during a down period, such as over a long holiday when the office is closed, or at least after office hours.

6. *Allow adequate time for start-up.* Initially, much data from existing records will have to be entered. This is an onerous and time-consuming task, but one that

# AMA COMPUTER CONFIDENTIALITY GUIDELINES

The utmost effort and care must be taken to protect the confidentiality of all medical records, including computerized medical records.

The guidelines below are offered to assist physicians and computer service organizations in maintaining the confidentiality of information in medical records when that information is stored in computerized data bases:

(1) Confidential medical information should be entered into the computer-based patient record only by authorized personnel. Additions to the record should be time and date stamped, and the person making the additions should be identified in the record.

(2) The patient and physician should be advised about the existence of computerized data bases in which medical information concerning the patient is stored. Such information should be communicated to the physician and patient prior to the physician's release of the medical information to the entity or entities maintaining the computer data bases. All individuals and organizations with some form of access to the computerized data bases, and the level of access permitted, should be specifically identified in advance. Full disclosure of this information to the patient is necessary in obtaining informed consent to treatment. Patient data should be assigned a security level appropriate for the data's degree of sensitivity, which should be used to control who has access to the information.

(3) The physician and patient should be notified of the distribution of all reports reflecting identifiable patient data prior to distribution of the reports by the computer facility. There should be approval by the patient and notification of the physician prior to the release of patient-identifiable clinical and administrative data to individuals or organizations external to the medical care environment. Such information should not be released without the express permission of the patient.

(4) The dissemination of confidential medical data should be limited to only those individuals or agencies with a bona fide use for the data. Only the data necessary for the bona fide use should be released. Patient identifiers should be omitted when appropriate. Release of confidential medical information from the data base should be confined to the specific purpose for which the information is requested and limited to the specific time frame requested. All such organizations or individuals should be advised that authorized release of data to them does not authorize their further release of the data to additional individuals or organizations, or subsequent use of the data for other purposes.

(5) Procedures for adding to or changing data on the computerized data base should indicate individuals authorized to make changes, time periods in which changes take place, and those individuals who will be informed about changes in the data from the medical records.

(6) Procedures for purging the computerized data base of archaic or inaccurate data should be established and the patient and physician should be notified before and after the data has been purged. There should be no mixing of a physician's computerized patient records with those of other computer service bureau clients. In addition, procedures should be developed to protect against inadvertent mixing of individual reports or segments thereof.

(7) The computerized medical data base should be on-line to the computer terminal only when authorized computer programs requiring the medical data are being used. Individuals and organizations external to the clinical facility should not be provided on-line access to a computerized data base containing identifiable data from medical records concerning patients. Access to the computerized data base should be controlled through security measures such as passwords, encryption (encoding) of information, and scannable badges or other user identification.

(8) Back-up systems and other mechanisms should be in place to prevent data loss and downtime as a result of hardware or software failure.

(9) Security:
   (a) Stringent security procedures should be in place to prevent unauthorized access to computer-based patient records. Personnel audit procedures should be developed to establish a record in the event of unauthorized disclosure of medical data. Terminated or former employees in the data processing environment should have no access to data from the medical records concerning patients.
   (b) Upon termination of computer services for a physician, those computer files maintained for the physician should be physically turned over to the physician. They may be destroyed (erased) only if it is established that the physician has another copy (in some form). In the event of file erasure, the computer service bureau should verify in writing to the physician that the erasure has taken place. (IV)

Issued prior to April 1977.
Updated June 1994 and June 1998.

**Figure 11-7**   Computer confidentiality guidelines. (Source: *Code of Medical Ethics Current Opinions with Annotations,* 1994 Edition, American Medical Association, copyright © 1998)

must be done with great accuracy. Do not expect the computer system to be 100 percent operational immediately. Allow time for medical records and other data to be entered and for staff to build confidence in their computer skills.

## THE SAFE USE OF COMPUTERS

In any environment where computers are routinely used, the concept of ergonomics must be considered. **Ergonomics** is the study of work environments; the purpose of the study is to effectively design work areas that both increase productivity and ensure worker safety and satisfaction.

Safety issues are of concern in computer environments because of documented adverse health effects. For example, low-level radiation has been correlated with increased incidence of miscarriages in women and increased incidence of leukemia. Other health and safety concerns relate to a category of problems classified as repetitive strain injuries. One of the most frequently encountered is carpal tunnel syndrome, which can be caused by excessive wrist strain. This syndrome is quite painful for the individual and may require surgical intervention for correction. Other health problems associated with routine computer use include increased stress, fatigue, eyestrain, and headaches.

To minimize the occurrence of health problems, computer equipment needs to be chosen, set up, and used properly so the medical assistant is protected from injury, strain, and discomfort (Table 11-1).

Posture is also critical in preventing injury. Figure 11-8 is a diagram of a recommended sitting posture for computer users developed by Gary Karp, Ergonomics Consultant of Onsight Technology Education Services of San Francisco, California.

### TABLE 11-1   PREVENTING COMPUTER INJURY

**General Prevention Methods**

- ☐ Maintain good health with proper diet, sleep, and exercise.
- ☐ Balance lifestyle—work, social, spiritual.
- ☐ Learn principles of ergonomics and the potential causes of injury.
- ☐ Do stretching exercises for hands, arms, shoulders and neck.
- ☐ Learn breathing and relaxation methods.
- ☐ Take ten-second "micro-breaks" several times each hour.
- ☐ Don't continue intense computer work when fatigued.
- ☐ Mix tasks to allow breaks from computing and the chance to get up and move around.
- ☐ Manage time to avoid unnecessary crises and times of stress.
- ☐ Keep temperature comfortable.
- ☐ Keep arms warm with long sleeves, sweaters, etc. Consider fingerless gloves.
- ☐ Promote a relaxed working atmosphere to reduce stress.
- ☐ Minimize loud noises, distracting sound in work environment.
- ☐ Streamline office processes and production systems to reduce stress.
- ☐ Don't allow jobs to be typically overloaded or overspecialized.
- ☐ Don't maintain "flattened" posture of hands when not actually keying.
- ☐ Reduce impact on fingers at the keyboards.
- ☐ Look away from monitor when waiting for printing, files opening, etc. Allow eyes to focus on distance or close them to rest.

**Workstation Setup**

**Chair**
- ☐ Chair back slightly reclined to carry body weight.
- ☐ Provide lumbar support to lower back.
- ☐ Optimize back height to conform to shape of back.
- ☐ Provide support to upper back—especially for those who sit for long periods.
- ☐ Thighs in optimal contact with seat pan, no contact behind knees.
- ☐ Thighs above knees without sense of sliding out of seat.
- ☐ Feet in firm contact with floor (use foot rest only if necessary).
- ☐ Armrests—if used—set so shoulders stay relaxed and arms are free to move.
- ☐ Ensure sufficient training in adjustment controls.

**Monitor**
- ☐ Top of screen just below eye level.
- ☐ Position close enough to allow sitting back in chair with head relaxed.
- ☐ Center in front of body to prevent turning trunk or head.
- ☐ Set optimal contrast and brightness.
- ☐ Position to prevent glare from windows, light fixtures.
- ☐ Keep clean of dust and smudges.

**Keyboard**
- ☐ Position so that wrists are straight, shoulders are relaxed, arms at side.
- ☐ Use "feet" of keyboard only if wrists are straighter.
- ☐ Do not allow wrists to be in contact with edge of desk or hard surfaces.
- ☐ Use wrist rest only if needed and comfortable.

*(continues)*

**TABLE 11-1**   *(continued)*

| General Prevention Methods | Workstation Setup |
|---|---|

**General Prevention Methods**

☐ Learn the computer and software properly to avoid frustration and stress.

☐ Take advantage of shortcuts, automated features, and efficiency utilities.

☐ Pay attention to your body. Do not ignore pain!

**Workstation Setup**

☐ Center in front of body to avoid twisting or bending wrists.

☐ Move hands and arms rather than stretching fingers or bending the wrist.

**Miscellaneous**

☐ Consider trackball, programmable mouse, or other alternative inputs.

☐ Headset telephone for people who talk while keying or writing.

☐ Keep oft-used objects close to avoid long reaches.

☐ Use document holders to prevent craning neck looking down to desk.

(Reprinted with permission from Gary Karp, Ergonomics Consultant, Onsight Technology Education Services, San Francisco, CA)

## *Sitting Diagram*

This is the general diagram of the recommended sitting posture for computer users. Keep in mind that fixed postures contribute to the risk of cumulative trauma injury. Variety of posture is crucial, as is the habit of standing up often. The body needs movement. Nothing counts more than comfort, and this illustration is simply a tool to understand what is happening in your body at the computer. Keep these principles in mind as you develop a repertoire of comfortable postures to use throughout the workday, knowing that slumped and leaning postures demand more work from the body leading to early fatigue.

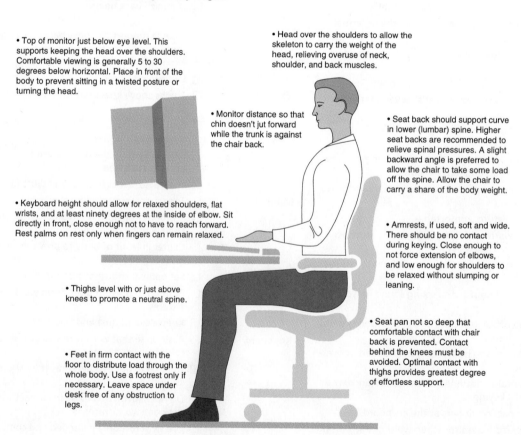

• Top of monitor just below eye level. This supports keeping the head over the shoulders. Comfortable viewing is generally 5 to 30 degrees below horizontal. Place in front of the body to prevent sitting in a twisted posture or turning the head.

• Monitor distance so that chin doesn't jut forward while the trunk is against the chair back.

• Head over the shoulders to allow the skeleton to carry the weight of the head, relieving overuse of neck, shoulder, and back muscles.

• Seat back should support curve in lower (lumbar) spine. Higher seat backs are recommended to relieve spinal pressures. A slight backward angle is preferred to allow the chair to take some load off the spine. Allow the chair to carry a share of the body weight.

• Keyboard height should allow for relaxed shoulders, flat wrists, and at least ninety degrees at the inside of elbow. Sit directly in front, close enough not to have to reach forward. Rest palms on rest only when fingers can remain relaxed.

• Armrests, if used, soft and wide. There should be no contact during keying. Close enough to not force extension of elbows, and low enough for shoulders to be relaxed without slumping or leaning.

• Thighs level with or just above knees to promote a neutral spine.

• Seat pan not so deep that comfortable contact with chair back is prevented. Contact behind the knees must be avoided. Optimal contact with thighs provides greatest degree of effortless support.

• Feet in firm contact with the floor to distribute load through the whole body. Use a footrest only if necessary. Leave space under desk free of any obstruction to legs.

**Figure 11-8**   Recommended computer operator position. (Courtesy of Gary Karp, Ergonomics Consultant, Onsight Technology Education Services, San Francisco, CA)

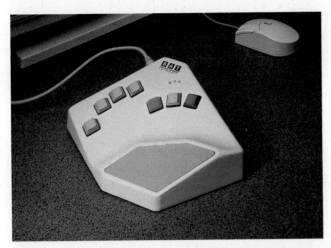
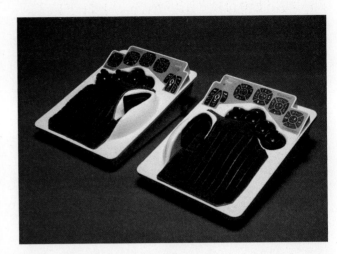

**Figure 11-9** A variety of alternative keyboards is available: (Left) The BAT keyboard (Courtesy of Infogrip, Inc.). (Right) Datahand (Courtesy of Industrial Innovations).

Other considerations include using alternative keyboards to reduce wrist strain (Figure 11-9), using screen glare protectors to deflect and reduce monitor glare, positioning monitors appropriately for the individual, and using chairs that offer comfortable lower back support to reduce fatigue. Medical assistants should organize their work so they take frequent breaks away from the computer. These recommendations do not represent a complete ergonomic solution as many other issues specific to the environment would need to be evaluated especially for those medical assistants who may be at computer terminals for most of the workday.

Once medical assistant Walter Seals received the go-ahead to order a computer system for Inner City Health Care, he immediately consulted a professional for advice on how to set up the workstations. As a health care professional, Walter firmly believes in preventive care and he wanted to ensure that staff members, especially those who might be using the computer extensively, did not develop some of the health problems associated with routine or prolonged computer use.

**11-1**

### CASE STUDY REVIEW

1. Imagine that you are helping Walter design a typical computer workstation. Make a list of how chair, monitor, and keyboard should be positioned. Sketch your diagram for a safe and effective workstation.

2. In addition to a proper workstation setup, what are other measures Walter should consider to ensure staff safety?

3. One of the center's medical assistants is reluctant to use the computer, not because of safety issues but because she feels intimidated by the process. How should Walter help her overcome her timidity of the computer?

Walter Seals, a CMA employed by Inner City Health Care, has been given approval to computerize the office. Walter is also concerned about confidentiality issues involved with a computerized medical office.

**11-2** ### CASE STUDY REVIEW

1. Identify the areas where confidentiality is most likely to be jeopardized.

2. Suggest possible solutions to protect confidentiality in each of these areas.

3. Write a one-page summary, and submit it to your instructor.

## SUMMARY

As the capabilities for networking and communications between computer systems continue to develop, the potential for increasingly sophisticated uses of computer systems is becoming a reality. We are entering the age of global computing where information is available almost as quickly as it is requested. As these changes occur, the role of the medical assistant will reflect the growing reliance of the medical practice upon the capabilities of computers.

It will become the responsibility of all medical assistants to be information managers, taking advantage of the wealth of resources available by computer that can enhance patient care.

Physicians will require assistance in retrieving information from medical databases that support diagnosis; office staff may need assistance in locating, accessing, and working with applications software.

The medical assistant's professional responsibilities will become even more challenging as computers become indispensable to the ambulatory care setting.

## REVIEW QUESTIONS

### Multiple Choice

1. Microcomputers:
   a. are the fastest and most powerful computers
   b. handle large amounts of processing and challenge the capabilities of older mainframe systems
   c. are widely used in today's health care facility
   d. are very expensive and complex
2. The CPU:
   a. is the brain of the computer system
   b. consists of electronic tablets with pointers, scanners, and touch screens
   c. is often referred to as memory
   d. frequently is referred to as a computer program
3. Documentation:
   a. performs a specific data processing function
   b. is a set of instructions that a computer follows to control computer hardware and to process data
   c. frequently is called the operating system
   d. consists of the manuals and documents that define how programs operate
4. Spreadsheets are used primarily in:
   a. document production
   b. financial analysis
   c. communications
   d. information retrieval
5. Formatting a document refers to:
   a. setting margins, tabs, and line spacing
   b. macro operations
   c. exporting features
   d. all of the above
6. Fields:
   a. are a collection of bytes
   b. can be logical, alphanumeric, numeric, memo, or date
   c. represent pieces of information or data categories
   d. all of the above

7. Importing and exporting data:
   a. save time when working with repetitive material
   b. allow users to carry a text file into another application program
   c. are keystrokes that have been saved separately so that the saved keystrokes may be inserted into any document
   d. allow the user to highlight and move blocks of text to another position within the document
8. Database management software may be used for all of the following *except:*
   a. employee information
   b. manage inventory systems
   c. tax and other financial reporting
   d. record the number of patient visits
9. All of the following apply to bytes *except:*
   a. they are the smallest unit of data a computer can process
   b. they are the equivalent of characters
   c. each byte that can be input from a keyboard can be translated into a unique code
   d. the above code is referred to as machine language
10. When going from a manual to a computerized medical office, it is important to do all of the following *except:*
    a. know what the office needs in a computer system
    b. install the operation during a down period
    c. work with a trusted, knowledgeable vendor
    d. expect the computer system to be 100% operational immediately

### Critical Thinking

1. Assume you work in an ambulatory care setting that operates on a manual system. Make a wish list of every function you would have a computer perform for the office.

2. The same office is now going to make the transition to a computerized system. What steps would you take to make the transition as smooth as possible?

3. Recall the four main types of computers and describe a situation in which each would be used.

4. What are the four components of a computer system? Discuss each component and its function.

5. If you were to create a file, what six functions would you perform in the process?

6. What are the major categories of applications software? What operations do they perform?

7. Your physician/employer has asked you to research a particular medical topic on the computer. How do you proceed?

8. Discuss the importance of patient confidentiality in medical computing. What measures could you take to ensure patient confidentiality?

9. Describe the study of ergonomics and give ten suggestions for preventing computer injury.

## WEB ACTIVITIES

 Go to a software provider's web site, such as www.microsoft.com, and list the name and purpose of each patch available for various system and application software programs.

## REFERENCES/BIBLIOGRAPHY

American Medical Association. (2000). E-5.07 confidentiality: Computers. [On-line]. Available: http://www.ama-assn.org

Computer-based Patient Record Institute. *Advancing electronic information systems for health care*. [On-line]. Available: http://www.cpri-host.org

Humphrey, D. D. (1996). *Contemporary medical office procedures* (2nd ed.). Albany, NY: Delmar.

Karp, G. (1996). *Preventing computer injury*. Adapted from paper presented at the Association of American Medical Transcriptionists, Baltimore, MD.

Kinn, M. E., & Woods, M. A. (1999). *The medical assistant: Administrative and clinical* (8th ed.). Philadelphia: W. B. Saunders Company.

# Chapter 12

# TELEPHONE TECHNIQUES

## KEY TERMS

Answering Services
Articulating
Automated Routing Unit (ARU)
Buffer Words
Cellular Telephones
Confidentiality
Diaphragm
Electronic Mail (E-mail)
Empathy
Enunciation
Ethical
Etiquette
Fax (Facsimile)
Fluent
Good Samaritan Laws
Jargon
Modulated
Obfuscation
Pagers
Posture
Pronunciation
Screen
Slang
Triage

## OUTLINE

**Basic Telephone Techniques**
   Telephone Personality
   Telephone Etiquette
**Answering Incoming Calls**
   Preparing to Take Calls
   Answering Calls
   Screening Calls
   Transferring a Call
   Taking a Message
   Ending the Call
**Types of Calls the Medical
   Assistant Can Take**
**Types of Calls Referred to the
   Physician**
**Special Consideration Calls**
   Referring Calls
   Emergency Calls
   Angry Callers

   Elderly Callers
   English as a Second Language
     Callers
**Placing Outgoing Calls**
**Placing Long Distance Calls**
   Placing Calls
   Time Zones
   Long-Distance Carriers
**Telephone Documentation**
**Using Telephone Directories**
**Legal and Ethical Considerations**
**Telephone Technology**
   Automated Routing Units
   Answering Services and Machines
   Facsimile (Fax) Machines
   Electronic Mail
   Cellular Service
   Paging Systems

## OBJECTIVES

*The student should strive to meet the following performance objectives and demonstrate
an understanding of the facts and principles presented in this chapter through written and
oral communication.*

1. Define the key terms as presented in the glossary.

2. Describe four useful rules for using proper telephone technique.

3. State at least five common telephone courtesies.

4. Discuss proper screening techniques.

5. Outline the proper procedure for answering incoming calls.

6. Describe the information every message should contain.

7. Name at least three calls the medical assistant can take, and state the
reasons why. Name three calls the medical assistant should refer to the
physician, and state the reasons why.

*(continues)*

155

8. Recall six questions that should be asked during telephone triage.
9. Elaborate on how calls from angry individuals should be handled in a professional manner, and give three steps to take when this type of call is received.
10. Outline the proper procedure for placing outgoing calls.
11. Discuss telephone documentation.
12. Identify ways to ensure patient confidentiality when using the telephone.
13. Recall four examples of telephone technology, and describe their functions.

## ROLE DELINEATION COMPONENTS

### ADMINISTRATIVE

**Administrative Procedures**

- Perform basic clerical functions
- Schedule, coordinate and monitor appointments
- Schedule inpatient/outpatient admissions and procedures
- Understand and adhere to managed care policies and procedures

### CLINICAL

**Patient Care**

- Adhere to established triage procedures
- Recognize and respond to emergencies

### GENERAL (TRANSDISCIPLINARY)

**Professionalism**

- Project a professional manner and image
- Adhere to ethical principles
- Demonstrate initiative and responsibility
- Work as a team member
- Prioritize and perform multiple tasks

*(continues)*

## SCENARIO

At a busy two-doctor family physician's office like Doctors Lewis and King, the telephone lines are rarely quiet. Yet, administrative medical assistant Ellen Armstrong has learned to maintain her composure when she is responsible for managing incoming calls. Ellen has in her favor a naturally warm telephone manner, but she has had to cultivate other traits so that she can represent the practice in a professional manner, help patients and other callers feel at ease, and efficiently screen or refer calls as necessary.

This is Ellen's first job since receiving her medical assisting certification, and initially she felt unable to properly screen calls. She was not sure when to refer them to the physician; she did not know when she should record a message. With some advice from Marilyn, the office manager, Ellen devised a simple system to keep herself and her thoughts organized throughout a hectic day of telephone communications. Every day before office hours, she gathers the materials she needs, including the appropriate message pad, a list of information needed to set a patient appointment, and any information she needs on prescription refills for patients. With these few measures, Ellen feels organized and prepared and thus able to focus her attention on interacting with the caller.

## INTRODUCTION

As in many office settings, the telephone is the lifeline of the ambulatory care setting. By means of telephone communication, which can also include fax and e-mail transmissions, patient appointments are scheduled, referrals made, critical information related, and the practice personality conveyed.

Medical assistants, more multiskilled than ever, have a wealth of knowledge to bring to their telephone communications. Over the telephone, they will welcome new patients, reassure current patients, collaborate with other organizations on patient care, and calmly and efficiently deal with emergencies. They will need to draw on their vast resource of administrative and clinical knowledge; they will also need to cultivate a telephone personality that is warm and accessible while also being efficient and organized.

In this chapter, medical assistants will come to understand the principles basic to successful telephone communications, whether initiating or

## ROLE DELINEATION COMPONENTS (*continued*)

**Communication Skills**
- Treat all patients with compassion and empathy
- Recognize and respect cultural diversity
- Adapt communications to individual's ability to understand
- Serve as a liaison
- Promote the practice through positive public relations
- Accommodate for cultural diversity (Adv.)
- Use professional telephone technique
- Use effective and correct verbal and written communications
- Recognize and respond to verbal and nonverbal communications
- Receive, organize, prioritize and transmit information

**Legal Concepts**
- Maintain confidentiality
- Practice within the scope of education, training and personal capabilities
- Document accurately
- Use appropriate guidelines when releasing information

**Operational Functions**
- Evaluate and recommend equipment and supplies
- Apply computer techniques to support office operations

answering calls; learn the extent and limits of their authority as medical assistants; discover how to prepare themselves for making or receiving calls; and be introduced to telephone systems and new technologies.

## BASIC TELEPHONE TECHNIQUES

The majority of patients seen in ambulatory care settings initiate their first contact with the office through the telephone. Medical assistants responsible for answering the telephone may be the first contact most people have with the practice. First impressions tend to be lasting ones, so both tone of voice and message content are important as communicators.

To create a positive impression, try to answer the telephone at the end of the first ring and always by the third ring. If your office has more than one incoming line and more than one telephone, it may be necessary to interrupt a conversation to answer another call. Some guidelines to follow in that instance include:

- Excuse yourself to the first caller by saying, "Excuse me, another line is ringing. May I put you on hold for a moment?"
- When the first caller has given permission to be put on hold, answer the second call. Ascertain who is calling, and determine if it is an emergency. If it is not an emergency, ask if you may put the person on hold or return the call when you have completed the first call.
- Return to the first caller, and thank the person for holding.

### Telephone Personality

First impressions are usually conveyed through verbal and nonverbal communication. (Refer to Chapter 4 for a review of these communication modes.) In telephone communications, however, personality and attitudes are conveyed only through the tone in which words are spoken and the words themselves. Remember, callers are not an interruption of your work but the reason for your job. Even in a large practice, it is rare that someone just answers the telephone and has no other duties. No matter what other duties are pressing, the primary responsibility of every employee in a physician's office is patient care; everything else is secondary. Whoever answers incoming calls should be prepared to give the caller complete attention.

Use a voice that is pleasant and well **modulated** (one that varies in pitch and intensity) and conveys interest in the callers' needs. Hold the handpiece correctly, about 1 to 2 inches away from the mouth, and project your voice *at* the mouthpiece not *over* it.

Volume, enunciation, pronunciation, and speed all have a profound effect on how you sound to the person on the other end of the line.

- Volume should be the same as when speaking conversationally.
- **Enunciation** implies speaking your words clearly and **articulating** carefully.
- **Pronunciation** involves saying the words correctly.
- Speed should be at a normal rate, neither too fast nor too slow.

**Posture**, the way the body is carried, also affects the voice. If slumped in a chair, the **diaphragm** (the muscle separating the abdominal and thoracic

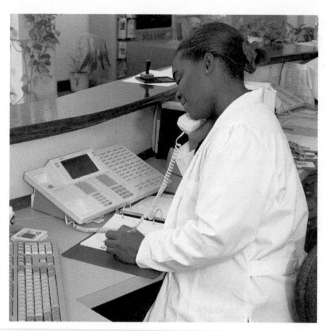

**Figure 12-1**    Practice proper posture and attitude when using a telephone in a professional setting.

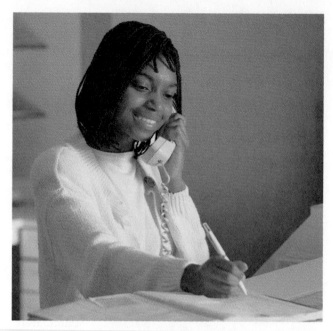

**Figure 12-2**    Tone of voice is able to put people at ease in a telephone conversation. People can hear an unpleasant mood, just as they can hear a warm smile.

cavities) is compressed and breathing may be restricted. This posture can make an individual sound tired and tense. Additionally, posture affects mood. Sitting up straight creates a professional and alert mood that comes across in the voice (Figure 12-1).

Being organized and prepared in advance for each telephone call enables the medical assistant to respond to each caller as if there is nothing else to do. By taking a breath before answering the telephone and putting a smile on one's lips, a pleasant vocal impression can be delivered to the caller.

Medical assistants who enjoy their work and want to be of assistance to patients communicate enthusiasm. Enthusiasm conveys interest to the caller and projects a sincere, caring attitude that can be "heard" over the telephone (Figure 12-2).

Though some callers will be upset, frightened, or even angry, the medical assistant must always be patient and in control. Some calls may be life-threatening emergencies; medical assistants need to remain calm to be of help to the caller, remembering their professional role as health care providers.

Medical assistants can concentrate on improving telephone communications by setting up a small tape recorder next to the telephone and setting it to record for an hour or two each day. At the end of the day, recorded calls will present an accurate representation of volume, articulation, and tone of voice. After using the tape as a self-improvement exercise, be sure to erase all messages in order to respect the confidentiality of callers.

## Telephone Etiquette

Telephone **etiquette**, as with all good manners, simply involves treating others with consideration. Medical assistants have chosen a profession in which care and concern for others are paramount, so it is especially important to keep the patient's feelings in the forefront at all times. Basic telephone courtesies should be kept in mind when answering any professional call.

### SPOTLIGHT ON AAMA ESSENTIALS THROUGH CAAHEP

- Answering the telephone with a smile on your face will help patients to "hear" what you are saying.

- Spending a few extra minutes talking to a patient on the telephone to find out how he or she is feeling often results in getting a clearer picture of what the patient's medical needs may be.

- Your tone of voice can either put someone at ease in a telephone conversation or cause the person to become angry and put off.

# ANSWERING INCOMING CALLS

Most calls received in an ambulatory care setting are from patients or prospective patients, though many are from other physicians or medical facilities. The remainder will be from family members, salespeople, and miscellaneous others. Personal calls should not be permitted in the medical office as they busy lines intended for business. Most physicians will tolerate occasional emergency calls from family members.

## Preparing to Take Calls

Before answering incoming calls or making outgoing calls, medical assistants should devise a simple system to keep organized throughout the hectic day of telephone communications. Collect pertinent materials, such as a message pad, information regarding scheduling of patients and prescription refills, internal and outside referral forms, listing of frequently used telephone numbers and extensions, and several sharpened pencils and working pens.

## Answering Calls

When answering incoming calls, the name of the facility should be clearly identified and with whom the caller is speaking. The name of the office is very important, as the caller wants to know the correct number has been reached. To avoid clipping off the office name, practice using **buffer words**. Buffer words are expendable words and may consist of introductory words, phrases, or statements. They allow a caller an opportunity to collect their thoughts and focus on what is being said.

Obtain the caller's full name and correct spelling, and ask if this is an emergency call. Determine how you can be of assistance, and complete the call efficiently by following all established office protocols. (Refer to Procedure 12-1.)

## Screening Calls

One of the medical assistant's responsibilities will be to **screen** incoming calls. The purpose of screening is twofold: 1) to be sure the caller talks to the person who

---

## TELEPHONE COURTESIES

- Always use callers' names and titles (for example, Mrs. O'Keefe or Dr. King) during the course of a conversation when confidentiality is assured; this shows interest in them as individuals.
- Do not use technical terms if simpler ones will convey the information adequately. Using professional jargon, or terminology, is an easy trap to fall into since this terminology is used daily with coworkers. Jargon only confuses people outside the profession; the goal in communication is mutual understanding, not obfuscation, which confuses people.
- Do not use slang or nonstandard terms in a business setting. Slang terms may have entirely different meanings to individuals from another generation or cultural background. Use of slang is not professional and tends to indicate a poor vocabulary range or lack of education. However, patients may use slang in their communications. It is important not to be offended by slang terms; also, be certain that patients who use slang understand any common medical terminology you may use.
- The "hold" button on the telephone is probably the most misused piece of equipment in the practice; always use it sparingly.
  Never put a caller on hold until you know who is calling and why. Never place an urgent or emergency call on hold. Never put a caller on hold without asking for and receiving permission to do so.

- No call should be left unattended for more than 20 to 30 seconds. If it is necessary to keep calls waiting longer, go back to the caller and give the option of continuing to hold or receiving a call back in a few minutes.
- When it is necessary to get additional information and call back later, let the person know when to expect the call. If for some reason the information is not available when the time for the call back arrives, call anyway to let the person know when to expect another call.
- When taking a message for someone in the office, give the caller an idea of when to expect a return call. If the person will be out of the office for an extended period, see if someone else can help or if the caller would rather wait to hear from that specific individual.
- Pay attention to what the person is saying and *how* they sound. Do not interrupt or finish sentences for slow talkers. The caller may have difficulty putting some things into words, but give the person a chance to explain the problem or question. Listen with empathy for the caller. Also listen to what the tone of voice expresses.
- Never talk to someone in the office while on an open line. This is confusing to the caller, and confidential information could inadvertently be overheard.
- Do not attempt to work on other things while talking on the telephone.
- Never eat or chew gum when talking on the telephone. This impedes enunciation and is distracting to the caller.
- Say "goodbye" when closing the call, and allow the caller to hang up first.

will be most helpful (this is not necessarily the person asked for); and 2) to ensure the physician's time with calls is efficiently managed.

Most people who call an ambulatory care setting will ask to speak to the doctor. Patients calling for appointments or with billing problems or insurance questions will frequently ask to speak to Dr. King, assuming she is the person in charge and therefore should answer any question or solve any problem. In most practices, this is not the case. Medical assistants and other administrative employees are equipped to deal with front-office functions; usually, physicians are not involved in these procedures and sometimes may not be aware of administrative routines.

**Proper Screening Techniques.** Screening is usually a simple process of asking the caller's name and the reason for the call. There are situations, however, that will require tactful persistence to get the information needed to properly direct the caller. Sometimes callers hesitate to give information because the questions are of a confidential and possibly even embarrassing nature.

Occasionally a caller flatly refuses to give any information or will just say, "I'm a friend." If it is a patient who refuses to give information after gentle prodding, respect the patient's privacy and take a message. If you do not know who the caller is and you are unable to get any information, take the message and give it to the physician. Frequently this type of caller is a salesperson. (Physicians are prime targets for all types of sales pitches.) If the physician does not know the person, he or she can decide whether to return the call. In any event, do not argue with the caller. Be polite and professional at all times.

## Transferring a Call

During the screening process, calls may mistakenly be directed to someone who is unable to assist the caller adequately. This call will need to be transferred to someone with more expertise in a particular area. Guidelines that ensure successful transfer of calls include:

- Get the caller's full name, telephone number, and any other situation-associated information before attempting to transfer the call.

- Determine who would be the best person to assist with this situation.

- Ask if you may place the caller on hold while you collect any pertinent data and make a call to see that the person best suited to assist is available.

- Return to the caller, thank him for holding, and give the name and extension of the person to whom you will be transferring the call.

- Follow your telephone system's procedure for transferring the call.

- Followup to be sure the call transferred correctly.

## Taking a Message

When taking messages, it is advisable to use a standard telephone message pad with a carbon that allows the office to maintain a record of all incoming calls (Figure 12-3). The information that should be recorded for *every* message includes:

1. Date and time call is received
2. Who the call is for
3. Caller's name and telephone number
4. When the caller can be reached
5. Nature and urgency of the call
6. Action to be taken (e.g., will call back, returned your call, please call back)
7. Message, if any
8. Your name or initials (in case there are questions)

Be sure to repeat the information back to the caller to verify that you have heard and copied it correctly. When taking a message, give callers an approximate time when they might expect to receive a call back. ("Dr. King will be returning calls between 4:30 and 5:00." "Ellen is out of the office today, but I'll ask her to call you before 10 A.M. tomorrow.")

Always attach a message from a patient to the patient's chart before placing the message on the physician's desk. The physician cannot discuss the patient's condition or answer questions without this information.

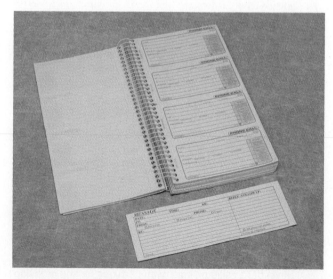

**Figure 12-3**   Message pads with a carbon allow the office to maintain a written record of all incoming calls.

## *Ending the Call*

Ending the telephone call is as important as answering the call promptly. Bring the conversation to a courteous closure, and repeat any pertinent information back to the caller. ("Your appointment is scheduled for Friday, January 12, at 9 A.M. with Doctor King.") Pause just a moment to see if the caller has any additional questions. If not, say "Goodbye." Never use slang terms such as *bye bye, see you later,* or *so long.* They do not reflect a positive professional image. You should always stay on the line until the caller hangs up. They might think of something else they wanted to ask or verify, and staying on the line gives the caller the opportunity to verbalize a thought rather than have to call back. Figure 12-4 summarizes four rules of proper telephone technique.

## TYPES OF CALLS THE MEDICAL ASSISTANT CAN TAKE

Keep in mind that, no matter how experienced, the medical assistant has definite limitations of authority and knowledge. The vast majority of calls can be handled by the knowledgeable medical assistant, but there are situations that only the physician should manage simply because the physician ultimately is responsible for what happens in the practice.

1. Established patients: When an established patient calls to set up an appointment, record the patient's name, daytime telephone number, and the reason for the appointment.
2. New patients: Require the same information as the established patient plus some additional information, including:

   - Address
   - Age/birthdate
   - Employer
   - Insurance carrier or HMO
   - Name of insured (self, spouse, or parent)
   - Name of referral source

   This information serves as a source for the establishment of the chart and may lead to a discussion regarding payment of fees. The information should be entered into the appointment book for both new and established patients. See Chapter 13 for more information on patient scheduling.

3. Scheduling appointments: A major portion of telephone communications will be spent scheduling patient appointments. See Chapter 13 for detailed information on patient scheduling and rescheduling.
4. Scheduling patient tests: Scheduling tests for patients can involve a great deal of coordination, for

*Rule 1. Callers are not an interruption of your work, but the reason for your job.*
Even in a large practice, it is rare that someone just answers the telephone and has no other duties. No matter what other duties are pressing, the primary responsibility of every employee in a physician's office is patient care; everything else is secondary. Whoever answers incoming calls should be prepared to give the caller complete attention.

*Rule 2. Always attach a message for the physician from a patient to the chart before putting it on the physician's desk; the physician cannot discuss the patient's condition or answer questions without that information.*
The information that should be recorded for every message will include: date and time the call is received; who the call is for; the caller's name and number; when the caller can be reached; and the nature and urgency of the call; and initials of person writing the message.

*Rule 3. When you take a message, give callers an approximate time when to expect to receive a call back.*
For example, "Dr. King will be returning calls between 4:30 and 5:00." "Ellen is out of the office today, but I'll ask her to call you before 10 A.M. tomorrow." This basic courtesy respects the caller's time.

*Rule 4. Complete patient confidentiality is an ethical and legal obligation.*
One of the most important issues in a medical setting is patient confidentiality. No information about patients should be discussed outside the office, even with family or friends, or with other patients. Violations of confidentiality leave the practice vulnerable to lawsuits. More importantly, violations of confidentiality erode patient trust. See Chapters 7 and 8 for more information on legal and ethical issues.

**Figure 12-4**   A summary of useful rules for the medical assistant to follow for using proper telephone technique.

often appointment times need to involve physician, patient, and the facility where a test may be conducted.

5. Patients' billing questions: Billing questions can be involved and complex and medical assistants should be prepared to answer questions by retrieving information on the patient's insurance and billing status.
6. Insurance information: Calls will come from patients about insurance as well as from insurance carriers and HMOs with questions about patients or their treatment. If the call is from an insurance company or HMO, be sure there is a signed "Release of Information" in the patient's chart before giving information.

7. Requests for prescription refills: If a patient or family member is requesting that a prescription be refilled, medical assistants may take the call. However, they may not authorize a refill or tell the patient that a prescription will be refilled without the physician's approval. Most offices ask that the patient call their refill requests into the pharmacy; the pharmacy then calls the physician's office for approval. Messages taken on these calls should be attached to the patient's chart and given to the physician for review and for permission to refill. When the physician approves the refill, the pharmacy may be called with an approval.

8. Receiving routine progress reports: Frequently physicians will ask patients to report on their progress. *If the patient is doing well*, it is acceptable for you to take that information on a message form to be given to the physician.

9. General information about the practice: People may call requesting information about hours, location, financial policies, or areas of practice.

10. Salespeople: The medical office will have policies regarding the scheduling of pharmaceutical representatives.

## TYPES OF CALLS REFERRED TO THE PHYSICIAN

1. Requests for test results: Only the physician should give this information. A seemingly simple report may frighten or confuse the patient; at the very least it will probably generate questions that medical assistants are not qualified to answer. Many physicians allow medical assistants to report on satisfactory test results.

2. Medical emergencies: There should be standard procedures for dealing with emergencies. The physician, when present, should be interrupted and notified of all emergency calls.

3. Medical questions: Medical assistants may not give medical advice without risking practicing without a license.

4. Other physicians: When other physicians call, always ask if they need to speak to the physician on staff immediately or if they would like a call back. Be sure to ask if the call is regarding a current patient; if so, pull the chart.

5. Patients who refuse information: If a patient will not provide information about a problem, take a message for the physician to call them back. Some patients are not comfortable discussing physical problems with anyone except the physician; they have a right to that privacy.

6. Complaints: In a medical office, all patient complaints should be viewed as potential malpractice suits. A patient with complaints about the office or the quality of care is best referred to the physician.

7. Poor progress reports: If a patient calls to report that a treatment regimen is not working, the information should be given to the physician immediately. Changes in the treatment or medication may need to be made or the patient may need to be seen right away. This is a medical judgment that medical assistants are not qualified to make.

8. Requests for patient information from a third party: Unless there is a signed release, patient information may not be given to anyone. Any such requests (other than from the patient's insurance carrier or HMO) must be referred to the physician.

9. Requests for referrals: (unless the physician has given the front office a list of specialists to use).

10. Requests for medication: (other than standard refills).

## SPECIAL CONSIDERATION CALLS

Working in an ambulatory care setting brings the medical assistant into contact with emergencies, angry callers, and people of all ages, ethnic backgrounds, and educational levels. As a professional, your goal is to treat every individual with courtesy and respect regardless of age, race, creed, or national origin.

### Referring Calls

Calls will often need to be referred to someone else in or out of the office—the physician, bookkeeper, insurance clerk, a hospital, laboratory, or other facility.

**Internal Referrals.** If it is necessary to transfer a caller to someone else in your office:

- Tell the caller to whom you are transferring the call and why.

- Call the party to whom you are transferring the call and tell them the caller's name and reason for the call in as much detail as the caller has provided.

  See the example of internal referral.

**External Referrals.** If it is necessary to refer the caller to someone outside the office, such as to a laboratory or another physician, be sure to tell the caller:

- Why they should speak to someone else

- The telephone number to call (be sure to include the extension and area code, if necessary)

- Who, specifically, to speak with at that number

- What information to have ready when they make the call

- When to call

● If your office should be called back after the call is made

See the example of external referral.

## Emergency Calls

Triage is the act of evaluating the urgency of a medical situation and prioritizing treatment. Keep in mind that most patients, when ill or injured or if a family member is ill or injured, feel the situation requires immediate med-

ical attention. Triage is one of the most important functions for the person answering the telephone. Triage takes skill and experience. Do not be afraid to ask questions of other professionals in the office. To determine if a call is truly a medical emergency, keep a list of questions near the telephone to assist in evaluating the situation. Standard triage questions can determine the nature of an emergency. Not all questions are appropriate to every call; suitable questions depend on the nature of the situation. (Refer to Procedure 12-2.)

---

### EXAMPLE: INTERNAL REFERRAL

Mrs. O'Keefe is calling about her account and asks specific questions regarding some tests done on her husband. You do not have access to the information she needs since Marilyn Johnson handles the bookkeeping and financial arrangements for the office.

#### Poor Technique

**Medical Assistant:** Oh, I don't do bills, hang on. *Dials Marilyn's extension.*

**Medical Assistant:** Marilyn, line 3 is for you." *Medical assistant hangs up. Marilyn picks up the telephone unprepared and has to put Mrs. O'Keefe on hold while she looks for the records. Once Marilyn has the records, Mrs. O'Keefe has to explain again why she is calling.*

#### Correct Technique

**Medical Assistant:** Mrs. O'Keefe, I would be happy to help you, but Marilyn has all the financial records in her office and is more knowledgeable about your account and better able to help you. If you would like to speak with Marilyn I can transfer you to her office." *When Mrs. O'Keefe acknowledges that she is willing to be transferred, you would then call Marilyn.*

**Medical Assistant:** Marilyn, I have Mary O'Keefe on the line and she wants to know why there are charges for three different blood tests on John's statement. Could you take the call? *This gives Marilyn the opportunity to pull the O'Keefe's ledger before she answers the phone. When Marilyn does answer, she can say,* "Hello, Mrs. O'Keefe, I have the information regarding John's lab charges in front of me. The receptionist tells me you have some questions about the charges for three blood tests on this last statement . . ." *Marilyn can then explain the reason for the charges.*

---

### EXAMPLE: EXTERNAL REFERRAL

Herb Fowler needs to have a glucose tolerance test done at the laboratory next door and make an appointment in your office for one week after the test is done.

#### Poor Technique

**Medical Assistant:** Mr. Fowler, you need to call Johnston Labs to arrange for those tests. We'll see you after the tests are done.

#### Correct Technique

**Medical Assistant:** Mr. Fowler, Dr. King has ordered a glucose tolerance test for you with Johnston Laboratory in Suite 516 of this building. Since you are working, we felt it would be better to have you call them yourself to make the appointment. If you have a paper and pencil, I'll give you the information you need.

The lab is open from 6:30 A.M. to 7 P.M. Monday through Friday. The phone number is 555-1234 and you should ask for Susan at Ext. 23; she makes the appointments. She will need your name, address, phone number, age, social security number, the name and address of your insurance company, and your insurance ID and Plan numbers.

After you make your appointment with Susan, please call me so we can make an appointment for you here for one week later. Dr. King will have your test results by then and will want to go over them with you at that time.

Do you have any questions or do you need any of the information repeated? Fine, I'll speak to you after you talk to Susan and we'll set up your appointment with Dr. King.

- What happened?

- Who is the patient? (Ask name and age.)

- Is the patient breathing?

- Is there bleeding? How much? From where?

- Is the patient conscious?

- What is the patient's temperature?

- If the patient ingested something:

  - What did the patient take?

  - How much?

  - Are there poison or overdose instructions on the bottle?

Triage does not only pertain to emergency calls. Triage techniques can also help determine when a patient with symptoms should be seen. By asking the caller questions such as:

- How long have you had the symptoms?

- Is there any fever?

- Are you taking any medications?

This information helps determine whether an appointment should be scheduled immediately or if it can wait a few days.

The practice should periodically review procedures for handling emergency calls. If an office situation involves a great deal of telephone triage, the staff should enroll in an advanced Red Cross first-aid course. This will enable all participants to more accurately give emergency instructions or to handle these calls if there is no physician in the office at that moment. Remember, **Good Samaritan laws** only protect persons rendering aid *within the areas of their training and expertise*. All ambulatory settings should also post a list of numbers to be used in case of emergencies, such as the poison control telephone number. See also Chapter 9 for more information on triage.

## Angry Callers

Medical assistants will probably have occasion to speak with callers who are angry or upset. Though these calls may eventually need to be referred to the office manager or the physician, medical assistants need techniques for managing problem calls.

The first priority is to diffuse the situation. This cannot be accomplished if you become angry or upset. As a professional, it is important to remain calm and in control at all times. Like most skills, diffusing a difficult situation becomes easier with practice. See Procedure 12-2.

## Elderly Callers

There are several issues that may arise when dealing with elderly patients: impaired hearing, confusion, and an inability to understand procedures or technical information.

Do not assume that all elderly people are senile or hard of hearing. This is a dangerous pitfall into which many people stumble.

If the individual has a hearing impairment, speak more slowly, more clearly, and a little louder than normal. Do not shout. If uncertain that the person has heard everything, ask if there are any questions or ask the person to repeat information back to you.

If the person has difficulty understanding you, simplify the information, ask frequently if there are any questions, and try to explain in simple, concrete terms. At times, if it is difficult to communicate with an elderly patient, someone from the patient's family should be given certain information. Discuss this option with the office manager or physician first.

## English as a Second Language Callers

 In any ambulatory care setting, it is possible to have contact with many patients whose primary language is not English.

It is extremely helpful to have at least one person in the office who is bilingual, particularly in an area such as the Southwest where many people speak a language other than English. For the non-bilingual medical assistant, certain techniques may help when communicating with all but totally non-English speaking patients.

- A patient who does not *speak fluent* English may still *understand* as well as anyone. Do not assume that individuals with strong accents cannot understand you.

- Speak at a normal volume; raising the voice does not increase the other person's ability to comprehend.

- If the other person has difficulty understanding, speak more slowly. Avoid complicated words when simple ones will express the meaning just as well.

- Ask the person if clarification is needed. Be willing to review the information again.

- Be patient.

If these techniques are not successful, it is the responsibility of your physician-employer to provide an interpreter (who may or may not be a member of the patient's family) if necessary.

## PLACING OUTGOING CALLS

When making calls for the medical office, whether to patients, health care facilities, or other physicians, know what information is needed and have it at hand before making the calls.

For example:

● If arranging for a patient to receive care at another facility, have the patient's chart and insurance information. Determine physician instructions as to the diagnosis and type of care (specific tests, x-rays, and so on) that need to be ordered.

● If calling insurance companies for claim follow-up, gather copies of all claim forms in question so you can answer specific questions regarding each claim.

● If scheduling meetings or outside appointments for office physicians, have their schedules in front of you.

Arrange to make outgoing calls from a telephone in a location that is not distracting. If the calls concern patients (whether bills, insurance, or care), it is mandatory that the calls be made from a telephone where you cannot be overheard by other patients or people in the reception area.

Always choose a time when calls can be made without interruption. Arrange for someone else to cover incoming calls during this period and to take messages on any calls that you need to handle personally.

It is best to establish a routine for making various types of outgoing calls. Most offices call the next day's patients to confirm appointments near the end of each day. Collection and insurance calls, as well as pharmacy callbacks, are usually done either before the office is open for patients in the morning, during the period from noon to 2 P.M. when the office is closed for lunch, or after the last patient has been seen.

Procedure 12-3 summarizes guidelines for placing outgoing calls.

## PLACING LONG DISTANCE CALLS

### Placing Calls

Most long-distance calls medical assistants make are likely to be direct dialing calls; that is, calls placed without the help of an operator. To direct dial a local long-distance call, which is a call within the area code but out of the local calling area, dial 1 plus the telephone number; in some parts of the country, it is no longer necessary to dial 1 before the seven-digit telephone number.

For long-distance calls out of the area code, dial 1 plus area code plus number. Nationwide area codes are usually listed in your telephone directory before alphabetical entries. When giving another party the medical office number, always include the area code.

When it is necessary to make an operator-assisted call, dial 0 plus area code plus number. Operator-assisted calls, many of which are automated, include collect calls, person-to-person calls, and occasionally credit card calls.

### Time Zones

When making a long-distance call out of the area code, it is likely that a time zone change may occur (Figure 12-5). When scheduling the day's calls, it is important to keep in

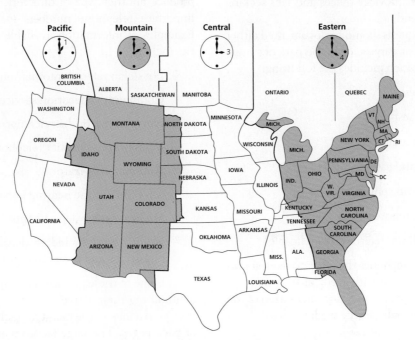

**Figure 12-5**    Time zone map.

mind the location of the call and plan accordingly. Time zones include Pacific, Mountain, Central, and Eastern times and usually span a three-hour difference. If it is noon in New York, it is 11 A.M. in Illinois, 10 A.M. in Arizona, and 9 A.M. in Washington state.

## Long-Distance Carriers

Many companies, some well-known, others new to the market, are competing for long-distance business. Judging the offers and services of long-distance companies can be a complex task, but a wise choice can save an ambulatory care setting hundreds of dollars a year or more in telephone charges. It is important to analyze the medical office long-distance requirements and then make comparisons among several long-distance companies. Company representatives are usually more than willing to discuss their services in light of specific needs to help you comparison shop.

## TELEPHONE DOCUMENTATION

Requests for medical information over the telephone should be discouraged. A physician or facility that needs the information to treat the patient usually places an emergency request. A "call-back" verification procedure should be implemented for this type of request. Request the caller's name and telephone number, and state that you will call back with the necessary information. Then call back to verify the identity of the caller, and provide or fax the information. It is important to follow this procedure during routine telephone interchanges that take place between facilities/provider offices and labs seeking test results or consult findings.

All telephone requests should be documented either in a log reserved for that purpose or in the patient's medical record. Documentation includes the following:

- Date of the request
- Name of the requestor
- The information requested
- Patient's name (and patient number)
- Name of the treating physician
- The information released
- To whom the call was referred (if applicable)

When a patient telephones the office to request prescription refills, is displeased with medical treatment, or expresses some form of a complaint, documentation of the call should always be recorded in the medical chart.

## USING TELEPHONE DIRECTORIES

The medical assistant should have on hand in the office a variety of telephone directories and be skilled in their use. The telephone directory contains an organized, accurate, and complete listing of the name, address, zip code, and area code with telephone number for most individuals with telephone service. Often, the pages within the directory are color-coded; residences listed on white pages, business numbers on blue, and advertisements on yellow pages. The front pages of many directories contain other very useful information such as:

- Information regarding emergency and nonemergency numbers.
- The Internet guide makes it easy to get on-line.
- Information guide and consumer tips provide a variety of free facts and answers about the things you want to buy and the services you need.
- Community pages provide attractions, events, and the general-interest information unique to a particular area. Often, maps are provided on these pages.
- Phone service pages answer questions you may have regarding your phone service.
- Government pages contain information about county, state, tribal, and federal government office as well as information regarding public schools and voter registration information.
- An index makes finding what you need easy.

Many metropolitan medical centers and hospitals produce another type of directory. These directories list important telephone numbers specific to that facility. Examples of information available within these directories include:

- Physician referral information
- Community education services
- Nurse counseling service/nurse line
- Main hospital/facility telephone number
- Automated operator
- TTY line for the hearing impaired
- Medical center departments
- Medical staff including department and photo of physicians and their names with credentials

Some of these publications list physicians no longer maintaining their active/associate privileges at the facility. Often a map of the facility is included within the front or back pages. The large facilities also may produce supplements to maintain current information.

## LEGAL AND ETHICAL CONSIDERATIONS

One of the most important issues in the medical setting is patient **confidentiality**, or right to privacy. Respecting the confidentiality of all patient information is a legal and **ethical** obligation. No information about patients is to be discussed outside the office, with family or friends, or with other patients. Violations of confidentiality leave you and your physician open to lawsuits. More importantly, they are violations of patient trust.

When calling patients, whether to discuss treatment or finances, do so with respect for the patient's privacy at all times. The front desk is certainly not the place to make collection calls when other patients are in the reception room. Either make calls from another location or choose a time when other patients cannot overhear you. Always be aware of the surroundings and who may be able to overhear conversations.

There are many situations when individuals will call the office to discuss a patient. Parents, spouses, grandparents, other relatives, significant others, employers, and friends often will have questions about a patient's condition or finances. Usually these people are asking questions out of genuine concern and a desire to help. The information they request may seem harmless, but discussing anything about a patient can turn into an ethical and legal issue.

See examples on this page.

To ensure patient confidentiality and practice sensible risk management, never discuss a patient with:

- The patient's spouse or family, without specific permission
- The patient's employer
- Insurance carriers, HMOs, or attorneys without a signed release
- Credit bureau/collection agency (reporting a patient to a credit bureau or collection agency is a violation of confidentiality)
- Other patients
- People outside the office (friends, family, acquaintances)

When necessary for medical or administrative reasons, you can discuss a patient with:

- Members of the office staff as necessary to the patient's care
- The patient's insurance carrier or HMO, if you have a signed release
- The patient's attorney (usually in accident or Worker's Compensation cases), if you have a signed release
- The patient's parent or legal guardian, except concerning issues of birth control, abortion, or sexually transmitted disease (check the laws in each state regarding minors' right to privacy)
- Another health care provider (physician, lab, or hospital) that is providing care to the patient under orders from the patient's physician
- Referring physician's office

## TELEPHONE TECHNOLOGY

Though much of this chapter has been dedicated to the interpersonal nature of telephone communications, astute medical assistants will also investigate and become knowledgeable about the technology of telephone communications.

Ongoing advances in telecommunications have had a tremendous impact on how the staff of a medical office communicates both within the office and with patients, hospitals, and others outside the office. These advances include telephone systems with automated routing units (ARUs); electronic transmissions (fax and e-mail); cellular telephones; and paging systems.

---

### EXAMPLES: LEGAL AND ETHICAL

#### Situation 1

A medical assistant called the home of a patient inquiring about the delinquent status of his account. The patient was not home, but his wife answered the phone. The medical assistant discussed the situation with the patient's wife, who wanted to know what the charges were for. Upon checking the file, it was discovered the patient had been tested for a sexually transmitted disease.

#### Situation 2

A patient's employer calls to find out "how Boris is doing and when he can come back to work. We really miss that guy!" The medical assistant, who just saw Boris in the reception area yesterday, responds without thinking, "Oh, he seems to be doing great, I'll bet you'll have him back in a few days." If he had checked the patient chart, he might have seen that Boris was filing a disability claim as well as a negligence suit against the employer for unsafe working conditions. He might also have seen that Boris is still in physical therapy and on pain medication or that he may have permanent problems as a result of the accident.

## Automated Routing Units

Many hospitals and larger ambulatory care settings have **automated routing unit (ARU)** telephone systems to manage heavy telephone traffic. The system answers the call and a recorded voice identifies departments or services the caller can access by pressing a specified number on the Touch-Tone telephone. If callers indicate they are having a medical emergency, the system can be programmed to immediately route calls to the medical assistant. This saves patients with immediate medical problems from waiting during busy telephone times.

Some automated telephone systems have electronic mailboxes so the caller can leave a message if the person they are calling is unavailable. In many ARU systems, selecting any of the numbered choices often gives the caller a second, third, or fourth menu of choices. If the caller does not select an option, the ARU will usually switch the call automatically to a "live" operator.

A disadvantage with ARU systems is that the recorded voice may be difficult to hear, especially for elderly or hearing-impaired patients. Many patients may not understand the recorded options. Offices with an ARU system should provide an information sheet to all patients explaining their options when calling the office and how to get through to the office quickly in an emergency.

## Answering Services and Machines

One responsibility of the office manager/medical assistant is to ensure that patient calls are answered after office hours, both on evenings and weekends. While in smaller ambulatory care settings it may not be possible to have staff on telephone duty twenty-four hours a day, nonetheless calls must be answered and messages taken. **Answering services**—typically staffed by a live operator—and answering machines are two methods of taking calls after hours.

Many ambulatory care centers favor answering services because a live operator is reassuring to patients and other callers. These services also can provide flexibility in routing calls and locating the physician for emergencies. Typically, fees for answering services are by the month or by the number of calls.

Answering machines are convenient but perhaps less reassuring for the caller. The machine must be checked frequently for messages should an emergency occur. Sometimes, the message may leave a telephone number where the physician can be reached, but this system is likely to be cumbersome, for too many nonemergency calls may be directed to the physician. If an answering machine is used, the message often contains a number, other than the physician's, that callers can use for emergencies. That call is answered by a live operator who then screens and refers the call appropriately.

## Facsimile (Fax) Machines

Fax machines are more and more common in the ambulatory care setting as they are used to send reports, referrals, insurance approvals, and informal correspondence. A **fax** is a **facsimile** transmission sent over telephone lines from one fax machine to another or from a modem to a fax machine. A fax document may contain data like typed characters, photographs, or line art.

 While fax machines are a great timesaver for the ambulatory care setting, confidentiality is a critical issue for fax machines are typically located in centralized areas where documents may be seen by unauthorized personnel. Before sending any document, be sure it will not violate confidentiality, have permission to transmit it by fax, and attach a cover sheet that stipulates the information is for the intended recipient only. Review fax machine information contained in Chapter 16.

## Electronic Mail

**Electronic mail (e-mail)** is the process of sending, receiving, storing, and forwarding messages in digital form through telephone lines. E-mail can save time and money. Instead of having to make personal or telephone contact, the sender can leave a message in an electronic mailbox via a computer where it can be retrieved by the receiver at a convenient time. Insurance inquiries lend themselves to this type of communication system. If a response is required, it can often be returned by the same system. If it is not retrieved within a certain amount of time, some electronic mail systems either send a printed copy of the message or delete the message from the system.

Another advantage of e-mail is flexibility. When computers are networked, electronic mail can substitute for the interoffice memo with one staff member composing information on the computer screen to be automatically transmitted to all members of a medical facility. Any message stored can be brought up on a computer screen and saved to a disk or printed.

It is possible to subscribe to an on-line computer information service that incorporates an e-mail system and communicate with any other users on the system around the world. Medical assistants, medical transcriptionists, medical billing services, and others subscribe to these services to network information to each other. These services also feature bulletin boards (electronic method of exchanging information publicly). Some of these computer information services are known as America On-Line, CompuServe, and Prodigy. Review the electronic mail section found in Chapter 16.

## Cellular Service

Since the 1980s **cellular telephones** have become very popular and are now available and used in all populated areas of the country. Cellular communication offers convenience and flexible communication. The telephones themselves are available in many models and sizes and some can even fit in the palm of the hand. Many physicians have car and/or portable phones allowing immediate verbal contact with their office or hospital staff.

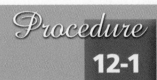 Cellular signals are not secure, which means that other people may be able to listen to the conversations with certain scanning radios. Therefore, staff and physicians should be very careful not to use patients' full names or reveal any confidential information over the cellular phone. Cellular phone usage is much more expensive than using traditional telephone lines, so calls should be kept brief and to the point.

## Paging Systems

Another telecommunication option available is the use of pagers or "beepers." Hospitals have used paging systems for many years both inside the hospital and for physicians on call. Several types of paging systems are available, and many physicians now use the same type of pagers available to individual consumers. Some paging system options include:

1. Voice alerts. The voice message is automatically heard by the person being paged. Not only does the person being paged hear the message but anyone in the vicinity will hear it as well.
2. Beep alerts. The pager emits a beeping sound or silent vibration that notifies the person being paged to call one designated phone number to obtain the message.

3. Digital message display.
   a. Alphanumeric display: displays the message on a digital screen. The message can include an entire typed message via a computer modem or through an operator who will input the message and transmit it to the receiver. The receiver can scroll through the text message and save or delete messages as needed.
   b. Numeric display: displays the callback telephone number on small screen. The number displayed is selected by the person initiating the page.

Pagers are not as convenient as cellular phones because they allow only one-way communication; cellular phones allow automatic two-way communication between caller and receiver. However, pagers are less expensive to use and typically have a set monthly charge while cellular phone bills include a monthly rate plus charges for each minute of phone use, whether the call is made or received by the user.

### DOCUMENTATION

In the log reserved for telephone documentation, the following entry could be made based on Case Study 12-2.

07/16/-- Claussen-Mason Laboratories requested previous laboratory findings from Qwik Lab in Nashville, Tennessee, for Juanita Hansen, patient number 306-30-7840. Juanita is a patient of Dr. King. The information was released to Janet Bailey, employee of Claussen-Mason Laboratories as directed by Dr. King. W. Slason 7/16/--.

## *Procedure*

### 12-1   Answering Incoming Calls

**PURPOSE:**
To answer telephone calls professionally, acquiring all necessary information from the caller, documenting it correctly, and properly acting on it.

**EQUIPMENT/SUPPLIES:**
Telephone
Message pad
Appointment calendar
Pen or pencil

**PROCEDURE STEPS:**
1. Be prepared. Have materials such as a message pad, notepad, appointment calendar, sharpened pencils, and working pens nearby. RATIONALE: Being ready for calls conveys professionalism and lets the caller know you are prepared to assist.
2. Answer the telephone promptly. The phone should not ring more than three times before it is answered. RATIONALE: Callers may become annoyed and hang up if a call is not answered within a reasonable time.

*(continues)*

# *Procedure*
## 12-1    *(continued)*

3. Answer the call with the preferred office greeting, speaking directly into the mouthpiece. The mouthpiece should be 1 to 2 inches away from the mouth. For example, "Good morning. Doctors Lewis and King. Ellen speaking." RATIONALE: Take a breath before answering the phone, put a smile on your lips, and use a pleasant tone of voice to convey a warm greeting. Holding the phone correctly and speaking directly into the mouthpiece aid the caller in hearing your message clearly.

4. Ask the name of the caller as quickly as possible, and determine if this is an emergency call. RATIONALE: Using the caller's name personalizes the call and acknowledges that you heard the name correctly. If this is an emergency call, follow emergency protocols.

5. Focus on the call. Concentrate on dealing with the call, and put aside other work. RATIONALE: This gives the caller a sense that you are listening attentively, and information will be transmitted correctly. You are less apt to have to ask the caller to repeat information or to record it incorrectly.

6. Repeat information back to the caller. RATIONALE: This technique confirms facts are complete and accurate. The caller also has opportunity to hear the message and confirm that it is accurate or may wish to modify the message meaning for clarity.

7. When using a multiline telephone as shown in Figure 12-6, it is helpful to keep a notepad by the telephone. When you answer the phone and have the caller's name, jot the name, which line the caller is on, and some quick notes about the content of the call. RATIONALE: Using this simple technique avoids problems if another line rings and you must put the first person on hold. No matter how many incoming lines there are, you will not forget who is on which line or what the call is about.

8. Ask if the caller has any other questions. RATIONALE: This saves you and the caller time. It is frustrating to have to place a second call because you forgot to ask something. It also ties up the telephone lines.

9. End the call courteously. Say "thank you" and "goodbye" (not "bye-bye"). RATIONALE: Saying goodbye conveys professionalism and leaves the caller with a positive image of the office.

10. Let the caller hang up before you disconnect. RATIONALE: Often callers think of questions just as they are ready to hang up. It is more time efficient to handle the question immediately rather than have the caller have to return a call.

11. Document information, and record any future actions necessary. RATIONALE: This procedure is necessary for legal reasons. Remember, a deed not documented is a deed undone in a court of law.

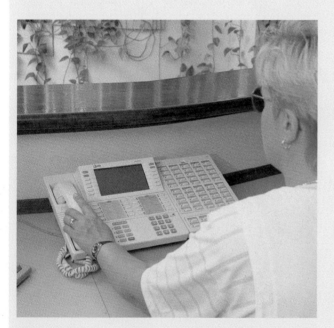

**Figure 12-6**    An example of a multiline telephone system.

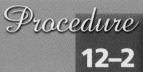

## 12–2    Handling Problem Calls

**PURPOSE:**
To handle calls in a positive and professional manner while providing necessary comfort, empathy, and information to the caller to resolve the problem.

**EQUIPMENT/SUPPLIES:**
Telephone
Message pad
Pen or pencil

**PROCEDURE STEPS:**

1. Remain calm and avoid becoming upset with an angry caller. Let the caller say what needs to be said without interruption (unless it is a medical emergency requiring immediate action). RATIONALE: This permits the caller to express concerns without having to repeat information or to forget something important.
2. Lower your voice both in pitch and volume. RATIONALE: This technique has a calming effect on an angry caller.
3. Listen to what the caller is upset about. Paraphrase information for verification that you have understood the problem. RATIONALE: This technique lets the caller know you are truly listening and have understood the problem.
4. Use the words "I understand" and show that you are interested in hearing the caller's concerns. RATIONALE: This does not necessarily mean you agree with the caller but that you are willing to empathize and at least accept that, from a particular point of view, there is a reason to be upset.
5. Do not take the call personally. RATIONALE: It is the situation that made the caller angry; you have not done so.
6. Offer assistance. RATIONALE: Ask what you can do to help, and then follow through.
7. Document the call accurately and properly. RATIONALE: Complete documentation promotes risk management and prevents lengthy litigation experiences.
8. When dealing with a frightened or hysterical caller, speak in a soothing voice; use a slower, lower tone than normal. RATIONALE: This often has a calming effect on the caller.
9. If the call is an emergency, begin triage procedures as needed. RATIONALE: Have a list of triage questions at hand to refer to or instruct the caller to dial 9-1-1. Be sure you have the name and telephone number for followup.
10. Always have the caller repeat instructions. RATIONALE: People who are upset may not hear or comprehend much of what is said. Your instructions may deal with an emergency situation, so it is important they are clearly understood.
11. Finalize and follow through on action to be taken, whether it is to confirm emergency medical personnel are on the scene or scheduling an emergency appointment. RATIONALE: Ensure quality patient care.
12. Always report problem calls to the physician or office manager at once. RATIONALE: This will ensure appropriate action is taken, and it is important for risk management purposes.

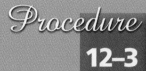

## 12–3    Placing Outgoing Calls

**PURPOSE:**
To place calls efficiently and effectively.

**EQUIPMENT/SUPPLIES:**
Notepad
Pen or pencil
All materials specifically applicable to the call

**PROCEDURE STEPS:**
1. Preplan the call by preparing all materials in front of you prior to making the call; for example, gather telephone number, chart, financial information, or appointment book. Also, have notes of questions you have or information you need to relay. RATIONALE: This technique uses time efficiently and conveys professionalism.
2. Make calls from a location and telephone that will not be disrupted with noise and distractions.

RATIONALE: This type of location permits you to concentrate on the call without distractions or interruptions.
3. Try to schedule specific times of the day for calls; for example, early morning before patients arrive, midday, or after the last patient has been seen. Be aware of the time zone you are calling, so you do not disturb people at inappropriate times. RATIONALE: Return calls to outside labs or consulting physicians may be done early in the morning before patients arrive and offices become busy with patient loads. Midday may be an appropriate time to call in prescription refills or reminders of appointments.
4. Use appropriate language and tone following proper telephone techniques. RATIONALE: Ensure that your message is conveyed clearly and understood accurately.

---

**12-1**

Audrey Jones, the young clinical medical assistant at Doctors Lewis and King, was on telephone duty on a busy Thursday afternoon. This was only the third or fourth time Audrey was responsible for answering incoming calls, but her energy and quick judgment saw her through some difficult situations when all the lines were ringing at the same time. Audrey just received a call; a young man is calling about his mother, a patient of Dr. Lewis, who is having trouble breathing.

### CASE STUDY REVIEW

1. What are the critical questions Audrey should ask the young man to triage the situation?
2. How will Audrey's training and background in Red Cross first aid help her assess the situation?
3. If Audrey needs to give medical information over the telephone, what limits should she respect?

---

**12-2**

Wanda Slawson, Clinical Medical Assistant at Inner City Health Care, receives a telephone call from Claussen-Mason Laboratories requesting medical information about patient Juanita Hansen. Wanda is told by lab personnel that the information is needed to perform the tests scheduled by Dr. King. Wanda is not familiar with this request and asks if she can check the chart and return a call to the lab (call-back verification procedure).

### CASE STUDY REVIEW

1. What information will Wanda need from Claussen-Mason Laboratories?
2. What is the purpose of the call-back verification procedure?
3. After the verification has been established, what should Wanda do?

## SUMMARY

Proper telephone techniques require the medical assistant to have excellent communication and listening skills. The ability to convey warmth and reassurance is vital to patient relationships. Efficiency and organization are also key elements in effectively managing the variety of telephone calls answered and placed in the ambulatory care setting. Medical assistants responsible for incoming and outgoing calls need to be able to perform telephone triage, screen calls, take messages, and refer calls professionally and efficiently.

Medical assistants also need to be aware of telephone technology in order to choose and productively use the office's telephone systems. An understanding of technology can result in savings of both time and money for the efficient ambulatory care setting.

## REVIEW QUESTIONS

### Multiple Choice

1. Positive first impressions are conveyed over the telephone by:
   a. using the hold button sparingly
   b. being authoritative with the caller
   c. not permitting the caller too much leeway to speak
   d. working while talking on the telephone
2. Basic telephone techniques involve:
   a. volume, enunciation, pronunciation, and control of speed
   b. being assertive with the caller
   c. not spending too much time talking
   d. referring all calls to the physician
3. Buffer words:
   a. are necessary for clarity
   b. confuse the caller
   c. are used to avoid clipping off the office name
   d. are not considered introductory words, phrases, or statements
4. Guidelines that ensure successful transfer of calls include all of the following *except:*
   a. determine who would be the best person to assist
   b. follow your telephone system's procedure for transferring the call
   c. followup to be sure the call transferred correctly
   d. getting the caller's name and telephone number is not necessary
5. Medical assistants should refer calls to the physician when:
   a. an appointment needs to be scheduled
   b. a patient has a billing question
   c. a salesperson is planning a call
   d. a patient requests test results
6. Triage:
   a. is the act of evaluating the urgency of a medical situation and prioritizing treatment
   b. is expressing oneself clearly and distinctly
   c. uses expendable words while answering the telephone
   d. is the ability to be objectively aware of and have insight into others' feelings, emotions, and behaviors
7. In handling a problem call, the medical assistant should:
   a. take it personally
   b. listen calmly to the upset person
   c. become upset to identify with the patient
   d. ask emotionally charged questions to calm down the patient
8. The "call-back" verification procedure:
   a. should never be documented
   b. should always be documented
   c. should sometimes be documented
   d. is not appropriate in the ambulatory office setting
9. ARU telephone systems:
   a. transmit over telephone lines via modem
   b. involve transmissions sent from one fax machine to another
   c. use a recorded voice that identifies departments or services the caller can access by pressing a specified number
   d. process messages in digital form through telephone lines
10. Pagers or beepers are:
    a. useful for calling back patients
    b. old technology
    c. capable only of one-way transmission
    d. now replaced by fax machines

### Critical Thinking

1. When is it acceptable to put a caller on hold?
2. What can you do to improve your sound on the telephone?
3. List six types of calls that must be referred to the physician.

4. Why should complaints be referred to the physician or office manager instead of managed by the staff?
5. What is triage?
6. List six questions you might ask to evaluate the urgency of a call.
7. What are the eight elements necessary to a proper telephone message?
8. When taking a message for someone, what information do you always give the caller?
9. When giving the physician a message from or about a patient, what should always be attached?
10. Describe how to properly transfer a call to someone else in your office.
11. How would you handle an angry caller?
12. If an individual is hearing impaired, what three changes do you make in the way you speak to them?

## WEB ACTIVITIES

 Using the World Wide Web, search for current information relative to legal and ethical considerations when using the telephone in the ambulatory care setting. Compile your information into a one-page report, and list your URL addresses for your instructor.

## REFERENCES/BIBLIOGRAPHY

Hosley, J. B., Jones, S. A., & Molle-Matthews, E. A. (1997). *Lippincott's textbook for medical assistants.* Philadelphia: Lippincott, Williams, and Wilkins.

Humphrey, D. D. (1996). *Contemporary medical office procedures* (2nd ed.). Albany, NY: Delmar.

Kinn, M. E., & Woods, M. A. (1999). *The administrative medical assistant* (4th ed.). Philadelphia: W. B. Saunders Company.

Saunders, J., & McGee, R. R. A. (1996). *Patient confidentiality.* Salt Lake City, UT: Medicode, Inc.

# PATIENT SCHEDULING

## KEY TERMS

Clustering
Double Booking
Established Patient
Matrix
Modified Wave
New Patient
No-Show
Open Hours
Practice-Based
Slack Time
Stream
Triage
Wave

## OUTLINE

**Tailoring the Scheduling System**
**Types of Scheduling Systems**
    Open Hours
    Double Booking
    Clustering
    Wave
    Modified Wave
    Stream
    Practice-Based
**Analyzing Patient Flow**
    Waiting Time
    Flexibility
**Legal Issues**
**Interpersonal Skills**
**Guidelines for Scheduling**
    **Appointments**
    Triage Calls
    Referral Appointments

Recording Information
Computer Scheduling
Patient Check-In
Patient Cancellation and
    Appointment Changes
Computer Cancellations
Reminder Systems
Scheduling Representatives
**Scheduling Materials**
    Appointment Books
    Appointment Sheets
    Daily Worksheets
    Computer Equipment
    Appointment Cards
**Establishing an Appointment**
    **Book**
**Informational Brochure**

## OBJECTIVES

*The student should strive to meet the following performance objectives and demonstrate an understanding of the facts and principles presented in this chapter through written and oral communication.*

1.  Define the key terms as presented in the glossary.
2.  Review six of the major scheduling systems.
3.  Describe the six considerations in scheduling appointments.
4.  Explain the importance of triage in scheduling patient appointments.
5.  Review proper cancellation procedures and explain the legal necessity of documenting cancellations.
6.  Recall three types of reminder systems.

(continues)

7. Choose an appropriate appointment scheduling tool and describe its advantages.

8. Establish a matrix for a new year and a new practice.

9. Prepare a daily appointment sheet. Describe how it differs from a daily worksheet.

10. Describe the purpose and content of a patient informational brochure.

## ROLE DELINEATION COMPONENTS

**ADMINISTRATIVE**

**Administrative Procedures**

- Schedule, coordinate, and monitor appointments
- Schedule inpatient/outpatient admissions and procedures

**CLINICAL**

**Patient Care**

- Adhere to established triage procedures

**GENERAL (TRANSDISCIPLINARY)**

**Communication Skills**

- Receive, organize, prioritize and transmit information
- Serve as liaison
- Promote the practice through positive public relations

**Legal Concepts**

- Document accurately

**Instruction**

- Explain office policies and procedures

**Operational Functions**

- Apply computer techniques to support office operations

## SCENARIO

At Inner City Health Care, medical assistant Walter Seals is responsible for efficient patient flow. Because Inner City is an urgent care center, patients are seen as walk-in appointments, on a first-come, first-served basis unless there is an emergency situation. Inner City also operates specialty care clinics, and these clinics require scheduled appointments. Walter has found that the clustering system is most efficient for these specialized care clinics, with certain days dedicated to certain procedures.

Because of the high volume of patients and the need to coordinate multiple physician schedules, Walter's job is not an easy one. However, Inner City is computerized, so paperwork is easy to generate as appointments are made, canceled, or rescheduled. And while Walter manages a smooth patient flow, he makes it a point to remain flexible to accommodate patient needs and keep stress to a minimum.

## INTRODUCTION

While patient appointment scheduling may seem like a routine function, a smooth patient flow often determines the success of a day in the ambulatory care setting. A variety of administrative skills are utilized in the performance of this vital office function. By effectively scheduling patients to fit a particular practice, it is possible to make profitable use of physician and staff time.

In addition, efficient patient flow is satisfying to the patient. A common patient complaint is the time spent waiting in the reception area. Most patients appreciate an office that recognizes the value of patients' time. Accordingly, these patients do not hesitate to advertise their experience (good or bad) to friends and families—a fact of great significance to any medical office.

In addition to the required administrative skills, medical assistants involved in scheduling patients must put into practice their interpersonal and communication skills. Scheduling an appointment may be the first contact patients have with the medical office. They remember and value the treatment they receive from the time of first contact. The personality of the ambulatory care setting is always reflected in the treatment and respect accorded to patients.

# TAILORING THE SCHEDULING SYSTEM

The schedule of each medical office will determine the best method for scheduling appointments. A surgeon's office will have a much different flow of patients than a pediatrician's office. The key is to customize the system to best accommodate the practice. Primary goals in determining this should include:

- a smooth flow of patients with a minimal amount of waiting time for the patients

- flexibility to accommodate acutely ill, STAT (or emergency) appointments, work-ins, cancellations, and no-shows

# TYPES OF SCHEDULING SYSTEMS

There are a number of methods for patient scheduling. The best method for a practice is the one that effects good patient flow and proper utilization of staff and physical facilities.

## Open Hours

In open hours scheduling patients are seen throughout a particular time frame; e.g., 9:00 A.M. to 11:00 A.M. or 1:00 P.M. to 3:00 P.M. Patients sign in and are seen on a first-come, first-served basis. Emergency rooms and many clinics frequently choose this method as they are able, by their nature, to maintain a steady flow of patients.

## Double Booking

With the double-booking method, two or more patients are given a particular appointment time. This method is limited to a practice where patients can be attended to more than one at a time. For instance, Maria Jover and Jim Marshal are both given a 9:30 A.M. appointment. Ms. Jover requires a complete checkup including lab tests, vitals, and so on. Mr. Marshal is being seen for suture removal. While the physician's staff conducts the lab tests on Ms. Jover, the physician can be seeing Mr. Marshal. Obviously, this method requires a precise accounting for time and rooms and adequate staff. A good rule to remember is that if patients are consistently having to wait for staff to attend to them, double booking is not a wise choice of method.

## Clustering

The clustering method utilizes the concept used in production line work, namely that performing only one step or process allows for efficient processing. In the ambulatory care setting, patients with similar problems are booked consecutively. Obstetricians and pediatricians commonly choose this method. A block of time, either hours or days of the week, is set aside for particular types of cases. For instance, an obstetrician might see only third trimester patients on Mondays and Fridays and gynecology patients on Tuesdays and Thursdays. A pediatrician's office might be organized for immunizations on Tuesday mornings and well-baby checkups on Monday and Friday afternoons.

## Wave

Wave scheduling is another method that can be used effectively in medical facilities that have several procedure rooms and adequate personnel to staff them. Using the wave scheduling system, patients are scheduled in the first half hour of each hour. This method takes into account the fact that there will be no-shows and late arrivals. It can also accommodate work-in appointments. However, it does require personnel who are able to triage patient problems precisely when establishing the appointments.

## Modified Wave

This is a variation of the wave method where patients are scheduled in "waves." In the modified wave method, two or three patients are scheduled at the beginning of each hour, followed by single appointments every 10 to 20 minutes the rest of the hour.

A variation of this method assesses major and minor problems (Figure 13-1). Major time-consuming problems are seen at the beginning of the hour; e.g., new patients. Minor problems are seen from 20 minutes past the hour to half past the hour; e.g., follow-ups, bandage changes, and other minor procedures, and walk-ins; e.g., a child with a 103° temperature, are accommodated at the end of the hour. Again, good triaging will determine the success of this method.

With both the clustering and wave methods, empty or unscheduled periods can be used for dictation or the processing of paperwork.

## Stream

Stream scheduling is perhaps the best known and most widely used scheduling system. When this system works as it should, there is a steady stream of patients at set appointment times throughout the workday; e.g., 30-minute appointment at 9:00 A.M.; 15-minute appointment at 9:30 A.M.; 15-minute appointment at 9:45 A.M. Each patient is assigned a specific time. This can best be

| TIME | TYPE OF APPOINTMENT |
|------|---------------------|
| 8:15 | Major |
| | |
| | |
| 8:20 | Minor |
| 8:50 | Work-in |
| 9:00 | Major |
| | |
| 9:20 | Minor |
| | |
| 9:50 | Work-in |
| 10:00 | Major |
| | |
| 10:25 | Minor |
| 10:40 | Work-in |
| | |
| 11:00 | Major |
| | |
| | |
| 11:25 | Minor |
| 11:45 | Minor |

**Figure 13-1** Modified wave variation. Major problems are scheduled at the beginning of the hour, minor problems scheduled 20 to 30 minutes past the hour, and work-ins toward the end of the hour.

accomplished by establishing time guidelines for particular types of appointments such as 60 minutes for returns, 15 minutes for immunizations, and 30 minutes for a hearing test.

## Practice-Based

As discussed earlier in this chapter, some ambulatory care settings find it necessary to develop a system unique to their patient load. In these customized systems (**practice-based**), the practice determines the schedule. An orthopedist might schedule cast removals on Mondays and Fridays using double booking and stream scheduling for new patients with each patient having a 60-minute appointment. A group of vascular surgeons might employ both a double-booking and a modified-wave system. They might double book patients for short rechecks and quick procedures, while using the modified wave for patients with pre- and postoperative checks and long specialty procedures.

There are many variations on these basic scheduling systems. Some offices use double booking for quick follow-ups and clustering for all new patients. Other facilities use

open hours for most patients but 15-minute interval appointments for follow-ups. Another system of double booking is to schedule follow-up calls in a two-column book while scheduling new patients for half-hour appointments. The medical assistant responsible for appointment scheduling will use the system that enables the ambulatory care setting to function smoothly and efficiently.

## ANALYZING PATIENT FLOW

When setting up a new practice or reviewing current scheduling practice, a simple analysis can maximize an office's scheduling practices. This entails looking at appointment times, patient arrival times, the actual time a patient is seen, and the time a visit is completed. A simple grid chart can be produced for a given period of time; e.g., one to two weeks (Figure 13-2). In addition, chart the number of no-shows and cancellations.

This analysis should provide a clear picture of patient flow and whether office personnel are being utilized efficiently. The data will assist in estimating how many patients to schedule and realistic time frames for particular problems or procedures. If the physician is scheduling return patients every 15 minutes yet the analysis shows these visits average 24 minutes, the scheduling method needs adjustment. This may mean either allowing 25 minutes for follow-up visits or building in slack time, or unscheduled time, where no appointments are made.

Develop a simple list of commonly scheduled visits with time estimates for each. This procedural sheet will be particularly useful when training new employees or when temporary help is utilized for scheduling (Figure 13-3).

## PATIENT FLOW ANALYSIS

February 2, 20—

| Patient Name | Length of Appt. | Appt. Time | Dr. King Time Seen | Time Out |
|--------------|-----------------|------------|--------------------|----------|
| Martin Gordon | 15 | 10:20 | 10:22 | 10:45 |
| Jason Jover | 45 | 11:20 | 11:20 | 12:30 |
| Nora Fowler | 30 | 1:00 | 1:25 | 1:45 |
| Jim Marshal | 15 | 1:30 | 1:50 | 2:10 |
| Herb Fowler | 60 | 2:45 | 2:15 | 3:25 |

**Figure 13-2** Patient flow analysis helps a practice determine realistic time frames for appointments.

## TYPICAL SCHEDULING TIMES FOR INTERNAL MEDICINE PRACTICE

New patients . . . . . . . . . . . . . . . . . . . . . . . . 30 minutes
Patients for consultation . . . . . . . . . . . . . . . 45 minutes
Patients requiring complete
   physical examinations . . . . . . . . . . . . . . . . 45 minutes
All other patients (minor illnesses,
   routine checkups, etc.) . . . . . . . . . . . . . . 15 minutes

**Figure 13-3** Most practices will have a list of typical visits with time estimates.

## Waiting Time

One of the most frequently voiced frustrations with physicians' offices is excessive waiting time. Obviously, emergencies and other unexpected interruptions cannot be anticipated. However, there are certain measures one can take when attempting to keep the schedule on target. If patients are kept waiting, it is a better strategy to explain the reason for the delay and give patients an estimate of how long the delay will be. *Never* ignore the delay hoping patients will not notice; this, in fact, seems to increase perceived waiting time. Find ways to make patients comfortable while they wait; e.g., providing an appropriate choice of reading materials (or in the case of children, activities). If a delay can be anticipated, e.g., the physician was called away for a delivery or surgery, attempt to contact patients before they leave home to reschedule the appointments.

If the delay is likely to be a half hour or longer, provide patients with options:

1. Offer patients the opportunity to run an errand, having them return at a specified time.
2. Offer to reschedule appointments for another day or later in the day.

In any case, remember that good customer relations dictate your willingness to acknowledge the inconvenience to the patients and attempt to provide an acceptable solution. Remember also that some patients simply will not appreciate any efforts to apologize for a delay, in which case you must continue to act professionally toward them.

## Flexibility

One principal above all else in scheduling is be *flexible*. Policies should be established to ensure effective patient flow; however, it is more important to meet the needs of patients. At times, patients cannot be scheduled according to the structured appointment times, and the medical assistant will need to decide how to best accommodate their needs.

In every ambulatory care setting, emergency patients must be seen. This situation can be handled in a variety of ways. After determining through triage that it is an emergency, the patient is most often told to come into the office and will be seen as soon as possible. (See Triage Calls in this chapter.) Some offices refer patients to the emergency room, thus minimizing disruption to other patients. Other offices let scheduled patients know of the emergency and offer them the opportunity of rescheduling or waiting until the emergency patient has been seen. A built-in slack time of 30 minutes in the morning and 30 minutes in the afternoon can provide some flexibility in last-minute scheduling.

## LEGAL ISSUES

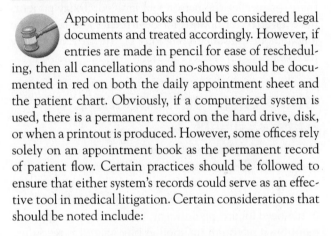

Appointment books should be considered legal documents and treated accordingly. However, if entries are made in pencil for ease of rescheduling, then all cancellations and no-shows should be documented in red on both the daily appointment sheet and the patient chart. Obviously, if a computerized system is used, there is a permanent record on the hard drive, disk, or when a printout is produced. However, some offices rely solely on an appointment book as the permanent record of patient flow. Certain practices should be followed to ensure that either system's records could serve as an effective tool in medical litigation. Certain considerations that should be noted include:

1. The Internal Revenue Service (IRS) can legally demand records from the beginning of a practice. While they generally do not go back more than three to five years, compared to other documents required for legal purposes, the space required for patient records seems minimal compared to the value these permanent records might have to IRS or litigation proceedings.
2. Many facilities make it a practice to keep appointment books in pencil because of the ease of making changes in the schedule. If this is the practice, ensure that there is a typewritten daily appointment sheet as a permanent legal record of each day's appointments.

Remember that anyone looking into a practice will be looking at the record of documentation. Taking the time to accurately and consistently document all aspects of patient care makes a statement about the physicians in the practice and their staff and reflects positively on the presumed quality of patient care.

## INTERPERSONAL SKILLS

Scheduling appointments requires interpersonal skills. Medical assistants convey a great deal to patients through attitude and actions. A hurried or disinterested manner communicates that the patient is not a priority. Because patients are often distraught or anxious when making appointments, it is extremely important to reduce rather than increase anxiety. Also, the medical assistant scheduling appointments may be the first contact a patient has with the office; patients do not easily forget rude or insensitive staff. A hurried, disinterested manner toward patients is more often the basis for legal action than is a negligent act.

The patient should always be made to feel worthy of attention. If scheduling a patient in the office and the phone rings, answer the call but excuse yourself first. Ask the caller to please hold for a moment. If on the telephone scheduling a patient and another patient walks in, acknowledge with a nod or signal that you will be right there—never let the person feel ignored. Today patients have a variety of options for health care and tend to be much more consumer-conscious of the treatment they receive.

## GUIDELINES FOR SCHEDULING APPOINTMENTS

Whether completed by manual methods or computer technology, the process of scheduling appointments for patients and other visitors to the ambulatory care setting involves a number of variables, including (1) the urgency of the need for an appointment; (2) whether the appointment has a referral from another physician, (3) recording methods for new and established patients; (4) implementation of check-in, cancellation, and rescheduling policies; (5) use of reminder systems; and (6) accommodating visits from medical supply and pharmaceutical company representatives.

Recently, the *Wall Street Journal* reported on physicians in some health maintenance organizations who are paid by a salary rather than by patient visit, experimenting with group scheduling. The group visits may be set up around patients with specific chronic ailments such as diabetes, hypertension, or geriatric complaints. While not yet widely accepted, it is one alternative to keep costs down while maintaining patient/physician relationships in providing health care.

### Triage Calls

Urgent calls will need to be triaged, or assessed, before they can be scheduled. In other words, the office personnel making the appointment will need to determine the actual urgency of that call and determine how the patient can best be scheduled. This requires a combination of both communication skills and medical knowledge.

Appropriate questions need to be asked to determine the actual urgency. Is the patient in immediate need of medical assistance? Is there any bleeding? Are there chest pains? The medical assistant needs to determine if this is a life-threatening matter or if the problem is "urgent" in the patient's eyes but not an emergency.

In triaging, also obtain information that will assist in determining the urgent nature of the call. How long have the symptoms/complaint been present? If there is bleeding or discharge, where is the origin? How profuse is it? If it is pain, how intense is it? Is it localized? Precise information will assist the physician in determining the critical or noncritical nature of the call.

In triaging the patient's urgency of care, be tactful in questioning and avoid making the patient feel that the need is insignificant. If questioning indicates this is a medical emergency, follow office policy for having the patient seen (whether it be an emergency appointment or referral to the emergency room). If it is determined that the situation is not an emergency, work the patient into the schedule as the situation warrants and time allows. Be sure to leave the patient with the understanding that you have done your best to address the situation. For more information on triage, see Chapters 9 and 12.

### Referral Appointments

One of the primary sources for a physician's practice base is physician referrals. This is especially true in a managed care climate, where patients usually must have a referral from their primary care physician and where physicians are part of an HMO network. It is important that these appointments be given special consideration and that referred patients be given an appointment as soon as possible.

Adequate information needs to be obtained to determine the urgency of scheduling. If the referring physician or office staff calls directly, the situation can be triaged at that time. However, if the referred patient calls, it is best to obtain necessary records and/or information from the referring physician to determine the urgency and appropriateness of an appointment. This can be done by obtaining general information from the patient and then scheduling an appointment after the physician's office is contacted for complete information regarding the patient's condition. Be polite and assure the patient of an appointment as soon as the referring physician is contacted.

### Recording Information

Patients can be sensitive to the amount of information they are required to provide to make an initial appointment. Keep the information as simple as possible and obtain only essential information. It should be tailored to fit the practice; e.g., an obstetrician and a pediatrician will have very different questions for the first-time patient.

Generally, these basic items should be obtained from a **new patient**, someone being seen for the first time in the office:

1. The patient's full legal name (with the correct spelling)
2. A daytime telephone number
3. The chief complaint or reason for the visit
4. The referring physician, if relevant.
   Repeat this information back to the patient to assure accuracy.

 Some offices today, particularly those with computerized scheduling and billing, will require a few additional items:

1. Date of birth
2. Type of insurance
3. Insurance number

The critical determination is whether the information is essential to the first contact or whether it could be obtained at the time of the visit.

An **established patient**, someone who has already been seen in the office, should require only:

1. Full legal name
2. Chief complaint or reason for the visit
3. A daytime telephone number

When the information is recorded, print it legibly and accurately in a manual system, and check for accuracy in the same manner when using a computer system for scheduling. Record the appointment as soon as it is made—never rely on memory.

When scheduling an appointment time, ask the patient what day and time would be most convenient for them and then make the appointment for the first available time stated. If possible, provide the patient with a choice of possible appointment times. Finally, confirm that the patient clearly understands the date and time of the appointment; be sure to repeat the date and time to ensure that both of you have recorded the same information. Spell the patient's name back if confidentiality is assured. If the patient is making the appointment in person, provide them with an appointment card (Figure 13-4).

Scheduling an appointment for the office's available times for a parent who works outside the home, serves in a carpool, and is a coach for the gymnastics or swim team can require a great deal of patience. If the patient requests a particular appointment and this is not possible, courteously offer an explanation.

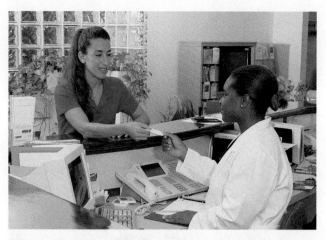

**Figure 13-4**   Provide patients with appointment cards neatly printed with the date and time of their next appointment.

## Computer Scheduling

 Typically, when using a computer system for scheduling, the program will search through a database of appointments, find an open appointment, and allocate an appointment time according to your instructions. These instructions can include finding an open appointment with a specific time length, on a specific day, or within a specified time frame. Once the appointment time is confirmed with the patient, patient data is keyed in and the appointment is automatically scheduled.

Software programs vary in their functions and capabilities; it is always advisable to network with other ambulatory care settings to discover their program likes and dislikes before choosing and purchasing scheduling software.

## Patient Check-In

Records of patient appointments serve a legal purpose. Establishing a procedure for checking in appointments simplifies tracking of the arrival of patients. (See Procedure 13-1.) This is particularly true in multiphysician settings or offices where a number of staff are attending to patients before, or instead of, seeing the physician.

There are offices where patients are required to sign a check-in list.

A word of caution here. The patient's right to privacy requires that patients do not see the names of other patients. Patients may be reluctant to sign in on such a list and it is within their legal rights to refuse. It is a better policy for the office staff to check the patients off on a list (Figure 13-5). When a patient checks in, a red √ or other appropriate mark should be used in the appointment book.

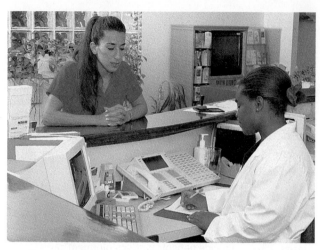

**Figure 13-5** The medical assistant/receptionist should be able to see patients as they enter the office. Patients may sign themselves in, or preferably check in with the medical assistant who will keep the patient check-in list current.

## Patient Cancellation and Appointment Changes

When using pencil on a manual appointment book system, a permanent record of no-shows should be designated on the appointment sheet with a red **X**. Cancellations should be marked through on the appointment sheet with a single red line (Figure 13-6). Computer scheduling will provide an area to indicate no-shows and cancellations also. No-shows and cancellations should always be noted in the patient's individual chart. Again, it is imperative that the physician's care of the patient be thoroughly documented. Should a patient develop complications and claim the physician was unavailable, the daily appointment sheet and chart should document the patient's failure to show.

Many offices have established firm policies for multiple no-shows and/or cancellations. The general rule is that after three no-shows and/or cancellations in a row, the physician will review the records. In order for the physician to adequately treat a patient, the patient's cooperation is necessary. A no-show pattern may indicate that the patient is not truly committed to assisting in treatment. If a patient routinely cancels or does not show, the physician will write a letter terminating services and explaining why the physician is discontinuing care. This should be sent by certified mail, return receipt requested, to ensure that the patient received the notice. See Chapter 9 for more information on termination of services and Chapter 15 for information on certified mail. Procedure 13-2 outlines the proper cancellation procedures.

| | | MONDAY, NOVEMBER 23 | |
|---|---|---|---|
| | | Dr. King | Dr. Lewis |
| 7 | 00 | | |
| | 15 | | |
| | 30 | | |
| | 45 | | |
| 8 | 00 | Hospital | |
| | 15 | | Surgery |
| | 30 | Rounds | |
| | 45 | | |
| 9 | 00 | Abigail Johnson - Black | Lenore |
| | 15 | Diabetes Check/466-2964 | McDonell |
| | 30 | Marge O'Keefe/CPE/296-7234 | |
| | 45 | | |
| 10 | 00 | | Joseph Ortiz/New Pt/462--1121 |
| | 15 | | |
| | 30 | Nora Fowler/Back Pain/466-2234 | Maria Tover/Stomach Problems/292-2104 |
| | 45 | | |
| 11 | 00 | Jim Marshal/CPE/763-2067 | Maria Tover/Stomach Problems/292-2104 |
| | 15 | | |
| | 30 | Partners | Partners |
| | 45 | | |
| 12 | 00 | | |
| | 15 | | |
| | 30 | | |
| | 45 | | |
| | | Lunch Meeting | Lunch Meeting |
| 1 | 00 | Matt. Hanes/Consultation/763-3284 | Boris Bolski/New Pt./466-8156 |

**Figure 13-6** Multiphysicians' office where physicians' commitments and no-shows are marked with a red "X" and cancellations are marked with a single red line. Other offices may have slightly different systems for tracking appointments, but in all offices all no-shows and cancellations should be marked in the patient's record.

## Computer Cancellations

While software programs differ, cancellations are typically performed by deleting the patient's name from the time slot: if the appointment is to be rescheduled, the name is then keyed in to the appropriate time. The first time opens for other appointments.

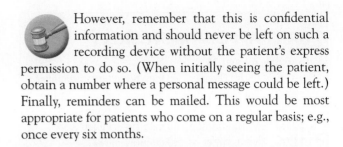

When canceling appointments by computer, be certain that the program maintains a list of canceled appointments including patient name, date, and time. This documentation is necessary for legal purposes; also record canceled appointments on the patient chart.

## Reminder Systems

Studies have shown that reminding patients of appointments results in a higher rate of fulfilled appointments. There are three ways of reminding patients of appointments. Appointment cards are the most obvious and perhaps the most widely used method. However, the card may be tucked in a wallet and forgotten. Many offices call patients in the afternoon to remind them of an appointment the next day. This can be particularly effective in this day and age with voice mail and message machines.

However, remember that this is confidential information and should never be left on such a recording device without the patient's express permission to do so. (When initially seeing the patient, obtain a number where a personal message could be left.) Finally, reminders can be mailed. This would be most appropriate for patients who come on a regular basis; e.g., once every six months.

## Scheduling Representatives

Every medical office needs to schedule time with representatives of pharmaceutical and medical supply companies. These representatives can provide a valuable service to physicians and patients and with clear guidelines regarding when and how often representatives can visit, a working partnership can develop. Most physicians set aside a specific time during the week to meet with these representatives; generally a time allotment of 15 to 20 minutes is sufficient for these appointments.

## SCHEDULING MATERIALS

Whether using a manual system for scheduling patients or a computer system, a thorough understanding of the manual system is helpful in understanding the whole process of patient scheduling. Materials needed for scheduling should be customized to the ambulatory care setting. For instance, a smaller practice may prefer a manual method involving appointment books; a large urgent care-type setting may use a computer program for patient scheduling. Increasingly, all appointment scheduling is done by computers. No matter what materials and which methods are used, the proper tools will enable patient scheduling to be a smoothly functioning, easily documented process.

## Appointment Books

An appointment book appropriate to the medical practice is essential to any ambulatory care setting. Each office has unique needs in its physical facilities and staff. This applies to the appointment book as well. In addition to the physical arrangement of the date pages, there are various combinations of time allotments. Some books have major headings for hours with minor spaces for 15-minute intervals. Others have 10-minute intervals, and others only hour intervals.

## Appointment Sheets

Another vital tool in efficient patient flow is a daily appointment sheet, which provides a permanent record for both legal risk management and quality management purposes. Figure 13-7 is a sample of a daily appointment sheet.

## DAILY APPOINTMENT SHEET

**Thursday, August 21**

| | | | |
|---|---|---|---|
| 9:15 | Chris O'Keefe | 30 minutes | Immunizations |
| 9:30 | Jim Marshal | 15 minutes | Blood pressure check |
| 10:00 | Martin Gordon | 60 minutes | PE/lab work |
| 11:00 | Nora Fowler | 30 minutes | URI |
| 2:00 | Maria Jover | 30 minutes | Suspicious rash |
| 4:00 | Joseph Ortiz | 30 minutes | Choking problems |

**Figure 13-7** Daily appointment sheet.

## DAILY WORKSHEET

**Thursday, August 21**

| | | | |
|---|---|---|---|
| 8:00 | Hospital Rounds | | |
| 9:15 | Chris O'Keefe | 30 minutes | Immunizations |
| 9:30 | Jim Marshal | 15 minutes | Blood pressure check |
| 10:00 | Martin Gordon | 60 minutes | PE/lab work |
| 11:00 | Nora Fowler | 30 minutes | URI |
| 11:30 | Lunch break | | |
| 12:30 | Dentist Appointment, Dr. Schleuter | | |
| 2:00 | Maria Jover | 30 minutes | Suspicious rash |
| 2:45 | Meet with drug rep regarding new beta-blocker agents | | |
| 4:00 | Joseph Ortiz | 30 minutes | Choking problems |

**Figure 13-8** Daily worksheet.

Using the daily appointment sheet, it is easy to check off shows, **no-shows**, and cancellations. If the sheet is double-spaced, walk-ins can easily be written in (in ink). For quality management purposes, check-in times can be indicated as well as check-out times. Perhaps more importantly, the daily appointment sheet assists the physician and staff and enables them to see the total scheme of the day's patient flow. If a physician works between two clinics or a hospital and office, it is helpful to have available a pocket-sized edition of the daily appointment sheet for easy referral. This is a simple task with today's reduction feature on many photocopiers—reduce the schedule and secure onto a 3 × 5 index card.

### Daily Worksheets

Some offices may also use daily worksheets that include not only patient appointments but also other physician commitments such as meetings and visits from pharmaceutical representatives. This is helpful in scheduling work-in and emergency appointments, as an empty section of time on a sheet with only patient appointments may in fact be booked for another purpose. Figure 13-8 is a sample of a daily worksheet.

### Computer Equipment

Although computers greatly simplify the scheduling process, the same guidelines as those required in a handwritten system will need to be employed. Obvious advantages are that appointments can be quickly changed and a daily list of appointments generated. There is also an easily accessible source of vital information on a patient without having to pull the chart.

There are a number of software programs specially designed for scheduling of appointments, such as *The Medical Manager*, published by Delmar Publishers. Many of them can be customized for individual office needs.

### Appointment Cards

In addition to the appointment book, offices should have available appointment cards. Studies show that fewer patients report at the wrong time or forget appointments when provided with an appointment card (Figure 13-9).

## ESTABLISHING AN APPOINTMENT BOOK

After selecting the type of appointment book that is most appropriate, the book must be readied for scheduling of patients.

Procedure 13-3 outlines the key steps in establishing the appointment **matrix**. Once these steps have been followed and information recorded, the appointment book is ready for patient scheduling. If done properly, the appointment book will serve as a valuable tool in effecting good patient flow and promoting satisfied clientele.

M _____

**HAS AN APPOINTMENT ON**

☐ MON. ☐ TUES. ☐ WED. ☐ THUR. ☐ FRI. ☐ SAT.

DATE _____ AM / PM

**LESLIE TRAYNOR D.D.S.**

500 WEST PARK AVENUE NEW YORK, NY 10012

TELEPHONE (202)555-9876

IF UNABLE TO KEEP APPOINTMENT KINDLY GIVE 24 HOURS NOTICE

**Figure 13-9** Sample appointment card.

# Inner City Health Care

*Meeting Families' Total Health Care Needs*

**C**ommitment to Patient Care

Our staff is committed to providing our patients with the best in medical care. We view your medical care as a team effort—providing you with qualified medical staff while encouraging you to be active participants in your total care. This brochure is designed to help you understand how our practice can best serve you. You are a very important part of our practice and we welcome your questions and comments.

**P**rofessional Staff

We are pleased to service the metropolitan area with a well-trained staff of physicians and support staff. Our team of physicians is available to meet your medical needs, assisted by our registered nurses, and certified medical assistants, lab technicians, and radiology technicians. Our urgent care clinic is an alternative to expensive emergency room visits and is open Monday through Saturday.

**S**ervices

We provide your family with complete medical facilities through our on-site diagnostic services, including X rays and clinical laboratory. In addition, we are located within five minutes of the local hospital should more extensive services be required. Our **triage line** is available 24 hours a day to assist in assessing problems.

**S**cheduling

To better serve you, we utilize different methods of scheduling your visits.

In our **Urgent Care Center**, no appointments are necessary. Patients will be seen on a first-come first-served basis, but patients with an urgent need for care will be attended to first. We do, however, request that you call the office first to let us know you are coming. The Urgent Care Center is best suited for problems that arise unexpectedly (fevers, flus, fractures, etc.).

Our **Clinics** require scheduled appointments. General medical appointments are made every day during regular hours. We make every attempt to see you as close to your scheduled appointment time as possible. Our **specialty clinics** utilize a clustering system so that we reserve certain days and times for particular types of appointments. These are as follows.

**Orthopedics**—Cast removals,
Mon/Wed 9 AM - 3 PM
Tues/Fri 11 AM - 7 PM
**Obstetrics**
Mon/Wed 9 AM - 2 PM   Friday 1 - 7 PM
**Gynecology**—Tues and Thurs, 9-7
**Pre-Surgery**—Mon-Fri, 9 AM - noon
**Vascular Lab**—Tues and Thurs, 1-7 PM

**C**ancellations

We request you provide 24 hours notice of an appointment cancellation. You will be billed $20 if you fail to show without notifying our office at least one hour in advance.

**P**ayment Plans

To assist you in obtaining proper medical care and minimizing your concerns for cost, we have established several methods of payment. We directly bill Blue Cross/Blue Shield, HMO Michigan, Shield Care, Care Michigan, and Medicare/Medicaid. Our **billing coordinator**, Karen Ritter, CMA, will be happy to assist you in setting up payment plans if you do not have insurance coverage. In addition, we accept pre-approved credit card payments.

**F**or More Information

Our staff is here to assist you with questions and concerns you may have. Please refer to the following phone numbers for quicker service with specific needs:

**Billing**
Karen Ritter, CMA, 555-7155, ext. 4

**Insurance Preauthorization**
Jane O'Hara, CMA, 555-7155, ext. 12

**Lab Results**
555-7155, ext. 22

**Appointment Scheduling**
555-7158

**Triage Line**
555-7159

**Clinic #1**
**Office Hours:**   Monday-Thursday, 9-7
Closed Friday

**Clinic #2**
**Office Hours:**   Monday, Wednesday, and
Friday, 10-7, Saturday, 10-3
Closed Tuesday and Thursday

**Dr. Brown's Hours:**
Clinic #1—Monday-Thursday, 9-2
Clinic #2—Monday & Wednesday, 2-7
Friday, noon-7, Saturday, 9-4

**Dr. Rice's Hours:**
Clinic #1—Monday-Thursday, 2-7
Clinic #2—Monday & Wednesday, 10-2,
Friday, 10-12

**Urgent Care Center**
**Office Hours:**   Monday-Friday, 9-8
Saturday, 9-2

**Dr. George's Hours:**
Monday & Wednesday, 9-5
Friday & Saturday, 9-2 every other week

**Dr. Woo's Hours:**
Monday and Wednesday, 1-8
Friday & Saturday, 9-2 every other week

**Dr. Reynolds' Hours:**
Tuesday, 1-8, Wednesday, 9-1, Thursday, 9-2,
Friday, 9-2

**Dr. Esposito's Hours:**
Monday, 9-8, Tuesday, noon-8, Wednesday, 4-8,
Thursday, 11-8, Friday, 3-8, Saturday, 9-2

**Dr. Whitney's Hours:**
Tuesday, 9-8. Thursday & Friday, 11-8,
Saturday, 9-2

**Figure 13-10**   Informational brochure.

## INFORMATIONAL BROCHURE

Informed patients make better clients. This is as true with scheduling as it is with procedural changes. A simple brochure on scheduling practices can elicit the cooperation of patients and reduce the time spent with explanations when efforts are required for other duties. See sample brochure in Figure 13-10.

In the facility brochure, list office hours. If a clustering system is used, explain to patients what this involves and why they may not be able to get an appointment for the particular day they desire. Provide simple instructions on what information is required by the medical office to make an appointment. Explain policies regarding cancellations and no-shows. In a tactful manner, emphasize to patients that their cooperation in observing scheduled times and cancellation procedures helps your office serve them better. For more information on developing patient brochures, see Chapter 22.

---

## *Procedure* 13-1     Checking in Patients

**PURPOSE:**
To ensure the patient is given prompt and proper care; to meet legal safeguards for documentation.

**EQUIPMENT/SUPPLIES:**
Patient chart
Required forms
Check-in list and/or appointment book

**PROCEDURE STEPS:**
1. The evening before or prior to opening the ambulatory care setting, prepare a list of patients to be seen and assemble the charts.
2. Check charts to see that everything is up to date.
3. When patients arrive, immediately acknowledge their presence. If you cannot assist them right away, acknowledge their presence, and then thank them for waiting.
4. Check the patient in, reviewing vital information such as address, telephone number, insurance, and reason for visit. **Be certain to protect the patient's privacy by reviewing this information where doing so cannot be overheard by others.**
5. Use a pen to check the patient's name off in the appointment book and/or day sheet if one is used for the permanent record.
6. Politely ask the patient to be seated and indicate the appropriate wait time, if any.
7. Following office procedures, place the chart where it will be used to route the patient to an appropriate location for the visit.

---

## *Procedure* 13-2     Cancellation Procedures

**PURPOSE:**
To protect the physician from legal complications; to free up care time for other patients; to assure quality patient care.

**EQUIPMENT/SUPPLIES:**
Appointment sheet
Pen (red)
Patient chart

*(continues)*

## *Procedure* 13-2 (continued)

**PROCEDURE STEPS:**

Develop a system so it is evident to staff making appointments that, due to cancellations, time is now open to schedule other appointments. Indicate on the appointment sheet all appointments that were changed, canceled, or failed to show by:

1. *Changes:* Note changes in the appointment sheet margin and directly in the patient's chart and indicate the new appointment time.

2. *Cancellations:* These should be noted also on both the appointment sheet and the patient chart. Draw a single red line through canceled appointments. Be sure to date and initial notations in the patient chart.

3. *No-shows:* These should be noted in both the appointment book and the patient chart. Be sure to date and initial notations in the chart. No-shows can be indicated with a red X on the appointment sheet.

## *Procedure* 13-3 Establishing the Appointment Matrix

**PURPOSE:**

To have a current and accurate record of appointment times available for scheduling patient visits.

**EQUIPMENT/SUPPLIES:**

Appointment book
Physician's schedule
Staff schedule
Office calendar

**PROCEDURE STEPS:**

1. Block off times in the appointment book when patients are not to be scheduled by marking a large "X" through these time slots. This establishes the matrix. Ideally the whole year can be mapped out to avoid scheduling patients when the physician has other commitments or when the office is closed.

2. Write in all vacations, holidays, and other office closures as soon as they are known. It may be helpful to indicate absences that might affect patient scheduling; e.g., the vascular lab tech is gone April 20–23 so no Dopplers will be scheduled.

3. Write in all physician meetings, hospital rounds, appointments, conferences, vacations, and other prescheduled physician commitments. If the physician has routine items, such as a Medical Society meeting that is always held on the first Thursday of the month at 7:00 P.M. or daily hospital rounds at 8:00 A.M., write these in.

4. If the office has a scheduling system for certain examinations or procedures; e.g., all cast removals are done in the morning before 10:30 A.M., these can be color-coded with highlighters. This way it is easily and quickly evident where particular types of appointments are available to be scheduled.

CASE STUDY 13-1

Rhoda Au has persistently canceled her appointments at Inner City Health Care; while she always reschedules, she has canceled the last four appointments. Today, she did not call to cancel nor did she show up for her fifth appointment. Walter Seals, CMA, who is responsible for scheduling and patient flow, is concerned that Rhoda is canceling because she is afraid to come in for some reason. Rhoda has been a patient for a few years now, and she was always responsible about keeping her appointments.

## CASE STUDY REVIEW

1. From the point of view of the urgent care center, why should Walter be concerned that Rhoda is canceling appointments? What action might be taken?

2. From the patient point of view, why should Walter be concerned?

3. How should Walter record these cancellations and no-shows if using a manual method of scheduling? If using a computer program?

## SUMMARY

Today's ambulatory care setting needs to function efficiently to provide quality care, ensure adequate patient flow, and maintain positive patient relationships. Proper scheduling of patients and other visitors is key to an efficient operation, and the well-organized medical assistant will design a system that meets with both physician and patient satisfaction.

There are at least six common methods of scheduling; ambulatory care settings should use the one that is most appropriate to their patient population, practice areas, and physician preferences. Scheduling methods can and should be customized to the setting, for this usually provides the most adaptable, workable system.

Patient scheduling tools, too, vary and can be tailored to facility needs. While all ambulatory care settings must carefully document appointments, cancellations, and no-shows, they may do so by either manual methods or computer technology. Whichever method is chosen, the goal is to use that tool wisely and consistently in all scheduling activities.

## REVIEW QUESTIONS

### Multiple Choice

1. Appointment books should always be:
   a. recorded only in pencil
   b. recorded only in red ink
   c. left out on the front desk where patients enter
   d. a current and accurate record and saved as documentation
2. Triaging:
   a. involves taking only emergencies
   b. is assessing the urgency of a call and need for appointment
   c. means sorting appointments by specialized procedure
   d. is only performed by physicians
3. Representatives from medical supply and drug companies:
   a. should only be seen as a last resort
   b. should not be scheduled, but seen only if the physician has time

   c. can provide a valuable service and should be scheduled for short visits
   d. have complex information to communicate and need one-hour appointments
4. The double-booking method:
   a. gives two or more patients the same appointment time
   b. keeps patients waiting unnecessarily
   c. is never the system of choice
   d. is purely for the physician's convenience
5. The stream method:
   a. gives patients appointments as they walk in
   b. schedules appointments at set times throughout the workday
   c. only works in one-physican offices
   d. refers to streamlining paperwork for each appointment
6. Daily appointment sheets:
   a. indicate when physicians and staff take lunch
   b. provide a permanent record for legal risk management and quality management

   c. are available only in computerized patient scheduling
   d. both a and b

7. Analyzing patient flow:
   a. can maximize an office's scheduling practice
   b. often reveals why patient flow is not efficient
   c. may indicate a change in pattern for patient scheduling
   d. all of the above

8. One principal above all else to be observed in scheduling is:
   a. always schedule in ink
   b. schedule for the patient's convenience
   c. be flexible
   d. referral patients are first

9. If a patient must wait for an appointment:
   a. it is best to say nothing about the delay
   b. explain the delay and offer options when possible
   c. find ways to make the patient comfortable
   d. both b and c

## Critical Thinking

1. Discuss the rationale and the procedure to follow for a canceled appointment and a no-show appointment.
2. Describe the following appointment systems: Stream; cluster; modified wave. Give examples of each.
3. Why is there no one best system of scheduling?

*Form small discussion groups and develop solutions to the following problems by (1) defining the problem, (2) describing the appropriate steps if required, and (3) developing a possible solution.*

4. Lenore McDonnell has called to cancel her appointment for the third consecutive time. (Background: Her last blood pressure reading in the office was 195/115, and there is a known history of stroke in her family.)
5. Dr. Lewis is running an hour behind schedule. It is now 1:00 P.M. He is just seeing a return patient. He has two new patients scheduled and has a surgery scheduled for 2:00 P.M. (Background: Return patients require 30 minutes and new patients 60 minutes.)
6. Your urology office has been using a double-booking system. Through tracking the patient flow, you find that patients are having to wait consistently half an hour or longer. (Background: There is one medical assistant and two examination rooms.)

7. You are using the modified-wave system. You have three appointments scheduled for 10:00 A.M., one for 10:50 A.M., and three for 11:00 A.M. The office closes at 11:30 for lunch so Dr. King can speak at a hospital luncheon. A patient calls and insists to be seen on an emergency basis. (Background: Dr. King's partner is unavailable to cover for her.)
8. Two patients are scheduled to be seen at 11:30. It is now 11:50 and Dr. Whitney has indicated that he will not be through with his current patient for another 20 minutes. (Background: Both patients waiting to see Dr. Whitney are for nonemergency problems.)

*For the following situations, briefly explain which type of appointment book and scheduling system you would choose and why.*

9. A four-physician practice has only two physicians seeing patients at any one time. There are three medical assistants sharing front and back office duties for all of the physicians.
10. An obstetrics practice specializes in problem pregnancies. There is one front and one back office medical assistant.

## WEB ACTIVITIES

 Research the World Wide Web for information related to the types of appointment books and/or computer software that might be appropriate to the ambulatory care setting for patient scheduling. What features might you especially want to have?

## REFERENCES/BIBLIOGRAPHY

Fordney, M. T., & Follis, J. J. (1998). *Administrative medical assisting* (4th ed.). Albany, NY: Delmar.

Humphrey, D. D. (1996). *Contemporary medical office procedures* (2nd ed.). Albany, NY: Delmar.

Martinez, B. (2000, August 21). Now it's mass medicine. *The Wall Street Journal*, p. B1.

Montone, D. (1997). *Power building in scheduling.* Philadelphia: W. B. Saunders Co.

3. Recall eight common supplies used in medical records management.
4. Name ten of the twenty rules described under Basic Rules for Filing.
5. Describe the five steps commonly used when filing any documentation.
6. State three advantages and three disadvantages of the alphabetic filing system.
7. Name the two other filing systems most often used in the ambulatory care setting.
8. Analyze the purpose of cross-referencing.
9. Recall four common documents filed in the patient's medical record.
10. Describe computer databases and their usefulness to the ambulatory care setting.

## ROLE DELINEATION COMPONENTS

**ADMINISTRATIVE**

**Administrative Procedures**

- Perform basic clerical functions

**GENERAL (TRANSDISCIPLINARY)**

**Legal Concepts**

- Maintain confidentiality
- Prepare and maintain medical records
- Document accurately

**Operational Functions**

- Apply computer techniques to support office operations

## SCENARIO

Consider a situation that might arise at the multiphysician Inner City Health Care. Patient Juanita Hansen was seen on Tuesday morning by Dr. Whitney for acute stomach pain. She was given a thorough examination and sent for appropriate testing that afternoon. She was then scheduled to return to Inner City on Friday to see Dr. Whitney.

After she was seen Tuesday morning, Juanita received an upper and lower GI series; the results were then sent to Dr. Whitney's office. However, because Karen Ritter, the medical assistant, could not locate Juanita's chart to file the test results, she just set them aside. Friday arrived and Juanita came back to Inner City for her appointment, anxious to know the results of her tests. Dr. Whitney found Juanita's chart, which was inadvertently left on his stack of dictation, and realized the patient's test results had not been filed.

This left Dr. Whitney with a very anxious patient. Karen Ritter is off today so the physician checks with the other medical assistants on duty. They have no knowledge of the test results. Two acts—not replacing the file and not promptly filing Juanita's test results—cause undue stress for the physician, medical assistants, and the patient.

## INTRODUCTION

With the vast number of medical records that must be maintained in the ambulatory care setting today, accurate filing of patient charts is the only method by which a facility can efficiently track information vital to patient care. Current medical litigation requires every health care facility to have an efficient filing system and staff who are experienced in using and maintaining medical records.

Medical assistants are often vitally involved in developing filing systems and maintaining accurate tracking of patient records.

Physicians provide the best care for patients when all pertinent data is readily accessible. The medical assistant in charge of filing and retrieving records must file information accurately and retrieve the file efficiently.

# THE IMPORTANCE OF ACCURATE MEDICAL RECORDS

Accurate medical records are essential to patient care in any ambulatory care setting. Patient files are critical to the facility's smooth functioning and are important when referring the patient to outside specialists with whom the facility may need to coordinate care. Each treating physician must be aware of tests, procedures, and diagnoses. Maintaining a conscientious record of patient care is also absolutely essential in controlling the costs of medical care.

Medical records management is also important due to the legal issues that every medical office and health care professional must face today. The standard in court is that if there is no written record of a temperature, a visit, a history or physical, a lab report, and so forth, it did not happen. To be prepared in the event of medical litigation, all medical treatment must be documented. No matter how competently a physician has performed treatment, if a written record cannot prove how and what was done, there is no basis for a defense in a court of law.

## EQUIPMENT AND SUPPLIES

There are three primary types of file cabinets used in medical offices. These include vertical, lateral, and movable file cabinets.

## *Vertical Files*

Vertical files are cabinets that have pull-out drawers where files are stored (Figure 14-1). Files are retrieved by

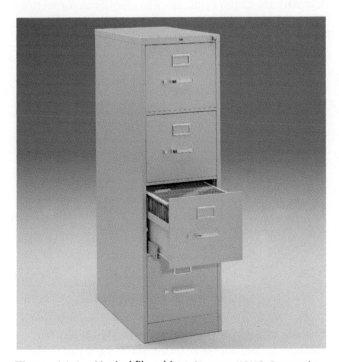

**Figure 14-1** Vertical file cabinet. (Courtesy HON® Company)

## SPOTLIGHT ON AAMA ESSENTIALS THROUGH CAAHEP

While the medical assistant should never share the contents of the patient's medical record, it is important to be sensitive to the patient's desire to know what is being written on the medical record and to share the patient's request for information with the physician.

● When obtaining subjective information from the patient, it is important not to allow your own biases to enter into the discussion, and to record only what the patient states in his or her own words.

● When recording the patient's history, always be careful not to allow the patient's responses to be overheard by others.

lifting the appropriate file up and out. These may be used for business records and documents.

## *Open-Shelf Lateral Files*

These are open file cabinets that make quick retrieval of files possible (Figure 14-2). The records are retrieved by pulling them out laterally from the shelf. They are used most often with color-coded filing systems where visual inspection makes it possible to ensure files are kept in the proper order.

## *Movable File Units*

Movable file units allow easy access to large record systems and require less space than vertical or lateral files. These units may be electrically powered to move on floor

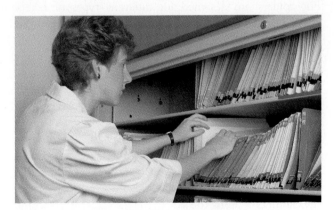

**Figure 14-2** Open-shelf lateral file cabinet.

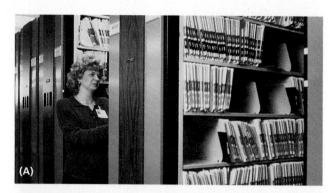

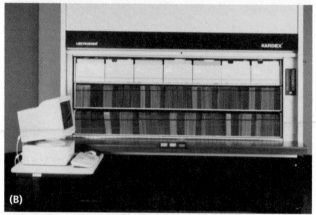

**Figure 14-3** Movable file units: (A) Kompakt movable shelving; (B) Lektriever vertical carousel with computer unit. (Courtesy of KARDEX Systems, Inc., Marietta, OH)

tracks or may be physically moved with an easy-to-turn handle mechanism. The movable shelving unit shown in Figure 14-3A is electrically powered to open aisles for accessing files or to close aisles when those files do not need to be accessed. There are also movable file storage units that will automatically travel on a computer-controlled carousel track moving files around until the required section reaches the operator, Figure 14-3B.

## File Folders

File folders are designed for different types of labels. Extending along the top edge (the edge that will be visible when filing) are tabs that are cut in varying sizes and positions to allow for different methods of labeling. Figure 14-4 shows the types of cuts, or tabs, found on file folders.

## Identification Labels

A variety of labels are used to display the information required to select the correct name or number designation for a particular file. The identification label is adhered either along the top of the file folder (top tab) in vertical file cabinets or along the side of the file folder (side tab) in lateral file cabinets.

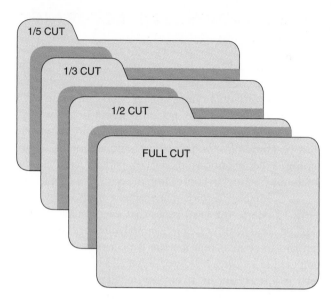

**Figure 14-4** Types of cuts, or tabs, on file folders.

## Guides and Positions

Guides are used to separate file folders. Guides are somewhat larger than file folders and are of heavier stock. Guides are described by the position of the tab, designated according to its location. For instance, a tab located at the far left would be in the first position, the next one to the right would be in the second position, and so forth. If using third-cut file folders, there are three positions of guides; if using fifth-cut file folders, there are five positions.

**Captions.** Captions are used to identify major sections of file folders by more manageable subunits (AA–AC, A, B, Office Supplies). Captions are marked on the tabs of the guides (Figure 14-5). These are denoted as single caption and double caption.

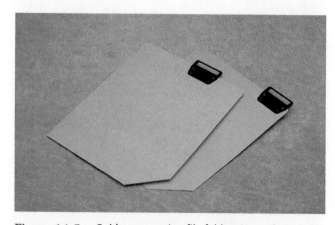

**Figure 14-5** Guides separating file folders into subsections. Captions such as A, B, C (single captions) or Ab–Be, Co–Dy (double captions) are placed on the tabs of the guides to identify the sections.

● **Single captions** contain just one letter, number, or unit:
  - A, B, C, D
  - Adams, Smith, Jones

● **Double captions** contain a double notation to denote a range of files:
  - Ab–Be, Co–Dy, Ho–Le
  - Appleston–Bertram, Cody–Devoe

## Out Guides

Out guides or out sheets are a device to help in tracking charts. An out guide is a cardboard or plastic/paper sheet kept in place of the patient chart when charts are removed from the filing storage (Figure 14-6).

## BASIC RULES FOR FILING

Regardless of the type of filing system used, alphabetizing is the key to organizing files and charts. It is easily recognizable that Adams would be filed before Benson, as A comes before B. In what order, though, are Winston Adams and Winston Alexandar Adams filed? What about Joseph Lee Masters, III and Joseph Lee Masters, Jr.? Is Northwest Diagnostic filed before or after North West Diagnostic? It is necessary to know more than just the alphabetic order of the letters A to Z. Thus, certain indexing rules have been developed to facilitate the alphabetic process in maintaining files in the medical office.

## Indexing Units

There must be an organized method of identifying and separating items to be filed into small subunits. This is accomplished with the use of what we call indexing units. A unit identifies each part of a name. In this process each unit is identified according to unit 1 (the key unit), unit 2, unit 3, and so forth, with each segment of the filing

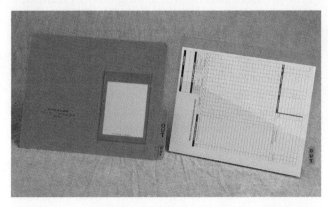

**Figure 14-6** An out guide indicating the name of the person who has possession of the file should always be put in place of a patient's record when it is removed from the file.

label identified. This process can be applied to individual names, organizations, or clinics. Accepted filing rules describe how to assign unit numbers to each element.

**Example.** Annette Barbara Samuels

| | |
|---|---|
| Unit 1 | Samuels |
| Unit 2 | Annette |
| Unit 3 | Barbara |

When working in a medical setting with patient charts the patient's legal name is always used for the chart rather than a nickname or abbreviation. If the office has a practice of calling patients by preferred names, a note of name preferences and nicknames may be noted on the chart. However, the filing label should use the proper name.

**Example.** The following items to be filed would be assigned units as illustrated:

| | Units Assigned | | |
|---|---|---|---|
| | **1** | **2** | **3** |
| Cole Blanche Little | Little | Cole | Blanche |
| Wayne Lee Elder | Elder | Wayne | Lee |
| Kelso Medical Supply | Kelso | Medical | Supply |
| GT Pharmacy | GT | Pharmacy | |

## Filing Patient Charts

**Rule 1.** The names of individuals are assigned indexing units respectively: last name (surname), first name, middle and succeeding names.

| | Units Assigned | | |
|---|---|---|---|
| | **1** | **2** | **3** |
| Jaime Renae Carrera | Carrera | Jaime | Renae |
| Lee Allen Au | Au | Lee | Allen |
| Bill Hugo Schwartz | Schwartz | Bill | Hugo |
| Dottie Marie Tate | Tate | Dottie | Marie |

**Rule 2.** Foreign language prefixes are indexed as one unit with the unit that follows. Spacing, punctuation, and capitalization are ignored. Such prefixes include *d, da, de, de la, del, des, di, du, el, fitz, l, la, las, le, les, lu, m, mac, mc, o, saint, sainte, san, santa, sao, st, te, ten, ter, van, van de, van der,* and *von der* (*st, sainte,* and *saint* are indexed as written).

| | Units Assigned | | |
|---|---|---|---|
| | **1** | **2** | **3** |
| Gerald Steven St. Simon | Stsimon | Gerald | Steven |
| Carol Louise del Rio | Delrio | Carol | Louise |
| Richard Saint Louis | Saint | Louis | Richard |

**Rule 3.** Titles are considered as separate indexing units. If the title appears with first and last names, the title is considered to be the last indexing unit. When dealing with patient charts, the first name always accompanies the title and last name.

**Units Assigned**

| | 1 | 2 | 3 | 4 |
|---|---|---|---|---|
| Dr. Marlene Elaine Smith | Smith | Marlene | Elaine | Dr |
| Prof. Marcia Tai Lewis | Lewis | Marcia | Tai | Prof |

**Rule 4.** Names that are hyphenated are considered as one unit.

**Units Assigned**

| | 1 | 2 | 3 |
|---|---|---|---|
| Adele Marie Johnson-Smith | Johnsonsmith | Adele | Marie |
| Ray Steven Reynolds-Martin | Reynoldsmartin | Ray | Steven |

**Rule 5.** When indexing names of married women, the name is indexed by the legal name. Remember that patient charts are legal documents, making this practice necessary (see cross-referencing to use husband's name).

**Units Assigned**

| | 1 | 2 | 3 | 4 |
|---|---|---|---|---|
| Amy Sue Sung (Mrs. John) | Sung | Amy | Sue | Mrs John |
| Tami Jo Strizver (Mrs. Todd) | Strizver | Tami | Jo | Mrs Todd |

**Rule 6.** Seniority units are indexed as the last indexing unit.

**Units Assigned**

| | 1 | 2 | 3 | 4 |
|---|---|---|---|---|
| James Edward Brown Jr. | Brown | James | Edward | Jr |
| Manuel Louis Garcia III | Garcia | Manuel | Louis | III |

**Rule 7.** Seniority units are filed in numerical order from first to last.

| | Matthew Earl Wallesz, Jr. |
|---|---|
| BEFORE | Matthew Earl Wallesz, Sr. |
| | Patrick James O'Neill, Jr. |
| BEFORE | Patrick James O'Neill, Sr. |
| | Virgil James Garcia, I |
| BEFORE | Virgil James Garcia, II |
| | Alex Curtis Jordan, I |
| BEFORE | Alex Curtis Jordan, II |

**Rule 8.** Numeric units are broken down such that numeric seniority terms are filed before alphabetic terms.

| | Edward Lee Kletka, IV |
|---|---|
| BEFORE | Edward Lee Kletka, Jr. |
| | George Lee Curtis, II |
| BEFORE | George Lee Curtis, Sr. |

## Filing Identical Names

When names are identical, the address may be used to order files. The address is indexed by:

| | |
|---|---|
| First: | City |
| SECOND | STATE |
| Third | Street Name |
| **Fourth:** | **Address #** |

Therefore, the following Acme Drug Supply files would be arranged from first to last as follows:

1. Acme Drug Supply, **839** *Kentucky Boulevard*, <u>Crawford</u>, MISSOURI
2. Acme Drug Supply, **683** *Wildflower Avenue*, <u>Fairbanks</u>, ALASKA
3. Acme Drug Supply, **1539** *Wildflower Avenue*, <u>Fairbanks</u>, ALASKA
4. Acme Drug Supply, **742** *Terminal Street West*, <u>Fairbanks</u>, ARIZONA
5. Acme Drug Supply, **731** *Terminal Street East*, <u>New York</u>, NEW YORK

Although this is the official indexing rule, most medical offices prefer alternative methods for filing identical charts. The primary consideration here is that patient addresses often change frequently. Therefore, preferred methods include date of birth or social security number.

## Filing Business and Organizational Records

When indexing businesses and organizations, the rules learned under filing individual names (Rules 1–8) will be used when individual names appear as part of the filing units. Rules for business and organizational records (Rules 9–20) do not apply to the filing of patient charts. However, they are used when filing business correspondence related to the running of the office, including correspondence for business equipment, maintenance contracts, medical equipment, and delivery services.

**Rule 9.** The order assignment of units for indexing businesses/organizations is as written.

| | Units Assigned | | |
|---|---|---|---|
| | **1** | **2** | **3** |
| Ace Bandage Supplies | Ace | Bandage | Supplies |
| Kent Memorial Hospital | Kent | Memorial | Hospital |

**Rule 10.** When *the* is the first unit of a business-organization, it is indexed as the last unit. The same would be true of *in, at,* and other prepositions and articles or words that do not provide a clearly identifiable key unit.

| | Units Assigned | | |
|---|---|---|---|
| | **1** | **2** | **3** |
| The Office Assistants | Office | Assistants | The |
| The Medical Specialists | Medical | Specialists | The |

**Rule 11.** Symbols such as &, ¢, $, #, and % are indexed as units, spelled out as words.

| | Units Assigned | | | |
|---|---|---|---|---|
| | **1** | **2** | **3** | **4** |
| Lawless & Krakoa, Attorneys | Lawless | and | Krakoa | Attorneys |
| # One Secretarial Service | Number | One | Secretarial | Service |

**Rule 12.** When indexing the $ sign before a number, the first unit is the number.

| | Units Assigned | | | |
|---|---|---|---|---|
| | **1** | **2** | **3** | **4** |
| $1 Quick Fax | 1 | Dollar | Quick | Fax |
| $5 Florists | 5 | Dollar | Florists | |

**Rule 13.** When punctuation marks are included as part of the indexing units, they are disregarded. Punctuation marks include: ." ' : ; - ! ? ( ).

| | Units Assigned | | | |
|---|---|---|---|---|
| | **1** | **2** | **3** | **4** |
| L. L. Transcription | L | L | Transcription | |
| M. E. Medical Equipment | M | E | Medical | Equipment |

**Rule 14.** When indexing numbers, the numbers are indexed as written.

| | Units Assigned | | |
|---|---|---|---|
| | **1** | **2** | **3** |
| Rx 2-Go | Rx | 2go | |
| Number Two Florists | Number | Two | Florists |

**Rule 15.** When indexing figures, the numbers are written as figures. *NOTE: d, nd, rd, st, and th are ignored when indexing.*

| | Units Assigned | | | |
|---|---|---|---|---|
| | **1** | **2** | **3** | **4** |
| 2nd Hand Office Supplies | 2 | Hand | Office | Supplies |
| 1st Rate Secretaries | 1 | Rate | Secretaries | |

**Rule 16.** When indexing numbers, if the number is written as a single word, it is indexed as a single unit.

| | Units Assigned | | |
|---|---|---|---|
| | **1** | **2** | **3** |
| Flowers 4 You | Flowers | 4 | You |

**Rule 17.** When indexing numbers, if the number is written with a word, it is indexed as one unit with the word.

| | Units Assigned | |
|---|---|---|
| | **1** | **2** |
| Flowers 4U | Flowers | 4U |

**Rule 18.** When indexing hyphenated numbers, they are indexed only by the number before the hyphen.

| | Units Assigned | | |
|---|---|---|---|
| | **1** | **2** | **3** |
| 8–4 Temporary Help* | 8 | Temporary | Help |

*If there happened to be an "8–4 Temporary Help" and an "8–5 Temporary Help," then the second number could be used.

**Rule 19.** When indexing alpha characters and numeric characters, the numeric characters are always filed before alpha characters.

| NAME | ORDER | FILE SECTION |
|---|---|---|
| 18th Street Pharmacy | First | Before any alphabetic sections—numeric* |
| 72nd Avenue Clinic | Second | Before any alphabetic section (72 follows 18)—numeric |
| Eighteenth Street Pharmacy | Third | The letter "E" section |

*The files could be set up with one file for all numeric designations followed by "A" to "Z" files/sections.

**Rule 20.** When indexing words that can be compound or two single words, the "as written" rule applies.

| | |
|---|---|
| | North West Rehabilitation |
| filed before | |
| | Northwest Rehabilitation |

## STEPS FOR FILING MEDICAL DOCUMENTATION IN PATIENT FILES

Before a discussion of the common filing systems, it is helpful to review procedural steps that accurately and efficiently process data sheets, laboratory requests, dictation, and so forth from the time they are generated to the time the file is returned to the medical records section. Efficiently following these steps will save considerable time in the ambulatory care setting.

### Inspect

Carefully inspect the report to identify the patient, subject, or file to whom the information belongs. Remove clips and staples. Make certain the information is complete.

### Index

Use the indexing process to determine how the chart would be located, properly identifying indexing units and their order.

### Code

Coding is the process of marking data to indicate how information is to be filed. If using a system other than a strict alphabetic system, determine the proper coding (numbers, Tab-Alpha, or other) for the chart so it can be retrieved. Otherwise, identify the indexed units by underlining or highlighting. This makes refiling more effective and assures that the item will always be filed in the same place. If a cross-reference is required, identify the cross-reference by double underlining and placing an "X" nearby. This chapter includes detailed information on coding and cross-reference.

### Sort

If there are a number of reports/documents to be filed, sort them into units according to the captions on the charts. This will eliminate wasted time in working back and forth through the alphabet or numbers.

### File

The papers are placed in the proper charts and the charts returned to their proper place in the medical records section. Be alert to the labels and refile any information or charts that have been misfiled.

## FILING TECHNIQUES AND COMMON FILING SYSTEMS

There are three major filing systems commonly used in the ambulatory care setting: alphabetic, numeric, and subject filing. The alphabet is intrinsic to all methods, and the basic rules for filing covered previously are used in all systems.

Color coding is used a high percentage of the time in all three systems to minimize filing errors. Another system, geographic, is seldom used in the ambulatory care setting unless there are multiple offices. Even then, a form of color coding may be used.

### Color Coding

Color coding is a technique often used in the three major filing systems. Color-coding methods most widely employed in medical facilities are Tab-Alpha® by Tab Products, Inc., Alpha-Z® by The Smead Manufacturing Company, and other variations of color coding methods. By working with these systems medical assistants will understand the principles behind the color-coding and be able to apply these principles to variations in any ambulatory care setting.

Color coding makes retrieval of files more efficient with the use of visible color differences that facilitate easier maintenance of the files. Color-coding filing systems utilize an alphabetic system in that after they are coded by color that designation is used to order the files alphabetically.

**Tab-Alpha System.** This system is designed primarily for filing systems that use vertical files where all individual charts are clearly visible in one unit.

Each alphabetic letter is assigned a different color. Each folder has a color-coded label. Only full-cut folders are used:

- Colored labels are applied over the edge of the full cut for the first two letters of the key indexing unit (Winston Paul Lewis: WI).

- A third white label is placed over the tab edge, which contains all of the indexing units (Winston Paul Lewis).

- In addition, some offices utilize a color-coded label to indicate the last year the patient was seen. This makes an efficient method for easily identifying active and inactive files.

- Any additional labels; e.g., allergies, last year seen, or industrial claim, are attached to the chart according to the office procedure.

**Alpha-Z System.** This particular system is designed for use with either open lateral files or vertical drawer files (Figure 14-7A). Alphabetic letters are utilized as the primary guides. Breakdowns of alphabetic combinations are added as determined by the needs of a particular facility.

A combination of thirteen colors is utilized in the Alpha-Z system with white letters on a solid colored background for the first half of the alphabet and white letters on a colored background with white stripes for the second half of the alphabet (Figure 14-7B).

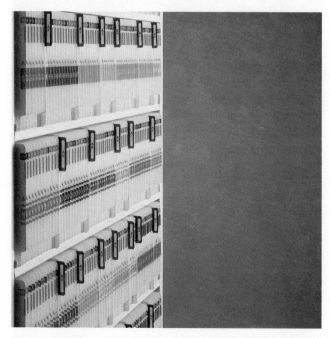

**Figure 14-7A** Alpha-Z Color-Coding Filing System uses open lateral shelving unit with color-coded files. (Courtesy Smead Manufacturing Company)

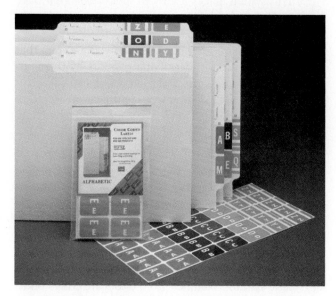

**Figure 14-7B** Alpha-Z Color-Coded Labels shown on top- and side-cut files.

The thirteen colors utilized are shown in Table 14-1. Folders have three labels:

● The first label contains the typed name, a color block, and the letter of the alphabet for the first letter of the first indexing unit:

**Winston, Lewis Paul YELLOW "W"**

● The second and third labels are color-coded to correspond to the second and third letters of the first unit:

**"I" on pink background and "N" on red striped background**

**Customized Color-Coding Systems.** Many offices utilize color systems to meet specific needs.

| TABLE 14-1 | THIRTEEN COLORS ARE USED IN THE ALPHA-Z SYSTEM | |
|---|---|---|
| **White Letter Colored Background** | **White Letter Striped Colored Background** | **Color** |
| A | N | Red |
| B | O | Dark Blue |
| C | P | Dark Green |
| D | Q | Light Blue |
| E | R | Purple |
| F | S | Orange |
| G | T | Gray |
| H | U | Dark Brown |
| I | V | Pink |
| J | W | Yellow |
| K | X | Light Brown |
| L | Y | Lavender |
| M | Z | Light Green |

*Colored File Folders by First Name.* One method color-codes the first letter of the first name. The folders then are filed alphabetically by last name.

**Example.** *A* is assigned red folders; *M* is assigned green folders; *S* is assigned blue folders

| | |
|---|---|
| Michael Taylor | Green Folder |
| Annette Samuels | Red Folder |
| Susan Boyer | Blue Folder |

Many small medical offices utilize this system and find it quite effective. In the multiphysician urgent care center, this would be quite time-consuming when locating files for patients of all physicians.

*Color File Folders by Last Name.* Another method utilizing this system assigns colored folders according to the first letter of the last name. The folders are then filed alphabetically.

**Example.** *S* is assigned pink folders; *B* is assigned gray folders.

| | |
|---|---|
| Bill Schwartz | Pink Folder |
| Corey Boyer | Gray Folder |

This system makes it easy to spot folders that have been misfiled under an incorrect first letter but does not break it down further for misfilings within the first-letter guides.

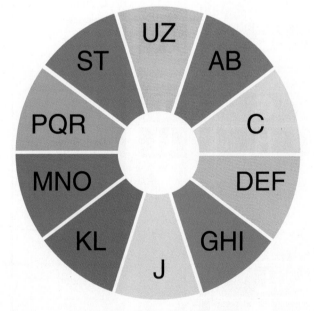

**Figure 14-8** Colorscan Color-Coded Filing System Color Wheel. (Courtesy of KARDEX System, Inc., Marietta, OH)

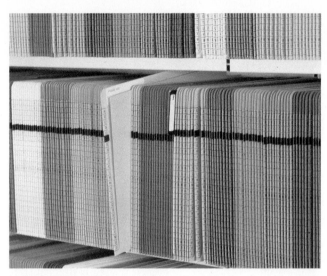

**Figure 14-9** Colorscan Color-Coded Filing System. Yellow file selected for "Carl"; "F" side tab selected for "Friend." (Courtesy of KARDEX System, Inc., Marietta, OH)

*Colorscan System.* The Colorscan Color-Coded Filing System by *KARDEX Systems, Inc.*, assigns color folders based on ten color groups (Figure 14-8). The color folder is assigned to a specific record based on the first letter of the second unit (usually patient's first name). Figure 14-9 shows that the yellow color file was selected because of the "C" in Carl. The files are further segmented by side tabs assigned to the first letter of the first unit (usually last name). In Figure 14-9, the side tab is assigned to the letter "F" for the patient's last name "Friend." All color folders would be used behind each alphabetic guide. If a record has only one unit, the first letter determines both position and color.

This system makes it easy to spot folders that have been misfiled under the incorrect first or second unit.

*Physician Coding.* In large clinics this is a system that many practices use for identifying patients by their primary care physician. Each physician is assigned a particular color of folder. This allows for identification of folders that have been misfiled under the incorrect physician. The folders themselves are filed under either the alphabetic or numeric system for each particular physician.

**Example.** Edith Leonard is a patient of Dr. Rice who has been assigned pink folders. Her chart is pink and is found under the "L's" as an alphabetic system is used.

*Color-Coded Numbers.* This system is utilized in a numeric filing system and operates in the same way as alphabetic systems. Numbers from 0 to 9 are color coded. The appropriate colored numbers are then placed on the tabs of the patient's folder.

## Alphabetic Filing

Strict alphabetic filing is one of the simplest filing methods, as files are strictly maintained by assigning a label to each file. The first letter of that label (e.g., Jones, Invoices, Pharmacies) is then used to alphabetize the files from A to Z. When a limited number of files is accessed, this is a very acceptable method of maintaining records.

## Numeric Filing

Numeric filing is organized by number rather than by letter. A key benefit of numeric filing is that it preserves patient confidentiality since the individual's name is not obviously apparent on the file folder.

Numeric filing systems are either consecutive (serial) or nonconsecutive.

### Consecutive or Serial. The consecutive or serial filing method is commonly used in handling invoices, sales orders, and requisitions. Each record is numbered and filed in ascending order.

**Example.**    576 93 or 57693

| Unit 1 | 5 |
| Unit 2 | 7 |
| Unit 3 | 6 |
| Unit 4 | 9 |
| Unit 5 | 3 |

### Nonconsecutive. The nonconsecutive filing system uses groups of two, three, or four or more digits; e.g., social security numbers or telephone numbers. Numbers are grouped and arranged in ascending order using the digits to the far right or the terminal digits. Each group of numbers is considered a unit (one number). To file the terminal digit files in numerical order, begin with strictly the terminal digit unit.

**Example.**    2108 23 879

| Unit 1 | 879 |
| Unit 2 | 23 |
| Unit 3 | 2108 |

**Components of Numeric Filing.** There are four essential components that are used with a numeric system, whether it is a manual or computerized system.

*Serially Numbered Dividers with Guides.* Consecutive numeric guides (5, 10, etc.; 50, 100, etc.) separate the individual file folders into smaller groups of files.

*Miscellaneous (General) Numeric File Section.* This is reserved for records that have not been assigned numbers. Patients should automatically be assigned a number on the first visit. However, there are occasions where patients cannot be assigned a number initially. The miscellaneous section is generally in front of all the numeric folders for ease of locating items. Files in the miscellaneous section are filed alphabetically by patient name. This is the best place for the miscellaneous file(s) for two reasons:

1.  They do not have to be moved each time a numbered file is added to the back of the order.
2.  In a large system of files, retrieval from the front is quick and easy.

*Alphabetic Card File.* This alphabetic file is necessary as a source to locate files or records.

A card contains name, address, and file number (or an M if located in the miscellaneous section); any cross-reference is here rather than in the numeric files.

The alphabetic card file and accession record in a manual system would be equivalent to the computerized record of the patient and whatever number is assigned to them in that computer record. If using a computerized system, the program generally will automatically cross-reference the number with the alphabetic list that was generated with the initial entry. If laboratory data come into the office on Leo M. McKay, there would need to be a method to know where to locate his chart to file the report; i.e., the alphabetic listing.

With a manual system, the alphabetic file is kept in an index card fashion. This file needs to contain the complete name and address (and any other information denoted by the office policy; e.g., insurance and emergency numbers).

Noted with this information there needs to be either an M for miscellaneous (for those items not assigned a number) or an assigned number (Figure 14-10 A and B).

If a cross-reference is required, prepare a cross-reference card and include an X next to the file number (or M) to indicate this is the cross-reference card and not the primary location (Figure 14-10C).

*Accession Record.* The accession record is a journal (or computer listing) where numbers are preassigned. Each new item to be assigned is written on the line next to the number (Figure 14-11). Each new entry for which a chart will be created must be assigned a number. A computerized system would have an accession record in its memory bank.

See Procedure 14-1 for numeric filing steps.

## Subject Filing

There are many reasons why material would be filed using a system of subjects in a medical office. If physicians are doing research, they might wish to index research according to diseases. Subject files are convenient for locating

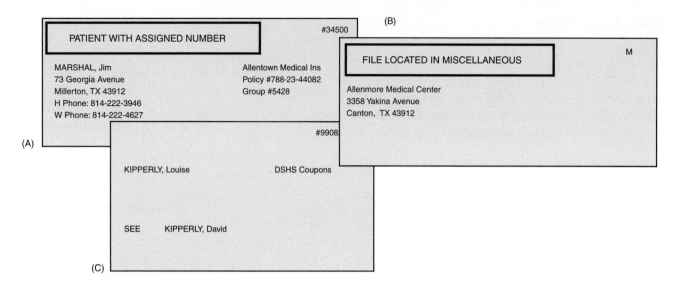

**Figure 14-10** Card files used in a numeric filing system: (A) Patient with an assigned number. (B) Patient record has not had a number assigned and is located in miscellaneous section. (C) Cross-reference card.

frequently used services or for filing reference materials for patient needs. Insurance company information also might be filed by subject.

When using a subject filing system, scan the material to determine the subject or theme. As with color-coding and numeric filing, an alphabetic file is necessary. This can be either a subject list or an index card file listing the subjects. Also, as with numeric filing, all cross-reference cards are done only with alphabetic file listings.

Within the folders, material can be arranged either alphabetically or chronologically; keep in mind the objective for maintaining the particular files. For instance, if using subject indexing for research projects physicians

have conducted, identify the subject category, and then in the material, code an item for reference to that specific material. See Procedure 14-2 for subject filing steps.

## Choosing a Filing System

To select a filing system, each office must decide what the primary objectives are with respect to storage of patient files, business records, and research files within the office. How will the charts be used primarily? Is there information that will need to be tracked by others not familiar with the records? It is often the case that more than one filing system will be utilized, such as alphabetic filing for patient charts, a numeric system for research subjects, and a subject system for miscellaneous correspondence (Table 14-2).

The number of documents to be filed seems to be one primary determinant in selecting an alphabetic or numeric system. Alphabetic filing is quite manageable when dealing with a relatively small number of patients. However, when the number of patients increases to several hundred or more, a numeric system becomes much more practical because there are an infinite set of numbers available. With the numeric system there is only one of each assigned designation. However, with an alphabetic system, there are a number of common names (e.g., Smith, Jones, Adams, and Johnson) that can have many

## ACCESSION LOG BOOK

| #   | File Name            |
| --- | -------------------- |
| 800 | CARRERA, Jaime       |
| 801 | AU, Rhoda            |
| 802 | TREMONT Drug Supply  |
| 803 |                      |
| 804 |                      |
| 805 |                      |
| 806 |                      |
| 807 |                      |

**Figure 14-11** Accession record or log sequentially lists numbers to be used to assign to numeric records. The next number available in this system is 803.

| TABLE 14-2 | ALPHABETIC OR NUMERIC FILING SYSTEM CONSIDERATIONS |
| --- | --- |

1. Consider the type, purpose, and use of the information.
2. Take into account the number of files or records.
3. Recognize the need for confidentiality.

multiples requiring additional sorting to narrow the search for the correct chart. In addition, with multiple charts of the same last name, the chances for misfiling increases. With the current trend in health care toward larger ambulatory care settings, there is likely to be an increase in the use of numeric filing over alphabetic filing. Confidentiality is another reason to select a numeric filing system. Confidentiality of charts is maintained more easily with numeric files as there is no visible name on the outside of the chart. Additionally, numerically referenced records can be utilized in research activities where random sampling and anonymity are required.

## FILING PROCEDURES

By adhering to some common principles in medical records management, any filing system will be more effective and enable the medical assistant to store, identify, retrieve, and maintain medical records efficiently.

### Cross-Referencing

In running an efficient medical office files must be stored for quick and accurate retrieval. If there is any doubt as to where a particular file would be located, cross-reference the file. Many offices fail to take the extra time it requires to do this. However, with the growing number of foreign names, hyphenated names, and stepfamilies, it is well worth the effort. When the office receives a letter and a release of information form inquiring about medical facts on Mr. David Kipperly's four stepchildren who were involved in an accident, how will these files be located? If they are cross-referenced under the stepfather's name, this will be a relatively easy procedure. However, if the medical assistant is unfamiliar with the family (as in a larger urgent care center with a large volume of patients), this may become a time-consuming job. Another scenario might involve insurance information on Janet Morgan. A search of the records does not produce a file for any Janet Morgan. The reason for this is that Janet Morgan is married and her chart has been filed under Janet Hill-Morgan. Time spent cross-referencing contributes to a more efficient method of retrieving information.

A cross-referencing system does not need to be elaborate. It is quite sufficient to use inserts with labels attached that are inserted in the appropriate place in the storage units. For instance, a plain piece of cardboard, rather than a file or chart, could be inserted for "Janet Morgan." This insert would simply have a label directing one to the location of the primary file.

The proper steps for cross-referencing along with several examples where cross-referencing might be used follow.

## Steps for Cross-Referencing

1. Identify the primary filing label.
2. Make a proper file to be used as the primary location for all medical records.
3. Identify one (or more) alternatives where one might find the file.
4. For the alternative filings, make a cross-reference sheet, card, or dummy chart that lists the primary reference and refers back to the location of the primary file.

**Example.** The patient, Jaime Renae Carrera, has made it known to the office that most of the correspondence received will refer to the name Renny Carrera as this is his preference. The SEE reference will identify where the primary file is located.

| | |
|---|---|
| PRIMARY FILE: | Carrera, Jaime Renae |
| X-REFERENCE FILE: | Carrera, Renny |
| | **SEE** Carrera, Jamie Renae |

**Rule 1. Married Women.** The primary file would be the patient's legal name with the cross-reference being listed under her husband's name.

| | |
|---|---|
| PRIMARY FILE: | Au, Rhoda A. (Mrs.) |
| | Lee Au |
| X-REFERENCE FILE: | Au, Mrs. Lee |
| | **SEE** Au, Rhoda A. (Mrs.) |

**Rule 2. Foreign Names.** The primary file would be located under the patient's legal name. It is important therefore that you identify the first, middle, and surname (last name) when the patient comes for the first visit. Unless people are familiar with a particular group of names, the first, middle, and surnames are often confused with one another. Again, your experience will teach you which cross-references should be set up.

| | |
|---|---|
| PRIMARY FILE: | Sing, Yange Teah |
| X-REFERENCE FILE: | Yange, Sing Teah |
| | **SEE** Sing, Yange Teah |
| X-REFERENCE FILE: | Teah, Yange Sing |
| | **SEE** Sing, Yange Teah |

**Rule 3. Hyphenated Names.** With the proliferation of hyphenated names, it is common for materials to be listed under different combinations of the hyphenated name. For instance, a married woman may have records under her maiden name, her husband's surname,

and her hyphenated name. Therefore, it is necessary to make two cross-references.

| | |
|---|---|
| PRIMARY FILE: | Krenshaw-Skiple, Rose Marie |
| X-REFERENCE FILE: | Skiple, Rose Marie |
| | **SEE** Krenshaw-Skiple, Rose Marie |
| X-REFERENCE FILE: | Krenshaw, Rose Marie |
| | **SEE** Krenshaw-Skiple, Rose Marie |

**Rule 4. Multiple Listings.** A great deal of correspondence is received with multiple listings of names. At times the medical office may receive correspondence from only one of the involved parties. Rather than keep a separate file for each, maintain a primary file as listed on the letter and then cross-reference file(s) for the individual names.

| | |
|---|---|
| PRIMARY FILE: | Olsen, Piper, and Dillard Associates |
| X-REFERENCE FILE: | Piper, Richard C., M.D. |
| | **SEE** Olsen, Piper, and Dillard Associates |
| X-REFERENCE FILE: | Olsen, Francis William, M.D. |
| | **SEE** Olsen, Piper, and Dillard Associates |
| X-REFERENCE FILE: | Dillard, Thomas E., M.D. |
| | **SEE** Olsen, Piper, and Dillard Associates |

## Tickler Files

Sticky notes and writing notes on the calendar are popular methods of reminding office personnel to follow up with some required action. However, a well-organized, efficient office will maintain what is known as a tickler file, a method that serves as a reminder that some action needs to be taken at a date in the future.

Many computer systems today have provision for establishing ticklers on files. However, a standard practice of using index cards for tickler files is easy to maintain (Figure 14-12).

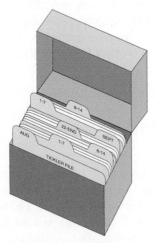

**Figure 14-12** Tickler files should be reviewed daily or weekly to follow up on activities and actions that must be taken.

The tickler card should contain the following information:

- Patient name
- Tickler date (when action should be taken)
- Required action (e.g., schedule surgery or mail reminder)
- Additional relevant information (telephone number)

If action is to be taken with a patient or on behalf of the patient; e.g., scheduling a hospital admittance or sending a reminder of a checkup visit, place the information on the tickler card as soon as possible so this task is not forgotten.

When filing records, be sure to look for such words as "on _____ date we will," "pending action," or "follow-up," indicating that some course of action needs to be taken.

## Release Marks

It is a good practice to use some type of release mark on every item that is filed (date stamp, initials, check mark). Ideally the physician should initial the document after it has been read. Then, if action is required by the medical assistant, a release mark is in a consistently identified place on every document. If no action is required after the physician has signed or initialed it, place a release mark on the document. A release mark on every piece of correspondence serves as an excellent quality control measure.

## Check-Out System

Many offices have developed dummy charts or cardboard files labeled "out sheets" or "out guides." Most of these guides are identified by an OUT label or metal holder, but they could be assigned a particular color; the key is that they stand out as different from the primary folders.

On the out guide there should be at the least:

- A record of when the chart was removed
- Where the chart can be located

Other information that is useful to note includes:

- Expected date of return
- Actual date the chart was returned
- Signature of the personnel checking out the record.
- Notation on what section of the chart file was borrowed, such as a lab report or specialty examination.

Some clinics prefer to have *temporary folders* rather than just an out guide. There are also out guides with pockets to file data in the absence of a chart. This allows for data storage on a temporary basis until the primary file is returned. The data can then be filed permanently when the primary folder is returned. If these folders are of a different color or have a different type of tab/label, they can be spotted easily so the staff can track the temporary files to be sure they do not become permanent folders.

## Locating Missing Files or Data

Misfiling can occur for a number of reasons. When this situation occurs, a specific procedure must be established to conduct a search for the missing information. By systematically searching, the missing data usually can be located. This systematic search can be aided by making a mental note of the particular items that commonly are misplaced; i.e., thin-paper lab reports, small lab slips, look-alike names such as "Ward" filed under "Wart" or "Adam" filed under "Adams." Make a note of what was misfiled and where the information was located to more easily locate similar items in the future.

To locate missing pieces of information when the correct file is located but not the particular item within that file:

- Check all of the items within the file.
- Check other files with similar labels.

To locate missing files:

- Check the folders filed before and after the proper location of the misplaced file.
- Look at folders with similar labels.
- Check the physician's desk, desk tray, and other office personnel.
- If using a color-coding system, look for folders with the same color-coding as the misplaced file.
- If using a numeric system, look for possible transposition of combinations of numbers.
- Check for transposition of first and last names.
- Check for alternative spellings of names or look-alike names.

Misplaced files can be very frustrating and time-consuming to locate. The best strategy is to check files for the proper filing order whenever returning or retrieving a file folder. When removing a file to answer a question, leave the file following it sticking out slightly to make its return easy and correct. Most importantly, when finished with a record, refile it immediately.

## Filing Chart Data

**Types of Reports.** The patient's chart is the key source of information relating to treatment. There are a number of reports kept in the chart, all serving to provide a total picture of patient care. Following are the most common documents that will be part of the patient's medical record:

*Clinical Notes.* These include documentation such as the medical history, the physical examination, and the follow-up notes. They track the patient's course of treatment.

*Correspondence.* This varies from office to office. Some offices file all types of correspondence together. Other offices file correspondence about the patient's treatment with the clinical notes.

*Laboratory Reports.* Included in this section are X-ray reports, CT scans, ultrasound reports, blood work, urinalysis, EEGs, ECGs, physical therapy-related reports, and pathology reports—information related to clinical data that assess the patient's condition.

*Miscellaneous.* This category includes insurance-related papers, requests for transfer of medical records, and personal notes from/to patients. In general, miscellaneous would encompass matters not related to direct treatment.

**Methods of Arranging Charts.** Just as the choice of a filing system is important to the efficient use of files, so too is the arrangement of materials within the charts. Again, the choice of method must be in accordance with how the information needs to be accessed and utilized for each individual office. No one method is correct.

*Problem-Oriented Medical Record (POMR).* The problem-oriented medical record (POMR) type of record-keeping uses a sheet, generally on the inside cover or other prominent location, which lists vital identification data, immunizations, allergies, medications, and problems. The problems are identified by a number that corresponds to the charting relevant to that problem number; i.e., bronchitis #1; broken wrist #2; and so forth. If the patient returns in nine months with recurring bronchitis, the same number (#1) is used.

The patient chart is then further built by adding a numbered and titled page for each problem the patient experiences; e.g., bronchitis #1; broken wrist #2.

Each problem is then followed with the SOAP approach for all progress notes:

S   Subjective impressions
O   Objective clinical evidence
A   Assessment or diagnosis
P   Plans for further studies, treatment, or management

This process makes the chart easier to review and helps in follow-up of all the patient's medical needs (Figure

**Figure 14-13    Example of POMR progress notes.** (Courtesy of Bibbero Systems, Inc., Petaluma, CA)

14-13). The SOAP approach also allows medical personnel to be aware of the patient's current medications. Starting and resolution dates for each problem also are noted on the tracking sheet.

Internists, family practitioners, and pediatricians use the POMR system more commonly than do specialists because they see their patients for a variety of problems over a long span of time.

*Source-Oriented Medical Record (SOMR).* The source-oriented medical record (SOMR) groups information according to its source; for example, from laboratories, examinations, physician notes, consulting physicians, and other sources. Many offices use this method as it makes different types of information quickly accessible. A fastener-folder is used that contains several partitions with their own fasteners. This allows for a separate section for lab reports, pathology, progress notes, physical examinations, and correspondence to be filed chronologically within each section. In the SOMR system, many physicians will use the SOAP method to record their chart notes.

*Strict Chronological Arrangement.* Using this method, data are filed strictly with the most recently charted materials to the top of the folder. For instance, a

patient is followed from 1963 to 1986. To locate information recorded in 1973, it would be necessary to flip through the chart until the material for the year 1973 was located. This method makes it difficult for a physician or medical assistant to quickly assess a patient's clinical picture.

*Shingling.* This method is generally used to file laboratory reports. Many of these reports are smaller than the standard size sheets of paper. Shingling ensures that medical personnel have quick access to the most recent data. In addition, it keeps small pieces of paper from being misplaced or lost within the medical record. Simply put, the sheets of paper are "shingled" either up or across the page, the most recent report placed on top of the previous one (Figure 14-14).

## Retention and Purging

As information accumulates, it is necessary to maintain files by the process known as purging. Purging can involve several forms of action.

**Record purging.** This process requires sorting through records and removing those not in active use. Each facility should establish a standard policy for control and processing of records.

States have different time requirements for retention of various types of records. See Table 14-3 for general guidelines. As a way of controlling risk and practicing responsible risk management, many facilities are choosing to maintain large inactive files rather than destroy records. Some keep them on optical disks or microfiche as discussed later in this chapter. Check with the Medical Practice Act in your state to determine record-keeping requirements.

**Active Files.** Active files include records that need to be readily accessible for retrieval of information.

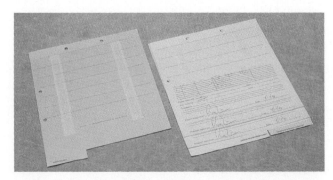

**Figure 14-14    Shingled lab reports:** (Left) shingling base form with sticky tape for attaching lab forms; (Right) shingled lab forms attached to base.

## TABLE 14-3 RECORDS FOR RETENTION

### Patient Index Files

These include appointment books or daily appointment sheets. They are kept for an indefinite period of time. They may be required for litigation and/or research.

### Case Histories

The length of storage depends on state requirements and individual practice requirements. Product liability cases have deemed long-term storage of these records necessary (20+ years). The records of minors must be retained at least until the age of majority. The statute of limitations is a deciding factor as well.

If records are to be destroyed due to death of physician or closure of a practice, the following procedure is required: Each patient should be notified of the circumstances and given the opportunity to have his or her records forwarded to another physician. After notification, the records must be retained for a "reasonable" period of time (determined by state regulations). A period of three to six months is generally determined to be a "reasonable" period of time. The records must be destroyed by burning or shredding to protect confidentiality.

### Personal/Professional Records

Professional licenses should be stored permanently in a secure location.

### Office Equipment Records

These records are generally kept until the warranties and/or depreciation are no longer valid. They should be kept in an easily accessible location if under maintenance contract.

### Insurance Records

Professional liability policies are kept permanently. Other policies are kept in active files while in force.

### Financial Records

Bank records are kept in active files for up to three years and then placed in inactive storage. Tax records must be retained permanently.

### Laboratory and X-ray Data

Originals should be retained permanently with the patient's case history.

**Inactive Files.** Inactive files consist of records that need to be retained for possible retrieval of information. Files not currently being accessed for information would thus become inactive. Often the type of practice will dictate the relevant time period when files are determined to be inactive (generally two to three years).

**Closed Files.** Closed files are those that are no longer required. Again, patient files are retained for significantly longer periods of time due to litigation and research considerations.

# CORRESPONDENCE

Most ambulatory care settings process a considerable amount of correspondence not directly related to patient care. Such items include employment applications, letters from/to pharmaceutical representatives, advertisements for medical supplies, magazine subscription information, and letters to/from other physicians on a variety of subjects. This correspondence is processed using alphabetic filing rules. However, an additional step is necessary to determine whether the correspondence is incoming or outgoing. The correspondence must be filed under some aspect that will be distinctly identifiable; i.e., what idea, subject, name would most likely be thought of if someone wanted to retrieve that correspondence or file additional relevant correspondence.

## Incoming Correspondence

This is defined as correspondence received *into* the office from an outside source. This type of correspondence is filed under the most important name—that is, the most likely name were someone to retrieve the correspondence. The key place to look for filing information is the letterhead name or the patient or item referenced in the letter.

## Outgoing Correspondence

Correspondence sent *out* of the medical office is considered outgoing correspondence. The key place to inspect here is the inside address or the patient or item referenced in the letter. Again, remember to identify the most probable place to locate the copy of this correspondence should it be needed for future use.

## Filing Procedures for Correspondence

Once it is determined whether correspondence is incoming or outgoing, follow the basic rules for filing. In addition:

- Remove paper clips and staple items together.
- Inspect to see if the item is ready to be filed; i.e., any appropriate action has been taken. If not, take care of copies, enclosures, and place note in the tickler file for future action before proceeding with the indexing.
- On incoming correspondence, be sure the letterhead is related to the letter.

**Example:** A personal letter written by a patient on hotel stationery—index the signature on the letter.

**Example:** When both the company name and the signature are important, index the company name. A letter from Preston

Industries written by the company president—index Preston Industries, not the president's name, which may change.

**Example:** If there is no letterhead and you have determined the material is not relevant to a patient, index the name on the signature line. A letter received from Carlton Fiske, RPT, advising your office of services his firm has to offer your patients—index Fiske.

● On outgoing correspondence, look at the inside address and the reference line.

**Example:** A letter to the District Court regarding Karen Ritter, an employee who is summoned to jury duty—index Karen Ritter rather than District Court.

**Example:** If the correspondence is relevant to a patient, index the patient's name. A letter RE: Wayne Elder—index under Elder.

**Example:** If the correspondence is not relevant to a patient, look to the inside address for the indexing information. A letter inquiring about cost estimates for redecorating the office reception room—index the firm in the inside address.

**Example:** When the inside address is relevant and contains both a company name and a person's name, index the company name. (This avoids the problem of personnel changes.) Cross-referencing would be done under the individual name. A letter to Marvin Fairchild, President of Brandex Pharmaceuticals—index Brandex Pharmaceuticals with a cross-reference for Morgan Fairchild, President, SEE Brandex Pharmaceuticals.

**Example:** If the letter is personal, the name of the person to whom the letter is written would be used for indexing purposes. Dr. Whitney writes a letter to Dr. Lewis, one of his colleagues, asking if he plans to attend an upcoming conference—index Dr. Lewis.

● On incoming or outgoing correspondence, code the indexing units of the designated label. If the correspondence is being cross-referenced, be sure to note the cross-referencing unit and place the X in a

visible place. You may find that the body of the letter contains an important name or subject.

● Create a miscellaneous folder for items that do not have enough in number (office policy will dictate this number, which can be from two to four pieces) to warrant an individual folder. Items in the miscellaneous folder are filed alphabetically first and then identical items are filed with the most recent piece on top. An individual folder is then created when enough pieces accumulate on a particular item.

## COMPUTER APPLICATIONS

While the majority of patient charts are still maintained manually, computers are playing an ever-increasing role in the management of records in the ambulatory care setting. Even offices that do not do a great deal of medical records management by computer find the basic database application of great assistance.

### Databases

Databases are exceedingly useful in a number of ways. A database is a tool for storing information in a form that allows easy retrieval of information related to a specific topic or element. Maintaining a list of patients with telephone numbers, addresses, family members, and insurance policies is perhaps the simplest use of a database. However, from this can spring a wealth of other information with which the medical office can form other databases; e.g., to retrieve information about patients in a particular locality, patients who are on a particular drug in the event of a drug recall, and general mailing lists for address labels that can be sorted by zip code, state, city, or patient name (Figure 14-15).

Any number of software programs are available to create databases. The steps involved are simple:

1. Design a form by designing the items of interest (called fields) such as patient name, address, date of birth, and sex.
2. Enter the data into each of these fields.
3. Name the database and save the file on the computer for future use.

Simple databases do not require an extensive knowledge of computers to be utilized effectively for routine office applications.

**Biomedical, Clinical, and Other Databases.** Because technology is changing so rapidly, physicians must stay up to date on medical and health developments.

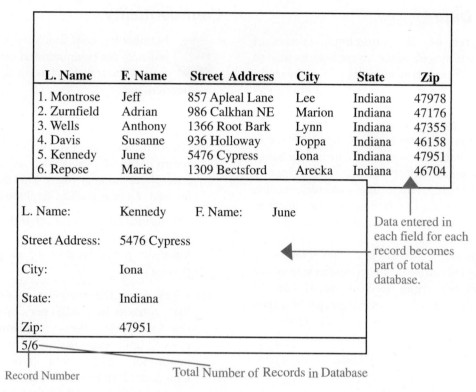

| L. Name | F. Name | Street Address | City | State | Zip |
|---------|---------|----------------|------|-------|-----|
| 1. Montrose | Jeff | 857 Apleal Lane | Lee | Indiana | 47978 |
| 2. Zurnfield | Adrian | 986 Calkhan NE | Marion | Indiana | 47176 |
| 3. Wells | Anthony | 1366 Root Bark | Lynn | Indiana | 47355 |
| 4. Davis | Susanne | 936 Holloway | Joppa | Indiana | 46158 |
| 5. Kennedy | June | 5476 Cypress | Iona | Indiana | 47951 |
| 6. Repose | Marie | 1309 Bectsford | Arecka | Indiana | 46704 |

L. Name:        Kennedy        F. Name:        June

Street Address:        5476 Cypress

City:        Iona

State:        Indiana

Zip:        47951

5/6

Data entered in each field for each record becomes part of total database.

Record Number        Total Number of Records in Database

**Figure 14-15** Patient information can be entered into a database once and then recalled to update, change, review, or manipulate order as needed.

A biomedical database, essentially a library of health information that can be accessed by a personal computer and modem, allows a physician to search available literature for a topic or combination of topics.

Medical assistants may be assigned the task of researching available databases before the physician subscribes to a particular database service or to search for specific pieces of information the physician requires. If so, look for a database that gives information from around the world. A good biomedical database should index at least 4,000 journals, including foreign journals.

Clinical databases are another aid in researching questions about drugs or chemicals. These databases index drugs and their interactions, poisons and their antidotes, emergency illnesses and their treatments, as well as scores of other clinically related topics. An ambulatory care setting seeking a service of this type should contact the local medical association, the American Medical Association, or a major vendor of medical software for names and addresses of the most widely used clinical database services. Poisindex™, Drugdex™, Emergindex™, and Identidex™ are typical information services. Each is offered by Micromex, Inc., in conjunction with the Rocky Mountain Poison and Drug Center and the University of Colorado.

Hospitals routinely use databases such as MedLine, Cumulative Index for Nursing and Allied Health Literature (CINAHL), GENONE (genetic information), and Micromedics. Users access these databases through networks such as Prodigy, CompuServe, Dialog, and Internet.

Nonmedical databases such as Nexus, which might occasionally be used in large medical offices, provide information on just about every imaginable subject, from travel schedules to financial information, art history, and physics.

Electronic databases work in the same way as magazine subscription services. A subscriber selects a particular database service, then pays a monthly fee. In addition, the subscriber pays long-distance telephone charges for the amount of time on-line each month with the database service.

## Archival Storage

Most physicians preserve patient medical records for at least the life of their practice. This obviously is a space-consuming prospect, particularly in today's large practices. Computers are helping to solve this dilemma through a process similar to microfiche and microfilm. Records can be copied with a laser beam onto what are called optical disks. This method not only eliminates the bulky storage problems encountered with traditional records but records can be retrieved and viewed almost instantaneously on a computer screen.

## Transfer of Data

Computers are also streamlining transfer of records from one office or medical facility to another. Faxing is an everyday part of the medical office. Gone are the days when it took a physician's office days to obtain information vital to treating a patient. Within minutes, a patient's entire medical record can be sent via a facsimile from one office to another. Refer to Chapter 12. Offices that are networked can also exchange information via e-mail (electronic mail) or computer modem (see Chapter 12). This requires a software program that allows one computer to communicate with another, sending information via the electronic network or telephone rather than via the post office. Scanners (optical character recognition) are devices that allow information to be converted to an image on the computer screen. For instance, a patient's entire medical record can be "scanned" by running this device over the pages; it is then recreated as a computer file just as it was in paper form.

## Confidentiality

Maintaining confidentiality is a major issue in utilizing the computer and on-line devices for storage and transfer of medical information. Key considerations are:

- Maintaining confidentiality with transmission of data. A cover sheet that advises the receiver of the confidential nature of the material, instructions for return to the medical office if received in error, and a telephone number where you (the sender) can be advised of a transmission error are critical.

- Precautions must be taken that the fax or computer receiving the information is in a location where the information will be accessed only by appropriate personnel.

- When using the computer to store and transfer data, consider how many personnel have access to that information. Security measures should be in place to limit access to only those with a legitimate reason for accessing the information. Refer to Chapters 12 and 15 for legal considerations when electronically transmitting patient information.

---

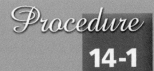

# Procedure 14-1

# Steps for Manual Filing with a Numeric System

**PURPOSE:**
To demonstrate an understanding of the principles of the numeric filing system.

**EQUIPMENT/SUPPLIES:**
Documents to be filed
Dividers with guides
Miscellaneous numeric file section
Alphabetic card file and cards
Accession journal if needed

**PROCEDURE STEPS:**
1. Inspect and index.
2. Code for filing units. Check the alphabetic card file for each piece to see if the card has already been prepared.
3. Write the number in the upper right-hand corner if the piece has been assigned a number.
4. If no number is assigned (i.e., it has an M for miscellaneous), check the miscellaneous file. If a miscellaneous item is ready to be assigned a number, make a card and note the number in the right-hand corner of the card file, cross out the M, and make a chart file.
5. If there is no card, make up an alphabetic card including a complete name and address, and then write either M or assign a number.
6. Cross-reference if necessary and file the card properly. You are then ready to file the document in the appropriate file folder/chart.
7. File in ascending order.

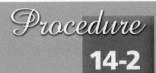

## Steps for Manual Filing with a Subject Filing System

**Procedure 14-2**

**PURPOSE:**
To demonstrate an understanding of the principles of the subject filing system.

**EQUIPMENT/SUPPLIES:**
Documents to be filed by subject
Subject index list or index card file listing subjects
Alphabetic card file and cards

**PROCEDURE STEPS:**
1. Review the item to find the subject.
2. Match the subject of the item with an appropriate category on the subject index list.
3. If the item contains information that may pertain to more than one subject, decide on the proper cross-reference.
4. If the subject title is written on the material, underline it.
5. If the subject title is not written on the item, write it clearly in the upper right-hand corner and underline ( ____ ) it.
6. Use a wavy ( ∿ ) line for cross-referencing and an X as with alphabetic and numeric filing.
7. Underline the first indexing unit of the coded units.

**CASE STUDY**

**14-1**

Karen Ritter, administrative medical assistant at Inner City Health Care, has been chiefly responsible for managing this urgent care center's medical records. However, since Karen is only part-time, the office manager feels she needs to delegate some of the responsibility of maintaining all office files to Liz Corbin, a medical assistant who also works part-time. Karen knows the system well and had a hand in designing an effective numeric filing method that both ensures patient confidentiality while meeting the needs of Inner City with its large volume of patients. Now she is trying to orient Liz, who has little experience of the filing system, to the intricacies of medical records management.

### CASE STUDY REVIEW

1. What is a good starting point for Liz Corbin's education in medical records management?
2. What are the basic procedures for filing any piece of documentation that Liz needs to learn?
3. Under the direction of the office manager, Inner City is gradually shifting to a computerized system for all operations. Eventually, patient files will be computerized. What can Karen and Liz do to prepare for this eventuality?

## SUMMARY

Records management plays an ever-increasing role in the ambulatory care setting today. With the need for thorough and proper documentation, a majority of interaction on the patient's behalf is concerned with proper information processing. It is imperative that medical records be managed efficiently and that the medical assistant possess the skills required for sorting, filing, retrieving, and maintaining information effectively.

A key aspect of managing patient records is selecting a filing system that achieves the goals of information access and storage. Once an alphabetic, numeric, or subject filing system is chosen, patient charts must be assembled and maintained accurately. Technology and computer applications will play a more prominent and varied role in the organization and utilization of files in the medical office.

## REVIEW QUESTIONS

### Multiple Choice

1. Maintaining order in files by separating active from inactive files is:
   a. indexing
   b. coding
   c. purging
   d. alphabetizing
2. A system used as a reminder of action to be taken on a certain date is called:
   a. accession log
   b. tickler file
   c. release mark
   d. purging system
3. To maintain an accurate filing system, select from the following list the tool used to ensure that records are tracked when borrowed:
   a. release mark
   b. out guide
   c. alphabetic card file
   d. cross-reference file
4. The correct indexing from first to last for assigning units to the name John Porter O'Keefe II would be:
   a. O'Keefe John Porter II
   b. John Porter O'Keefe II
   c. II O'Keefe John Porter
   d. the "II" would be disregarded
5. Of the four systems of filing, the best for every ambulatory care setting is:
   a. the numeric system
   b. the color-coding system
   c. the one that is customized to the needs of the office
   d. the alphabetic system
6. Three main primary types of file cabinets used in medical offices are:
   a. vertical, horizontal, and movable
   b. vertical, open-shelf lateral, and movable file units
   c. vertical, horizontal, and lateral
   d. none of the above
7. Out guides:
   a. are used when the staff is out of the office
   b. are devices to help track charts
   c. may be cardboard or plastic/paper sheets kept in place of a patient's chart
   d. both b and c
8. The first indexing unit for Jayne Carol Warden-Bloomberg is:
   a. Carol
   b. Jayne
   c. Warden
   d. Wardenbloomberg

9. When identical names are being indexed, which system is preferred in medical offices:
   a. index street address next
   b. index using a social security number
   c. index by city
   d. index by state
10. The preferred order for steps in filing medical documentation is:
    a. code, index, sort, inspect, file
    b. inspect, code, index, sort, file
    c. sort, inspect, index, code, file
    d. inspect, index, code, sort, file

### Critical Thinking

1. Discuss the importance of maintaining accurate records with regard to the two key issues involving the management of a patient's medical records identified in the text.
2. Discuss briefly two considerations for choosing a filing system for a particular medical office.
3. Briefly outline the differences between the Alpha-Z and the Tab-Alpha color-coding systems.
4. Discuss the significance of the alphabetic card file in a numeric filing system.
5. Provide an example of a subject for subject filing and define five divisions for using this system for a physician working in communicable diseases.
6. Determine the correct filing order for the following pharmaceutical companies from first to last:
   a. Ledsoe-Watson Pharmaceuticals, 789 North Fifth Street, Beckwood, Alabama
   b. Ledsoe-Watson Pharmaceuticals, 345 Ninth Avenue, Little Rock, Arkansas
   c. Ledsoe-Watsen Pharmaceuticals, 893 North Eighth Street, Minneapolis, Minnesota
   d. Ledsoe-Watson Pharmaceuticals, 621 Tenth Street, Shreveport, Louisiana
7. If a chart cannot be located, discuss strategies for locating the missing file.
8. Review the use and capabilities of the computer in regard to medical records management.
9. Properly index and cross-reference (if necessary) your own name. Using the Alpha-Z system, color code your name. Color code your name using the Colorscan Color-Coded Filing System.
10. Research the Statute of Limitations in your state for medical records to determine how long a medical record should be kept. The statute will also tell you what "triggers" activity on a medical file that might dictate it be kept longer than normally indicated.

11. When determining the type of equipment to purchase for storage of medical records, identify a minimum of three indicators to keep in mind.
12. It has been said that filing records is the easiest task the medical assistant will perform; yet it is often the most difficult. What reasons can you give for this statement?

## WEB ACTIVITIES

 Research the World Wide Web for information that relates to how patient records can be kept confidential in an age of electronic transfer of data. From this information determine what steps you might take to assure patients of their privacy.

## REFERENCES/BIBLIOGRAPHY

Fordney, M. T., & Follis, J. J. (1998). *Administrative medical assisting* (4th ed.). Albany, NY: Delmar.

Humphrey, D. D. (1996). *Contemporary medical office procedures* (2nd ed.). Albany, NY: Delmar.

Johnson, J. (1994). *Basic filing procedures for health information management*. Albany, NY: Delmar.

Kalles, N. F., & Johnson, M. M. (1992). *Records management* (5th ed.). Cincinnati: South-Western Publishing Co.

Montone, D. (1998). *Power building in documentation*. Philadelphia, PA: W. B. Saunders Company.

Seare, J. G. (1996). *Medical documentation*. Salt Lake City, UT: Medicode.

LEWIS & KING, MD
2501 CENTER STREET
NORTHBOROUGH, OH 12345

NORTHBOROUGH
FAMILY MEDICAL GROUP

**Date Line**

January 12, 20___   (approximately 15th line)

**Inside Address**

Jeremy Brown, MD   (approximately 20th line)
111 S Main
Blossom, UT 10283-1120
   (double-space)

**Salutation**

Dear Dr. Brown:
   (double-space)

**Subject Line**

Blossom Medical Society Meeting
   (double-space)

Thank you for inviting me to speak at the Blossom Medical Society Meeting June 15, 20___. As requested, my topic will describe the use of the MRI in assisting physicians to make a more accurate diagnosis without resorting to invasive procedures. The exact title of my speech will be sent by next Friday.
   (double-space)

Please have your office manager send information regarding the number of participants expected, time of meeting, location, and any other details that will assist me in preparing my speech.

I will write or call if I have any additional questions.
   (double-space)

**Complimentary Closing**

Yours truly,

*Winston Lewis, MD*   (4–5 line spaces)

**Keyed Signature**

Winston Lewis, MD
   (double-space)

**Reference Initials**

WL:jg
   (double-space)

**Enclosure Notation**

Enclosure: Handout on MRI

**Figure 15-3**   Sample full block style letter; all elements start at the left margin.

address, complimentary close, or keyed signature. When using the full block style, all lines begin flush with the left margin. This style is suggested when desiring a contemporary-looking efficient letter. Figure 15-3 illustrates a full block style letter.

## Modified Block

In the **standard modified block** style letter, all lines begin at the left margin with the exception of the date line, complimentary closure, and keyed signature, which usually begin at the center position or a few spaces to the right of center. Figure 15-4 illustrates a modified block style letter without indention.

The assistant may choose to use the **indented modified block** style letter. In this format, paragraphs may be indented five spaces. Figure 15-5 illustrates a modified block style letter with indented paragraphs.

## Simplified

The **simplified letter** style omits the salutation and complimentary closure. All lines are **keyed** (input by keystroke) flush with the left margin. The subject line is keyed in capitals three lines below the inside address. The body of the letter begins three lines below the subject line. The signature line is keyed in all capital letters four lines below the body of the letter. The Administrative Manage-

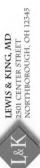

LEWIS & KING, MD
2501 CENTER STREET
NORTHBOROUGH, OH 12345

NORTHBOROUGH
FAMILY MEDICAL GROUP

January 12, 20___    (approximately 15th line)

January 12, 20___    (approximately 20th line)

Jeremy Brown, MD    (approximately 20th line)
111 S Main
Blossom, UT 10283-1120

Dear Dr. Brown:

Blossom Medical Society Meeting

Thank you for inviting me to speak at the Blossom Medical Society Meeting June 15, 20___. As requested, my topic will describe the use of the MRI in assisting physicians to make a more accurate diagnosis without resorting to invasive procedures. The exact title of my speech will be sent by next Friday.

Please have your office manager send information regarding the number of participants expected, time of meeting, location, and any other details that will assist me in preparing my speech.

I will write or call if I have any additional questions.

Yours truly,

*Winston Lewis, MD*

Winston Lewis, MD

WL:jg

Enclosure: Handout on MRI

**Figure 15-5**   Sample modified block style letter with indented paragraphs; this format is the same as the standard modified except that the subject line and paragraphs are also indented.

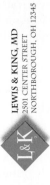

LEWIS & KING, MD
2501 CENTER STREET
NORTHBOROUGH, OH 12345

NORTHBOROUGH
FAMILY MEDICAL GROUP

January 12, 20___    (approximately 15th line)

January 12, 20___    (approximately 20th line)

Jeremy Brown, MD    (approximately 20th line)
111 S Main
Blossom, UT 10283-1120

Dear Dr. Brown:

Blossom Medical Society Meeting

Thank you for inviting me to speak at the Blossom Medical Society Meeting June 15, 20___. As requested, my topic will describe the use of the MRI in assisting physicians to make a more accurate diagnosis without resorting to invasive procedures. The exact title of my speech will be sent by next Friday.

Please have your office manager send information regarding the number of participants expected, time of meeting, location, and any other details that will assist me in preparing my speech.

I will write or call if I have any additional questions.

Yours truly,

*Winston Lewis, MD*

Winston Lewis, MD

WL:jg

Enclosure: Handout on MRI

**Figure 15-4**   Sample standard modified block style letter; all elements start at left margin except date, complimentary closing, and keyed signature.

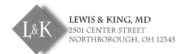

LEWIS & KING, MD
2501 CENTER STREET
NORTHBOROUGH, OH 12345

NORTHBOROUGH
FAMILY MEDICAL GROUP

January 12, 20___    (approximately 15th line)

Jeremy Brown, MD    (approximately 20th line)
111 S Main
Blossom, UT 10283-1120

(triple-space)

BLOSSOM MEDICAL SOCIETY MEETING

(triple-space)

Thank you for inviting me to speak at the Blossom Medical Society
Meeting June 15, 20___. As requested, my topic will describe the use of
the MRI in assisting physicians to make a more accurate diagnosis
without resorting to invasive procedures. The exact title of my speech
will be sent by next Friday.

Please have your office manager send information regarding the number of participants expected, time of meeting, location, and any other
details that will assist me in preparing my speech.

I will write or call if I have any additional questions.

*Winston Lewis, MD*    (4 line spaces)

WINSTON LEWIS, MD

WL:jg

Enclosure: Handout on MRI

**Figure 15-6**    The simplified style letter has no salutation or complimentary closing. The subject line and keyed signature are all upper case.

ment Society recommends this style of letter. However, in medical offices this style is most often employed when sending a form letter. Figure 15-6 illustrates a simplified style letter.

## SUPPLIES FOR WRITTEN COMMUNICATION

The paper should be **bond**, of good quality, and at least 20–24 pound stock with a watermark. A **watermark** is legible when paper is held to the light. Choose a shade of white, cream, or grey.

Although colored paper may be more eye-catching, it does not display a professional image. Also be sure that the paper stock is compatible with printers used in the ambulatory care center.

### *Letterhead*

The letterhead style and design is usually chosen by the physician(s) and may include a specially designed logo for the practice. The physician/practice name, street address and/or post office box number, city, state and zip code, and telephone number with area code are usually printed on the letterhead. Many offices also add their fax number and e-mail address. Letterhead information may be placed at either side or in the center of the paper.

## Second Sheets

When an order is placed for letterhead, the medical assistant should order additional plain paper of the same stock as the letterhead to be used for second page sheets. The number of sheets will vary from office to office. If physicians normally dictate long letters, this must be taken into consideration when ordering quantities.

## Envelopes

The stock and quality of the envelopes should match the stationery used in the office. With the use of **ZIP+4** and City State Files, mail is processed more efficiently and effectively. The address should be standardized so it contains all delivery address elements. The correct name, city, state and ZIP+4 codes must be used.

**Example:**

JEREMY BROWN MD
1111 S MAIN
BLOSSOM UT 10283-1120

If Dr. Brown uses a post office box for the delivery of his mail, that address should be used. The postal service delivers to the last line before the city, state, and zip code.

**Example:**

JEREMY BROWN MD
PO BOX 1453
BLOSSOM UT 10283-1120

Place the intended delivery address on the line immediately above the city, state, and ZIP+4 code. The other address may be placed on a separate line above the delivery line.

**Example:**

JEREMY BROWN MD
1111 S MAIN
PO BOX 1453
BLOSSOM UT 10283-1120

This letter would be received at the post office box, not the street address.

### General Standards for Addressing Envelopes.
For successful processing by **optical character readers (OCRs)**, the United States Postal Services suggests that the address on letter mail needs to be machine-printed, with a uniform left margin. It should be formatted in a manner that allows an OCR to recognize the information and find a match in its address files.

Optical character readers are used by the post office to scan an address. This scanner reads the zip code on the bottom line and prints a bar code in the lower right corner of the envelope.

Envelopes that are handwritten cannot be read by the OCR. Envelopes with handwritten addresses are "spit-out" by the automatic mail sorter. These letters must wait for more costly and slower manual sorting.

New encoding facilities have been established at various sites in the United States. A picture of the handwritten address is taken by a high-speed camera. This picture is transmitted by telephone line to the encoding center. The operators translate the handwritten address into an electric bar code. This code is printed on the envelope, which allows for automatic sorting.

The United States Postal Service publishes several pamphlets and booklets that describe the format to be used when sending any mail. Check with the postal service regarding the latest publications. Service and deliverability will be improved if these standards are used.

To conform to standards, eliminate all punctuation in the envelope address with the exception of a hyphen in the ZIP+4 code. Leave a minimum of one space between the city name and two character state abbreviations and the ZIP+4 code. The OCR can read a combination of uppercase and lowercase characters in addresses but prefers all uppercase characters. See Procedure 15-2.

Dark ink on a light background using uppercase letters is the suggested method in preparing a keyed address. There should be a uniform left margin on all lines of the address. An imaginary rectangle which extends ⅝ inch to 2¾ inches from the bottom of the envelope with one inch on each side should contain the address. The lower right edge should be kept free of any marks. This area will contain the bar code whether it is preapplied or printed by an OCR. The bar code area is ⅝ inch from the bottom and 4½ inches from the right side of the envelope.

### Types of Envelopes.
Number 6¾ and number 10 are the envelopes most often used. A window envelope may also be used, especially when mailing statements.

| Number | Size |
| --- | --- |
| 6¾ | 6½″ long × 3⅝″ wide |
| 10 | 9½″ long × 4⅛″ wide |
| 7 | 7½″ long × 3⅞″ wide |

The address on the statement need only be keyed once. The entire address is capitalized with no punctuation. Only one space should be used between the state abbreviation and the zip code. When this statement is folded with the address in view, it may be inserted into a window envelope. Make certain that the entire address is visible through the window. To prepare envelopes for mailing, lay all envelopes facing upward in a row with the flaps displayed. Moisten all the envelopes with a sponge. With the dominant hand, seal the flap and with the non-dominant hand, push the envelope aside while the next flap is closed. This method will speed the process. Procedure 15-3 illustrates letter folding and placement of envelopes for moistening prior to closure.

## OTHER TYPES OF CORRESPONDENCE

Other specialized types of correspondence the medical assistant may be involved in preparing include memoranda, meeting agendas and meeting minutes, and travel itineraries.

### Memoranda

A type of interoffice correspondence is the **memorandum** or **memo** for short. The use of memos permits messages to be sent quickly and without labor intensive preparation. The memo format may already be preformatted on your computer software. If not, it is easy to design your own memo format.

The side margins should be set for 1 inch. Begin to key the memo heading 2 inches from the top of the page (line 13). The heading includes the words *date, to, from,* and *subject,* which should be emboldened and capitalized. The words should each be keyed on a separate line with a double space between each word. By setting a tab stop 10 spaces in from the left margin, you will be able to tab to each entry and clear the headings to add the appropriate information. Triple space after the entry for the subject heading.

The body of the memo may begin at the left margin or may be set 10 spaces in so that the text starts directly beneath the typed headings. No salutation is required in a memo. Figure 15-7 provides a sample memo.

### Meeting Agendas

Most meetings operate by following *Robert's Rules of Order, Newly Revised,* as their parliamentary authority. The outlined order of business is as follows:

- Reading and approval of the minutes
- Reports of officers, boards, and standing committees
- Reports of special committees (ad hoc)
- Special orders
- Unfinished business and general orders
- New business
- Date and time of next scheduled meeting

The **agenda** lists the specific items that the group plans to discuss at the meeting under each of the abovementioned divisions. The medical assistant preparing the agenda must determine the topics that are to be discussed. Copies of the agenda should be sent to each group member before the meeting date and extra copies should be taken to the meeting for those who may have misplaced or forgotten to bring the agenda with them to the meeting. Figure 15-8 provides a sample meeting agenda.

---

**DATE:** August 25, 2001 (key heading 2 inches from top of page, line 13)

**TO:** Staff of Doctors Lewis & King (embolden and capitalize headings and double space between them)

**FROM:** Walter Seals, Office Manager

**SUBJECT:** Vacation Schedule (triple space after the subject)

Doctors Lewis & King will be on vacation January 1–15. Please do not schedule appointments during that time for either doctor. Office personnel should report to work as usual. During this two-week period, we will be preparing for the annual audit.

**Figure 15-7** Sample memorandum.

---

**AGENDA**
**STAFF MEETING**
**Tuesday, September 1, 2001**
**Location–Conference Room**

Reading and approval of last months' minutes
Reports
    Risk Management Committee
    Personnel
Unfinished business
    Purchase of new X-ray machine
New business
    Doctors Lewis & King vacation January 1–15
    Annual Audit
Date and time for next meeting
Adjournment

**Figure 15-8** Sample meeting agenda.

## Meeting Minutes

A written record of what transpired during a meeting is called the **minutes**. The minutes should record what business actions were taken during the meeting, who made each motion and what it was, who seconded the motion, any pertinent discussion, and whether the motion was passed or not.

The first paragraph of the minutes should contain the following information:

- Kind of meeting (regular, special, emergency)
- Name of the group or association
- Date, time, and place of the meeting
- Who officiated at the meeting and names of members present and absent
- If the previous meeting minutes were read and approved

The body of the minutes should include a paragraph discussing each subject matter or each item listed on the agenda. All motions should be recorded including the exact wording of the motion, the name of the person making the motion, the person seconding the motion, and if the motion passed or failed. If the meeting had a guest speaker, the speaker's name and title and the subject of the presentation may be included in the minutes.

The last paragraph should contain the next meeting date, time, and place, and the time of adjournment for this meeting. The person recording the minutes should sign them, and a copy of all minutes should be maintained in a notebook designated for that purpose. Corporations are required to have regular meetings with recorded minutes for legal purposes. Figure 15-9 provides a sample of recorded minutes.

---

### STAFF MEETING MINUTES

The monthly staff meeting of Doctors Lewis & King was held Tuesday, September 1, 2001, in the conference room. The meeting was called to order by Walter Seals, Office Manager. Those members present included: Dr. Lewis, Dr. King, Marilyn Johnson, Ellen Armstrong, Jane O'Hara, Wanda Slawson, and Bruce Goldman.

The previous meeting's minutes were read and approved as published.

Marilyn Johnson, CMA heading the Risk Management Committee reported that a thorough walk through of the clinic had taken place to assess for safety issues. It was determined that the pull cords on the blinds could pose a potential hazard to small children. Marilyn made a motion that the blinds be upgraded with new vinyl louvered blinds with the plastic rod-type louver adjuster. Wanda Slawson seconded the motion. After discussion, a unanimous vote was cast to replace the blinds at the earliest time possible.

Walter Seals, Human Resource Manager, announced that he would be posting an opening for a CMA to work in the lab. All staff personnel were asked to share information about this opening with professionals who might be interested in working with Doctors Lewis & King.

Discussion was presented by Doctors Lewis & King regarding the purchase of a new X-ray machine. A committee consisting of Wanda Slawson, Bruce Goldman, and Marilyn Johnson was appointed to investigate the specific needs of the clinic and to locate appropriate vendors. They will present their findings at the next scheduled staff meeting.

New Business items include the fact that Doctors Lewis & King will be on vacation January 1–15, 2002. We are asked to not schedule appointments during that time.

Walter Seals discussed preparations for the annual audit during the vacation period of Doctors Lewis & King. He will provide a schedule and timeline at the next staff meeting.

The next scheduled meeting will be October 3 at 12:30 p.m. in the conference room.

The meeting adjourned at 1:45 p.m.

*Ellen Armstrong*

**Figure 15-9** Sample meeting minutes.

# PROCESSING INCOMING AND OUTGOING MAIL

The management of written communications also involves developing procedures for sorting, distributing, and otherwise processing incoming mail. It also includes posting and shipping outgoing items by the most cost- and time-effective method.

## Incoming Mail and Shipments

All mail should be sorted by type prior to opening. Incoming mail includes telegrams, faxes, certified or registered letters, personal letters, e-mail, checks from patients, insurance forms, invoices, medical journals, newspapers, magazines for the reception area, and advertisements regarding equipment and supplies.

Once it is categorized, incoming mail is directed to the appropriate personnel in the office. Checks from patients and invoices may be distributed to the bookkeeper, insurance forms to the insurance clerk, medical journals and advertisements can be placed on the physician's desk, and magazines and newspapers can be placed in the reception area. Personal or confidential letters should not be opened unless the medical assistant has been given this responsibility by the physician or office manager.

Use a letter opener to open all mail before taking out the contents and reading the document. After removing the contents:

- Stamp the date it was received in the office.

- If the address is not included on the letter, write the address on the letter, as identified on the envelope or on the bank check (if patient is making a payment).

- When a colored reply envelope is sent with the statement to the patient, payments returned in these envelopes can speed the sorting process.

- Look into the envelope to make certain that all contents have been removed.

- Attach the letter to the envelope with a paper clip, preferably on the left side.

Reply promptly to all requests, answering letters according to date of arrival; emergency situations need to be managed immediately.

## Outgoing Mail and Shipments

Before placing postage on outgoing mail, weigh the item to be mailed, using a manual or electronic scale. A manual scale will read ounces. The assistant will then affix the appropriate postage, either stamps or postal meter. An electronic scale will automatically display the correct postage. If your office has a postal meter, this should be used to expedite mail. Metered mail does not have to be canceled or postmarked at the post office.

A postage meter is leased or purchased from a manufacturing company recommended by the postal service. However, the postage meter must be taken to the post office to purchase postage. The meter is locked for the amount of postage purchased. Ambulatory care centers that send a large volume of mail may purchase a postage meter.

See Procedure 15-4 for preparing outgoing mail.

## Postal Classes

Check with the local post office to determine anticipated delivery turnaround to specific destinations. Common postal classes include:

1. *First-class mail.* Correspondence and statements are usually sent first class. All single-piece letters weighing less than 11 ounces are included in first-class mail. A postal card may be sent via this method if the card is not larger than 4¼ inches by 6 inches. The card may not be smaller than 3½ inches by 5 inches. If the recipient has moved, first-class mail may be forwarded at no additional cost.

2. *Priority mail.* Mail weighing more than 11 ounces and up to 70 pounds may be sent via priority mail. Check your postal service for current cost. The fee is based on weight and destination. Use the free priority mail stickers available from your local post office.

3. *Second-class mail.* Only newspapers and periodicals that have been authorized second-class privileges are sent by this manner.

4. *Third-class mail* (*bulk mail*). Circulars, books, catalogs, and other printed material and merchandise weighing less than 16 ounces can be sent via this method. Regular and special bulk rates are available only to authorized mailers. A minimum of 200 pieces of mail is required to utilize the bulk rate, and an annual fee must be paid to send via this classification. All mail must be sent from one post office.

5. *Fourth-class mail* (*parcel post*). Fourth-class mail must weigh more than 16 ounces (1 pound) and not more than 70 pounds.

6. *Certified mail.* This service provides proof that a letter has been received. For example, if a physician dismisses a patient from the practice due to non-compliance of orders, a letter should be sent by certified mail, return receipt requested. When the receipt of acceptance of the letter is returned to the office, make certain that this receipt is filed in the patient's medical record. This provides legal protection for the physician. Other examples of mail that should be certified include birth certificates, marriage licenses, and deeds to property.

7. *Registered mail.* When an item has an intrinsic (real) value it should be sent via registered mail. Receipts are provided to identify the individual who accepted this mail. The sender declares a value on the item. A signature is required prior to delivery being made. Examples of items that should be sent by registered mail include clothing and jewelry.

8. *Express mail.* This service is available seven days per week for mailing items up to 70 pounds and 108 inches in combined length and girth. Express mail may be sent for noon delivery on the next day between major business markets.

## Formats for Efficient Processing

Certified, registered, and special delivery markings should be placed below the stamp or approximately nine lines from the right top edge of the envelope. "Personal" or "confidential" notation should be keyed in all caps three lines below the return address. Adherence to other regulations will ensure accurate, timely delivery.

**ZIP+4.** ZIP+4 consists of the basic five ZIP code digits followed by a hyphen and four additional digits. The use of ZIP+4 will expedite the delivery of mail. If the envelope has been prepared properly to be read through OCR, the digits will be converted to a bar code. This piece of mail then goes to the bar code sorter which rapidly sorts for the final destination.

**Abbreviations.** When addressing mail, use the abbreviations for states and United States possessions (Figure 15-10) and official postal service abbreviations for street suffixes, directionals, and locators (Figure 15-11).

## International Mail

Classes of international mail include letters and letter packages, postcards and postal cards, aerogrammes, printed matter, direct sacks of printed matter, matter for the blind, small packets, and parcel post. Special services such as insurance, recorded delivery, registered mail, restricted delivery, return receipt, special delivery, COD mail, and certified mail are also available. For the most current information on rates and services, inquire at the local postal service.

## TECHNOLOGIES

In recent years, many new technologies such as fax and e-mail have changed the way written communications are sent. Also see Chapters 11 and 12 for more information on these technologies.

## Facsimile (Fax)

A facsimile, or fax, is the transmission of a written document through a telephone line using a fax machine both at the sender's and receiver's end. A fax can be sent as easily as putting the document in the machine similar to the way a document is put in a copy machine and dialing the receiving telephone number. See Procedure 15-5. There are

| AL | Alabama | NE | Nebraska |
|---|---|---|---|
| AK | Alaska | NV | Nevada |
| AS | American Samoa | NH | New Hampshire |
| AZ | Arizona | NJ | New Jersey |
| AR | Arkansas | NM | New Mexico |
| CA | California | NY | New York |
| CO | Colorado | NC | North Carolina |
| CT | Connecticut | ND | North Dakota |
| DE | Delaware | MP | No. Mariana Islands |
| DC | Dist. of Columbia | OH | Ohio |
| FL | Florida | OK | Oklahoma |
| GA | Georgia | OR | Oregon |
| GU | Guam | PA | Pennsylvania |
| HI | Hawaii | PR | Puerto Rico |
| ID | Idaho | RI | Rhode Island |
| IL | Illinois | SC | South Carolina |
| IN | Indiana | SD | South Dakota |
| IA | Iowa | TN | Tennessee |
| KS | Kansas | TX | Texas |
| KY | Kentucky | TT | Trust Territory |
| LA | Louisiana | UT | Utah |
| ME | Maine | VT | Vermont |
| MD | Maryland | VI | Virgin Islands, U.S. |
| MA | Massachusetts | VA | Virginia |
| MI | Michigan | WA | Washington |
| MN | Minnesota | WV | West Virginia |
| MS | Mississippi | WI | Wisconsin |
| MO | Missouri | WY | Wyoming |
| MT | Montana | | |

**Figure 15-10** Abbreviations for states, territories, and District of Columbia. (Courtesy United States Postal Service)

| AVE | Avenue | PL | Place |
|---|---|---|---|
| BLVD | Boulevard | RD | Road |
| CT | Court | STA | Station |
| CTR | Center | ST | Street |
| CIR | Circle | TPKE | Turnpike |
| DR | Drive | VLY | Valley |
| EXPY | Expressway | APT | Apartment |
| HTS | Heights | RM | Room |
| HWY | Highway | STE | Suite |
| IS | Island | PLZ | Plaza |
| JCT | Junction | | |
| LK | Lake | N | North |
| LN | Lane | E | East |
| MTN | Mountain | S | South |
| PKY | Parkway | W | West |

**Figure 15-11** Abbreviations for street suffixes, directionals, and locators. (Courtesy United States Postal Service)

| TABLE 15-4 | ADVANTAGES OF THE FAX |
|---|---|
| Speed | The document is transmitted immediately or within minutes of sending. |
| Cost | Cost of a fax is the approximate cost of the telephone call. For long-distance faxes, this can be many times less than the cost of an overnight service. |
| Patient Care | Patient care could be enhanced, especially in emergency situations where the receiver may need to make decisions based on information in the document. |
| Legality | The receiver has the "hard copy" document versus relying on verbal information if the information is needed immediately. |

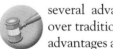 several advantages to using the fax machine over traditional postal or carrier services. These advantages are listed in Table 15-4.

There are other issues involved in using the fax, especially when sending patient information. Figure 15-12 provides insight on several legal and confidentiality issues that should be considered before sending any communications via the fax. See Chapter 11 for additional guidelines related to fax use.

## Electronic Mail (E-Mail)

 Medical information previously communicated via mail, telephone, or fax may now be sent from computer to computer using **e-mail**. Just as business communication requires proper use of written language, so does e-mail.

Composing e-mail is similar to composing any written communication. Just as a letter or memo has a particular format, the e-mail transmission should also follow a format style. The subject line should be brief and clearly identify the content of the e-mail body.

If your message is in response to another piece of e-mail, your e-mail software will probably preface the subject line with *Re:* (for regarding). If your e-mail software

---

## DON'T FAX YOUR WAY INTO A LAWSUIT

One of the cornerstones of the doctor/patient relationship is professional confidentiality. But quality care often depends on sharing patient information, swiftly and accurately, with other medical professionals.

About the fastest and most accurate way to transmit medical information is by fax. But faxed records can all too easily fall into the wrong person's hands.

In this lawsuit-driven age, all of us know why we must never fax confidential records, but in our convenience-driven culture, we also know that confidential records are being faxed every day, all across America. So the question becomes: How can we keep faxed records as confidential as mailed, messengered, or verbally-summarized-over-the-phone records?

The answer is to set up a *Fax Security System*, as follows:

### Fax Security System

1. Make sure you have an Authorization To Release Records form, dated and signed by the patient or legal guardian, before you fax any information (just as you'd make sure you had a signed release if you wanted to send records any other way).
2. Never fax financial information. You can justify (in court) the faxing of medical information on the basis of medical necessity; but you cannot justify (anywhere) the faxing of financial data that the patient deems confidential.
3. Before you fax, ask yourself: "Is this really necessary? Or are we better off mailing or messengering these records?"
4. After you answer yourself, ask your office manager: "Will you sign an approval to fax these records? You will? I'll do

it right away. You won't? Thanks for taking the decision off my back."
5. Only fax to telecopiers located in physician offices, nursing stations, or other secure areas. Do *not* fax to machines in mail rooms, office lobbies, or other open areas unless they are secured with passwords. When in doubt about the machine's exact location, "Hold your fax 'til you see the whites of their thermal paper."
6. Use a cover sheet that contains the warning: "The following material is strictly confidential; all persons are advised that they may be prosecuted under federal and state law for sharing this information with unauthorized individuals."
7. If your fax has a display showing the phone number being faxed to, make sure the displayed number corresponds to the number you want to fax to.
8. After faxing, call the faxee and confirm that the fax was received. If not, use your "recall" to find the last number dialed (your manual should show you how). Fax an urgent alert to that number and ask "all persons of goodwill to immediately and effectively destroy all documents received in the previous transmission."

Photocopy this Fax Security System and post it right above your fax machine. Make sure every staff member reads and understands it.

Oh? You say you can't be bothered with all this "security stuff"? That's all right; there's a much easier item to post for practices that aren't all that security-conscious: Your lawyer's telephone number.

**Figure 15-12**    Don't fax your way into a lawsuit. (Copyright © 1994 The Doctor's Office. Reprinted with permission.)

does not do this, it would be polite to key in "RE:". If your message is time critical, starting with "URGENT" is appropriate. If you are referring to previous e-mail, you should explicitly quote that document to provide context.

If your message is being addressed to several parties, list the e-mail addresses in "bcc" which stands for **blind copies**. This procedure protects the privacy of your audience. "Cc" permits all recipients to view the full list of addresses. It is a good practice to put your own e-mail address at the top of the list, as a quality check, so you can see what everyone else is receiving and/or maintain a copy for the file.

The body of the message should contain short and clear sentences. In trying to be brief and to the point, however, it is important to not leave out important facts or information. Remember also that some e-mail software only understands plain text. Italics, bold, and color changes should be used sparingly. Some software will also recognize **URLs (Uniform Resource Locators,** or web site addresses) in the text and make them "live." Since different software recognizes different parts of the address, if you include a URL in your e-mail, it is much safer to use the entire address, including the initial http://.

The advantages of using e-mail as a means of communication include:

- Asynchronous communication—both parties need not be available at the same time for communication to take place
- Physicians and patients can prepare, leave, read, and respond to messages at times that are convenient
- Can be used to automate certain tasks such as sending out appointment reminders or reports of lab results
- Creates a documentation trail of interactions between physician and patient
- Some patients may be more forthcoming using e-mail than in face-to-face discussion

The disadvantages of e-mail communications include:

- Lack of real-time interaction and feedback
- Lack of body language or vocal inflection, which may lead to misunderstanding
- Reimbursement for the time spent responding to patient messages and receipt of messages from non-patients may not be defined
- May not be suitable for time-sensitive material since determination of when the message will be delivered or read can not be assessed

## LEGAL AND ETHICAL ISSUES

Written communication, no matter what form is used, must take into consideration legal and ethical issues. A

 copy of all written communication should be maintained in the patient chart or in office files should it be needed at a later date.

It is important to include e-mail in your office's confidentiality policy. Confidentiality issues must be considered if the ambulatory care office sends or receives **clinical e-mail** from a computer that can be used by more than one person. Many offices use a privacy disclaimer to establish boundaries and ground rules for e-mail messages. The following is an example of such a disclaimer:

This message is a privileged and confidential clinical communication intended solely for the person to whom it is addressed. If you are not the intended recipient, please be advised that any dissemination, copying, or distribution of this message is strictly prohibited. If you received this message in error, please forward it back to the sender.

Clinical e-mail to or from patients should be treated the same as telephone messages or letters. That means that they should be printed out and filed in the chart. It is important to remember to file both the initial message and any reply.

Before your office begins to use clinical e-mail, a written agreement of understanding should be designed for signature by the patients. In addition to obtaining the patient's permission for you to use clinical e-mail, key elements to include in such an agreement may include:

- E-mail will be exchanged with established patients only.
- E-mail from the patient will include the patient's full name and number.
- The physician is not responsible for e-mail that is not received or responded to in a timely manner.
- E-mail may not be private and confidential.
- E-mail may be read by others, intercepted, or mis-addressed.
- E-mail will be filed in the chart.
- E-mail will not be permanently stored on the computer system.
- Urgent issues need to be handled by telephone or in person.

Examples of appropriate uses of e-mail in the ambulatory care setting include:

- Appointment requests
- Prescription refill requests
- Reminder notices
- Insurance or billing questions
- Managed care referrals

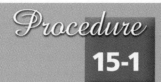

# Preparing and Composing Business Correspondence Using All Components

**15-1**

## PURPOSE:

Prepare and compose a rough draft and final-copy letter using appropriate language and letter style to convey a clear and accurate message to the recipient.

## EQUIPMENT/SUPPLIES:

Computer or word processor and printer; or typewriter
Printed letterhead and plain second sheet
Dictionary
Thesaurus
Medical dictionary
Style manual

## PROCEDURE STEPS:

1. Organize key points to be addressed in a logical sequence. RATIONALE: To assist in writing an effective letter.

2. Compose a rough draft of the letter. With time and experience, these outlining steps may be eliminated before drafting the letter. RATIONALE: Business correspondence should be clear, concise, courteous, and accurate. A draft letter aids in checking that the letter is logical and achieves the intended purpose.

3. Use language that is easily understood. State the reason for the letter in the first paragraph and encourage action in the last paragraph. RATIONALE: For communication to take place, both parties must understand the message. The letter must be written so that the recipient understands the language and responds appropriately.

4. Read the draft for obvious errors in grammar, spelling, and punctuation. Use the appropriate reference material (dictionary, style manual, and so on) to check any inaccuracies. Read again for content; is the message accurate, logical, and organized appropriately? Lay the letter aside and read it a third time at a later time. RATIONALE: Reading several times allows you to concentrate on different elements of the letter. Errors may "jump" out when reading the third time.

5. Choose the letter format that is customary to the ambulatory care setting. RATIONALE: The letter style should be efficient to prepare and professional in appearance and content in order to represent the physician/employer in a professional manner.

6. Begin keying the letter, referring to the chosen format. Key the date on line 15 or two to three lines below the letterhead. The date should be completely written out; i.e., January 15, 20__, rather than 1/15/__. RATIONALE: Using the component parts of a business letter ensures that the letter is professional in appearance and represents the physician/employer in a professional manner.

7. Key the recipient's name and address flush with the left margin beginning on line 20. RATIONALE: Using the component parts of a business letter ensures that the letter is professional in appearance and represents the physician/employer in a professional manner.

8. On the second line below the recipient's address, key the salutation flush with the left margin. Follow the salutation with a colon unless you are using open punctuation. RATIONALE: Using the component parts of a business letter ensures that the letter is professional in appearance and represents the physician/employer in a professional manner.

9. Key the subject of the letter on the second line below the salutation flush with the left margin, if the subject line is being used. RATIONALE: Using the component parts of a business letter ensures that the letter is professional in appearance and represents the physician/employer in a professional manner.

10. Begin the body of the letter on the second line below the salutation or subject line. The body format will depend upon the style of letter used. For example, if the full block format is used, paragraphs will begin flush with the left margin. Single-space within paragraphs; double-space between paragraphs. RATIONALE: Using the component parts of a business letter ensures that the letter is professional in appearance and represents the physician/employer in a professional manner.

11. Key the complimentary closure on the second line below the body of the letter. Capitalize only the first letter of the first word of the complimentary closure; e.g., Respectfully yours. RATIONALE: Using the component parts of a business

*(continues)*

## Procedure 15-1 (continued)

letter ensures that the letter is professional in appearance and represents the physician/employer in a professional manner.

12. Key the signature four to six lines below the complimentary closing. RATIONALE: This ensures that the recipient will be able to determine who sent the letter.

13. If reference initials are used, key the initials two lines below the keyed signature; e.g., WL: jg. RATIONALE: Using the component parts of a business letter ensures that the letter is professional in appearance and represents the physician/employer in a professional manner.

14. Key the enclosure or carbon copy notation one or two lines below the reference initials. RATIONALE: Using the component parts of a business letter ensures that the letter is professional in appearance and represents the physician/employer in a professional manner.

15. Proofread the document and make corrections as necessary. RATIONALE: All information contained in the letter must be accurate and written in a clear and concise manner with logical organization. The grammar, spelling, punctuation, and capitalization must be correct to ensure a professional appearance and represent the physician/employer in a positive manner.

16. Prepare the envelope. Place the envelope flap over the letter and attach it with a paper clip. RATIONALE: Prepare the envelope using United States Postal regulations to ensure delivery in a timely manner. Proofread to be sure the address is accurate to ensure deliverability. By placing the envelope flap over the letter and attaching it with a paper clip the two will not become separated.

17. Place the letter on the physician's desk for review and signature. RATIONALE: The physician's signature signifies the letter is accurate, sends the intended message, and represents the office in a professional manner.

## Procedure 15-2 Addressing Envelopes According to United States Postal Regulations

**PURPOSE:**
To address envelopes according to United States Postal Service regulations to ensure timely delivery.

**EQUIPMENT/SUPPLIES:**
Computer or word processor and printer with envelope tray; or typewriter
Envelopes
United States Postal Service Publication 221, *Addressing for Success*

**PROCEDURE STEPS:**
1. Insert the envelope in the typewriter or select the envelope format from the software program. When using a word processor or computer, labels may be used rather than printing directly on the envelope. The label is then adhered to the envelope. RATIONALE: United States Postal regulations suggest that the address on letter mail should be machine-printed, with a uniform left margin.

2. Visualize an imaginary rectangle on the envelope. The rectangle extends ⅝ inch to 2¾ inches from the bottom of the envelope, with 1 inch on each side. The address is placed within this rectangle (Figure 15-13). RATIONALE: United States Postal regulations suggest that the address on letter mail should be machine-printed, with a uniform left margin.

*(continues)*

*Procedure*

## 15-2   *(continued)*

3. Key the address in uppercase letters. Be sure to maintain a uniform left margin on all lines. Eliminate all punctuation in the address except the hyphen in the ZIP+4 code. Leave a minimum of one space between the city name and the two-character state abbreviation and the ZIP+4 code. RATIONALE: A scanner reads the Zip code on the bottom line and prints a bar code in the lower right corner of the envelope. The OCR prefers all uppercase characters.

4. If you are not using preprinted envelopes, key the return address in uppercase letters in the upper left corner of the envelope. Include the name on the first line, address on the second line, and city, state, and ZIP+4 code on the third line. RATIONALE: The return address should be printed in the upper left corner of the envelope should the letter need to be returned to the sender for any reason.

5. Proofread the envelope, make corrections as necessary. RATIONALE: When all information is correct, processing will take place efficiently and correctly.

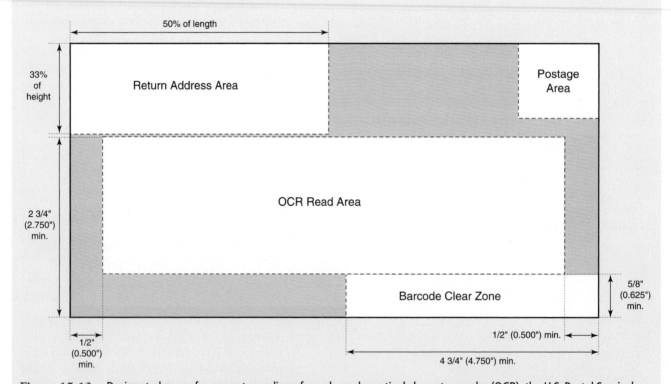

**Figure 15-13**   Designated zones for accurate reading of envelopes by optical character reader (OCR), the U.S. Postal Service's computerized scanner. (Courtesy United States Postal Service)

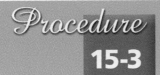

## Folding Letters for Standard Envelopes

### 15-3

**PURPOSE:**
To fold and insert letters into envelopes so that the letters fit properly in the envelopes.

**EQUIPMENT/SUPPLIES:**
Letters to be mailed
Number 6¾ envelope
Number 10 envelope
Window envelope

**PROCEDURE STEPS:**

1. To fit a standard-size letter into a number 6¾ envelope, fold the letter up from the bottom, leaving ¼ inch to ½ inch at the top, and crease it. Then fold the letter from the right edge about one-third the width of the letter. Fold the left edge over to within ¼ inch to ½ inch of the right-edge crease. Insert the left creased edge first into the envelope (Figure 15-14A). RATIONALE: Ensures a proper fit of the letter into the envelope with a minimum of folds. The last crease made enters the envelope first. This enables the recipient to begin to read the letter with minimum effort.

2. To fit a standard-size letter into a number 10 envelope, fold the letter up about one-third the length of the sheet and crease it. Then fold the top of the letter down to within ¼ inch to ½ inch of the bottom crease, and crease the top. Insert the top creased edge first into the envelop (Figure 15-14B). RATIONALE: Ensures a proper fit of the letter into the envelope with a minimum of folds. The last crease made enters the envelope first. This enables the recipient to begin to read the letter with minimum effort.

3. To fit a standard-size letter into a window envelope, turn the letter over and fold the top of the letter up about one-third the length of the page

*(continues)*

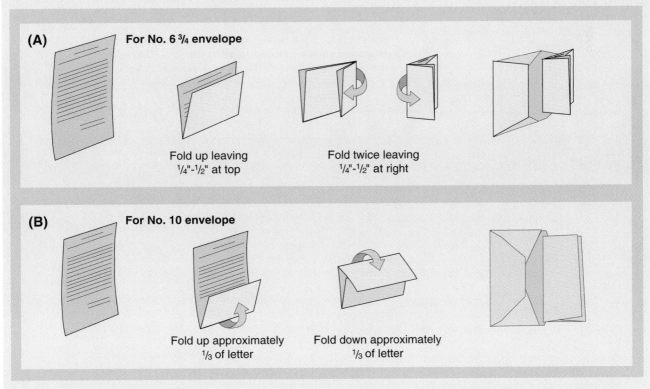

**(A)**  **For No. 6 ³/₄ envelope**

Fold up leaving
¹/₄"-¹/₂" at top

Fold twice leaving
¹/₄"-¹/₂" at right

**(B)**  **For No. 10 envelope**

Fold up approximately
¹/₃ of letter

Fold down approximately
¹/₃ of letter

**Figure 15-14**  Proper letter folding procedures for various envelope types (A–C) and bulk placement of envelopes for moistening prior to closure (D).

## *Procedure*
## 15-3 *(continued)*

so that the address is facing you. Then fold the bottom of the letter back to the first crease. Insert the letter into the envelope bottom first (Figure 15-14C). You should be able to read the entire address through the window. RATIO-NALE: Ensures that the entire address can be

read through the window envelope and be delivered correctly.

4. Place envelopes as shown in Figure 15-14D to moisten prior to sealing. RATIONALE: Efficient method of sealing multiple letters for mailing.

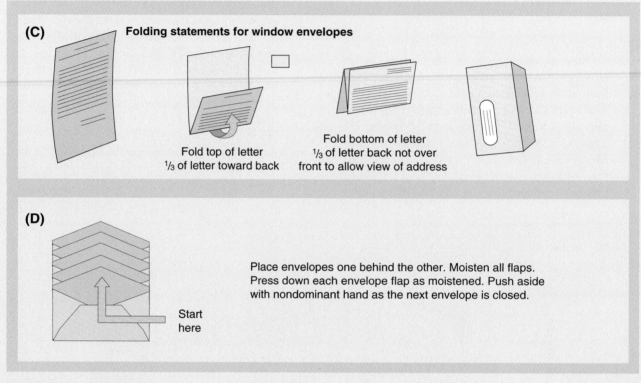

**(C)**    **Folding statements for window envelopes**

Fold top of letter
1/3 of letter toward back

Fold bottom of letter
1/3 of letter back not over
front to allow view of address

**(D)**

Start
here

Place envelopes one behind the other. Moisten all flaps.
Press down each envelope flap as moistened. Push aside
with nondominant hand as the next envelope is closed.

**Figure 15-14** *(continued)*

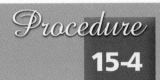

# Preparing Outgoing Mail According to United States Postal Regulations

**15-4**

**PURPOSE:**
To prepare outgoing mail for expeditious delivery.

**EQUIPMENT/SUPPLIES:**
Manual or electronic scale
Postage meter or stamps
Envelope or package to be mailed

**PROCEDURE STEPS:**
1. Sort the mail according to postal class. For example, all single-piece letters that weigh less than 11 ounces are included in first-class mail. Correspondence and statements are sent in this classification. RATIONALE: Sorting by postal class expedites processing at the Post Office.
2. Using the manual or electronic scale, weigh the item to be mailed. If you are using a manual scale, read the weight in ounces and compute the amount of postage due. If you are using an electronic scale, the correct postage will be displayed on the scale. RATIONALE: Correct postage on each postal item is essential to ensure faster delivery service.
3. Using a postal meter or stamps, affix the appropriate postage to the piece to be mailed. Use of a postal meter expedites delivery of mail because metered mail does not have to be canceled or postmarked at the post office. RATIONALE: Correct postage on each postal item is essential to ensure faster delivery service.
4. Place the prepared mail in the area of the office designated for outgoing mail or deliver the mail to the post office according to office policy. RATIONALE: Ensures that all mail going out is centrally located and that the postal worker can pick up outgoing and deliver incoming mail efficiently.

# Preparing, Sending, and Receiving a Fax

**15-5**

**PURPOSE:**
To send and receive information quickly and accurately by fax (facsimile).

**EQUIPMENT/SUPPLIES:**
Fax machine
Telephone

**PROCEDURE STEPS:**
*To send a fax:*
1. Prepare a cover sheet or use a preprinted cover sheet for the document to be faxed. Include the names of the sender and receiver, the number of pages being sent and whether this includes the cover sheet, and a short message if necessary. RATIONALE: A cover sheet aids in the correct delivery of a fax to the designated person. It also provides a disclaimer should the fax be received in error and what to do if it is misdelivered.

**CAUTION:** Fax machines may be located in areas where unauthorized personnel may see confidential material. Always include a notice of confidentiality on the cover sheet and always ask the receiver for permission to fax a confidential document.
2. Place the document face down in the fax machine, similar to the way a document is put into a copy machine. RATIONALE: Ensures that content will be read for transmission.
3. Dial the telephone or dedicated fax number of the receiver. If your fax machine has a display showing the number being faxed to, check to be sure the number you dialed is correct. Then press start. RATIONALE: Verify number to be sure fax is being transmitted to correct phone.

*(continues)*

*Procedure*

**15-5** *(continued)*

4. After the document passes through the fax machine, press the button requesting a receipt. Some fax machines automatically issue a report. RATIONALE: A receipt is your documentation of the date, time, and where the fax was sent.

5. Remove the document from the machine and, when necessary, call the recipient to be sure the fax was received. RATIONALE: Maintains confidentiality and verifies fax was received by intended recipient.

*To receive a fax:*

6. Be sure that the fax machine is turned on and that the telephone line to the machine is not being used. Most offices will have dedicated fax lines. RATIONALE: Enables you to receive a fax.

7. Remove the document from the machine after it is received and immediately deliver it to the addressee. RATIONALE: Maintains confidentiality and enables recipient to take action immediately if necessary.

**15-1**

When she was assembling the style manual for all written communications generated by the office of Doctors Lewis & King, office manager Marilyn Johnson wanted it to be as comprehensive as possible. Therefore, she gathered research over a period of months, noting problems the office had experienced in written communications, such as letters going out without the physician's signature; she became very familiar with proofreading devices that would ensure letter-perfect correspondence; and she developed source materials on the different classes of mail and the services of the United States Post Office.

## CASE STUDY REVIEW

1. Marilyn is ready to outline the manual. Review the chapter information and create an outline indicating major topic headings for the Lewis & King style manual.

2. Because a few of the medical assistants are not comfortable with composing, what writing tips can Marilyn include to make them more confident?

3. Marilyn wants all letters to look alike. What information should she include to educate the manual users about the components of a standard letter?

**15-2**

Doctors Lewis & King are considering adopting the use of clinical e-mail since many of their patients have home computers and use e-mail in their day-to-day communications. Office manager Marilyn Johnson is concerned about maintaining patient confidentiality and appropriate use of clinical e-mail. She has decided to develop a written agreement of understanding and plans to ask each patient to sign the agreement before transmission of any clinical e-mail is instituted. Marilyn also feels a privacy disclaimer could be of legal value to the office.

## CASE STUDY REVIEW

1. Marilyn is developing the agreement of understanding. What are some key elements that should be included in the agreement?

2. Responding to patients using e-mail correspondence is different than social communication. What are some guidelines for e-mail correspondence that will be helpful to remember?

3. List several advantages and disadvantages to using e-mail in the ambulatory health care setting.

## SUMMARY

Communication is vital in any ambulatory care setting, and the proper management of written communications ensures both a professional image and an efficient operation. Because of our ability to write letters, send reports, transcribe physician notes, and otherwise communicate with others, the quality of patient care is enhanced, for communication is at the core of much patient treatment.

As well as becoming knowledgeable about the techniques of written communication, it is important for the medical assistant to become comfortable with the act of composition and writing. Proper techniques in letter formatting and proofreading ensures quality control and the maintenance of high administrative standards. Ease in writing and communicating on paper ensures that information is accurate, reliable, and capable of being held up in a court of law if this becomes necessary.

The administrative medical assistant must be skilled in the use of technologies and understand and follow confidentiality and legal policies and procedures.

## REVIEW QUESTIONS

### Multiple Choice

1. When proofreading a letter, you should:
   a. never read it against the document
   b. proof it on the computer screen
   c. read long documents a section at a time
   d. always finish the job no matter how tired you may be
2. Form letters should be used:
   a. for all patients
   b. for all referring physicians
   c. only for pharmaceutical salespeople
   d. with individualized addressing when possible
3. Of the four major letter styles, which is the most contemporary?
   a. full block
   b. modified block, standard
   c. modified block, indented
   d. simplified
4. Form letters may be written for each of the following *except*:
   a. letters containing laboratory and/or diagnostic results
   b. letters announcing new insurance or HMOs accepted
   c. letters to announce new staff
   d. letters to order supplies or subscriptions
5. The subject line is keyed:
   a. on line 15 or two to three lines below the letterhead
   b. on the second line below the inside address
   c. four lines below the complimentary closing
   d. on the second line below the salutation

6. When keying a second page, all of the following apply *except*:
   a. always use a second-page heading
   b. when dividing a paragraph at the bottom of a page, keep one line on the bottom of the page and one line at the top of the next page
   c. a minimum of three lines should be keyed on the second page of a letter
   d. never use a letterhead page as a second page
7. After removing the contents from incoming mail, what should you do?
   a. stamp the date it was received in the office
   b. look in the envelope to make certain that all contents have been removed
   c. if the address is not included on the letter, write it on the letter as it appeared on the envelope
   d. all of the above
8. In the ambulatory care setting, the postal class likely to be used most frequently is:
   a. express
   b. first class
   c. bulk rate
   d. second class
9. The body of an e-mail communication should:
   a. contain short and clear sentences
   b. be written in italic, bold, and color for emphasis
   c. be brief and to the point but contain all pertinent information
   d. answers a and c only
10. To establish boundaries and ground rules for e-mail messages, many offices are developing:
    a. privacy disclaimers
    b. written agreements of understanding
    c. itineraries
    d. agendas

## Critical Thinking

1. Recall the five writing tips for more effective communication. Now write a letter using these points.
2. With a group of students, organize a spelling bee of commonly used medical words. Include some of the words that are often misspelled.
3. Identify the four major letter styles. Compose and key a letter using each of these styles.
4. List the component parts of any business letter. Give a brief description of the placement of each component part.
5. State at least eight of the guidelines of letter composition.
6. Use those guidelines to revise a letter. Work from an existing draft that needs corrections, then rewrite, rekey, and proofread the revised letter.
7. In a small group, exchange the original and revised letters produced in number 6. Make comments on how (and whether) the letters are improved.
8. Address an envelope with all address elements in proper format for expeditious handling by the United States Postal Service.
9. Prepare a document with a cover sheet for faxing. Before you fax the document, however, recall the eight points from Figure 15-16. Does your document meet these guidelines?
10. Discuss legal and ethical issues regarding the use of clinical e-mail.

## WEB ACTIVITIES

Use the Internet to research additional information pertaining to confidentiality and legal issues related to faxing medical records or electronic mail to transmit medical information. Follow instructor's instructions on completing and turning in your results.

## DOCUMENTATION

Clinically related e-mail to or from patients should be treated the same way as telephone messages or letters. That means they should be printed out and filed in the chart.

| | |
|---|---|
| **From:** | Elizabeth J. Parker |
| **Sent:** | Tuesday, July 20, 20__ 8:55 AM |
| **To:** | Dr. King [King@doctor.com] |
| **Subject:** | Prescription refill |

Please call in a prescription refill for my thyroid medication. The pharmacy is Inner City Pharmacy and the phone number is 890-271-2600. The prescription number is RX6437350 and I have enough pills for three days.

## REFERENCES/BIBLIOGRAPHY

Humphrey, D. D. (1996) *Contemporary medical office procedures* (2nd ed.). Albany, NY: Delmar.

Kinn, M. E., & Woods, M. A. (1999). *The medical assistant: Administrative and clinical* (8th ed.). Philadelphia: W. B. Saunders.

Pearce, F. (1999). *Business netiquette international.* [On-line]. Available: *http://www.bspage.com/inetiq/Netiq.html*

Physicians Insurance 2000. March/April 2000. *Physician's risk management update.* (Vol. XI, No. 2.) Author.

Robert, H. M., III, Evans, W. J., Honemann, D. H., Balch, T. J. (2000). *Robert's Rules of Order Newly Revised* (10th ed.). Cambridge, MA: Perseus Publishing.

Sherwood, K. D. (1998). *A beginner's guide to effective e-mail.* [On-line]. Available: *http://www.webfoot.com/advice/email.top.html.*

Tessier, C. (1995). *The AAMT book of style for medical transcription.* American Association for Medical Transcription.

United States Postal Service. (1995). *Addressing for Success* (Pub. 221). Washington, DC: Author.

Virtual mail center not your ordinary sort. (1995, October 16). *Tulsa Daily World.*

# Chapter

## 16

# TRANSCRIPTION

## KEY TERMS

American Association for Medical
Transcription (AAMT)

Breach of Confidentiality

Certified Medical Transcriptionist (CMT)

Chart Notes

Chief Complaint (CC)

Confidentiality

Confidentiality Agreement

Consultation Report

Continuing Education (CE)

Continuous Speech Recognition (CSR)

Digital Dictation

Editing

Flag

Freelance MTs

History of the Present Illness (HPI)

History and Physical Examination
(H&P) Report

Home-Based MTs

Index Counter

Joint Commission on Accreditation of
Healthcare Organizations (JCAHO)

Medical Transcriptionist (MT)

Medical Transcriptionist Certification
Program (MTCP)

Privileged

Progress Notes

Proofreading

Quality Assurance (QA)

Recertification

Review of Systems (ROS)

Risk Management

Split Keyboard

STAT

Transcriber

Wrist Rest

## OUTLINE

History of the American
Association for Medical
Transcription
  AAMT Membership

The Medical Transcriptionist's
Career
  Attributes of the Medical
    Transcriptionist
  Job Description
  Employment Opportunities
  Certification for Medical
    Transcriptionists

Transcription Tools
  Equipment
  Ergonomics
  Facsimile Machines
  Photocopy Machines

Transcription Guidelines

Proofreading and Making
Corrections
  Proofreading Skills
  Where Errors Occur
  Editing
  Making Corrections

Medical Reports
  Chart Notes and Progress Notes
  History and Physical Examination
    Reports
  Consultation Reports
  Correspondence

Turnaround Time

Ethical and Legal Issues
  Confidentiality
  Risk Management

New Technology
  Continuous Speech Recognition
  Integrating Digital Photographs
    into Medical Transcription

## OBJECTIVES

*The student should strive to meet the following performance objectives and demonstrate an understanding of the facts and principles presented in this chapter through written and oral communication.*

1. Define the key terms as presented in the glossary.

2. Briefly describe the history of medical transcription.

3. List a minimum of ten benefits of membership in AAMT.

4. Describe the two major categories of attributes of the medical transcriptionist.

5. Compare and contrast the various types of work environments for the medical transcriptionist.

*(continues)*

241

## OBJECTIVES (*continued*)

6. Describe the certification and recertification process for the medical transcriptionist.
7. List important considerations when setting up a workstation ergonomically.
8. Describe the process of flagging and its significance.
9. Discuss the proper ways to make corrections within medical record transcription.
10. Differentiate between chart notes, history and physical examination reports, consultation reports, and medical correspondence.
11. Describe turnaround time and its importance.
12. Discuss ethical and legal issues as they apply to medical transcription.

## ROLE DELINEATION COMPONENTS

**ADMINISTRATIVE**
**Administrative Procedures**
- **Perform basic clerical functions**

**GENERAL (TRANSDISCIPLINARY)**
**Legal Concepts**
- **Document accurately**

## SCENARIO

Inner City Health Care, a multispecialty clinic, employs two full-time medical transcriptionists. Marilyn Johnson, CMA, is the office manager and has former training and experience as a medical transcriptionist. This experience provides her with the basic understanding necessary to manage the medical transcription and medical records department of the clinic. Marilyn has involved the transcriptionists in the ergonomic set up of workstations and in the selection of state-of-the-art equipment and latest reference resources to create a safe work environment and one that encourages quality documents in a timely manner.

## INTRODUCTION

In early times, when only a few people could read and write, scribes copied and interpreted the spoken word. Often the scribes transcribed legal and sacred orations into written documents that became the principles and rules by which society was governed. The word *transcription* is composed of two word elements: *trans* and *scriba*. *Trans* is a prefix meaning across, beyond, through, or so as to change. *Scriba* means official writer. Translated, transcription means to change the spoken word to a written record.

Ancient cave writings testify to the beginning of patient care documentation. Hieroglyphics changed to papyrus and parchment using berries to produce ink, to paper using typewriters, and most recently to computer-generated medical records. Until the twentieth century, physicians were both providers of medical care and scribes maintaining their own records. With the standardization of medical data for research purposes after 1900, medical stenographers replaced physician scribes by taking their dictation in shorthand. The career of medical transcription came into being with the development of dictation equipment during World War I. Today medical transcriptionists use computers to transmit patient records electronically to distant locations. Future technology includes incorporating digital images into medical records and the use of continuous voice recognition systems.

# HISTORY OF THE AMERICAN ASSOCIATION FOR MEDICAL TRANSCRIPTION

The **American Association for Medical Transcription (AAMT)** began in 1978 as a nonprofit organization incorporated in California. One of the greatest desires of AAMT's founders was that **medical transcriptionists (MTs)** be appropriately recognized for the important contribution they make in health care. As a direct result of AAMT's continued efforts to promote the profession, medical transcription is a respected profession, with practitioners recognized as medical language specialists.

The definition of a medical transcriptionist according to the *AAMT Model Job Description* is "a medical language specialist who interprets and transcribes dictation by physicians and other healthcare professionals regarding patient assessment, workup, therapeutic procedures, clinical course, diagnosis, prognosis, etc., in order to document patient care and facilitate delivery of healthcare services." (AAMT, 1990)

For someone seeking education and training, advertisements for medical transcription education programs appear in many places. Here are four ways to evaluate the advertising:

1. The advertising should accurately represent the profession as a medical language specialty requiring a substantial educational investment.
2. When describing a home-based transcription business opportunity, the advertising should indicate the need for additional training in accounting procedures and management protocols for operating a business.
3. A reference source for the income should be cited within the advertising if potential income is discussed.
4. If certification is referenced, it should clearly state that a certificate will be granted upon completion of the educational course. Certification, or the recognized professional credential of **certified medical transcriptionist (CMT)**, can be obtained only through successful completion of both parts of the core certification exam administered by the **Medical Transcriptionist Certification Commission (MTCC)** at AAMT.

At the present time AAMT does not accredit or approve educational programs. A complete checklist for the evaluation of medical transcription schools and education programs is included on AAMT's web site: http://www.aamt.org.

## AAMT Membership

AAMT offers individual membership for professional development, and corporate or institutional membership for visibility and promotion. Other types of membership include practitioner, associate, and student. Student membership is available to any person who is not working as a transcriptionist and is verified as being enrolled in a nine-month or two-semester (defined as 15 to 18 weeks) medical transcription program that includes a student-instructor relationship. Student application requirements include (1) obtain a signed letter from your instructor on school letterhead, indicating enrollment date and length of the program and (2) enclose the letter with an AAMT membership application and your annual payment of $50.

Membership benefits include:

- One-year subscription to *Journal of the American Association for Medical Transcription* (JAAMT)
- AAMT *Desk Companion* (updated annually)
- Information on state-of-the-art technology
- Networking opportunities
- Continuing education
- Access to professional assistance
- Membership help desk (e-mail, fax, or toll-free)
- Discounts on AAMT programs, products, and services
- Professional development opportunities
- Peer recognition
- Pride of accomplishment
- Insurance programs available: errors and omissions, group life and income disability insurance, and equipment insurance
- Optional benefits (from outside companies): discounted travel services and car rental, and no-fee credit card

# THE MEDICAL TRANSCRIPTIONIST'S CAREER

Medical transcription is a prosperous industry that offers the educated and experienced transcriptionist opportunities for employment around the world. Diverse work settings and a variety of specialty areas and complexity levels make medical transcription an engaging occupation. The MT career continues to evolve, offering the opportunity for continued learning experiences, rewards in excellent salary packages, and self-actualization. The following paragraphs describe the attributes of a transcriptionist, job description, employment opportunities, and certification.

## Attributes of the Medical Transcriptionist

The attributes of the medical transcriptionist may be broken into two major categories: personal attributes and acquired skills developed specific to the career itself. These two categories are key elements to being successful as an MT.

Personal attributes include the love of words. It is not uncommon to find medical transcriptionists working on crossword puzzles and involved with various word games. They have an innate ability to listen closely to what others say and the skill for hearing and understanding different accents and languages. They enjoy detective work and are curious; if terminology is new to them, they use references to research and learn more. MTs are self-disciplined, detail-oriented, independent, and are usually perfectionists. They are dedicated to professional development and enthusiastically committed to learning. They are not afraid to ask questions. They have a genuine caring attitude and an interest in patient care from a medical record point of view. MTs possess integrity and understand the importance and legal implications of medical confidentiality.

Medical transcriptionists must have excellent keyboarding skills. Entry-level positions may require 60 words per minute, while experienced MTs may transcribe more than 80 words per minute. Today's MT must be able to operate a variety of software programs efficiently and maintain continued learning as new programs are developed. Excellent language skills and above-average spelling skills are mandatory. It is recognized that the MT must understand the anatomy and physiology of the human body, have knowledge of surgical terms, equipment, instruments and anesthesia, and directional and body plane terms. A background in common laboratory tests, radiology techniques and terms, drug names and their uses, both brand and generic, common signs and symptoms of diseases and treatment modalities is also required.

New technology, breakthroughs in medicine, and new medications are recognized daily as researchers explore ways in which to treat disease and to produce longevity. MTs must remain current with new medical developments to maintain their professionalism.

## Job Description

The *AAMT Model Job Description* is a practical, useful compilation of the basic job responsibilities of a medical transcriptionist. It is designed to assist human resource managers, department managers, supervisors, and others in recruiting, supervising, and evaluating individuals in medical transcription positions. It is also useful for prospective medical transcriptionists as a checklist for employment readiness. The complete *AAMT Model Job Description* may be downloaded from the following web address: http://www.aamt.org/model.htm.

## Employment Opportunities

Medical transcriptionists may seek employment in a variety of settings—hospitals, multispecialty clinics, solo physician practices, transcription services, home-based offices, research facilities, radiology clinics, pathology laboratories, tumor boards or registries, law offices, and/or veterinary hospitals. MTs may work as employees, supervisors, managers, or teachers, or may be self-employed or freelancers.

Hospitals, multispeciality clinics, and solo physician practices generally offer competitive salary and benefit packages. Payment for professional membership and/or registration fees for continuing education opportunities may also be included in the benefit package. Some offices will also include money to purchase reference materials. A wide range of dictation types, including a variety of medical specialties, dictator styles and dialects, and a vast degree of complexities are transcribed in these facilities. State-of-the-art equipment is often available, and opportunities for advancement into supervisory positions may be a possibility. A stable work schedule and job security are experienced for those who perform to their standard and have a positive work ethic.

The disadvantages of working in hospital and multispeciality clinics are the inflexible work schedule, low wages, facility politics, and the prospects of a supervisor who is unfamiliar with the needs of transcriptionists. The impacts of managed care and its associated cost-cutting efforts lead more of these facilities to out-source their medical transcription.

Transcription service employees often enjoy competitive pay rates. They transcribe a variety of accounts (physician offices, specialty offices, and so on), so there is a vast difference in the complexity and length of the documents. The work environment is usually quite comfortable and flexible scheduling is a primary advantage. Disadvantages may include the absence of immediate feedback concerning questions regarding dictation and compensation. Often in these types of settings compensation is based on production. If there is a lack of tapes available for transcription, or if the MT experiences an off-day, it will be reflected in the paycheck.

Transcription services often employ **home-based MTs** who transcribe exclusively for those employers. The employer may provide the equipment and the MT works directly under the supervision of the employer. The disadvantages of a home-based business include the fact that larger facilities frequently out-source dictation that is difficult because of the specialty or has been dictated by a foreign-speaking physician. It has been estimated that seven out of ten dictating physicians are foreign-born today. If you do not have an ear and an aptitude for dialects, it may be impossible to service these accounts and maintain a livable wage.

The entrepreneurial MT may opt to establish a freelance business. **Freelance MTs** function as independent contractors. Often they transcribe hospital overflow. The advantages of freelance are a sense of accomplishment and independence, and opportunity to work flexible hours. If you have been employed specifically for medical offices, clinics, or other specialties and feel well qualified, it is best to concentrate your independent transcription work within your field of expertise. Generally, independents are paid by production—by the line, page, or character count. Your earnings will probably be excellent *if* you are highly productive, transcribe accurately, and remain focused on building the business. The disadvantages of freelance include having to handle all areas of a business including bookkeeping, pickup of dictation and delivery of completed work, and finding other MTs to cover during illness, vacation or overload periods. Another disadvantage is the unpredictable income; income is dependent on someone else's need. Some freelance MTs feel isolated and never free to get away from their work.

Insurance companies and law offices also may employ MTs. In these environments the MT analyzes discrepancies in health records and translates medical language in a chart into lay language for attorneys. Other opportunities for MTs include teaching within hospitals, community colleges, or vocational/technical schools, preparing manuscripts for research documentation, or authoring textbooks for MTs.

## Certification for Medical Transcriptionists

A qualified MT, described as one with a minimum of two years' experience in performing medical transcription in a variety of medical and surgical specialties, may apply for the certification examination through the Medical Transcriptionist Certification Commission (MTCC). The MTCC is the credentialing program of the AAMT. MTCC offers a voluntary two-part certification exam to individuals who wish to become certified medical transcriptionists (CMTs).

The purpose of MTCC's core examination is to assess core knowledge and skills needed to practice medical transcription. This is accomplished by demonstrating competence to interpret and transcribe routine patient care documentation in a wide variety of work settings and across a broad range of specialty areas.

Part I of the test is written. It includes 120 multiple-choice questions (only 100 of which are scored) in six major content areas:

1. Medical terminology, 30%
2. English language and use, 25%
3. Anatomy and physiology, 20%
4. Disease processes, 15%
5. Health care record, 5%
6. Professional development, 5%

The test is given electronically on touch-screen computers with a time allocation of three hours. No reference materials are permitted while testing. The test is available year-round at testing centers across the United States. For details about exam content and instructions on scheduling an exam, request the *MTCC Candidate Handbook* from AAMT's web site: http://www.aamt.org/certinfo.htm. Anyone who feels ready to take the exam after self-assessing skills and knowledge based on the content outline may apply. The cost is $150, and test results are available immediately. A passing score of 85 (not a percentage) is required.

Part II of the test is practical. About 15 minutes of dictation representing a variety of report types and specialties must be transcribed, proofread, and printed within two hours. Reference materials, notes, spellcheckers, and abbreviation expanders are permitted. The examination sites and an appropriate proctor to administer the examination are chosen by the candidate. The third weekend in February, June, and October, and a choice of Thursday evening, or Friday or Saturday morning test administration are test options.

Individuals who have passed Part I within the previous two years are eligible for Part II of the test. Products from MTCC and AAMT are available to help assess readiness and supply information regarding the application/registration process. Application/registration materials must

### SPOTLIGHT ON AAMA ESSENTIALS THROUGH CAAHEP

- When transcribing medical records, maintain confidentiality and never discuss the contents of the medical record with the patient.

- Encouraging the physician to explain the contents of the transcribed medical record to the patient helps to alleviate the patient's confusion and distress about what has been said in the record.

- Respect for the medical information being transcribed into the patient's medical record is just as important as maintaining confidentiality and providing good patient care.

be postmarked seven weeks before exam dates. Results are available within ten weeks and a passing score of 85 (not a percentage) is required. The cost is $150.

Recertification is through continuing education (CE) activities. The purpose of recertification is to maintain competency in the field of medical transcription and must be done every 3 years. Recertification is accomplished by accruing at least 30 CE credits (at least 20 of which must be in the medical science category) over a 3-year cycle. The recertification fee is $60 or $45 by early-bird deadline. CE guidelines for CMTs are updated annually and provide details about credit-worthy activities and recertification procedures.

CMTs are not required to be members of AAMT, but membership is encouraged because of the opportunities and benefits that result from professional commitment and involvement. For additional information regarding certification, check AAMT's web site: http://www.aamt.org/certinfo.htm.

## TRANSCRIPTION TOOLS

Machine transcription came into its own in the 1950s replacing written shorthand as a method of recording physician notes. Carbon paper and manual typewriters produced the required copies for record management. A few years later analog dictation and electronic typewriters came into use. During the end of the 1960s, self-correcting typewriters were the newest technology. Word processors evolved during the 1970s making production and storage of reports possible in an electronic environment. Cassette tapes were the dictation medium of choice in hospitals and physician offices for years. Personal computers with word-processing software were developed in the 1980s. Magnetic tape was still the most common method of recording dictation; however, transcribing machines were improved. In the 1990s, digital dictation—dictation recorded directly into computers and managed by computers—was developed. Digital dictation can be transferred over telephone lines via computer modems, transcribed live, re-recorded for later transcription, and even transferred by waveform audio format (WAV) file. Using file transfer protocol (FTP), encrypted WAV files can be transferred between computers that are connected via the Internet, eliminating long-distance costs involved with telephone transfers.

### Equipment

The transcriber is a device that makes it possible to transform voice recordings into a transcript or printed documents. Index counters measure the length of dictation on a cassette. The index counter is useful to scan cassettes or to find the correct dictation location. The auto

playback/auto rewind feature allows you to replay a word or a phrase. Some repeat at the beginning is helpful to ensure that you have not missed any words. The speaker button permits you to listen to dictation out loud or to play the tape for someone. The eject button opens the cassette door. The speed control feature allows you to increase or decrease the speed at which the words are spoken. If the speed is decreased too much, the words will become distorted and difficult to recognize. A normal speaking rate is suggested for the best results. The volume control feature permits you to increase or decrease the volume to compensate for dictators having a soft or loud voice. The tone feature is similar to the treble/bass feature in your car radio. It mutes or accentuates consonants for nasal tones or a stuttering style of dictation. Finally, the erase feature allows you to clear or erase the tape once you have completed the transcription.

Earphones plug into the transcriber and allow you to hear what has been dictated. Earphones should be cleaned with rubbing alcohol after each using. Use a cotton swab to reach into small areas.

Standard cassette transcribers play standard audio tapes. When inserting the cassette, be sure the side you want to play is top side up. There are also microcassette and minicassette transcribers. You will need to use the correct audio tape size when using these transcribers.

The foot pedal frees your hands to use the keyboard. Pushing the foot pedal causes the transcriber to play, and releasing the pedal stops the transcriber. In most cases, the center of the foot pedal is the position to press for play; fast forward is on the left; and rewind is on the right. Study the foot pedal manual to learn how to use your particular model correctly.

### Ergonomics

Working at a computer for long periods of time can produce sore muscles, headaches, eyestrain, tension, and fatigue. Carpal tunnel syndrome is soreness, tenderness, and weakness of the muscles of the thumb caused by pressure on the median nerve at the point at which it goes through the carpal tunnel of the wrist. If conservative therapy fails, surgical relief of tension is required. Wearing softFLEX Computer Gloves™ may relieve wrist resting syndrome, which is the true cause of carpal tunnel syndrome symptoms in most keyboard users. The gloves are biomedically engineered and developed by a hand surgeon. They are said to be comfortable and effective, and work without restricting hand motion.

Careful thought should be taken when setting up your workstation, and an emphasis on developing specific habits to prevent injury should be instituted. Take short, frequent breaks and focus on distant objects to relieve eye strain. Wear tinted glasses to reduce glare from the screen.

Arrange the monitor so that it is away from windows; or use drapes, blinds, or an antiglare screen. Adjust the contrast and brightness levels to satisfy eye comfort level. Select a screen color that is restful to your eyes. Practice blinking as it has been documented that computer workers blink at one-fifth the normal rate while they are watching the screen. This causes dry, scratchy eyes.

Prevent ear infections by keeping earphones clean and not allowing others to use them. As much as possible, work in a relatively quiet area.

Keyboards are being redesigned to decrease carpal tunnel syndrome and other repetitive motion injuries. The **split keyboard** is slanted to accommodate the natural position of the hands as opposed to a straight, flat keyboard that does not support the wrists. **Wrist rests** may be purchased for use with the straight, flat keyboard for wrist support. These two devices may also alleviate back pain caused by tensing the muscles around the shoulders. Taking frequent breaks and exercising are recommended for preventative measures.

Adjust the workstation for your individual body. Raise or lower the chair and provide support for the lower back with a lumbar cushion, a rolled up towel, or a small, thin, firm pillow. Use a footrest if you are short-legged. Adjust the table or desk height if possible. Time spent setting up a comfortable, personalized workstation will pay in productivity and decreased health risks. See Chapter 11 for additional ergonomic information.

## Facsimile Machines

Facsimile (fax) machines are used in the medical community today to transmit various documents within the facility, to distant communities, and internationally. It is important to note that fax machines print on plain, thin paper or thermally treated paper. Exposure to sunlight quickly fades the printed material, and some paper does not produce clear images. A photocopy of important documents using bond paper will preserve the contents. It is a courtesy to send a hard copy of any important faxed document. Review Chapters 11 and 15 for additional information regarding fax machine use and confidentiality in the medical setting.

## Photocopy Machines

Medical offices use photocopy machines in a variety of ways on a daily basis. A photocopy machine should be selected that will satisfy the office needs, produce copies that closely resemble the original, represent the office professionally, and be relatively maintenance free. When disposing of unwanted or extra copies, remember confidentiality. Many offices shred unwanted pages to protect confidentiality and prevent litigation issues.

## TRANSCRIPTION GUIDELINES

Punctuation creates more problems than any other aspect of document preparation for the transcriptionist. Authorities disagree with one another, and on occasion there may be more than one correct way to punctuate a sentence. Basic capitalization rules should be followed in medical transcription. The purpose of capitalizing a word is to give it emphasis, distinction, authority, or importance.

The MT must have a clear understanding of when a number should be keyed as a figure, keyed in spelled-out form, or keyed as a roman numeral. Knowledge of the use of symbols and abbreviations commonly found in medical documents is also contradictory.

Guidelines for these specifics may be found in AAMT's *Book of Style*. Your instructor will provide you with additional instructions regarding the actual rules that apply to the transcription of documents.

## PROOFREADING AND MAKING CORRECTIONS

**Proofreading** is the process of checking a document for spelling, sentence structure, punctuation, capitalization, style and format, accuracy, and sense. While transcribing the document, it is a good idea to proofread as you look at the screen and key the information. Many software programs identify spelling and grammar errors making it easy to locate and make corrections as you go.

### Proofreading Skills

Proofreading is easier said than done. It has been proven that errors are more often missed while proofreading on the computer screen than proofing a printed copy. The beginning MT should first proof for accuracy by listening to the dictation again while reading the transcribed document. A second reading should be done to identify any misspelled words, incorrect grammar usage, punctuation errors, and inconsistencies in style and format. When time permits, the document should be read a third time after it has been set aside for a period. Errors often "jump out" after being away from the document for awhile.

Transcription departments and services often employ **quality assurance (QA)** reviewers. These individuals check a percentage of each MT's work against dictation. Quality assurance measures documents to be sure they are accurate, complete, consistent in health care documentation, and prepared in a timely manner. Every reasonable effort should be made to resolve inconsistencies, inaccuracies, risk management issues, and other problems.

### Where Errors Occur

Examples of where errors occur within dictation include incomplete and run-on sentences, subjects and verbs that do not agree, and dictated spelling and/or punctuation that is incorrect. These types of errors are easily corrected without changing the dictator's style or meaning.

Sound-alike words are another area in which errors may occur. Examples of sound-alike words include ilium/ileum, right/write, site/cite, and aural/oral. Be aware of your personal errors and take steps to avoid them.

## Editing

Editing is the process of reviewing the transcribed document for accuracy and clarity. It is important to remember that you must not change the dictator's style or meaning when editing. If the MT encounters a term that cannot be interpreted or something new that cannot be referenced, they should ask other MTs or QA personnel. If the question cannot be resolved, the document should be flagged to alert the dictator something needs to be corrected or resolved. The flagged message may indicate the doctor was cut off, what the term sounds like, or the message is incomprehensible. Provide as much information as you can to assist the dictator in recalling the dictated area in question.

Flagging procedures vary from one facility to another. In large facilities, flagged documents may be referred to QA personnel. The notation may be incorporated into the computerized document using a color code approach with a flag message. The correct information can then be added to the document and the color coding removed. In-house flagging may simply consist of a sticky note or a preprinted flag attachment.

Up-to-date reference materials, adequate equipment, adequate dictating methods and equipment, continuing education, an ergonomically and psychologically safe work environment, and supervision by qualified MTs are essential conditions for successful QA in medical transcription.

## Making Corrections

Errors that are made while keying the document should be corrected before the document is printed. Errors that are found in handwritten chart notes are corrected by drawing a single line through the error. The correction is made either just above or just below the error, and if space is available add your initials and the date. Identify the location of correct information as a cross-reference when possible. This procedure gives credibility to the record. Entries into the medical record should always be made using black ink. Black ink is considered more permanent and produces clear, dark writing that photocopies better when necessary.

When errors are found on self-adhesive typing strips, make the corrections as if the document had been handwritten. If the strip is not legible, or if it looks too messy once the corrections have been made, rekey a new strip and place it below the original. Be sure to identify it as "corrected for keying errors." The physician should sign the original and the corrected copy.

## MEDICAL REPORTS

Physicians employed in all types of medical specialties including oral surgeons, dentists, and veterinarians dictate numerous types of medical reports. The transcribed medical report is a legal document and is formatted in a variety of styles similar to business correspondence. Medical reports frequently dictated by ambulatory care facilities include:

- Chart or progress notes
- History and physical examination reports
- Consultation reports
- Correspondence

Hospitals and large medical centers dictate numerous medical reports including:

- History and physical examination reports
- Consultations
- Operative reports
- Discharge summaries

Physicians employed in specialty departments within hospitals dictate specialized medical reports. Examples may include:

- Pathology reports
- Radiology reports
- Autopsy reports
- Psychiatric reports
- Medicolegal reports

Medical records become part of the patient's permanent medical record and are vital to continued patient care. Other physicians, attorneys, insurance companies, or the court may review the medical records in part, or entirety. Therefore, the medical record must be neat, accurate and complete. *Neat* refers to a medical record that is legible and assembled to permit easy access to information as needed. *Accurate* means that the dictation has been transcribed as dictated, and *complete* indicates that the document has been dated correctly and signed or initialed by the dictator. If the medical record is subpoenaed for evidence in court, the signed or initialed document indicates that the content was true and correct at the time it was written.

Complete documentation of medical records is also important for payment and/or reimbursement of services for which the physician expects to be paid. The billing and diagnosis codes reported on the health insurance claim form must be supported by the documentation contained with the medical record.

## Chart Notes and Progress Notes

**Chart notes** are also known as **progress notes** or follow-up notes. They may be formal (keyed) or informal (handwritten) notes taken by physicians when they meet with or examine a patient in the office, clinic, ambulatory care center, or hospital setting. Chart notes are a concise description of the patient's present problem, the physician's physical findings, and the treatment plan. Laboratory test results may also be included within the chart note. Figure 16-1 is a sample chart/progress note.

## History and Physical Examination Reports

The **history and physical examination (H&P) report** includes information relating to the patient's main reason for encounter. The report is divided into two sections. The first is the history, which includes the **chief complaint (CC)**, a description of symptoms, problems, or conditions that brought the patient to the office; **history of the present illness (HPI)**, a chronological description of the development of the patient's illness; past medical and surgical history; family history; and social history. The second section is the **review of systems (ROS)**, an inquiry about the system directly related to the problems identified in the HPI. The physician determines the extent of the examination performed and documented based on the problems presented. The findings of the actual physical examination make up the documentation for the physical examination section of the report.

## Consultation Reports

When one physician requests the services of another physician in the care and treatment of a patient, a **consultation report** is generated. The information may be disseminated in the form of a report or within the body of a letter. The contents of the consultation report/letter usually contain all of the elements of an H&P with a focused history of the patient's illness and the body system directly related to the consultant's area of specialty. The consultant also includes within the report/letter the findings, supporting laboratory data, diagnosis, and suggested course of treatment. Figure 16-2 is a sample consultation.

## Correspondence

It is important for the MT to remember that medical correspondence also is considered medical documents and must be transcribed with the same care as any other medical record would. Review Chapter 15 for information regarding various styles and formats for business correspondence. Figure 16-3 is a sample of medical correspondence.

## TURNAROUND TIME

Specific time limits are often established for completion of medical reports. Turnaround time is a term used to indicate the specific time period in which a document is expected to be completed from the time it is received by the transcriptionist until it is back for the physician to sign and made a part of the permanent medical record. Examples include:

**STAT**: means immediately. Used frequently with radiology, pathology, and laboratory reports. These reports should be reported within 12 hours or less.

**Current**: H&Ps, consultations, and operative reports. These reports should be turned around within 24 hours.

```
1/4/20__                                    HANSEN, HENRY

RV following treatment for fx of the left wrist. The cast was removed
last week. The skin texture and turgor are returning to normal. Range
of motion has increased with physical therapy, and strength is slightly
improved at -4/5. PLAN: Continue whirlpool and ROM exercises. RV 4 weeks.
                                                              AE/rf
```

**Figure 16-1** Sample chart/progress note.

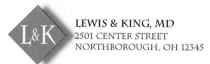

**LEWIS & KING, MD**
2501 CENTER STREET
NORTHBOROUGH, OH 12345

NORTHBOROUGH
FAMILY MEDICAL GROUP

January 4, 20___

Margaret Holly, MD
Metroma Medical Center
900 Union Street, Suite 208
Metroma, MI 11666

RE: MARY O'KEEFE

Dear Dr. Holly:

Thank you for referring Mary O'Keefe to our clinic. She presented
today stating that she recently relocated to Clinton with her husband
and children to be closer to her parents. Mary has been experiencing
symptoms suggestive of pregnancy and is here for evaluation. Over the
past three weeks, she has noticed increased tenderness of her breasts,
fatigue, and a feeling of being bloated. A home pregnancy test was
positive.

Her past medical history is positive for the usual childhood diseases
and the births of two children, following normal pregnancies. She has a
negative past surgical history.

She has no allergies to medications and takes Tylenol for occasional
headaches. She is married and has two children, ages 3 years and 12
months. She is employed part-time in an insurance office. She does not
smoke or drink.

The family history is noncontributory.

On review of systems, her complaints are limited to those described
above. She has had no nausea or vomiting, and no change in bowel habits.
She has no dizziness, no fevers, and no urinary symptoms.

Physical examination revealed a 32-year-old white female in no acute
distress. HEENT normocephalic, atraumatic. PERRLA, EOMI. The thyroid
was not enlarged, and there was no cervical adenopathy. The lungs were
clear. The heart had a regular rate and rhythm. The abdomen was soft
and nontender. Bowel sounds were normal. The extremities revealed trace
ankle edema. The neurological examination was within normal limits.
Pelvic examination confirmed a gravid uterus, compatible with a very
early pregnancy.

An abdominal ultrasound has been ordered and a beta HCG was drawn.

I believe Mary is pregnant and I will put her on our OB regimen starting
with monthly visits. Thank you for your kind referral.

Sincerely,



Elizabeth M. King, MD

EMK/lmb

**Figure 16-2**   Sample consultation.

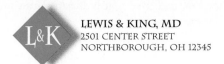

**LEWIS & KING, MD**
2501 CENTER STREET
NORTHBOROUGH, OH 12345

NORTHBOROUGH
FAMILY MEDICAL GROUP

January 4, 20___


Susan Smith, Coordinator
Special Project Division
American Drug Company
90058 Northover Road
Welfond, PA 44578

Dear Ms. Smith:

It is my understanding that your department oversees the Aid for
Patients program, which provides Glucogenasin for indigent patients.
I am interested in learning more about this.

I have a 74-year-old female patient who would be greatly helped by this
medication. She suffers with hypertension, adult onset diabetes mellitus,
and moderate angina. Medication compliance has been a problem; however,
we feel that this new drug, with its q.d. dosage, will be easy for her
to deal with.

Any information you could forward would be appreciated.

Yours truly,


Winston Lewis, MD

WL/bk

**Figure 16-3** Sample medical correspondence.

**Old**: Discharge summaries and emergency department notes. These reports should be turned around within 72 hours.

## ETHICAL AND LEGAL ISSUES

You will remember from Chapter 8 that ethics are not laws but rather standards of conduct. These standards vary from state to state so you will want to research your specific state's standards. The AAMT adopted a Code of Ethics for professional MTs and CMTs who are employed in hospital settings and/or are self-employed. Health Professions Institution in Modesto, California, has established Medical Transcription Industry Alliance Code of Ethics and Standards for MTs employed by transcription services.

The **Joint Commission on Accreditation of Healthcare Organizations (JCAHO)** is a commission established to improve the quality of care and services offered in health care settings through a voluntary accreditation process. Their accreditation standards are published in the *Accreditation Manual for Hospitals* (AMH). Legal aspects of the medical record applicable to the MT are not addressed by AMH; however, standards are given pertaining to medical record format. The MT is responsible only for the accuracy of the transcribed medical report and for seeing that it remains confidential.

The JCAHO requires that each hospital submit a list of abbreviations and symbols along with their meaning for approval. The approved abbreviations and symbols are the only ones that may be used by the MT for a specific hospital. Each hospital's approved list will vary, so it is important for the MT to review the list before beginning work.

The date the material was dictated, not the date it was transcribed, is the date used on a document. This is extremely important because statements within the document could reference this date. In case of litigation in which the document was entered as evidence, the physician's credibility could be questioned if dates are inconsistent.

The physician dictating the document must sign the report. If the physician is away from the office after dictating a report, and the report is urgent, the MT has two options. The MT may opt to sign the physician's name with the MT's initials after it, or to send a photocopy of the report and state that a signed original will be forwarded upon the physician's return.

### Confidentiality

**Confidentiality** means treating the patient's medical information as private and not for publication. The patient has a right to privacy, and as such medical information is **privileged**. Privileged information may only be communicated with the patient's permission or by court order. The MT must learn to follow the motto: *What you see here and what you hear here, must stay here when you leave here.*

The institution of **confidentiality agreements** has been established in many transcription businesses today. A signed confidentiality agreement signifies that the MT is committed to keep all patient information confidential. A **breach of confidentiality**, the unauthorized release of confidential information, is one of the few areas in which the MT can be held liable.

### Risk Management

The AAMT explains **risk management** as follows: "Healthcare institution activities that identify, evaluate, reduce, and prevent the risk of injury and loss to patients, visitors, staff, and the institution itself" (1990). Medical transcriptionists are vital in this area because of their commitment to quality and their awareness of dictated data that may indicate risk management problems. The MT should immediately report this information to the appropriate designated personnel. Appropriate personnel may include the risk management manager, the office manager, a supervisor, or your employer's attorney. The MT falls under the jurisdiction of *respondeat superior*, meaning "let the master answer." In actuality, this means that the physician/dictator is liable in certain cases for the wrongful acts of the MT.

## NEW TECHNOLOGY

Technology is continually changing especially in the areas involving computerized systems. The following items are areas of new technology that hold promise of significant impacts on the MT.

### Continuous Speech Recognition (CSR)

**Continuous Speech Recognition (CSR)** is the process of direct conversion of spoken documentation into a written text (electronic) version using a computer equipped with voice recognition software. Some proponents of this advance in technology wrongly predict that when perfected, CSR will spell transcription's demise. Nothing could be further from the truth for the foreseeable future. CSR, once it is perfected, will constitute one of the most significant advances in the history of patient care delivery; but it will not replace the MT. It will, however, have a significant impact on the productivity of the MT.

CSR is currently not refined to the point where it is sufficiently accurate to be used without the MT acting as the quality control interface. The rate at which CSR software is being improved will continue to accelerate; however, it has been predicted that 10 to 20 percent of all clinical processes and records of health care delivered will never be fully converted using CSR due to complex rapidly changing vocabularies.

Accents, pronunciation, grammar, and other aspects of the clinician's personal style are difficult and costly for the CSR software to address. The MT adjusts to accents, dictation speed, and individualized pronunciations to overcome difficulties without requiring the clinician to change habits.

In most specialties it is desirable to standardize the content of patient records and ensure that critical information is included. The MT normally performs this function by cutting and pasting sections together to maintain a standardized format, and filling in gaps in sentences and information to preserve meaning without altering clinical information. CSR technologies cannot be expected to restructure reports and emphasize critical information in the foreseeable future.

CSR will become an important tool of the MT, not a replacement. It will increase productivity, and reduce the time between dictation of the oral patient record and availability of the electronic record for use by others in the health care network.

## Integrating Digital Photographs into Medical Transcription

A new trend in transcription is the integration of digital images directly into the transcribed record. The response to inputting digital images (photographs, scans, and x-rays) has been very positive from both the local health care community as well as patients themselves. This is attributed to easier understanding of a picture by patients and more precise presentation using both pictures and written text to medical professionals.

The tools required for integrating digital images into word processing is already available to most MTs in their current Microsoft Word® or Corel WordPerfect® software packages. They only have to obtain a disk containing digital images from their physician/employer. If the transcribed record is included in the computer-based electronic record, also known as the electronic chart, digital images can be attached allowing other clinicians to view, enlarge, and manipulate the images at will.

---

## DOCUMENTATION

*right Marilyn Johnson 9/12/01 See entry dated 8/28/01 CXR shows perihilar infiltrate.*

---

### 16-1

Erin Saunders is a recent graduate from a reputable junior college offering a two-year program in medical transcription. Erin was an excellent student and graduated at the top of her class. She is investigating types of employment opportunities available and has put her resume together. Erin's long-range goal is to become a CMT.

### CASE STUDY REVIEW

1. List the types of work environments available for MTs and briefly describe the transcription with which each would be involved.

2. Review the CMT test content and determine which work environments would best prepare Erin for the examination. Provide the rationale for your decision.

---

### 16-2

At the offices of Doctors Lewis and King, the medical transcriptionist has just completed the following content in a document: "This patient developed a persistent lesion on the inner aspect of the left upper lip. This lesion was at the junction of the vermilion and mucous membrane. A punch biopsy was obtained of this 1 cm lesion and was read as a probable verrucous squamous cell carcinoma of the lower lip."

### CASE STUDY REVIEW

1. What inconsistencies, if any do you find within this document?

2. What should the MT do to verify inconsistencies and/or inaccuracies?

3. How should these inconsistencies and/or inaccuracies be corrected?

## SUMMARY

Medical transcription is a vital part of patient health care. Without appropriate medical documentation it is impossible to provide quality health care, to bill insurance carriers properly to ensure physicians are reimbursed for services rendered, and to support and protect the physician should records be subpoenaed. The MT must keep all patient information strictly confidential and may be asked to sign a confidentiality agreement. A breach of confidentiality is one of the few areas in which the MT can be held liable.

Professional MTs often become CMTs and recertify every three years. A current credential indicates the active involvement in continuing education activities that keep the transcriptionist knowledgeable of new technologies, techniques, procedures, and drugs being used. Medical transcriptionists will continue to be medical language specialists. Their role and job description may change, however, with the innovation and use of new technology.

## REVIEW QUESTIONS

### Multiple Choice

1. AAMT student membership is available to:
   a. anyone working as an MT who has completed training
   b. anyone not working as an MT and currently enrolled in a two-year program
   c. anyone not working as an MT and currently enrolled in a nine-month or two-semester student-instructor related course
   d. anyone not working as an MT and currently enrolled in a correspondence course

2. Acquired skills developed specific to MTs include:
   a. minimum keyboarding speed of 60 words per minute
   b. love of words
   c. ability to listen and understand different accents and languages
   d. self-disciplined, detail-oriented, and independent

3. The MT who is employed by a transcription service but works from the home is known as a(n):
   a. home-based MT
   b. freelance MT
   c. associate MT
   d. self-employed MT

4. The credentialing program of AAMT is known as the:
   a. JCAHO
   b. AAMA
   c. MTCC
   d. CSR

5. Examples of ergonomics include all of the following *except:*
   a. split keyboards
   b. lumbar cushions
   c. footrests
   d. straight, flat keyboards

6. Quality assurance measures documents for all of the following *except:*
   a. line length of document
   b. accuracy and completeness
   c. consistency in health care documentation
   d. timely preparation

7. MTs with a question that cannot be resolved should:
   a. guess at what is being dictated
   b. edit the document and exclude what cannot be understood
   c. flag the document
   d. refuse to transcribe documents for that physician

8. Types of documents transcribed in ambulatory care settings include all of the following *except:*
   a. chart notes
   b. HPI
   c. H&Ps
   d. consultation reports

9. Turnaround time for most laboratory reports should be:
   a. STAT
   b. current
   c. within 12 hours
   d. both a and b

10. Continuous speech recognition:
    a. cannot restructure reports and emphasize critical information
    b. involves the integration of digital images into the transcribed document
    c. operates on the premise that a picture is worth a thousand words
    d. is available with MS Word® and Corel WordPerfect® software packages

## Critical Thinking

1. List the personal attributes and acquired skills specific to the medical transcription career, and discuss why these are important.
2. Read through the section on employment opportunities again. Now use the World Wide Web for additional research and develop a work environment in which you personally would feel comfortable as an employee. Discuss with classmates your discoveries, and explain why you arrived at them.
3. Design a workstation on paper, and list a minimum of 10 ergonomic considerations.
4. Discuss the meaning of QA and its implications on insurance billing.
5. Identify possible legal issues that could arise if medical records are not corrected appropriately.
6. Discuss the importance of turnaround time and its legal implications.
7. Discuss the requirements of JCAHO and the use of abbreviations within medical records.

## WEB ACTIVITIES

 Using the World Wide Web, locate the AAMT web site, and search through the web pages to locate the *Medical Transcriptionist's Bill of Rights*. Download this item. Discuss it with a classmate, or follow your instructor's directions related to this activity.

## REFERENCES/BIBLIOGRAPHY

American Association for Medical Transcription. (1990). *AAMT Model Job Description: Medical Transcriptionist.* Modesto, CA: Author.

American Association for Medical Transcription. *A medical transcriptionist's bill of rights* [On-line]. Available: http://www.aamt.org/billorts.htm

American Association for Medical Transcription. *MTCC Disciplinary Policy and Procedures* [On-line]. Available: http://www.aamt.org/certcode.htm

American Association for Medical Transcription. *Student membership* [On-line]. Available: http://www.aamt.org/stu.htm

Burns, L., & Maloney, F. (1997). *Medical transcription and terminology: An integrated approach.* Albany, NY: Delmar.

Diehl, M. O., & Fordney, M. T. (1997). *Medical keyboarding, typing, and transcribing techniques and procedures* (4th ed). Philadelphia: W. B. Saunders Company.

Ettinger, B., & Ettinger, A. G. (1997). *Medical transcription.* St. Paul, MN: Paradigm Publishing, Inc.

Kinn, M. E., & Woods, M. A. (1999). *The medical assistant: Administrative and clinical* (8th ed). Philadelphia: W. B. Saunders Company.

*The medical transcription workbook* (1999). Modesto, CA: Health Professions Institute.

Shaha, S. (1999). The future of transcription with continuous speech recognition. *Journal of the American Association for Medical Transcription, 18*(6), 12–14.

Tessier, C. (1995). *AAMT Book of Style for Medical Transcription.* Modesto, CA: Author.

Tossey, K. L. (1998). The integration of digital photographs into medical transcription. *Journal of the American Association for Medical Transcription, 17*(6), 19–21.

# MANAGING FACILITY FINANCES

# Chapter 17

# DAILY FINANCIAL PRACTICES

## KEY TERMS

Accounts Payable
Accounts Receivable
Adjustments
Balance
Cashier's Check
Certified Check
Charges
Charge Slip
Credit
Currency
Day Sheet
Disbursement
Ledger
Money Market Account
Notary
Payee
Pegboard System
Petty Cash
Petty Cash Voucher
Posting
ROA
Superbill
Traveler's Check
Usual, Customary, and Reasonable (UCR)
Voucher Check
Write-It-Once System

## OUTLINE

**Determining Patient Fees**
 Usual, Reasonable, and Customary Fees
 Discussion of Fees
 Adjustment of Fees
**Credit Arrangements**
 Payment Planning
**The Bookkeeping Function**
 Managing Patient Accounts
 The Importance of Good Working Habits
 The Pegboard System
 Computerized Systems
**Banking Procedures**
 Types of Accounts
 Types of Checks

 Deposits
 Accepting Checks
 Lost or Stolen Checks
 Writing and Recording Checks
 Reconciling a Bank Statement
**Purchasing Supplies and Equipment**
 Preparing a Purchase Order
 Verifying Goods Received
 Preparing the Invoice for Payment
**Petty Cash**
 Establishing a Petty Cash Fund
 Tracking, Balancing, and Replenishing Petty Cash

## OBJECTIVES

*The student should strive to meet the following performance objectives and demonstrate an understanding of the facts and principles presented in this chapter through written and oral communication.*

1. Define the key terms as presented in the glossary.
2. Understand the importance of communication in regard to establishing patient fees.
3. Develop a knowledge of various credit arrangements for patient fees.
4. Differentiate between manual and computerized bookkeeping systems.
5. State the advantages of the pegboard system.
6. State the advantages of computerized systems.
7. Demonstrate a knowledge of banking procedures, including types of accounts and services.
8. Show proficiency in preparing bank deposits, writing checks, recording checks, and reconciling accounts.

*(continues)*

257

9. Explain the process of purchasing equipment and supplies for the ambulatory care setting.
10. Demonstrate proficiency in establishing and maintaining a petty cash system.

## ROLE DELINEATION COMPONENTS

**ADMINISTRATIVE**

**Administrative Procedures**

- Perform basic clerical functions

**Practice Finances**

- Apply bookkeeping principles
- Document and maintain accounting and banking records
- Manage accounts receivable
- Manage accounts payable
- Develop and maintain fee schedules (advanced)

**GENERAL (TRANSDISCIPLINARY)**

**Legal Conceps**

- Document accurately

## SCENARIO

At the offices of Doctors Lewis & King, many different types of patients are seen: most have some kind of insurance, either a traditional plan or an HMO-type plan, some are on Medicare, a few on Medicaid, and occasionally a patient does not have any insurance or any financial resources to pay for treatment. Whoever schedules the first patient appointment also opens a frank but courteous discussion with the patient about physician fees and the patient's anticipated method of payment. Initiating this discussion of fees at the beginning of the physician-patient relationship keeps patients informed of their responsibility for payment and helps the medical assistants at Doctors Lewis & King make any necessary credit arrangements with the patient before treatment begins.

## INTRODUCTION

Ambulatory care settings are primarily designed to serve the patient. However, without sound financial practices, patient care will suffer and the office will not thrive and grow. The health care industry has become more complex in recent years with the explosion of managed care. The impact of managed care has been tremendous and it affects not only the way patients receive treatment but the manner in which the ambulatory care center is administered from a financial point of view.

Of course, this discussion of fees is only a small part of the ambulatory care setting's daily financial practices. Selecting an appropriate bookkeeping method, taking responsibility for banking, managing the purchase of supplies, and establishing a petty cash system are all vital to the smooth functioning of today's ambulatory care setting.

## DETERMINING PATIENT FEES

**MC** In today's managed care climate, ambulatory care settings have many different arrangements with insurance carriers and with their patients. Often, the office or urgent care center will have a contract with HMO-type insurance carriers in which they agree to a specific fee for certain procedures. In this instance, the physicians of the center are usually known as participating providers. In some plans, the patient pays what is known as a copay amount for each visit. In other situations, the patient is liable for a certain percentage of the fee. This is usually known as coinsurance. Ambulatory care centers may also accept Medicare and Medicaid patients, usually for a predetermined fee.

The situations for payment are numerous and varied, and subsequent chapters in this unit will examine them in greater detail. Of critical importance at the onset of the patient relationship, however, is that both patient and physician have an understanding of their fiscal responsibility to each other. The patient must also be made aware of any fees imposed for missed appointments, telephone consultation, and other charges the patient may not anticipate. It is not unethical to charge for these, but it is not recommended without prior notification to the patient. Insurance carriers will not reimburse missed appointment charges. If the office plans to implement charges, they need to have a signed waiver from the patient. The waiver explains that you have notified the patient in advance that these charges will be added to their account.

## Usual, Customary, and Reasonable Fees

A fee schedule often used by Medicare and some insurance carriers is referred to as usual, reasonable, and customary fees. Usual refers to the fee typically charged by a physician for certain procedures; customary is based on the average charge for a specific procedure by all physicians practicing the same specialty in a defined geographic region; and reasonable refers to the midrange of fees charged for this procedure. Also see Chapter 18.

## Discussion of Fees

The manner in which billing is done and fees established will vary depending on the type of medical facility, the needs of the practice, and the professional services rendered. Years ago, personnel in medical facilities would typically ask patients at the end of their visits if they would like to pay then or be billed later. It is now customary and in some offices mandatory to request payment at the time of service. Today, the fee for the visit is simply stated, and if a person does not have cash or a check, the option of credit card payment is often provided. If a patient is a member of an HMO, and the ambulatory care setting is a member of that HMO, then the patient is typically responsible only for any established copay amount.

Inherent to the total billing process (see Chapter 20) is the necessity of initially establishing a fee schedule and informing patients of charges and exactly what portion of the bill they are expected to pay. Ideally, the patient should be told the approximate cost of the procedures at the start of treatment. For Medicare and Medicaid patients, this must be in writing and should indicate the type of procedure(s), the total responsibility of the patient, and the reason why this is the patient's responsibility. This form is officially known by Medicare as an Advanced Beneficiary Notification, or by Medicaid as a waiver. These forms are the only legal means an office has to collect payment on charges not allowed by Medicare or Medicaid. Charges for some daily routine visits may be submitted to the insurance carrier, and the office may not know what portion is covered until information is received from the carrier. The facility may accept numerous insurance plans and participation in these plans determines the amount that the patient owes. Many misunderstandings will be prevented and subsequent collection of delinquent accounts expedited when the office staff is well informed about insurance reimbursement and carefully explains fees to the patients.

## Adjustment of Fees

If an office accepts assignment with Medicare and Medicaid, they are mandated to charge every patient the same amount for similar services rendered. If an office extends a professional courtesy, it is considered insurance fraud. The office would then be billing insurance an increased rate than what they charge others. More specifically, deductibles are to be collected from the patient; this is part of their premium expectation. Unless you follow government guidelines for establishing when a patient is financially unable to pay their portion of the bill, you cannot give discounts to patients for cash payments.

Adjustments may be made for patients with limited income. For example, if a patient had been going to the ambulatory care center for many years, but recently lost a job or ran into unfortunate financial circumstances, the physician may "write off" a portion of the bill. This sum will be written off against the physician's income, and the patient will not have to pay any amount or will pay a reduced amount according to what is affordable. This courtesy usually applies to only existing patients and is not offered to new patients.

Adjustments also may occur with Medicare, Medicaid, Blue Shield, and private health insurance patients. Physicians who accept assignment in these programs agree to accept as payment in full what the insurer allows. For instance, a fee of $150 may be charged, but $95 is accepted as payment in full by the provider. The remainder of the bill, $55, is written off so that the patient is not responsible for this remainder of the fee.

Medical assistants must be aware, however, of the pitfalls of adjusting or reducing fees. It is difficult to accept all hardship cases and still remain a viable practice. It is always a helpful resource to patients who cannot pay to be given the names and telephone numbers of local health care clinics that may be able to accept them as patients on a sliding scale or no-fee basis.

## CREDIT ARRANGEMENTS

If the patient will need to pay a substantial out-of-pocket amount, it is helpful to make the patient aware of this and discuss different credit arrangements that can be made. Many ambulatory care settings will work out installment payments, usually without finance charges, to spread the cost of services over a pre-agreed period of time. This eases the financial burden on the patient and also makes it more likely that the office will be able to collect monies due.

### Payment Planning

Medical assistants can help patients plan for anticipated medical expenses (having a baby, surgery, extensive therapy). When patient and physician know in advance that there will be costly medical expenses, the medical assistant should review the patient's insurance coverage. It is also helpful to prepare an estimate sheet, which will give the patient an idea of the cost of the medical services for the planned treatment. The estimate may also include the cost of anesthetist, consultants, and hospital charges.

More recently, ambulatory care settings have begun to accept credit cards as a means of payment. It must be remembered that this is strictly for the convenience of the patient. According to the AMA Code of Ethics, physicians should not increase their charges for patients who wish to use credit cards nor encourage patients to use credit cards. Physicians, therefore, may offer the service, but not actively encourage its use.

The one advantage to the ambulatory care setting that accepts credit cards is that monies for fees charged are usually available within 24 hours or so. Also, the physician is relieved of the responsibility of collection. However, credit card companies do assess a fee for every charge made, which the ambulatory care center must pay.

When a patient decides to use a credit card, it is extremely important that confidentiality be maintained to the fullest extent possible. When writing a description of the services on the credit card receipt, the medical assistant should be as vague as possible to preserve patient confidentiality. For example, medical services versus STD testing.

## THE BOOKKEEPING FUNCTION

Daily financial management in the ambulatory care setting is most important to the functioning of the office as it

### SPOTLIGHT ON AAMA ESSENTIALS THROUGH CAAHEP

- Portraying a positive attitude when dealing with the patient regarding his or her financial obligations will help the patient maintain a positive relationship with all members of the health care practice.

- Positive communication between members of the staff responsible for daily financial practices and those responsible for caring for the patient's needs is paramount to the efficiency of a smooth-running and financially stable practice.

- Members of the staff responsible for the practice's daily financial duties must maintain a high level of integrity and honesty; the physician-employer must be able to depend upon them for his or her livelihood and for the livelihood of those employed at the practice.

directly affects overall accounting and bookkeeping procedures. Accounting generates financial information for the ambulatory care setting and is defined as a system of monitoring the financial status of a facility and the specific results of its activities. Accounting provides financial information for decision making. (See Chapter 21.) Bookkeeping, the actual daily recording of the accounts or transactions of the business, is the major part of this accounting process. This chapter deals with daily bookkeeping (or recording) functions necessary to manage the income and expenses of an ambulatory care setting.

### Managing Patient Accounts

All businesses must keep careful records of income and expenses for tax and legal purposes. One aspect of this recordkeeping in a medical practice is maintaining patient accounts. Since few patients are able to pay in full each time they are seen by the physician, it is necessary to maintain account records for each individual or family as opposed to simply keeping a record of cash received as is done in many other types of business. The money owed to the office by patients is known as **accounts receivable**, and must be carefully monitored to assure that the physician is paid for services provided and that patients are properly credited for payments made.

There are various ways to track patients' balances. In this chapter we will discuss the two most common methods:

● The **pegboard** system (also known as the **write-it-once** method)

● Computerized systems

Though many practices are fully automated, all except the newest ones probably started with some sort of manual system (generally pegboard). Converting from manual to computerized record-keeping is initially expensive, requires thorough retraining of staff, and takes a great deal of time at the beginning. However, it offers great versatility and reduces the need to record and re-record entries.

However, it is necessary for a well-prepared medical assistant to be fully versed in both bookkeeping systems.

## The Importance of Good Working Habits

In managing the day-to-day finances of the ambulatory care setting, always observe two guidelines:

1. Always work with care and accuracy; it is extremely easy to transpose numbers (i.e., writing 23 instead of 32) or make other posting errors. A moment of carelessness can result in hours spent trying to find the mistake.
2. The work must be kept current or it may become an overwhelming chore.

Also, develop these habits:

● Form your numerals and letters carefully with good penmanship.

● Use a consistent ink color.

● Align your columns.

● Be careful when carrying decimal points.

● Double-check your math.

● If a mistake is found, neatly cross out the incorrect figure and write the correct figure above it.

## The Pegboard System

A complete pegboard or write-it-once system consists of day sheets, ledger cards, charge slips, and receipt forms. The forms are designed to work together to simplify the task and to avoid costly and embarrassing mistakes in patient accounts. All forms will have matching columns

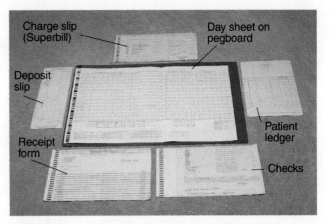

**Figure 17-1** An example of the pegboard system and possible overlays.

that align and are held in place on the pegboard when the system is in use (Figure 17-1). The forms are generally carboned or on NCR© paper (no carbon required), which permits entering of **charges**, credits or **adjustments**, or **posting**, onto the day sheet, charge slip, or receipt and the patient's ledger card simultaneously. Some major advantages of the pegboard system include:

● The system is efficient and timesaving—by only having to enter information once, it is impossible to enter incorrect information on one of the forms due to copying errors or errors of omission. (This can also be a major disadvantage when an error made and entered appears on *all* forms.)

● The **day sheet** provides complete and up-to-date information about accounts receivable status at a glance.

● A pegboard system is relatively inexpensive.

Several companies produce pegboard systems, all with slight variations. Though the information and method of use are the same, it is not usually possible to "mix and match" forms from different companies since even a slight difference in column width or location will make the forms incompatible.

**Day Sheets.** The day sheet is used to list or post each day's charges, payments, credits, and adjustments: the daily financial transactions. This is an important part of the overall bookkeeping process, so legibility and absolute accuracy are critical. At the close of each business day, the day sheet will be balanced to provide a complete picture of all patient financial activity for that day. Those balances carried over from day to day will provide the accumulated data needed for month-end closing.

The day sheet consists of five sections (Figure 17-2), the first three of which are used when posting transactions

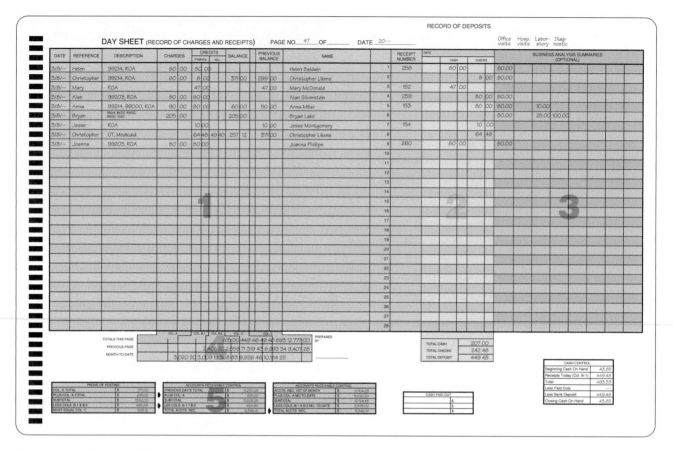

**Figure 17-2**    Pegboard day sheet with major sections.

and the last two of which are for balancing, proof of posting, accounts receivable control, and accounts receivable proof.

- *Section 1* is where individual transactions are posted, using the ledger card and charge slips, or receipt forms. The information here includes the date, patient name, description of transaction or service, charges, credits, and previous and current balances. This is the write-it-once portion of the day sheet.

- *Section 2* is the deposit portion (some companies make this part detachable to be used as an actual deposit slip). If a transaction includes a payment, the payment amount will be listed under the appropriate right-hand column showing method of payment after the ledger portion is posted.

- *Section 3* is for business analysis. These columns might be used for recording payments or charges to be credited to different physicians or they are often used as a breakdown for types of service (i.e., office examination, hospital visit, surgery, and so on). The use of this area will vary from practice to practice.

- *Section 4* is where transactions are totaled and balanced at the end of the day. (See Procedure 17-5 later in the chapter.)

- *Section 5* is used to verify the daily balances and to balance and track cumulative accounts receivable figures. The total accounts receivable figure shows how much is owed to the practice by all patients to date, allowing the physician or administrator to see the total outstanding balance at a glance without having to add hundreds of individual balances.

**Ledger Cards.** It is, of course, necessary to maintain a record of services provided and charges and payments for each individual seen in the office or hospital. This is accomplished by creating a separate ledger for each patient household. In order to easily keep track of patient accounts, there should be a responsible party for each family whose name and address will appear in the mailing window at the top of the ledger card (Figure 17-3). In a case where both spouses are employed and each is covered by employer-provided insurance, there may be more than one responsible party. It is also possible to have more than one responsible party for a household if one child is from a

**STATEMENT**

**LEWIS & KING MD, PC**
2501 CENTER STREET
NORTHBOROUGH, OH
(312) 824-6925

| DATE | REFERENCE | DESCRIPTION | CHARGES | CREDITS | | BALANCE |
|------|-----------|-------------|---------|---------|--|---------|
| | | BALANCE FORWARD → | | | | |

RB40BC-2                                    PLEASE PAY LAST AMOUNT IN BALANCE COLUMN

THIS IS A COPY OF YOUR ACCOUNT AS IT APPEARS ON OUR RECORDS

**(A)**

| TELEPHONE | SPOUSE NAME | DATE OF BIRTH | SOC. SEC. NO. | DRIVERS LIC. NO. |
|-----------|-------------|---------------|---------------|------------------|

EMPLOYER: CITY - STATE - PHONE          SPOUSE EMPLOYER: CITY - STATE - PHONE

NAME - ADDRESS - PHONE OF NEAREST RELATIVE          OTHER PROF. SERVICE USED: CITY - STATE - PHONE

CREDIT/INSURANCE INFORMATION

OWN ☐  RENT ☐
COMMENTS

USE LEAD PENCIL - FELT TIP MARKER - TYPEWRITER

**(B)**

**Figure 17-3**    Patient ledger card: (A) Front of ledger. (B) Back of ledger.

spouse's prior marriage and the responsible party is the noncustodial parent. Services or payments for any other members of the family seen in the office or hospital will be entered on the same ledger and the patient's first name (or coded number) will be written in the space provided (reference space columns). If the office is doing insurance billing or receiving insurance payments, it is extremely important that charges and credits be applied to the correct family member, so never omit this step when making entries.

The columns on the front of the ledger card will show the date of activity, name of patient, a clear description of type of activity, amount of charge or credit, adjustments (if any), and the family's total balance due.

The back of the ledger card in Figure 17-3 includes all pertinent patient and insurance information needed for collection purposes.

The ledger is placed under the charge slip or receipt, directly on the day sheet, and aligned prior to posting. *Never* post any patient entry without the patient's ledger in place. This prevents recording information on the day

sheet and thus omitting it inadvertently from the patient's ledger.

**Charge Slips and Receipts.** The charge slip (or superbill) shown in Figures 17-1 and 17-4 is a three-part form that:

1. Provides patients with a record of account activity for the day
2. May eliminate the need for separate insurance forms
3. Provides the office with a copy of that day's services, which will be filed in the individual's chart

Charge slips can be ordered to fit the practice. Information on the charge slip includes not only the amount of the day's transaction, but procedure codes and diagnosis codes (see Chapter 19) that satisfy the requirements for most insurance companies to reimburse the patient or physician. When the slips are ordered, the office will indicate the most common services provided, which will be printed on the form with the applicable procedure codes

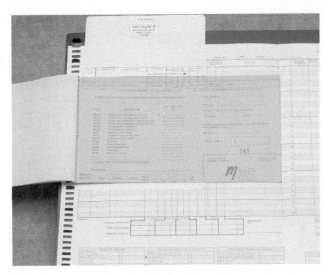

**Figure 17-4**    Pegboard with day sheet, ledger card, and charge slip.

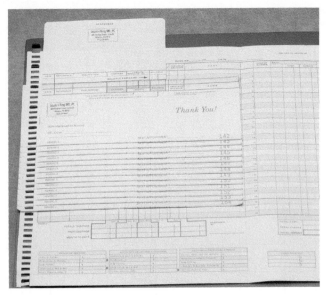

**Figure 17-5**    Pegboard with day sheet, ledger card, and receipt.

(and some blank lines for infrequently used procedures). After seeing the patient, the physician places a check mark beside the services rendered. In addition, there is an area for the diagnosis code to be filled in by the physician at the same time. The charge slip is printed with the name, address, and telephone number of the practice.

Unlike charge slips, the receipt forms (Figures 17-1 and 17-5) used for payments on account are not customized other than to have the name, address, and telephone number of the practice preprinted. The receipt form is only used when someone makes a payment on account and no services are rendered that day. There is only one copy of this form, which is given to the patient after the payment is recorded. Like many charge slips, the receipt form may include a space to write in the date of the patient's next appointment. It is not necessary to keep any other record of the transaction, since it is entered on the day sheet and ledger card at the time the receipt is filled out using the write-it-once procedures.

### Recording Information: Charges, Credits, and Adjustments.
Procedures 17-1, 17-2, 17-3, and 17-4 provide step-by-step details on posting and recording activities.

### Adjustments.
These are entries made to change the patient's balance but do not represent charges or payments. The adjustment column is a credit column, and therefore entries here normally reduce the balance due. When making an adjustment intended to increase the balance, a negative entry (in parentheses) is made to show that you will reverse the function when you balance (add instead of subtract the amount).

As noted earlier in this chapter, adjustments are frequently made to show a reduction in fee for service granted by the physician, a write-off to the account if the physician has agreed to accept insurance as payment in full, or to correct an error in posting. For example, Edith Leonard had surgery for which the physician agreed to reduce his fee by half of the balance remaining after insurance has paid. At the time of the surgery a charge of $2,500 was entered on her ledger and the day sheet. Today payment is received from her insurance company in the amount of $2,000, which would normally leave a balance of $500. However, since the physician agreed to write off half of that amount ($250), you would enter $250 in the adjustment column when posting the insurance payment. Since the adjustment column is a credit column, this amount, along with the payment received, is subtracted from the previous balance to arrive at the new balance of $250.

### Balancing Day Sheets.
In any bookkeeping function balancing is done to be certain all entries are correct. Day sheets are always balanced at the end of each workday. Occasionally, in a busy practice, more than one day sheet will be required to record all of the transactions for a full day. If that happens, balance each day sheet as if it were the end of the day and carry the standard information forward to the next sheet just as if it were a new day. The day sheet will have a place to enter the page number if more than one page is needed for posting transactions for a single day (i.e., Page 1 of 2). Be sure to number and date all pages.

Most medical assistants will be entering an established practice, where there is a financial history and previous accounts receivable balance and work with the first and second day sheets of a new month. This means that there will be a figure on the line of "Accounts Receivable

Control" and the "Accounts Receivable Proof" boxes showing the accounts receivable balance from the end of the preceding month. Since the first day sheet being balanced is for the first working day of the month, the column boxes marked "Previous Page" will all contain a zero that can be entered at the same time as the information carried forward at the beginning of the day. See Procedure 17-5 for steps in balancing day sheets. NOTE: When balancing any financial information, always use a calculator with the print function turned on to create a tape of the calculations. These tapes will be an invaluable timesaver if the initial balance is incorrect and you need to search for mistakes.

**Month-End.** When the last day sheet for the month has been balanced, it is then necessary to verify that the month-end figures on the day sheet agree with patients' ledgers. Though this may be a time-consuming process, it will find mistakes before they grow into major accounting or collection problems.

Reconciling the month-end sheet to the patient ledgers is accomplished by adding all the open balances on the ledger cards and verifying that the total agrees with the end-of-month accounts receivable balance on the last day sheet of the month. When these figures agree, the accounts receivable balance is correct.

By following these procedures of "checks and balances," it is likely that all monies have been properly credited to patient accounts and deposited and that all charges shown as outstanding on the day sheet agree with the outstanding balances of the individual patient accounts. If a payment is somehow misplaced, the deposits will not agree with the credits or with the patient ledgers and it will be known immediately that money is missing. Not only does

this catch errors, it also eliminates the possibility of undetected theft of funds, for when a mistake is caught immediately, the payer can stop payment on the missing check or credit card slip and a new payment can be made.

## Computerized Systems

With increasing numbers of medical facilities turning to computers for word processing, patient records, and bookkeeping, there is an ever-increasing number of medical practice software packages on the market. These ready-made systems are available for both single or dual physician offices and large group practices. Often, a consultant is hired to design a customized program, though this is far more expensive than purchasing mass-produced software. When selecting and using any computer bookkeeping software:

- Be sure the system will meet not only current needs but future needs as well (some packages can be expanded to grow with the practice).

- The hardware (computer system) must be powerful enough to run the program.

- To use the automated system, it is necessary to understand the workings of the manual procedures on which the computerized accounting is based.

**Computerized Patient Accounts.** A software management program offers many advantages in managing patient accounts. The program automatically creates a charge slip at the time of each patient's visit. After the physician's examination, the program calculates the charges for the monthly billing statement (Figure 17-6). The management program also creates and updates the

| | | | | | | |
|---|---|---|---|---|---|---|
| **L&K** LEWIS & KING, MD 2501 CENTER STREET NORTHBOROUGH, OH 12345 | | STATEMENT DATE PATIENT NUMBER PREVIOUS BALANCE | 08/29/-- 113 $0.00 | | OFFICE PHONE: (404) 555-0078 | |

| DATE | CODE | DESCRIPTION | AMOUNT | | STATEMENT DATE   08/29/-- | |
|---|---|---|---|---|---|---|
| 02/12/-- | 00000 | BALANCE FORWARD | 23.00 | | CURRENT | 0.00 |
| 02/16/-- | 71020 | CHEST X RAY, 2 VIEWS | 40.00 | | OVER 30-DAYS: | 52.00 |
| 03/14/-- | 81000 | URINALYSIS | 20.00 | | OVER 60-DAYS: | 75.00 |
| 04/22/-- | 85022 | CBC | 12.50 | | OVER 90-DAYS: | 1.85 |
| 06/13/-- | 99221 | INIT. HOSP. EXAM, EXTENSIVE | 75.00 | | BALANCE DUE | $128.85 |
| 07/05/-- | 93040 | RHYTHM STRIP | — | | | |
| 07/26/-- | 93000 | ELECTROCARDIOGRAM | 52.00 | | | |
| 08/29/-- | PMT | PERSONAL CHECK | -93.65 CR | | | |
| | | | | | | |
| | | BALANCE DUE | $128.85 | | **THANK YOU FOR YOUR PAYMENT.** | |
| | | | | | **113** | |
| OFFICE CLOSED SEPTEMBER 5TH. NEW CHARGES HAVE BEEN SENT TO YOUR INSURANCE CARRIER(S). | | | | | MARTIN GORDON 107 KNOWLEDGE DRIVE NORTHBOROUGH, OH 12345 | |

**Figure 17-6**   Computerized patient bill.

PATIENT LEDGER
=============

Patient #218                    O'KEEFE, MARY                        Date:    06/24/--
                                43 KINGSBORO AVENUE
                                NORTHBOROUGH, OH 12345               PHONE: (404) 555-6123

            Insured #1                              Insured #2

            SAME                                    O'KEEFE, JOHN
                                                    43 KINGSBORO AVENUE
                                                    NORTHBOROUGH, OH 12345

    Insurance #1:  PRUDENTIAL       Policy #:  987654321       Group #:  987700
    Insurance #2:  BLUE CROSS       Policy #:  321654907       Group #:  123456987

============================================================================

01/26/--      59400      TOTAL OBSTETRICAL CARE                        1200.00
01/26/--      99202      INTERMEDIATE EXAM, NEW PT.                       30.00
01/26/--      88150      PAPANICOLAOU SMEAR                               18.50
01/26/--      PMT            DEPOSIT OB CARE                            -250.00
02/18/--      PMT            Insur. Pmt.   01/26/-- 90015                -20.00
02/18/--      ADJ            Adj. Cat.  #1 01/26/-- 90015                -10.00
02/25/--      85022      CBC                                             12.50
02/25/--      99212      LIMITED EXAM, ESTAB. PT.                        15.00
02/25/--      PMT            Cash Pmt.  01/26/-- 94000                   -75.00
04/26/--      85022      CBC                                             12.50
04/26/--      99212      LIMITED EXAM, ESTAB. PT.                        15.00
04/26/--      76805      DIAGNOSTIC ULTRASOUND                           55.00
04/26/--      88150      PAPANICOLAOU SMEAR                              18.50
                                                                      ---------
                         Balance for MARY O'KEEFE                    $1,022.00

**Figure 17-7**    Computerized patient ledger card.

ledger card, adds new names to the list of patients and to the daily log, and transfers data to produce insurance forms, statements, a list of checks received each day, and deposit slips. In addition, the program automatically ages accounts at each billing cycle and creates billing statements. As a result, when patient accounts are computerized, practice collections usually increase.

**Computerized Patient Ledger.** The computerized patient ledger contains personal information about each patient, including the name, address, and telephone number, the person responsible for payment, and all insurance carriers (Figure 17-7). The ledger also lists all previous office visits and the procedures, procedure codes, charges, payments, and adjustments for each visit. Most account management software can be customized to meet the special needs of the individual ambulatory care setting.

As information is entered from the charge slips, the computer automatically updates the ledger by adding a description of each procedure and procedure code and each diagnosis and diagnosis code (see Chapter 19 for coding information). It automatically posts the charges and calculates the balance after credits and adjustments are entered.

Although the ability to view a patient's account is fairly accessible, once charges and/or payments have been entered they are not easily removed or changed. This is important as it ensures that monies are not removed from receivables credited to a previous month. This procedure would cause the practice year-end balance to be off.

As useful and efficient as a computerized bookkeeping system can be, it is important to recognize that an inadequate manual system will not get better once computerized. Also, it takes far more time than predicted to move to a computerized system, train personnel, and enter patient data. A manual and computer system may need to run concurrently for several months.

## BANKING PROCEDURES

Understanding banking accounts and services, making deposits, writing checks, and reconciling accounts are all a part of daily financial practices. While many banking services are similar from one bank to another, it is a good idea for the medical assistant in charge of maintaining daily accounts to investigate the banking resources of the local community. In an effort to secure new business, many banks compete for customers by offering special services that can be of utility to the ambulatory care setting.

### Types of Accounts

Checking and savings accounts are the two primary types of accounts.

**Checking Accounts.** The checking account is the primary account type the medical assistant will use in the ambulatory care setting. Stated simply, a checking account allows the depositor to write checks against money placed in the account. Today, there are many variations on checking accounts; in the event that the medical assistant is responsible for establishing a new account, it is worthwhile to investigate features of different checking accounts both within the same bank and at competing banks.

Some features that may differ include:

- Interest paid
- Monthly fees
- Per check fees
- Automated teller machine (ATM) access and fees
- Initial deposit and balance requirements
- Fees for checks
- Special services extended free of charge such as **notary**, cashier's checks, traveler's checks, balance reconciliation, and services designed expressly for small businesses.

When selecting an account, do not only choose the account with the lowest fees. Also consider convenience, the relationship possible with a given bank, number of bank locations, and other factors.

**Savings Accounts.** Savings accounts were initially distinguished from checking accounts because they paid interest on the money deposited. However, many checking accounts also pay interest now as well. In either case, the interest is usually minimal on accounts that give immediate access to the deposit. Some **money market savings accounts** pay a higher rate of interest, although they require a higher initial deposit and maintenance of a higher balance, usually around $2500. Access to the account is limited; often the depositor is permitted to write three checks a month on the account. Savings accounts are useful when money is not needed on demand or when putting monies aside for long-term goals.

## Types of Checks

For the most part, the ambulatory care setting will use a standard business check. However, for special purposes, it is useful to understand the other check types available:

- A **cashier's check** is often used when a check must be guaranteed for the amount in which it is written. Because a cashier's check is the bank's own check drawn against the bank's accounts, the recipient has the assurance that the check will clear.

Cashier's checks are obtained at the bank by paying the bank representative cash or sometimes a personal check for the amount of the cashier's check.

- A **certified check** is the depositor's own check which the bank has "certified" with a date and signature to indicate that the check is good for the amount in which it is written.

- Money orders are available from banks and the United States Postal Service. They are purchased with cash and are used in ways similar to cashier's checks.

- A **voucher check** is a type of check with a stub attached to it which can be used to indicate invoice dates, services provided, and so on. Many payroll checks are written on voucher checks; the voucher check is also frequently used in the ambulatory care setting for accounts payable.

- **Traveler's checks** are available in most banks and are convenient and safer to use than cash when traveling. They are written in specific denominations ($10, $20, $50) and require a signature when purchased and when used.

## Deposits

Deposits are usually made daily since they serve as another proof of posting and because it is unwise to leave large sums of money in the office overnight. The office should have a rubber endorsement stamp from the bank; use it to immediately imprint the back of all checks received directly from patients and in the mail. Before depositing them, be sure all checks are stamped.

Because the endorsement transfers rights to whoever holds the check, it is important to take certain precautions. A blank endorsement consists of a signature only (whether in pen or with a stamp) and presents a danger in that, if the check is lost or stolen, someone else could endorse the check below the signature and cash it. A restrictive endorsement should be used on all checks received in the ambulatory care setting. Restrictive endorsements include the signature as well as the words "for deposit only" or "pay to the order of (include the name of bank and account number. Additionally, all possible payees' names should be listed under the company name, with the practice address)." This restricts the use of the check should it be lost or stolen.

Most business accounts use a deposit slip similar to the one in Figure 17-8. They are always filled out in duplicate—one copy to accompany the deposit, one to be retained for office records. As shown, these deposit slips are longer than those generally used for personal accounts and have room for more entries and more information. If

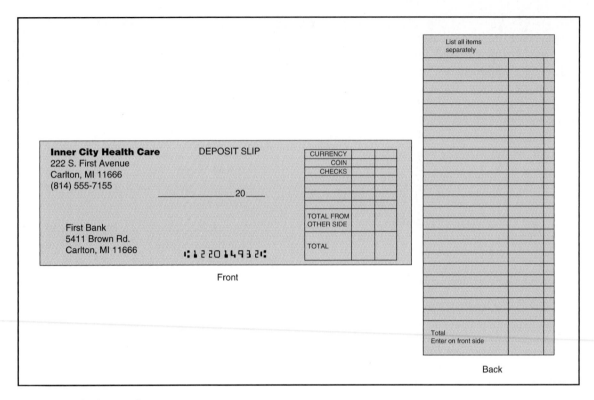

**Figure 17-8**    Sample deposit slip.

your day sheet has a built-in duplicate deposit slip, it will have been completed during posting (see Day Sheets in this chapter).

Procedure 17-6 outlines the steps in preparing a deposit.

## Accepting Checks

When accepting checks from patients and other individuals, take a few minutes to inspect the check; this may eliminate checks returned from the bank for various reasons:

- Inspect the check for correct date, amount, and signature.

- Do not accept a third-party check (a check written to the patient from another person or company) unless it is from the insurance carrier.

- If a deposited check is returned marked "insufficient funds," call the bank that returned it and verify availability of funds. If funds are available, immediately redeposit the check for processing. If the check is returned again, add any fees the bank may charge your office to the patient's account. Be sure to adjust the checking account balance accordingly. Follow office procedure for notifying the patient that the check was returned.

## Lost or Stolen Checks

In the event that a check is missing and is thought to be lost or stolen, report this to your bank immediately. In some cases, you may be advised to stop payment to prevent unauthorized cashing of the check. In other situations, the bank may place a warning on the account, advising bank representatives to be especially careful about checking signatures to detect any attempt at a forged signature.

## Writing and Recording Checks

Part of daily financial practices includes writing checks to pay bills (accounts payable), refunds of overpayment, and replenishment of petty cash. It is important that checks be typed or written legibly to avoid bank errors. Checks should be dated and must include the name of the payee and the amount of payment entered both in figures and in words. It is also advisable to complete the "memo" line on the check indicating what the check is for or, in some cases, an account number and/or invoice number for reference purposes. Most medical practices use computerized accounting software packages such as Quickbooks™ or Quickbooks Pro™. These software packages enable you to write checks and keep a running register. They also have the ability to run payroll with tax tables automatically loaded.

In addition, business checking accounts need to make reference to the **disbursement** of the funds. Disbursement accounts are numbered accounts that break all expenditures into categories (i.e., salaries, rent, supplies) in the general ledger. At the end of the year, the accounts in this ledger will provide the figures for all tax-deductible expense. When the accountant completes the tax form for the practice, the information from the disbursement accounts is then easily transferred to the tax forms.

Before preparing the actual check, complete the check stub, which is the only record of payments made from the account. The stub should include the same information entered on the check as well as the disbursement account name or number for the accountant. Remember, it is critical for tax purposes that each check stub contain disbursement information so the bookkeeper can post the information to the correct accounts in the general ledger.

When the checks have been prepared, verify that the check amounts agree with the amounts written on the stubs, then subtract those amounts from the checkbook balance (Figure 17-9).

**Rules for Writing Checks.** Follow these few rules to assure that checks are properly written and recorded:

- Check that the numerical and written amounts agree.

- Check that everything is spelled correctly.

- Determine that the check has been signed by an individual with signature privileges.

- Follow office procedure for having the physician or office manager approve all expenditures and/or sign all outgoing checks.

- Check that it is payable to the correct payee and that the current date is used.

## Reconciling a Bank Statement

Each month the bank will send a statement for the checking account (Figure 17-10). The statement will show the account balance according to the bank's records, a listing of all checks that have cleared the bank, deposits received by the bank, and any service charges deducted from the account. It is necessary to reconcile the entries in the checkbook against this statement to be sure there are no errors either in the checkbook or in the bank's records. Your bank statement is another means of ensuring that the accounts receivable is accurate for the previous month. If you use an accounting software package, this will also have a computerized option for reconciling.

Procedure 17-7 details the steps involved in reconciling the statement.

## PURCHASING SUPPLIES AND EQUIPMENT

It is important to ensure proper control over purchasing of supplies and equipment for several reasons:

1. To avoid purchase of unnecessary items
2. To avoid duplication of items purchased
3. To prevent employees from ordering items for personal use
4. To provide a system for payment of only those items properly ordered and received

In order to accomplish these things, the first rule of purchasing should be that nothing is ordered or paid for without a purchase order or purchase order number. A copy of the purchase order is sent to the supplier and a copy is retained by the office for verification of shipment and payment of invoice.

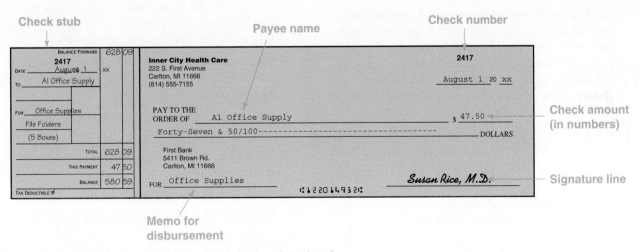

**Figure 17-9** Sample of a properly completed check and check stub.

Summary of Account Balance                Closing Date 1/15/02

Account # 1257-164013                     Ending Balance $8,347.62

| | | |
|---|---|---|
| Beginning Balance | $7,152.18 | |
| Total Deposits and Additions | $8,643.86 | |
| Total Withdrawals | $7,433.21 | |
| Service Charge | $ 15.24 | |

| Number | Date | Amount | Number | Date | Amount |
|---|---|---|---|---|---|
| 201 | 12/18/01 | 173.82 | 234 | 1/4/02 | 96.31 |
| 223* | 12/18/01 | 44.12 | 235 | 1/4/02 | 73.48 |
| 224 | 12/20/01 | 586.00 | 236 | 1/6/02 | 325.40 |
| 225 | 12/21/01 | 24.15 | 237 | 1/7/02 | 40.00 |
| 226 | 12/22/01 | 33.90 | 238 | 1/8/02 | 66.77 |
| 228* | 12/23/01 | 1250.00 | 241* | 1/9/02 | 15.55 |
| 229 | 12/24/01 | 11.75 | 242 | 1/10/02 | 12.45 |
| 230 | 12/24/01 | 19.02 | 243 | 1/10/02 | 4441.25 |
| 231 | 1/2/02 | 43.80 | 244 | 1/10/02 | 64.55 |
| 232 | 1/3/02 | 39.00 | | | |
| 233 | 1/4/02 | 71.50 | | | |

*Denotes gap in check sequence

| Date | Deposit Amount | Date | Deposit Amount |
|---|---|---|---|
| 18-Dec | 361.75 | 4-Jan | 825.00 |
| 19-Dec | 586.00 | 5-Jan | 1286.71 |
| 20-Dec | 918.21 | 7-Jan | 608.00 |
| 21-Dec | 201.00 | 8-Jan | 811.15 |
| 2-Jan | 475.00 | 9-Jan | 1092.68 |
| 3-Jan | 1478.36 | | |

Front

1. Enter Ending Balance from the front of this statement
$ 8,347.62

2. Enter deposits not shown on this statement
$ 3,162.50

3. Subtotal (add 1 & 2)
$ 11,510.12

4. List outstanding checks or other withdrawals here

| Check # | Amount |
|---|---|
| 222 | 37.89 |
| 227 | 161.15 |
| 239 | 11.50 |
| 240 | 92.12 |
| 245 | 835.17 |
| 246 | 21.75 |
| 247 | 586.00 |

5. Total outstanding checks
$ 1,745.58

Balance (subtract #5 from #3)
$ 9,764.54

This should equal your checkbook balance

Back

**Figure 17-10** Sample bank statement.

## Preparing a Purchase Order

Purchase order forms are available from office supply companies or can be ordered from a printer and customized to the needs of the ambulatory care setting. Figure 17-11 shows a typical purchase order form properly completed, which will be reviewed section by section.

The purchase order form can vary greatly; some have more or less information. The form shown in Figure 17-11 contains the usual information required. The important thing is that the purchase order is used consistently.

- *Purchase order number.* A preprinted number that is used on invoices and statements from the supplier and on the check used to pay the invoice. It is also important for tracking the status of the order. In smaller practices, the purchase order number may simply be the name of the person ordering with the date the order was placed immediately following.

- *Bill to address.* Generally used when items are to be shipped to an address different from the address where the supplier will send the bill for goods or services.

- *Ship to address.* When items are to be sent by supplier; this must always be completed.

- *Vendor information.* Name and address of supplier where purchase order is to be sent.

- *Req. By.* States which individual or department has requested the item(s).

- *Buyer.* States the individual in the office who is authorized to issue a purchase order.

- *Terms.* Agreement between buyer and seller as to when payment is due.

- *QTY.* Quantity of item being ordered (number of units).

- *Item.* Vendor's catalogue part or item number.

- *Units.* How the item is sold—individually (ea.), by the box, case, or dozen. Many suppliers will not split units (i.e., sell less than a full case).

- *Description.* Brief description of item (helps as a cross-check for vendor in the event that an item number is entered incorrectly).

- *Unit Price.* How much *one* unit (ea., box, case, dozen) costs.

- *Total.* Cost of one unit multiplied by the number of units being ordered.

- *Subtotal.* Sum of the "Total" column.

- *Tax.* Sales tax required by the state.

- *Freight.* How much the customer must pay to have the order delivered (not always applicable).

# PURCHASE ORDER

NO. 1742

| Bill To: | Ship To: | Vendor: |
|---|---|---|
| **Inner City Health Care**<br>222 S. First Avenue<br>Carlton, MI 11666<br>(814) 555-7155 | **Inner City Health Care**<br>222 S. First Avenue<br>Carlton, MI 11666<br>(814) 555-7155 | **AZ Medical Supply**<br>4721 E. Camelback Rd.<br>Phoenix, AZ 85252<br>(602) 555-3246 |

| REQ BY | BUYER | TERMS |
|---|---|---|
| Karen Ritter | Walter Seals | Net 30 |

| QTY | ITEM | UNITS | DESCRIPTION | UNIT PR | TOTAL |
|---|---|---|---|---|---|
| 10 | 427A | Box | Surgical Gloves - Sz 7 | 6.75 | 67.50 |
| 1 | 327DC | Case | 2" gauze pads | 42.75 | 42.75 |
| 5 | 1943C | Box | Tongue Depressors | 4.00 | 20.00 |
| 15 | 7433 | Ea | Examination Table paper (roll) | 5.75 | 86.25 |
| | | | | | |
| | | | | | |
| | | | | | |
| | | | | | |
| | | | SUBTOTAL | | 216.50 |
| | | | TAX | | 14.07 |
| | | | FREIGHT | | Prepaid |
| | | | BAL DUE | | 230.57 |

**Figure 17-11** Purchase order form.

● *Bal. Due.* The sum of the subtotal, tax, and freight charges—this is how much the office will be billed.

## Verifying Goods Received

Proper purchasing procedure does not stop with the completion and mailing of the purchase order. When goods are received, it is necessary to verify that the correct items and quantities were shipped by the vendor. All packages include a packing slip either on the inside of the box or attached to the outside. This packing slip should be attached to the office copy of the purchase order that is later attached to the invoice. Sometimes this packing slip serves as the original invoice as well.

As each item is unpacked, the item number and quantity received are checked against the office copy of the purchase order. If any discrepancies are noted between what has been received and what was ordered, they should be indicated on the office copy of the purchase order and the vendor should be contacted immediately and arrange-

ments made to ship any missing items or provide return procedures for any incorrect or overshipped items.

## Preparing the Invoice for Payment

When an invoice is received from the vendor (it may be included in the shipment or mailed later), it is necessary to confirm that charges are correct for the items ordered and the shipment received.

The invoice should be compared to the original purchase order to verify quantities, unit prices, and other charges. If there are discrepancies, contact the vendor's accounts receivable department to have the errors corrected before you send payment.

Once the invoice and purchase order are reconciled, the purchase order number is noted on the invoice (if not already printed there by the vendor) and the invoice is marked as "OK to pay." The invoice is then forwarded to the accounts payable department in the office for payment.

# PETTY CASH

**Petty cash** is money kept in the office for minor, routine, or unexpected expenses such as postage-due mail or coffee supplies and cash back for patients paying their co-payments. Keeping this cash on hand eliminates the necessity of the physician or office manager having to sign checks for such items. Petty cash is not used to pay bills or make large routine purchases.

The amount of cash on hand for this purpose is small, usually $75 to $100, and is usually kept in small denominations such as ones and fives and only a few tens. However, records must be as carefully maintained as for any other financial transactions and balanced weekly.

## Establishing a Petty Cash Fund

If your office does not already have a petty cash fund or if you are in a new practice and one has not yet been established, the physician or office manager will need to decide how much the fund should be and write a check to "Cash" for that amount.

## Tracking, Balancing, and Replenishing Petty Cash

**Tracking.** Keep a supply of **petty cash vouchers** on hand for tracking how petty cash was used (Figure 17-12). When money is taken from petty cash, a voucher must always be completed and the receipt from the purchase attached. Vouchers and receipts are kept in the petty cash box with the money until the fund is replenished.

---

**PETTY CASH VOUCHER**

Amount: $16.98                     *December 18, 20__*

For:   *Coffee filters, coffee, creamer, sugar*

Account:   *Office supplies*

Approved By:                     Received By:

*Jane O'Hara*                     *Karen Ritter*

**Figure 17-12**    Petty cash voucher.

**Balancing and Replenishing.** When the fund gets low, write another check to "Cash" to bring it back up to the original amount. To determine the amount of the check, it is necessary to first balance the account. After the account is balanced, list how funds were spent in such a way that the bookkeeper can disburse the check properly.

Procedure 17-8 outlines the steps involved in balancing a petty cash account.

---

## DOCUMENTATION

Financial and ongoing billing records should not be maintained in the patient's chart. Keep financial information separate from medical information to ensure that the physician's care is not influenced by the patient's ability to pay.

---

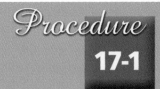

## 17-1    Preparation for Posting a Day Sheet

### PURPOSE:
To ensure that the medical assistant in charge of recording patient transactions prepares the day sheet before patients arrive.

### EQUIPMENT/SUPPLIES:
Pegboard
Quantity of new charge slips and receipt forms
New day sheet
Ledger cards of patients scheduled for the day

### PROCEDURE STEPS:
1. At the start of the day, a new day sheet and strip of charge slips are placed on the pegboard. RATIONALE: Prepares the day sheet for a new day's transactions.
2. Information at the top of the day sheet (date and page number) is filled in. RATIONALE: Establishes the sequential order of the business' daily financial record throughout the year.

*(continues)*

# Procedure

## 17-1 (continued)

3. Balances forwarded from the previous sheet are carefully entered in Section 4, "Previous Page" columns A–D and the "Previous Day's Total" and "Accts. Rec. 1st of Month" in the Accounts Receivable Control and Accounts Receivable Proof boxes. Now the day sheet is ready to use. RATIONALE: Provides information for the month-end closing.

4. The ledger cards for all scheduled patients are pulled from the storage file and kept at the front desk in the order in which patients will be seen. RATIONALE: Ensures efficiency when patients arrive for their appointment.

5. A strip of receipt forms is kept at hand in case someone comes into the office to make payment on account. RATIONALE: Allows efficient use of time when patient makes a payment on their account.

# Procedure

## 17-2 Recording Charges and Payments Requiring a Charge Slip (Patient Visits)

### PURPOSE:

To record information pertaining to a patient's visit to the physician on the patient's ledger and the day sheet and to provide a charge slip for insurance billing.

### EQUIPMENT/SUPPLIES:

Patient ledger card
Day sheet
New charge slip

### PROCEDURE STEPS:

*When a patient comes in for an appointment:*

1. Place the ledger under the next charge slip and turn back the first two pages of the slip. RATIONALE: Takes complete advantage of the write-it-once system.

2. Write the date, responsible party's name and the patient's name (often entered in the "Reference" column), and any previous balance on the charge slip in the spaces provided. The information automatically transfers to the ledger through the carbon strip on the last page of the charge slip and to the day sheet through the NCR© paper. RATIONALE: Documents appropriate information.

3. Remove the charge slip from the pegboard and clip it to the front of the patient's chart to be given to the physician. RATIONALE: Allows physician to indicate appropriate procedure and diagnosis codes.

4. When the physician has completed treatment or examination, the spaces for procedures will be checked, the diagnosis filled in, and the physician will sign the bottom of the form. The form is then given to the patient to carry to the receptionist. RATIONALE: Physician marks the appropriate codes and signs the charge slip indicating it is correct.

*When the patient returns the form to the front desk:*

1. Enter the charge next to each procedure and write in the total on the front of the slip. RATIONALE: Completes the form.

2. Replace the charge slip on the pegboard, carefully lined up with the patient's name on the day sheet, and insert the ledger card under the last page of the charge slip. CAUTION: Be sure to align the *first blank line* of the ledger with the entry strip on the charge slip. RATIONALE: Uses the write-it-once system to record charges and any payment on the ledger card.

*(continues)*

## *Procedure* 17-2 *(continued)*

3. Turn back the first two pages of the charge slip and enter the total charge and any payment the patient makes in the correct columns. RATIONALE: Uses the write-it-once system to record charges and any payment on the ledger card.

4. To arrive at the final balance, simply look at the day sheet at the column that shows previous balance, add the day's charge, and subtract payment made. RATIONALE: Provides the final balance on the day sheet.

*Most day sheets have additional columns to the right of the charge slip. Information recorded here usually includes:*

1. Receipt number (if your system uses numbered charge slips and receipts). RATIONALE: May be used to trace charges or payments related to specific patient transactions.

2. The method of payment (columns are provided for cash, by check, or credit card payments). RATIONALE: Provides a current record of cash, checks, or credit card totals after each entry.

3. Business analysis to be used as outlined by office procedure. RATIONALE: Business analyses require specific records as designed by the office. CAUTION: Be sure to complete the posting of each transaction all the way to the far right and on the same line of the day sheet as instructed by office procedure.

4. When posting is complete, keep the first copy of the charge slip for filing in the patient's chart, keep second copy for submission for insurance reimbursement, and give third copy to the patient. RATIONALE: Ensures a record is distributed to all parties involved.

## *Procedure* 17-3 Receiving a Payment on Account Requiring a Receipt

### PURPOSE:
To record a payment on the day sheet and patient's ledger card and to provide a receipt to the patient.

### EQUIPMENT/SUPPLIES:
Day sheet
Patient ledger card
New receipt form

### PROCEDURE STEPS:
*When someone comes into the office to make a payment:*

1. Receipt forms are placed on the pegboard in place of the charge slips. RATIONALE: A receipt documents the payment.

2. The patient's ledger is pulled and placed under the receipt form with the *first blank line* of the

ledger under the carbon strip. RATIONALE: Takes advantage of the write-it-once system.

3. The following information is then entered along the top of the receipt: date, reference, description, payment amount, previous balance. RATIONALE: Ensures correct patient is referenced and credited the correct amount.

4. The new balance is calculated by subtracting the payment amount from the previous balance. RATIONALE: Indicates the new balance.

5. The receipt is given to the person making payment. RATIONALE: Proof of payment.

NOTE: No copy of the receipt is needed for the office since the information has been recorded on both the patient's ledger and the day sheet.

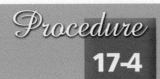

## Recording Payments Received Through the Mail

**PURPOSE:**
To record payments received in the mail on the day sheet and patient ledger card. Payments received through the mail include payments from patients and from insurance companies on the patients' behalf. Both payments are handled in the same manner.

**EQUIPMENT/SUPPLIES:**
Day sheet
Patient ledger cards

**PROCEDURE STEPS:**
*If a patient mails in a payment or if payment is sent by an insurance company:*

1. Pull the appropriate ledger card and place it directly on the day sheet. RATIONALE: Utilizes the write-it-once system.
2. Temporarily remove the strip of charge slips from the pegboard. RATIONALE: Charge slip is not needed when recording a mail payment; patient should never send cash and would have canceled check or money order receipt.
3. Enter the patient's previous balance on the day sheet (your ledger card does not extend to this column). RATIONALE: Indicates previous balance since ledger card does not extend to the column.
4. Post directly onto the ledger card the date, reference (patient name), description*, and payment amount. RATIONALE: Provides accurate information, including differentiating ROA and ROA ins.
5. Calculate the new balance as you did with personal payments. RATIONALE: Provides the new balance.

NOTE: No receipt forms or charge slips are used when posting payments received through the mail.
*ROA = Received on Account
*ROA Ins = Received on Account from insurance company

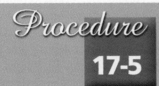

## Balancing Day Sheets

**PURPOSE:**
To verify that all entries to the day sheet are correct and that the totals balance.

**EQUIPMENT/SUPPLIES:**
Day sheet
Calculator

**PROCEDURE STEPS:**

1. *Column Totals.* The first step in balancing a day sheet is to total columns A, $B_1$, $B_2$, C, and D and enter the total for each column in the boxes marked "Totals This Page." The column totals are then added to the figures entered in the "Previous Page" column boxes to arrive at the "Month to Date" totals which provide the total charges, credits, and so forth entered from the first working day of the month to the present. RATIONALE: Establishes column totals.
2. *Proof of Posting.* This box is used to verify that entries have been made correctly and that the column totals are accurate. *All figures entered here are taken from the "Totals This Page" column boxes.*

   a. Enter today's column D total which shows the sum of all the previous balances entered when the transactions were posted.
   b. Added to this is the column A total of all charges for that day to arrive at a subtotal and enter the amount where indicated in the box.

*(continues)*

## Procedure

### 17-5    (continued)

c. Since columns $B_1$ and $B_2$ are both credit columns which reduce balances, they are added together, entered in the box labeled "Less Cols $B_1$ and $B_2$," and the total of credits is subtracted from the subtotal. If all entries and addition are correct in the posting area, the result should equal the amount in column C and the transactions for that day are balanced. RATIONALE: Verifies entries have been made correctly and that the totals are accurate.

*Overview:* When an individual transaction is entered, the patient's previous balance (D) is added to the charges for the day (A). If there are any payments or adjustments made at that time, they are entered in the B columns and subtracted from the A + D amount to achieve the new balance (C). Since each transaction is actually D + A – B = C, the column totals of D + A – B will always equal the C total.

$$
\begin{array}{ccccc}
D & A & B & C \\
10 & + \; 5 & - \; 2 & = \; 13 \\
2 & + \; 7 & - \; 1 & = \; 8 \\
\end{array}
$$

**Column Totals**    12 + 12 – 3 = 21

3. *Accounts Receivable (A/R) Control.* This box simply adds the previous day's Accounts Receivable balance to the current day's totals to include the current day's business and arrive at the new A/R total.
   a. The column A and column B totals are carried straight across from the Proof of Posting box to the corresponding blanks in the A/R Control box.
   b. Add the amount already entered in the Previous Day's Total space to the Column A amount to arrive at a subtotal.
   c. Subtract the amount carried over from the "Less Columns $B_1$ and $B_2$" box to find the new Accounts Receivable amount. RATIONALE: Determines new accounts receivable balance.

4. *Accounts Receivable Proof* verifies, or proves, the A/R balance in the A/R Control box. *The figure entered on the first line of this box will not change during a calendar month* as it shows how much the A/R balance was on the first working day of the month. *All other figures entered will be taken from the "Month-To-Date" column boxes.*

   a. Enter the amount from column A (month-to-date) where shown.
   b. Add the column A amount to the "A/R 1st of Month" figure and enter the sum in the subtotal space.
   c. Enter the $B_1$ and $B_2$ month-to-date amounts and subtract from the subtotal. This amount goes in the Total Accounts Receivable space.

If all posting and addition are correct, the Total Accounts Receivable amounts in the A/R Control and A/R Proof boxes will match and the day is balanced. RATIONALE: Verifies the accounts receivable balance in the accounts receivable control box.

5. *Deposit verification* involves totaling the columns in Section 2 and entering the sum of the columns in the space marked "Total Deposit."

NOTE: The total deposit and the total of payments received in column $B_1$ should match. RATIONALE: Verifies deposit total.

6. *Business Analysis Summary.* If this section is used, total each column in the summary section.

NOTE: If the Business Analysis Summary is used to break out charges by type or by physician, the sum of the columns should equal today's column A total. If it is used to credit payments to different physicians, the sum of the columns will equal today's payment column. RATIONALE: The total deposit and the total of payments received in column $B_1$ should match to prove totals.

7. *After the Day Sheet is Balanced,* there is one step remaining: the transfer of balances.
   a. Take out a new day sheet for the next day.
   b. Transfer the "Month-To-Date" column totals to the "Previous Page" columns boxes on the new sheet.
   c. Enter the Total Accounts Receivable amount from the last day sheet in the "Previous Day's Total" space of the A/R Control box on the new day sheet.
   d. Enter the Accounts Receivable 1st of Month Amount in the A/R Proof box on the new sheet. RATIONALE: Transfers balances to prepare a new day sheet for the next day's activities.

The new day sheet is now ready for posting.

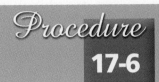
## 17-6    Preparing a Deposit

**PURPOSE:**
To create a deposit slip for the day's receipts.

**EQUIPMENT/SUPPLIES:**
New deposit slip
Check endorsement stamp
Calculator
Cash and checks received for the day

**PROCEDURE STEPS:**
1. Separate all checks from **currency** (paper money). RATIONALE: Each must be entered as a separate total.
2. Count all currency to be deposited and enter the amount in the space provided. Gather bills in order; i.e., fifties, twenties, tens, and so on. RATIONALE: Follows bank procedure.
3. Count all coins to be deposited and enter the amount in the space provided. Coins may need to be wrapped. RATIONALE: Follows bank procedure.
4. On the back of the deposit slip list each check separately. Include the patient name in the left-hand column and enter the amount of the check in the right-hand column. RATIONALE: Follows bank procedure.
5. Total the checks listed and copy the total on the front where it is indicated to place the total from

the other side. RATIONALE: Follows bank procedure.
6. The sum of currency, coins, and checks should always equal the total in the "payments" column on that day's day sheet. RATIONALE: Proof of accuracy.
7. Attach the top copy of the deposit slip to the deposit, leaving the carbon on the pad. RATIONALE: Provides the office and bank with record of deposit.
8. Enter the date and amount of the deposit in the space provided on the checkbook stubs. RATIONALE: Keeps checkbook register current with money in account.
9. Add the amount of the deposit to the checkbook balance. RATIONALE: Keeps checkbook register current with money in account.
10. Deposit at the bank, either in person or at the night deposit. In either case, be sure a record of deposit is received (it will be mailed if the night deposit is used). It is not recommended that deposits be made through automated teller machines (ATMs); currency should never be deposited in an ATM. RATIONALE: Proof bank processed the deposit as indicated.

## 17-7    Reconciling a Bank Statement

**PURPOSE:**
To verify that the balance listed in the checkbook agrees with the balance shown by the bank.

**EQUIPMENT/SUPPLIES:**
Checkbook
Bank statement
Calculator

**PROCEDURE STEPS:**
1. Make sure the balance in the checkbook is current (all deposits and checks entered have been added or subtracted). RATIONALE: Ensures totals are accurate.
2. If there is a service charge listed on the statement, subtract that amount from the last balance listed in the checkbook. RATIONALE: Reconciles current balance.

*(continues)*

## Procedure 17-7 *(continued)*

3. In the checkbook, check off each check listed on the statement and verify the amount against the check stub. RATIONALE: Verifies accuracy.
4. In the checkbook, check off each deposit listed on the statement. RATIONALE: Verifies accuracy.
5. The back of the statement contains a worksheet to be used for balancing.
6. Copy the ending balance from the front of the statement to the area indicated on the back.
7. Go through the check stubs and list on the back of the statement in the area provided any checks that have not cleared and any deposits that were not shown as received on the statement.
8. Total the checks not cleared on the statement worksheet.
9. Total the deposits not credited on the worksheet.
10. Add together the statement balance and the total of deposits not credited.
11. Subtract the total of checks not cleared. This amount should agree with the balance in the checkbook. If so, the checkbook is balanced and the statement should be filed in the appropriate place. RATIONALE: Following procedure steps 5–11 completes verification of accuracy.

## Procedure 17-8  **Balancing Petty Cash**

**PURPOSE:**
To verify that the amount of petty cash is consistent with the beginning amount less expenditures shown on receipts.

**EQUIPMENT/SUPPLIES:**
Petty cash box
Vouchers
Calculator

**PROCEDURE STEPS:**
1. Count the money remaining in the box. RATIONALE: Verifies amount of cash and coin remaining in petty cash.
2. Total the amounts of all vouchers in the petty cash box. RATIONALE: Determines amount of expenditures.
3. Subtract the amount of receipts from the original amount in petty cash. This should equal the amount of cash remaining in the box. RATIO-NALE: Proves that the amount of expenditures deducted from the beginning amount equals the amount left in the box.
4. When the cash has been balanced against the receipts, write a check *only for the amount that was used.* RATIONALE: Brings dollar amount back to original petty cash amount.

**PETTY CASH CHECK DISBURSEMENT:**
1. Sort all vouchers by account.
2. On a sheet of paper list the accounts involved.
3. Total vouchers for each account, and record individual totals on the list.
4. Copy this list with its totals on the "memo" portion of the stub for the check written to replenish petty cash.
5. File the list with the vouchers and receipts attached, after noting the check number on the list.

At the offices of Doctors Lewis & King, office manager Marilyn Johnson, CMA, is training a new administrative medical assistant in the practice's bookkeeping functions. The new medical assistant, Joann Crier, is a recent medical assistant graduate. This is her first position since earning her credentials. Joann has a basic interest in bookkeeping but wants Marilyn to instruct her, if possible, in the range of daily financial practices she may eventually be responsible for at Doctors Lewis & King.

## CASE STUDY REVIEW

1. Suppose Marilyn were to give Joann a broad overview of every activity involved in Doctors Lewis & King's daily financial practices. What topic areas would she include?

2. Marilyn is very proficient in the pegboard system but knows little about computerized bookkeeping systems. Joann has current information on computer systems because she is a recent graduate; however, she is not really sure of herself with pegboard accounting. How can Marilyn and Joann use their complementary skill areas to help one another?

3. Joann will be helping Marilyn with accounts payable. What does she need to know and what rules should she observe?

## SUMMARY

In this chapter we have discussed the daily financial duties in a medical office: patient bookkeeping, working with the checkbook, purchasing supplies and equipment, and petty cash. By becoming proficient in these functions, you will be prepared to handle the day-to-day financial aspects of any ambulatory care setting.

Patient bookkeeping involves not only a responsibility to the physician/employer (you are keeping track of income), but also to the patient to be certain that charges for services rendered are correct and that payments are properly credited. The pegboard system is a comprehensive manual system to post and track this data. Computerized bookkeeping offers advantages of speed, high accuracy, and elimination of some routine tasks.

It is also important to maintain a scrupulous accounts payable system to ensure that bills are paid on time and that payments are properly documented for tax purposes. To accomplish this, checks must be written properly and on time and recorded on the check stubs to effectively track expenditures.

Whether working with a pegboard or computerized system, accuracy is important at all times. To ensure maximum accuracy in all bookkeeping functions, observe a few rules: record all charges and receipts immediately; make deposits of checks and currency the same day they are received; always verify and recheck totals of all deposits and expenditures; stay current with all checking account duties such as account reconciliation; be prompt with all accounts payable.

## REVIEW QUESTIONS

### Multiple Choice

1. "Usual" refers to:
   a. the fee based on the average charge for a specific procedure by all physicians practicing the same specialty in a defined geographic region
   b. the fee typically charged by a physician for certain procedures
   c. the midrange of fees charged for this procedure
   d. the fee based on the physician's decision

2. The use of credit cards by patients to pay for services in ambulatory care settings is:
   a. never done
   b. highly unethical
   c. sure to compromise the integrity of the office
   d. a credit arrangement that can be used with discretion

3. The first section of the day sheet is used:
   a. to record deposits
   b. for business analysis

c. to post individual transactions

d. to total transactions

4. Good working habits for bookkeeping functions include:

   a. always using pencil

   b. always using red ink

   c. being meticulous about aligning columns

   d. relying on a calculator only

5. When moving from a manual to computerized bookkeeping system:

   a. it can be expected to be up and running within a week or so

   b. the manual and computer systems may need to run concurrently for a few months

   c. it is not necessary to understand manual bookkeeping systems

   d. accuracy will be assured in the computerized system

6. Charge slips (or superbills):

   a. may be ordered to fit the practice

   b. is a separate ledger for each patient household

   c. lists common services provided, procedural code, and diagnosis code

   d. only a and c are correct

7. Posting is the process:

   a. that increases or decreases patient accounts not due to charges incurred or payments received

   b. that decreases balance due

   c. that records financial transactions into a bookkeeping or accounting system

   d. that increases the balance due

8. When accepting checks from patients, all of the following are true *except:*

   a. always accept third-party checks

   b. always inspect the check for correct date

   c. always inspect the check for correct amount in numbers and written portion

   d. always inspect the check for the signature

9. A check with an attached stub for recording information is called a:

   a. certified check

   b. cashier's check

   c. voucher check

   d. money order

10. It is important to ensure proper control over purchasing of supplies and equipment for all of the following reasons *except:*

    a. to avoid purchase of unnecessary items

    b. to avoid duplication of items purchased

    c. to permit employees to order items for personal use

    d. to provide a system for payment of only those items properly ordered and received

11. Petty cash:

    a. is usually $25 to $50

    b. is usually $75 to $100

    c. usually consists of small denominations

    d. only b and c are correct

12. To balance petty cash do all of the following *except:*

    a. count the money remaining and total the amounts of all vouchers

    b. subtract the amount of receipts from the original amount of petty cash

    c. write a check for only the amount that was used (bringing the petty cash back to original amount)

    d. in the checkbook, check off each check listed on the statement and verify the amount against the check stub

## Critical Thinking

1. List the three functions of a charge slip. How can charge slips be customized?

2. What is the primary advantage of a pegboard system of bookkeeping? Discuss the forms required for a complete pegboard system.

3. Explain the necessity of maintaining ledger cards.

4. What is the purpose for "running a tape" on the calculator whenever you are working on bookkeeping tasks?

5. Describe the five sections of a day sheet and the function of each.

6. What is the procedure for preparing a new day sheet?

7. Explain the difference in procedure between receiving a payment in person versus a payment that has been mailed to the office.

8. Why are bank deposits usually done daily?

9. When should the checkbook be balanced? Why?

10. Explain the purpose of petty cash.

## WEB ACTIVITIES

Utilize the World Wide Web to gather information on several different computerized accounting programs and compare the advantages and disadvantages of each. Follow your instructor's instructions for additional information regarding this activity.

## REFERENCES/BIBLIOGRAPHY

Andress, A. A. (1996). *Manual of medical office management.* Philadelphia: W. B. Saunders Company.

Humphrey, D. D. (1996). *Contemporary medical office procedures* (2nd ed.). Albany, NY: Delmar.

# Chapter 18

# MEDICAL INSURANCE

## KEY TERMS

Assignment of Benefits
Bar Code
Basic Insurance
Beneficiary
Birthday Rule
Capitation
Catchment
Claim
Coinsurance
Coordination of Benefits (COB)
Copayment
Deductible
Diagnosis Code
Diagnosis-Related Groups (DRGs)
Direct Payment
Drug Formulary
Elective Procedures
Envoy
Exclusion
Exclusive Provider Organization (EPO)
Fiscal Intermediary
Health Care Financing Administration (HCFA)
Health Maintenance Organization (HMO)
Integrated Delivery System
*International Classification of Diseases, 9th Revision, Clinical Modification (ICD-9-CM)*
Major Medical Insurance
Managed Care Organization (MCO)
Medicare Allowable
Medicare Assignment
Medicare Part A
Medicare Part B
Medigap Policy                    *(continues)*

## OUTLINE

**The Evolution of Medical Insurance Coverage**
  Changes in Health Insurance Today
  Screening for Insurance
**Medical Insurance Terminology**
  Terminology Specific to Insurance Policies
  Terminology Specific to Billing Insurance Carriers

**Types of Medical Insurance Coverage**
  Traditional Insurance
  Managed Care
  Medicare
  Other Types of Coverage
**Prospective Payment Systems and Diagnosis-Related Groups**
**Legal and Ethical Issues**

## OBJECTIVES

*The student should strive to meet the following performance objectives and demonstrate an understanding of the facts and principles presented in this chapter through written and oral communication.*

1. Define the key terms as presented in the glossary.
2. Describe the history of medical insurance in this country and its evolution in recent years.
3. Define the terminology necessary to understand and submit medical insurance claims.
4. Recall at least five examples of medical insurance coverage and discuss their differences.
5. Explain the significance of diagnosis-related groups.
6. Describe six primary managed care organization models.
7. Discuss legal and ethical issues related to medical insurance and the physician office.

## KEY TERMS (*continued*)

Nonavailability Statement
Physician-Hospital Organization (PHO)
Preauthorization
Pre-Existing Condition
Preferred Provider

Preferred Provider Organization
(PPO)
Primary Care Physician (PCP)
Proof of Eligibility (POE)
Prospective Payment

Resource-Based Relative Value Scale
(RBRVS)
Usual, Customary, and Reasonable (UCR)
Utilization Review Organization
Waiting Period

## ROLE DELINEATION COMPONENTS

### ADMINISTRATIVE

**Administrative Procedures**

- Understand and apply third-party guidelines
- Obtain reimbursement through accurate claims submission
- Monitor third-party reimbursement
- Understand and adhere to managed care policies and procedures

### GENERAL (TRANSDISCIPLINARY)

**Legal Concepts**

- Document accurately

**Instruction**

- Explain office policies and procedures

**Operational Functions**

- Apply computer techniques to support office operations

## SCENARIO

At Inner City Health Care, a multidoctor urgent care center in a large city, medical assistant Jane O'Hara, CMA, is responsible for all patient billing procedures. While she delegates much of the responsibility for encoding claim forms to her two assistants, Jane oversees the process. Inner City participates in a number of insurance plans, so Jane must stay abreast of policy changes regarding reimbursement, preauthorizations, and claims filing. She also tries to become acquainted with the conditions of each patient's insurance coverage and helps patients understand their responsibility, if any, for payment. Finally, Jane holds periodic meetings with her assistants to update them; she continually stresses to them the importance of timeliness in filing claims and the need for absolute accuracy in diagnosis and procedure codes, which must always reflect services actually performed.

## INTRODUCTION

An understanding of medical insurance and proper coding techniques is absolutely critical to the survival of the ambulatory care setting. In recent years much has changed in medical insurance coverage: more patients are choosing HMO and other managed care options, and even traditional insurance carriers like Blue Cross and Blue Shield are modifying their insurance plans to include some aspect of managed benefits.

In some ways, managed care coverage has simplified the patient's responsibility for payment, but it is more important than ever for the medical assistant to be accurate, timely, and conscientious in both filing insurance claim forms and understanding—and helping the patient understand—the conditions of individual insurance policies.

The increasing complexity of health insurance today means that medical assistants must continually update their base of information. This chapter will provide the groundwork for understanding the role of insurance, its terminology, and its various forms, and will give the medical assistant the confidence to take responsibility for claim filing in the ambulatory care setting.

# THE EVOLUTION OF MEDICAL INSURANCE COVERAGE

The first medical insurance contract began in 1929 when a group of Texas teachers made an agreement for each member to pay Baylor University Hospital the amount of $6 a year to cover any of the group for hospitalization up to 21 days if that should become necessary.

Prior to this time, there was no formal medical insurance as we know it today. Then, if someone became ill, the family had to pay hospital, physician, and any related medical bills. If no family members were available to help, or if the family did not have adequate resources to pay these fees, the patient sometimes had to work for years to repay the debt. The physician sometimes gave the patient a reduced bill for office services.

In today's medical insurance, most carriers pay for hospitalization due to illness, accident, or disease. If a patient wishes to undergo an elective procedure (e.g., face-lift or abdominoplasty), most carriers will not pay the costs associated with that procedure. Not all insurance carriers cover the same exposures equally and none of the carriers pays at the same rate. Similarly, not many of the carriers charge the same premiums to policyholders. Some insurance companies cover individuals, families, or employee groups through work or through groups such as American Association of Retired Persons (AARP). Some premiums reflect an insured's past medical history and the company's exposure in covering the person. Premiums may be lower if the insured selects a higher annual deductible. Other premiums represent the rate that a group is able to obtain based on the group's claim history.

## Changes in Health Insurance Today

There is much discussion today about changes in the health care insurance industry. Foremost is the idea that health care insurance should be available to all citizens of the United States. At this time, health insurance is usually tied to the employment package that covers the employee, spouse, and dependent children. One problem with work-related coverage is that some part-time employees are not eligible for health insurance and thus often go uninsured. Another problem is if an employee takes a position elsewhere, medical benefits may not transfer equally. If a family member is ill with an ongoing disease like cancer, or diabetes mellitus, the new insurance policy may not cover that disease or condition for at least one year. This is an **exclusion** known as a pre-existing condition. Current changes in the law prevent insurance companies from penalizing a patient with a pre-existing condition.

Another controversial aspect of health insurance is refusal to provide coverage for certain procedures because they are not sufficiently proven to be effective. In the early 1990s, bone marrow transplants were being performed on patients with breast cancer, at that time an experimental treatment for breast cancer. Because most insurance carriers will not extend coverage to experimental treatment, family and friends of patients often gathered for fund-raising drives to ensure that medical costs would be covered.

## Screening for Insurance

Until universal coverage becomes a reality, it is the responsibility of the medical assistant to screen all new patients for their insurance. Clear all the insurance hurdles (authorizations, referrals) before giving treatment. If not cleared in advance, these hurdles may be insurmountable when trying to collect for fees for physician services.

Always ask:

- Is the patient covered by insurance?
- Is this procedure covered by the insurance?
- Is the primary care provider performing the procedure?
- Is a referral required? Is an authorization number or authorization code required? Has evidence of qualifying been received?

If the ambulatory care center does not participate in a particular plan and a patient with that plan does not have a referral to the physician, tell the patient in advance that there must be a referral or insurance will not pay. Requesting a referral when scheduling the first appointment should be routine practice and makes the billing process much easier for patient and office.

When screening patients for insurance, it is important to understand the philosophy of the medical office. Some may see patients regardless of ability to pay; responsible medical assistants will investigate all avenues for reimbursement first. Some situations may include the patient who is eligible for Medicaid but has not yet applied, or the patient who has applied for Medicaid but has not yet received notification of qualification.

The medical assistant should investigate and verify that all avenues have been taken to achieve the **proof of eligibility (POE)** that the office will need to receive reimbursement from Medicaid. This may include calling the Medicaid office to verify eligibility, or going on-line and printing a POE directly from the Medicaid system. This electronic data exchange system is called an **envoy**. POE cards are distributed to recipients and are in effect for at least one year. However, the most common avenue to ensure that services will be reimbursed is not to see any patient that does not have proof of Medicaid coverage. Medicaid sends their eligibility statements (medical coupons) to the patient the first day of the month. This coupon guarantees the ambulatory care center payment for the services provided. The majority of offices will not schedule Medicaid patients, unless it is an emergency, before the fifth of each month. This allows ample time for the beneficiary to receive the medical coupon. If the patient presents for their appointment without a medical coupon and proof of eligibility cannot be determined elsewhere, it is common practice to have that patient reschedule the appointment. The exception would be in the instance of an emergency.

Medical assistants with responsibility for billing are one key to a thriving ambulatory care center. Billing the insurance carriers promptly, completing claim forms properly, billing patients as needed, and keeping track of aging accounts will do much to ensure there is a flow of adequate income. In all insurance matters, be available to patients with questions regarding their insurance or accounts, for a friendly attitude helps patients feel positive about the care they receive and establishes a long-term relationship.

There are many hurdles to pass before the idea of universal health care, or coverage for all U.S. citizens, becomes reality. Many people believe that universal coverage will give everyone equal access to health care, regardless of their ability to pay. Others are of the opinion that universal health care will overload the system and result in delayed availability of health care to most people. Which point of view is correct is open to debate.

## MEDICAL INSURANCE TERMINOLOGY

Before discussing the types of insurance coverage, one must understand the language used by the insurance industry. The terminology is specific in meaning and has been tested in courts of law to further define its meanings.

### Terminology Specific to Insurance Policies

A policy is an agreement between the insurance company and the insured or beneficiary, the person covered under the terms of the policy. The insured person may include as beneficiaries the spouse and dependent minor children and others if related by blood and dependent upon the insured for more than 50 percent of their support. The insurance carrier pays a percentage (coinsurance) of the cost of the services covered under the policy in exchange for a monthly premium or charge. This premium is paid by the insured, the employer, or shared by both.

At the inception or beginning of the policy, the insured is given an identification card, which must be presented before receiving medical treatment (Figure 18-1). This card contains the insured's name, identification number, group number, and any copayment amount or restrictions for treatment. The back of the insurance card contains an address where claims should be submitted and telephone numbers needed to receive prior authorization for treatment.

**Deductible.** The language of the policy spells out the terms of the coverage. Usually there is an annual deductible, or an amount of money that the insured must incur for medical services before the policy begins to pay. This deductible can range from $100 to $1,000 or an even greater amount depending upon the language of the policy. The deductible must be met by medical charges that are incurred after the inception or anniversary date of the policy.

For instance, if Boris Bolski went to the physician on January 22 and incurred $258 in charges but his policy did not go into effect until February 1, none of these charges would apply toward his deductible. If, however, he returned to the doctor on February 3 and incurred another $85, this amount could be applied against his deductible.

**Coinsurance.** After the application of the deductible to the submitted bills, the insurance policy pays a percentage of the remaining amount. This percentage or coinsurance can vary from 50 percent to 100 percent depending upon the language in a specific policy. Most companies pay 80 percent.

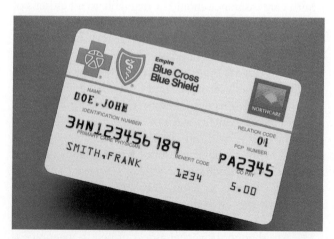

**Figure 18-1** Example of a Blue Cross/Blue Shield insurance identification card. (Courtesy of Empire Blue Cross/Blue Shield)

**Copayment.** Some insurance policies, especially health maintenance organizations (HMOs) and other managed care policies, require the patient to make a payment of a specified amount, for instance $5 or $10, at the time of treatment. This is usually done in place of a coinsurance being applied to the claim. This payment must be collected at the time of the office visit. Some policies have both a copayment and coinsurance clause.

**Pre-Existing Condition.** The example of Boris Bolski presents another problem. If a person had an illness, disease, or injury prior to the inception of the insurance whether or not treatment was received, there is a good chance that most insurance policies will not cover any charges related to that specific illness, injury, or disease because it is considered a pre-existing condition. Most policies have a specific waiting period before coverage is extended to those pre-existing conditions. This waiting period can be a matter of months, years, or the lifetime of the policy. If the person had a previous insurance policy that was not as inclusive as the new policy, often the new policy would still consider this a pre-existing condition and will deny payment until the waiting period is met. However, if the new policy has similar benefits and the person had no lapse in coverage, legally, the company must cover those conditions without applying a pre-existing condition or waiting period to the policy.

**Exclusions.** Exclusions are an important part of a policy. Some policies exclude elective procedures (procedures that are not medically necessary) such as cosmetic surgery, where other policies may allow some elective procedures. Other examples of exclusions might be pre-existing conditions, dental services, chiropractic services, or routine eye examinations. Not every policy has the same exclusions.

**Coordination of Benefits.** When more than one policy covers an individual, the policy language provides for coordination of benefits (COB). This is determined by the policy language and coordinates payments between the policies so that the final total benefit is not greater than the original charge. Policy language again determines which of the two policies is primary or will pay first.

The employee's policy will pay first for the employee. For instance, if John O'Keefe is covered by an insurance policy where he works and is also covered by his wife's medical coverage, the policy Mr. O'Keefe gets from his employer will pay benefits first for him. The coverage under his spouse's policy will pay second because John is considered a dependent under that policy.

If one policy has coordination of benefits and the other policy does not, the policy *without* coordination of benefits will pay first.

When children of undivorced parents are covered under both parents' policies, often the birthday rule will be used to determine which policy is primary. This rule simply states that the policy of the parent with the birthday falling earlier in the year is primary. Thus, if the father's birthday is October 17 and the mother's birthday is May 12, the mother's policy will be primary. The year of the birth date is not relevant.

If the parents share the same birthday, then the policy with the earlier inception date is primary. If John and Mary both have birthdays on July 12, and the policy for John started August 1, 2001, and the policy for Mary started December 1, 2000, Mary's policy would be primary for their dependent children.

For children of divorced parents who are covered under both parents' policies, the policy of the custodial parent is usually primary.

## Terminology Specific to Billing Insurance Carriers

There is specific terminology that one must understand when submitting insurance claims for medical benefits. Most ambulatory care settings will bill all appropriate insurance carriers to ascertain that the claim is made and the physician receives payment.

Many policies require preauthorization before certain procedures or before a visit can be made to a specialist or even a physical therapist. In these cases, the medical assistant must contact the insurance carrier with all of the diagnosis information and the proposed course of treatment. For instance, in a patient with a diagnosis of cholecystitis, preauthorization requires notification and approval before referring that patient to a surgeon for possible cholecystectomy. If this is not done, the surgery may not be covered.

A claim occurs when patients, having received treatment, wish to receive reimbursement under their insurance policies for charges for treatment. The patient (or the center's billing office) sends the claim to the insurance carrier for the amount of the treatment. This is done via a claim form, the most common of which is the HCFA-1500 (12-90) (Figure 18-2). This form was developed by the Health Care Financing Administration (HCFA) and is available with or without the bar code feature.

The claim form contains all of the identification information that the insurance company will need to process, or analyze, the claim for payment. The patient's name, address, telephone number, and, if they differ, the insured's name, address, and telephone number, social security number, group number, and member number are contained in the upper portion of the claim form. The lower portion of the form includes an area for up to four diagnosis codes, the procedure and visit codes, and the charges for those. Finally, the bottom section of the claim form includes the physician's name, address, telephone number, Internal Revenue Service (IRS) number, and Physician Identification Number (PIN).

All of the diagnoses as well as the visit types and procedures are coded. This coding will be discussed in Chapter 19. The completed claim form is sent to the insurance carrier either by mail, electronically, or through

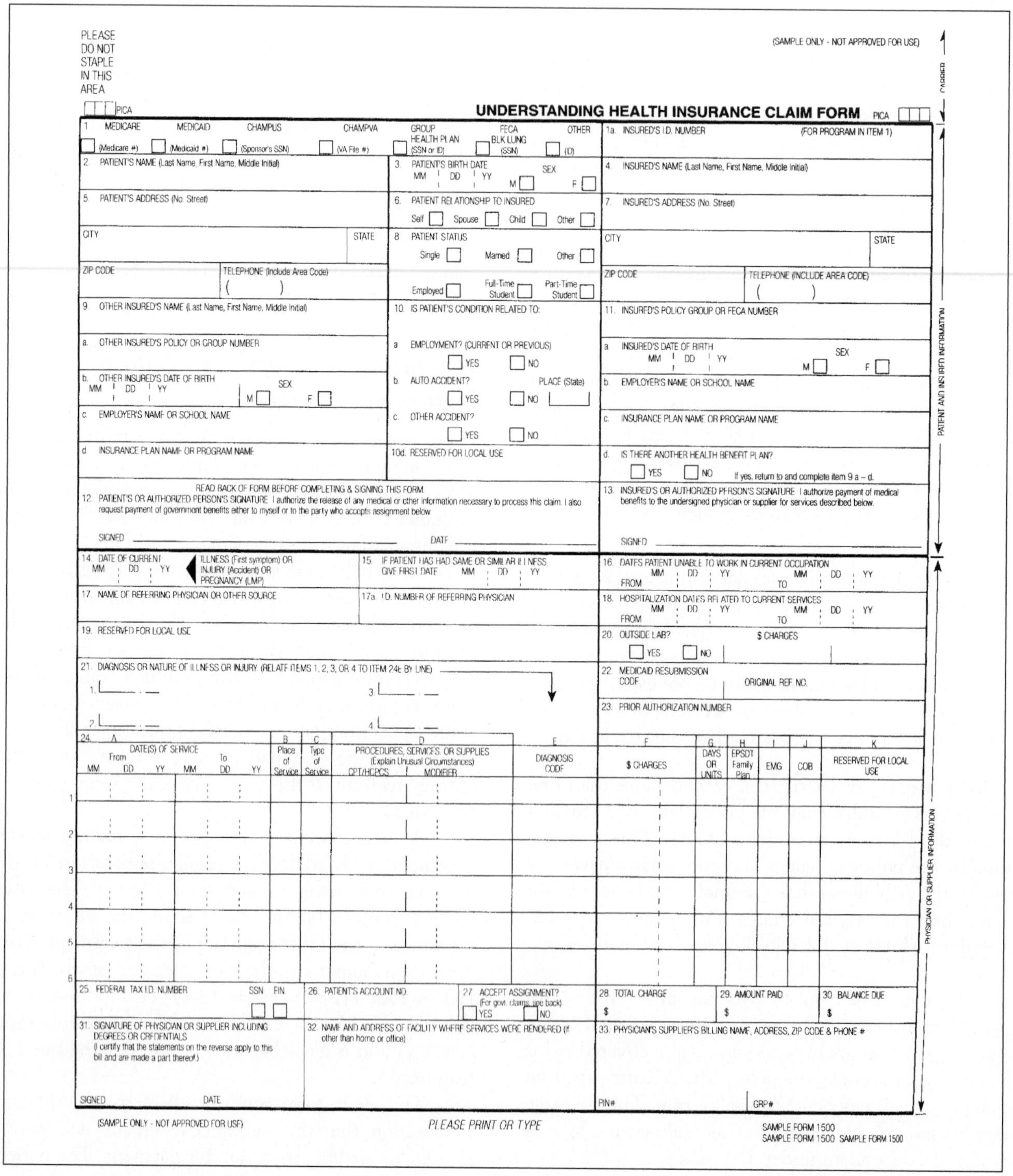

PLEASE DO NOT STAPLE IN THIS AREA

(SAMPLE ONLY - NOT APPROVED FOR USE)

CARRIER

PICA

UNDERSTANDING HEALTH INSURANCE CLAIM FORM PICA

1. MEDICARE (Medicare #) MEDICAID (Medicaid #) CHAMPUS (Sponsor's SSN) CHAMPVA (VA File #) GROUP HEALTH PLAN (SSN or ID) FECA BLK LUNG (SSN) OTHER (ID)

1a. INSURED'S I.D. NUMBER (FOR PROGRAM IN ITEM 1)

2. PATIENT'S NAME (Last Name, First Name, Middle Initial)

3. PATIENT'S BIRTH DATE MM DD YY SEX M F

4. INSURED'S NAME (Last Name, First Name, Middle Initial)

5. PATIENT'S ADDRESS (No. Street)

6. PATIENT RELATIONSHIP TO INSURED Self Spouse Child Other

7. INSURED'S ADDRESS (No. Street)

CITY STATE

8. PATIENT STATUS Single Married Other Employed Full-Time Student Part-Time Student

CITY STATE

ZIP CODE TELEPHONE (Include Area Code) ( )

ZIP CODE TELEPHONE (INCLUDE AREA CODE) ( )

9. OTHER INSURED'S NAME (Last Name, First Name, Middle Initial)

10. IS PATIENT'S CONDITION RELATED TO:

11. INSURED'S POLICY GROUP OR FECA NUMBER

a. OTHER INSURED'S POLICY OR GROUP NUMBER

a. EMPLOYMENT? (CURRENT OR PREVIOUS) YES NO

a. INSURED'S DATE OF BIRTH MM DD YY SEX M F

b. OTHER INSURED'S DATE OF BIRTH MM DD YY SEX M F

b. AUTO ACCIDENT? PLACE (State) YES NO

b. EMPLOYER'S NAME OR SCHOOL NAME

c. EMPLOYER'S NAME OR SCHOOL NAME

c. OTHER ACCIDENT? YES NO

c. INSURANCE PLAN NAME OR PROGRAM NAME

d. INSURANCE PLAN NAME OR PROGRAM NAME

10d. RESERVED FOR LOCAL USE

d. IS THERE ANOTHER HEALTH BENEFIT PLAN? YES NO If yes, return to and complete item 9 a – d.

READ BACK OF FORM BEFORE COMPLETING & SIGNING THIS FORM.

12. PATIENT'S OR AUTHORIZED PERSON'S SIGNATURE I authorize the release of any medical or other information necessary to process this claim. I also request payment of government benefits either to myself or to the party who accepts assignment below.

SIGNED DATE

13. INSURED'S OR AUTHORIZED PERSON'S SIGNATURE I authorize payment of medical benefits to the undersigned physician or supplier for services described below.

SIGNED

PATIENT AND INSURED INFORMATION

14. DATE OF CURRENT: MM DD YY ILLNESS (First symptom) OR INJURY (Accident) OR PREGNANCY (LMP)

15. IF PATIENT HAS HAD SAME OR SIMILAR ILLNESS, GIVE FIRST DATE MM DD YY

16. DATES PATIENT UNABLE TO WORK IN CURRENT OCCUPATION MM DD YY FROM TO

17. NAME OF REFERRING PHYSICIAN OR OTHER SOURCE

17a. I.D. NUMBER OF REFERRING PHYSICIAN

18. HOSPITALIZATION DATES RELATED TO CURRENT SERVICES MM DD YY FROM TO

19. RESERVED FOR LOCAL USE

20. OUTSIDE LAB? YES NO $ CHARGES

21. DIAGNOSIS OR NATURE OF ILLNESS OR INJURY (RELATE ITEMS 1, 2, 3, OR 4 TO ITEM 24E BY LINE)

1. 2. 3. 4.

22. MEDICAID RESUBMISSION CODE ORIGINAL REF. NO.

23. PRIOR AUTHORIZATION NUMBER

| 24. A DATE(S) OF SERVICE From MM DD YY To MM DD YY | B Place of Service | C Type of Service | D PROCEDURES, SERVICES, OR SUPPLIES (Explain Unusual Circumstances) CPT/HCPCS MODIFIER | E DIAGNOSIS CODE | F $ CHARGES | G DAYS OR UNITS | H EPSDT Family Plan | I EMG | J COB | K RESERVED FOR LOCAL USE |
|---|---|---|---|---|---|---|---|---|---|---|
| 1 | | | | | | | | | | |
| 2 | | | | | | | | | | |
| 3 | | | | | | | | | | |
| 4 | | | | | | | | | | |
| 5 | | | | | | | | | | |
| 6 | | | | | | | | | | |

25. FEDERAL TAX I.D. NUMBER SSN EIN

26. PATIENT'S ACCOUNT NO.

27. ACCEPT ASSIGNMENT? (For govt. claims, see back) YES NO

28. TOTAL CHARGE $

29. AMOUNT PAID $

30. BALANCE DUE $

31. SIGNATURE OF PHYSICIAN OR SUPPLIER INCLUDING DEGREES OR CREDENTIALS (I certify that the statements on the reverse apply to this bill and are made a part thereof.)

SIGNED DATE

32. NAME AND ADDRESS OF FACILITY WHERE SERVICES WERE RENDERED (If other than home or office)

33. PHYSICIAN'S SUPPLIER'S BILLING NAME, ADDRESS, ZIP CODE & PHONE #

PIN# GRP#

PHYSICIAN OR SUPPLIER INFORMATION

(SAMPLE ONLY - NOT APPROVED FOR USE)

PLEASE PRINT OR TYPE

SAMPLE FORM 1500
SAMPLE FORM 1500 SAMPLE FORM 1500

**Figure 18-2** HCFA-1500 claim form (revised 12-90).

a holding system that batches and transmits claims at timed intervals, usually weekly. The most common and expeditious method for submitting claims is electronically. Only a few carriers do not accept electronic billings. This is generally when the HCFA-1500 form will be used. Additionally, the HCFA-1500 would be used when additional documentation will be needed to expedite the claim processing. Depending upon the policy language and the **assignment of benefits**, payment is sent either directly to the physician (known as **direct payment**) or to the patient/insured but payable to both the insured and the physician (known as indirect payment). With Medicaid, payment is made to the insured and the physician must collect from the insured.

# TYPES OF MEDICAL INSURANCE COVERAGE

In today's health care environment, medical assistants will need to be aware of the different types of medical insurance policies.

## Traditional Insurance

Traditional policies include coverage on a fee-for-service basis. There is usually a deductible and a coinsurance amount. Bills are submitted to the insurance carrier and if the annual deductible has been met, the coinsurance is applied to the difference. Payment is made either to the physician directly or to both the insured and physician.

Usually these policies pay only when there are diagnoses of illness, disease, or injury. Generally, they will not cover examinations to diagnose or to treat fertility problems; only a few carriers cover routine physicals or preventative health care.

Medical insurance policies often defined two types of coverage: basic insurance and major medical insurance. **Basic insurance** covers a specific dollar amount for physician fees, hospital care, surgery, and anesthesia.

**Major medical insurance** was developed to cover the costs of catastrophic expenses from illness or injury.

Many of the traditional insurance policies require that each policyholder, or insured, choose a **primary care physician (PCP)**, and to coordinate all of their medical care through that primary care physician.

### Blue Cross and Blue Shield. While many traditional policies are offered by commercial carriers, the "Blues" are a well-known type of traditional insurance company. The 1929 Baylor University Hospital insurance agreement was the beginning of what we know today as Blue Cross. Over the years it has grown and matured into a nonprofit organization providing basic and major medical

coverage. In most parts of the United States, Blue Cross and Blue Shield work in conjunction with each other. Blue Cross normally covers the hospitalization, radiology, and other basic coverages under the health plan. Blue Shield steps in as the major medical portion, picking up physicians' fees, medications, and other charges not covered on the basic portion of the plan. Blue Cross and Blue Shield plans usually have a large network of participating providers. In addition to the traditional Blue Cross and Blue Shield plans, they also offer several HMO-type plans that feature managed benefits and managed care options.

## Managed Care

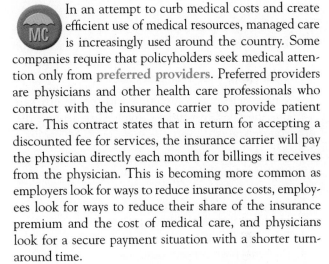 In an attempt to curb medical costs and create efficient use of medical resources, managed care is increasingly used around the country. Some companies require that policyholders seek medical attention only from **preferred providers**. Preferred providers are physicians and other health care professionals who contract with the insurance carrier to provide patient care. This contract states that in return for accepting a discounted fee for services, the insurance carrier will pay the physician directly each month for billings it receives from the physician. This is becoming more common as employers look for ways to reduce insurance costs, employees look for ways to reduce their share of the insurance premium and the cost of medical care, and physicians look for a secure payment situation with a shorter turnaround time.

**Managed care organizations (MCOs)** have multiplied with concentrations varying widely across the United States. Figure 18-3 illustrates these concentrations. The major principles of MCOs are to offer health insurance programs that ensure cost-effective services by employing case managers or PCPs to save dollars. To accomplish this, MCOs:

- Use PCPs or case managers.

- Utilize preauthorization for medical services, prospective and retrospective view of treatment plans, and significant discharge planning.

- Use specific treatment guidelines for high cost chronic disorders.

- Place emphasis on outpatient care versus hospitalization.

- Use a **drug formulary**, or list of medications that may be prescribed without preapproval.

- Place emphasis on health education and preventive care.

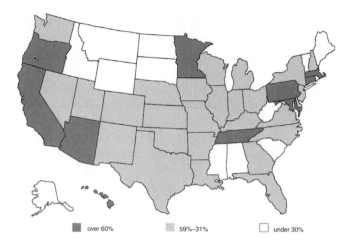

| ■ over 60% | ▨ 59%–31% | ☐ under 30% |

**Figure 18-3**    National managed care concentrations.
(Source: Rowell, 1998)

● Place emphases on patient/family collaboration with health care providers to improve patient's compliance with treatment regimen.

● Utilize selective contracting with all health care providers and institutions involved to achieve discounted rates.

Six primary MCO models operate across the country. They include:

1. Integrated delivery systems
2. Health maintenance organizations
3. Exclusive provider organizations
4. Preferred provider organizations
5. Physician-hospital organizations
6. Utilization review organizations

**Integrated delivery systems** are groups of affiliated provider sites that operate under single ownership to offer full service/specialty services to their subscribers. The affiliated providers may include physician offices/clinics, hospitals, ambulatory surgery sites, and other ancillary allied health facilities. The patient's health record may be accessed at any affiliated site through a common computerized medical record system.

Health maintenance organizations (HMOs) are another type of managed care facility. In a total departure from the philosophy of the traditional insurance, HMOs cover a large group of people for a monthly premium and a small copayment from the patient at each time of service (usually $5 or $10). Sometimes, physicians are employed by the HMO and are paid according to the number of members enrolled (**capitation**) rather than the number of visits. Two types of HMOs are available: HMOs "with walls" and HMOs "without walls." HMOs "with walls" are facilities that offer all types of services under one roof. For

example, physicians in a variety of specialty areas, x-ray and laboratory departments, physical therapy, and pharmacy facilities are all in one building. HMOs "without walls" establish a network of preferred providers. Each provider may be located in its own building and location. Ideally, members can have all their medical needs met by the HMO. Members cannot see a physician outside the HMO setting unless they pay out-of-pocket for services rendered or only in those instances when the HMO refers the patient outside the HMO, in which case the treating specialist bills the HMO for the treatment and services rendered.

See Table 18-1 for common differences between traditional and managed care policies.

An **exclusive provider organization (EPO)** often requires the provider to work exclusively for the EPO organization. Subscribers receive no benefits if they choose to receive care from a provider who is not associated with the EPO.

A network of physicians and hospitals that have contracted together with insurance companies to provide health care at a discounted fee is known as a **preferred provider organization (PPO)**. Usually, PPOs do not have contracts for laboratory or pharmacy services, but they do offer reduced-rate contracts with specific hospitals. Patients have a greater out-of-pocket fee if they choose to receive health care from a non-PPO. The advantage of a PPO is that the fee-for-service is lower than HMOs; however, the disadvantage is that the premiums, deductibles, and copayments are usually higher than an HMO.

A hospital and selected physicians may form an entrepreneurship known as a **physician-hospital organization (PHO)**. Their primary function is to contract with MCOs to provide health care to their subscribers.

| TABLE 18-1 | DIFFERENCES BETWEEN TRADITIONAL AND MANAGED CARE POLICIES |
|---|---|
| **Traditional** | **Managed Care** |
| Usually can go outside physician network | Usually must stay inside physician network |
| Coinsurance | Copay each visit |
| Annual deductible | No annual deductible |
| Illness or injury only | Preventive treatment as well as illness and injury |
| Premium paid monthly to company by employer or subscriber | Premium paid monthly to company by employer or subscriber |
| MD paid by fee for service | Physician paid by capitation |

**Utilization review organizations** are also known as third-party administrators. They supervise funds set aside to cover medical expenses to employees under self-insured plans. The utilization review organization determines medically necessary treatments, approves/denies payment of health care claims for these services, and completes a retrospective utilization review.

## Medicare

In 1965 the United States Congress created Title 18 of the Social Security Act giving all senior citizens (age 65 and above) access to health care coverage. Congress recognized that with advancing age, the likelihood of illness and the need for health care increases. Medicare was created to give continuing medical coverage to senior citizens, most of whom had retired and had only limited, if any, access to health care coverage through their former employers. Many Medicare recipients also buy supplementary insurance policies through private carriers, which are known as **Medigap policies**.

Medicare is administered by the Health Care Financing Administration (HCFA). Claims are handled locally by a **fiscal intermediary**, or insurance carrier that has signed a contract with Medicare to handle all claims for a particular area. Recently, in some areas of the country, Medicare has contracted with managed care companies to administer benefits.

When a physician agrees to accept **Medicare assignment**, **Medicare's allowable** charge is accepted as payment in full for that particular service. Medicare pays 80 percent of that amount and the patient pays the remaining 20 percent. The difference between the physician's charge and the Medicare allowable charge is adjusted or written off by the physician. The benefits to the physician are that Medicare makes a direct payment to the physician, and the fee schedule is 5 percent higher for physicians who accept assignment than for those who do not.

Medicare has two parts: **Medicare Part A** covers hospitalization, home health care, and hospice care. This part has a monetary deductible as well as a limit to the number of days per hospitalization and the number of hospitalizations per year that a person may have. Part A involves just these services, so the hospital or agency responsible bills for the services.

**Medicare Part B** covers outpatient services including physicians' fees, physical therapy and occupational therapy charges, diagnostic tests, lab tests, radiological studies, ambulance services, and charges for durable medical equipment such as walkers and wheelchairs.

Currently, an annual deductible of $100 must be paid by the patient before Medicare will begin to pay its share of the bills. The rate at which Medicare then reimburses is 80 percent of the Medicare fee schedule for medical care and 100 percent for laboratory fees, which was adopted in 1992 and is based on the **resource-based relative value scale (RBRVS)**. The RBRVS was developed using values for each medical and surgical procedure based on work, practice, and malpractice expenses and factoring for regional differences.

For instance, if a patient goes to the physician for an office visit and the fee is $75, the patient will submit the bill to Medicare through the local Medicare fiscal intermediary to apply against the deductible. At the next visit, the bill is $50. This bill will also be submitted to Medicare. Total bills submitted: $125. Ideally, Medicare will subtract the $100 deductible, apply the 80 percent coinsurance to the amount in excess of the deductible, or $25, and pay $20. The patient would be responsible for the difference (20 percent coinsurance) or $5, plus the $100 deductible.

| **Example:** | |
|---|---|
| Office visit | $ 75.00 |
| Return visit | + 50.00 |
| **Total Charges** | $125.00 |
| Less deductible | −100.00 |
| Subtotal | $ 25.00 |
| Apply 80% coinsurance | × 80% |
| **Insurance Payment** | $ 20.00 |
| **Patient Owes** | $ 5.00 |

The example shows how the worksheet would look if there were no exclusions or deductions. Medicare, however, as well as many other insurance companies, uses a fee schedule based upon **usual, customary, and reasonable (UCR)** fees. *Usual* refers to the fee that the specific physician charges most of his patients for the same treatment. *Reasonable* refers to the midrange of fees charged for this type of procedure or visit. *Customary* is based on the average charge for a specific procedure by all the physicians practicing the same specialty in a specific geographical location. Also see Chapter 17 for a discussion of fees.

Based on the Medicare fee schedule, Medicare might decide it will only consider $70 of the first bill and $45 of the second bill or a total of $115. From this amount Medicare subtracts $100 (the deductible), which leaves an amount of $15 on which to base payment. Now the 80 percent coinsurance is applied resulting in a payment of $12. The patient is left owing one of the following amounts in addition to the $100 deductible: $3 if the physician accepts Medicare assignment or $13 if the doctor does not accept assignment ($3 plus the $10 disallowed by Medicare).

| Example: | Total Charges | Allowed Charges |
|---|---|---|
| Office visit | $ 75.00 | $ 70.00 |
| Return visit | + 50.00 | 45.00 |
| **Total Charges** | $125.00 | $115.00 |
| Less deductible | −100.00 | −100.00 |
| Subtotal | $ 25.00 | $ 15.00 |
| Apply 80% coinsurance | × 80% | × 80% |
| **Insurance Payment** | $ 20.00 | $ 12.00 |
| **Patient Owes** | $ 5.00 | $ 3.00* |

*(or $13.00 if physician does not accept assignment)

## Other Types of Coverage

In addition to the coverages described, there are other insurance coverages for persons unable to work due to illness or life circumstances (Medicaid), for dependents of persons serving in the Armed Forces (CHAMPUS and CHAMPVA), and for workers who are injured on the job (Workers' Compensation or State Industrial Insurance).

**Medicaid.** Medicaid was created in 1965 by Congress under Title 19 of the Social Security Act to provide funding for medical care for qualifying persons. It is federally funded but administered through each state's department of human services. People who are on Aid for Families with Dependent Children and Supplemental Security Income (SSI), single women who are pregnant and whose income is at or below the national poverty level, and people who for many reasons due to physical, emotional, or mental difficulties are unable to work may qualify for this program. The recipient is given an identification card which is presented to the medical provider at the time of the office visit. A claim form is then completed and the identification card or a copy of the card is attached to the form and mailed to the administrator's address. Some states have a requirement for a copayment by the recipient at the time of service but collection cannot be enforced.

Many medical practices accept Medicaid but when referring a patient to a specialist or another provider, it is wise to ascertain whether that provider accepts Medicaid patients. A referral form usually must be completed by the primary care or referring physician prior to the visit with the specialist.

Billings to Medicaid are considered only after all other insurance payments have been made. When a person has both Medicare and Medicaid, charges are submitted first to Medicare and last to Medicaid. Both are federal programs and errors in billing could be construed as fraud, for which there are criminal penalties. It is therefore imperative that all billing practices conform to the legal requirements of these programs.

**CHAMPUS and CHAMPVA.** Military personnel are covered by the medical personnel in the Armed Services. However, their dependents (spouse and children) often are not able to receive medical care on the base, or in many cases they live outside the catchment area of a 40-mile radius of the assigned base. When these dependents need medical care and no military medical care is easily available to them or they need emergency medical care, they may seek medical care from nonmilitary medical providers without prior authorization. CHAMPUS, the Civilian Health and Medical Program for Uniformed Services, covers the dependents of active duty personnel, retired personnel, dependents of retired personnel, and dependents of personnel who died while on active duty.

CHAMPVA, the Civilian Health and Medical Program of the Veteran's Administration, covers the spouse and unmarried dependent children of a veteran with permanent total disability from a service-related injury and the surviving spouse and children of veterans who died of a service-related disability.

As in all the previous insurance plans, each person covered by CHAMPUS or CHAMPVA will have an identification card showing name, identification number, and program covered. A person cannot be covered by both CHAMPUS and CHAMPVA.

CHAMPUS and CHAMPVA are billed after all other insurance coverages except Medicaid. Preauthorization is required for patients living within a catchment area for treatment. Patients living outside the catchment area do not need preauthorization. Preauthorization is obtained using a nonavailability statement. This form is completed and submitted to the local CHAMPUS office. If treatment is rendered and payment is denied, an appeal process is available to the patient and physician.

**Workers' Compensation or State Industrial Insurance.** When an on-the-job accident or illness results in injury and/or disability, workers' compensation insurance pays the medical bills and a significant portion of the lost wages if the patient was covered by a workers' compensation policy.

In most states, the employer pays a premium to an insurance carrier for a policy known as Workers' Compensation insurance. This premium is rated upon the number of workers employed and the degree of risk a job entails. A few states provide coverage through a statewide fund, often called State Industrial insurance, which is funded by premiums paid to the state by employers. Again, the premiums are based upon the number of employees and the job risk.

When a claim is made, a workers' compensation claim form is completed and sent to the insurance carrier or to the state fund for reimbursement (Figure 18-4). The injured worker receives no bills, pays no deductible or coinsurance, and is covered 100 percent for medical expenses related specifically to that injury.

**Self-Insurance.** Many larger companies, nonprofit organizations, and state and county governments choose to self-insure in an attempt to reduce the costs of medical insurance and to gain more control over their finances. In self-insured plans, special accounts are established and, rather than paying premiums to an insurance carrier, the entity makes payments into the plan. Each self-insured plan will differ in its organization and claim filing requirements; if a patient is covered by a self-insured plan, call the plan administrator before scheduling a patient appointment.

## PROSPECTIVE PAYMENT SYSTEMS AND DIAGNOSIS-RELATED GROUPS

In an effort to control the costs of hospital care for Medicare patients, in 1983 the Health Care Financing Administration (HCFA) adopted a plan called **diagnosis-related groups (DRGs)**. DRGs, a concept that originated at Yale University, is a method of **prospective payment** in which hospitals are paid a flat fee for Medicare patients. The fee is based on an *average* cost of service, not the *actual* cost of service for a particular patient. With the DRG plan, patients are classified into categories based on principal diagnosis, principal procedure, and discharge status. All patients in the same DRG are predicted to respond in a clinically similar way.

While the DRG system of pricing is typically applied in a hospital setting, the medical assistant in the ambulatory care setting will benefit from an awareness of how this system works. The forty-seven DRG categories are derived from the *International Classification of Diseases, 9th Revision, Clinical Modification* (ICD-9-CM), which contains all standard **diagnosis codes** used to encode a claim form. If responsible for filing any Medicare claim based on the DRG, the medical assistant should note that, like all claim filing, accuracy is essential

and assignment of the correct DRGs helps to ensure maximum financial reimbursement in the processing of medical insurance claims.

## LEGAL AND ETHICAL ISSUES

It is critical that the medical assistant be well versed on various insurance plans carried by patients. Explanations regarding insurance submission policies and patient financial responsibilities are often part of the day's work. It is essential that signatures to authorize insurance billing and supply information to insurance carriers be secured. Without the signature, release of information is illegal.

Many Medicare claims are now submitted electronically and private payers in growing numbers are also using electronic claims submission. In a computerized system, everything related to billing and reimbursement is computerized and transmitted electronically. If the office is participating in HCFA's Electronic Data Interchange (EDI), they will be assigned a unique identifier number that constitutes their legal electronic signature. Be cautious with this electronic signature as the office is responsible for any and all claims made with it. The Health Insurance Portability and Accountability Act of 1996 (specifically title II, subtitle F) regulates the security and privacy of transmitted health care information.

EVERY QUESTION MUST BE ANSWERED AND FORM SIGNED

**INSTRUCTIONS**

1. Type answers to All questions and file original with the Workers' Compensation Commission within 72 hours after first treatment.
2. DO NOT FAIL to forward to the Workers' Compensation Commission PROGRESS REPORTS and FINAL REPORT upon discharge of patient.

| | DO NOT WRITE IN THIS SPACE |
|---|---|

# WORKERS' COMPENSATION COMMISSION
### 6 NORTH LIBERTY STREET, BALTIMORE, MD. 21201-3785
### SURGEON'S REPORT

WCC CLAIM #

EMPLOYER'S REPORT Yes ☐ No ☐

This is First Report ☐  Progress Report ☐  Final Report ☐

| 1. Name of Injured Person: Maureen A. Santega | Soc. Sec. No. 610-98-7432 | D.O.B. 7/19/69 | Sex M ☐  F ☒ |
|---|---|---|---|

2. Address: (No. and Street) 905 Raymond Lane  (City or Town) Atlanta  (State) GA  (Zip Code) 30385-8893

3. Name and Address of Employer: Majors Concrete Company, 238 Leaf Lane, Atlanta, GA  30342-3329

| 4. Date of Accident or Onset of Disease: 4/9/__ | Hour: A.M. ☒ P.M. ☐ | 5. Date Disability Began: 4/9/__ |
|---|---|---|

6. Patient's Description of Accident or Cause of Disease:
Concrete truck struck and backed over patient's foot while she was pouring concrete at the job site.

7. Medical description of Injury or Disease:
massive bruising to left foot, no broken bones, great deal of pain associated with bruises

8. Will Injury result in:
(a) Permanent defect? Yes ☐ No ☒  If so, what?  (b) Disfigurement Yes ☐ No ☒

9. Causes, other than injury, contributing to patients condition:
None

10. Is patient suffering from any disease of the heart, lungs, brain, kidneys, blood, vascular system or any other disabling condition not due to this accident?
Give particulars: No

11. Is there any history or evidence present of previous accident or disease? Give particulars:
No

12. Has normal recovery been delayed for any reason? Give particulars:
No

| 13. Date of first treatment: 4/10/__ | Who engaged your services? patient |
|---|---|

14. Describe treatment given by you:
Darvon, 100 mg q4h prn for pain

| 15. Were X-Rays taken? Yes ☐ No ☒ | By whom? — (Name and Address) | Date 4/10/__ |
|---|---|---|

16. X-Ray Diagnosis:

| 17. Was patient treated by anyone else? Yes ☐ No ☒ | By whom? — (Name and Address) | Date |
|---|---|---|

| 18. Was patient hospitalized? Yes ☐ No ☒ | Name and Address of Hospital | Date of Admission: <br> Date of Discharge: |
|---|---|---|

| 19. Is further treatment needed? Yes ☐ No ☒ | For how long? | 20. Patient was ☒ will be ☐ able to resume regular work on: <br> Patient was ☐ will be ☐ able to resume light work on: | 4/14 |
|---|---|---|---|

21. If death ensued give date:  22. Remarks: (Give any information of value not included above)

| 23. I am a qualified specialist in: orthopedics | I am a duly licensed Physician in the State of: Georgia | I was graduated from Medical School (Name) Emory | Year 1967 |
|---|---|---|---|

Date of this report: 6/21/__   (Signed)  *John N. Sparks, M.D.*

(This report must be signed PERSONALLY by Physician)

Address: 8504 Capricorn Drive, Atlanta GA 30312   Phone: (404)544-0078

**Figure 18-4**  Sample workers' compensation claim form.

## DOCUMENTATION

Documentation must support all claims submitted. Failure to document a service translates into nonperformance of that service, from the perspectives of quality patient care, legal safeguards, and reimbursement issues. In other words, a deed not documented is a deed not done.

**CASE STUDY 18-1**

Jane O'Hara, CMA, is responsible for all patient insurance billing procedures. Jane has the following information:

|  | Total Charges | Allowed Charges |
|---|---|---|
| Office visit | $85.00 | $80.00 |
| Return visit | $65.00 | $55.00 |

Deductible has not been satisfied.

### CASE STUDY REVIEW

1. Calculate the correct billing if the physician accepts assignment.
2. Calculate the correct billing if the physician does not accept assignment.

## SUMMARY

An understanding of medical insurance terminology and various types of coverage is vital to a thriving ambulatory care setting. The astute medical assistant will perceive the challenges involved in understanding the role in the management of medical office insurance. The medical assistant must be able to explain insurance procedures to the patient and know how to make contact with appropriate representatives to determine eligibility and coverage questions.

## REVIEW QUESTIONS

### Multiple Choice

1. The most common avenue to ensure that services will be reimbursed is:
   a. not see any patient that does not have proof of Medicaid coverage
   b. complete an envoy
   c. go on-line and print a proof of eligibility directly from the system
   d. ask the patient if they are covered
2. The most common insurance claim form is the:
   a. UB92 form
   b. ICD-9-CM
   c. HCFA-1500 form
   d. CPT
3. Medicare:
   a. was created by Title 19 of the Social Security Act
   b. was created in 1965
   c. is designed to cover prescriptions
   d. is handled separately by each state

4. If the charge is $150 and the deductible has not been met, Medicare will pay:
   a. $20
   b. $40
   c. $120
   d. 80 percent of UCR after $100 deductible
5. There are _____ primary MCO models operating across the country.
   a. four
   b. three
   c. six
   d. eight
6. EPOs:
   a. often require the provider to work exclusively for that organization
   b. are groups of affiliated provider sites that operate under single ownership
   c. are paid according to capitation
   d. are also known as third-party administrators

7. Medicaid:
   a. was created by Title 19 of the Social Security Act
   b. is designed to cover prescriptions
   c. is handled separately be each state
   d. accommodates only military personnel
8. CHAMPUS:
   a. is a type of HMO
   b. is a type of EPO
   c. is a civilian health and medical program of the Veteran's Administration
   d. stands for Civilian Health and Medical Program for Uniformed Services

## Critical Thinking

1. What is the difference between basic insurance and major medical insurance?
2. What is the difference between copayment and coinsurance?
3. Explain the birthday rule and when it is used.
4. What are four insurance considerations to keep in mind when treating a patient?
5. Compare the traditional approach of insurance companies to HMOs.
6. Dr. Lewis accepts Medicare assignment. What does this mean to Dr. Lewis? What does this mean to Abigail Johnson, one of Dr. Lewis' Medicare patients?
7. If a patient lives six miles from an Army hospital, will a preauthorization for treatment be needed by a specialist in the nearby city? Why or why not?

## WEB ACTIVITIES

Use the Internet to locate the Intermediary-Carrier Directory for Medicare. Determine the Medicare Part A intermediaries and the Medicare Part B carriers for the state or region in which you live. Follow instructor guidelines to submit your findings.

## REFERENCES/BIBLIOGRAPHY

HCFA. (2000). *Medicare Part B basic billing manual.* Noridian Mutual Insurance.

Humphrey, D. D. (1996). *Contemporary medical office procedures* (2nd ed.). Albany, NY: Delmar.

Keir, L., Wise, B. A., & Krebs, C. (1993). *Medical assisting: Administrative and clinical competencies* (3rd ed.). Albany, NY: Delmar.

Kinn, M. E., & Woods, M. A. (1999). *The medical assistant: Administrative and clinical* (8th ed.). Philadelphia: W. B. Saunders Company.

Rowell, J. C. (1998). *Understanding medical insurance* (4th ed.). Albany, NY: Delmar.

Spock, M. (2000). *The coding answer book.* Rockville, MD: Physician Practice Coder.

# 19

# MEDICAL INSURANCE CODING

## KEY TERMS

Breach of Confidentiality
Charge Slip
Claim
Claim Register
Current Procedural Terminology (CPT)
Diagnosis Codes
E Codes
Explanation of Benefits (EOB)
Fraud
HCFA-1500 (12-90)
HCFA Common Procedure Coding System (HCPCS)
Insurance Abuse
International Classification of Diseases, 9th Revision, Clinical Modification (ICD-9-CM)
Point-of-Service (POS) Device
Procedure Codes
Subrogation
Superbill
Uniform Bill (UB92)
V Codes

## OUTLINE

**Insurance Coding Systems**
Procedure Coding
Diagnosis Coding
**Coding the Claim Form**
Completing the HCFA-1500 (12-90)
**Overseeing the Claims Process**
Point-of-Service Device
Maintaining Claim Register or Diary

The Insurance Carrier's Role
Explanation of Benefits
Following Up on Claims
**The Computerized Claims Process**
**Legal and Ethical Issues**

## OBJECTIVES

*The student should strive to meet the following performance objectives and demonstrate an understanding of the facts and principles presented in this chapter through written and oral communication.*

1. Understand the process of procedure and diagnosis coding.
2. Code a sample claim form.
3. Explain the difference between the HCFA-1500 and the UB92 forms.
4. Describe the way computers have altered the claims process.
5. Discuss why claims follow-up is important to the ambulatory care setting.
6. Discuss legal and ethical issues related to coding and insurance claims processing.

**Administrative Procedures**

- Understand and apply third-party guidelines
- Obtain reimbursement through accurate claims submission
- Monitor third-party reimbursement
- Understand and adhere to managed care policies and procedures

**Practice Finances**

- Perform procedural and diagnostic coding

### GENERAL (TRANSDISCIPLINARY)

**Professional**

- Project a professional manner and image

**Communication Skills**

- Treat all patients with compassion and empathy
- Recognize and respect cultural diversity
- Use effective and correct verbal and written communication
- Use medical terminology appropriately
- Receive, organize, prioritize, and transmit information
- Serve as liaison

**Legal Concepts**

- Maintain confidentiality
- Document accurately
- Use appropriate guidelines when releasing information

*(continues)*

## SCENARIO

At Inner City Health Care, a multi-doctor urgent care center in a large city, medical assistant Jane O'Hara, CMA, is responsible for all patient billing procedures. While she delegates much of the responsibility for encoding claim forms to her two assistants, Jane oversees the process. Jane and the assistants must be acquainted with the requirements of each patient's insurance coverage and help patients understand their responsibility—if any—for payment. Finally, Jane holds periodic meetings with her assistants to update them; she continually stresses to them the importance of timeliness in filing claims and the need for absolute accuracy in diagnosis and procedure coding which must always reflect services actually performed and documented within the patient's chart.

## INTRODUCTION

Coding is the basis for the information on the claim form. Medical coding is mandatory for the accurate transmission of procedures and diagnosis information between health care providers and various agencies that compile health care statistics and the insurance companies that act as third-party payers for health care services rendered to patients. In order to code accurately, the medical assistant must have a good understanding of medical terminology, especially of those medical specialties found in the ambulatory care setting.

The issue of who owns the medical record, health care provider or patient, has been debated for decades. Generally, it is considered that the health care provider is responsible for maintaining and preserving the patient record, but the patient has a right to access and copy the information contained within the record upon appropriate request. It is extremely important to maintain confidentiality when dealing with physician/patient privilege. Before releasing any information to a third party, a medical release must be obtained from the patient.

## INSURANCE CODING SYSTEMS

The process of converting descriptions of diseases, injuries, and procedures into numerical designations is termed coding. **Current Procedural Terminology (CPT)** was developed by the American Medical Association (AMA) to convert commonly accepted, uniform descriptions of medical, surgical, and diagnostic services rendered by health care providers into five-digit numeric codes. The **International Classification of Diseases, 9th Revision, Clinical Modification (ICD-9-CM)** was compiled by the World Health Organization (WHO). It is designed for the classification of patient morbidity (sickness) and mortality (death) information for statistical purposes and for the indexing of hospital records by disease and operation for data storage and retrieval. Medical assistants employed in ambulatory care facilities will use procedure codes and diagnosis codes on a regular basis.

### Procedure Coding

**Procedure codes** for procedures done and for visits of all kinds—office, hospital, nursing facility, home services—is found in *Current Procedural Terminology* (CPT). This volume is updated annually and is divided into seven sections:

## ROLE DELINEATION COMPONENTS (*continued*)

**Coordinate and oversee compliance with federal, state, managed care, and regulatory agencies**

- Medicare/Medicaid (advanced)
- Third-party payers (advanced)
- Managed care (advanced)

1. Evaluation and Management
2. Anesthesia
3. Surgery
4. Radiology, Nuclear Medicine, and Diagnostic Ultrasound
5. Pathology and Laboratory
6. Medicine
7. Index

**Evaluation and Management Section.** The Evaluation and Management section takes every possible combination of visits into consideration and assigns each its own number. For instance, Mary O'Keefe, a new patient, is seen for a period of 45 minutes during which the physician takes a detailed history, examines the patient, and makes a medical decision of moderate complexity. The CPT code for this visit (99204) is found by looking under office services, new patient, time and service provided. In another instance, Abigail Johnson, an established patient, is seen in the hospital for several days. These visits (99231, 99232, or 99233) would be found under hospital services, subsequent hospital care, and the time and service provided. Codes for any type of evaluation and/or management are found in this section. In many offices the physician will determine the level or charge for visits; however, the medical assistant must be very familiar with all of the codes to make certain that billings are correct and that codes match the physician's documentation.

**Anesthesia Section.** The Anesthesia section includes all codes for anesthesia required for any procedure. The codes begin with the head and continue down the body to the legs and feet, concluding with anesthesia for radiological procedures. If you want to find the correct code for anesthesia during a total hip replacement, you will find "Anesthesia" in the index, look for "hip" and refer to the codes listed: 01200–01214. When you refer back to the Anesthesia section, you find:

| | |
|---|---|
| 01200 | Anesthesia for all closed procedures involving hip joint |
| 01202 | Anesthesia for arthroscopic procedures of hip joint |
| 01210 | Anesthesia for open procedures involving hip joint; not otherwise specified |
| 01212 | hip disarticulation |
| 01214 | total hip replacement or revision |

As you read through the codes, you see that the correct code is 01214.

**Surgery Section.** The section on Surgery divides codes according to system. It begins with the skin, subcutaneous and areolar tissues, and continues through subsequent systems ending with ocular and auditory systems. The codes are very specific. For instance, a simple laceration repair is found as:

| | |
|---|---|
| 12001* | Simple repair of superficial wounds of scalp, neck, axillae, external genitalia, trunk and/or extremities (including hands and feet): 2.5 cm or less |
| 12002* | 2.6 cm to 7.5 cm |
| 12004* | 7.6 cm to 12.5 cm |
| 12005 | 12.6 cm to 20.0 cm |
| 12006 | 20.1 cm to 30.0 cm |
| 12007 | over 30.0 cm |

Thus, the exact length of the laceration and complexity of repair can be found and coded correctly on the claim form. The * signifies a surgical procedure for which a charge is made that does not include pre- or post-operative visits.

**Radiology, Nuclear Medicine, and Diagnostic Ultrasound Section.** Coding in the Radiology section covers each procedure done and each specific alteration to the procedure. For instance,

| | |
|---|---|
| 75889 | Hepatic venography, wedged or free, with hemodynamic evaluation, radiological supervision, and interpretation |
| 75891 | Hepatic venography, wedged or free, without hemodynamic evaluation, radiological supervision, and interpretation |

Radiological procedures are not often done in the physician's office, although they may be in larger urgent care centers. Occasionally chest X rays are done or, in an orthopedic specialty, many skeletal X rays may be done. More often, though, radiological studies are ordered by the physician through a local facility which bills the insurance company directly, using the diagnosis the physician has provided.

**Pathology and Laboratory Section.** The Pathology and Laboratory section includes every test and combination of laboratory tests that can be ordered as well as a section on surgical pathology. This latter section includes specimens sent for examination, such as Pap smears, analysis of biopsy tissue from surgical sites, and tissue typing. Following is an example of a laboratory procedure code for hepatitis B and illustrates the complete selection of tests that may be ordered:

| | |
|---|---|
| 87340 | Hepatitis B surface antigen (HBsAg) |
| 86704 | Hepatitis B core antibody (HBcAb); IgG and IgM |
| 86705 | IgM antibody |
| 86706 | Hepatitis B surface antibody (HBsAb) |
| 87350 | Hepatitis Be antigen (HBeAg) |
| 86707 | Hepatitis Be antibody (HBeAb) |

The medical assistant should be aware of laboratory codes because when a lab test is ordered, the lab may call to clarify the order. If the coding is correct, the lab should have no questions.

For surgical pathology, the codes are different. The level of examination for the item determines the code. The physician usually determines these levels or the charge for these services.

**Medicine Section.** The section of the CPT entitled Medicine includes codings for immunizations, injections, dialysis, allergen immunotherapy, and chemotherapy, as well as ophthalmologic, cardiovascular, pulmonary, and neurological procedures, to name a few. As in the earlier sections, there is a comprehensive breakdown of each procedure. Under Cardiography, for example:

| | |
|---|---|
| 93000 | Electrocardiogram, routine ECG with at least 12 leads; with interpretation and report |
| 93005 | tracing only, without interpretation and report |
| 93010 | interpretation and report only |

Under Chemotherapy Administration:

| | |
|---|---|
| 96408 | Chemotherapy administration, intravenous, push technique |
| 96410 | infusion technique, up to one hour |
| 96412+ | infusion technique, one to 8 hours, each additional hour |
| 96414 | infusion technique, initiation of prolonged infusion (more than 8 hours), requiring the use of a portable or implantable pump |

The plus symbol indicates that the procedure is an add-on to a previously described procedure. For example, 96410 would be used to describe the service and the time administered up to one hour. Anything over one hour would use the add-on code of 96412 for each additional hour administration took place.

**Index.** The final portion of the CPT is a comprehensive index listing every procedure alphabetically. The proper use of the CPT involves looking for the procedure in the index and then checking the number given to determine the precise code.

Each code found in the CPT has five numerical digits. Note that there are no letter codes and no decimal points in these codes. Each five-digit code stands for a specific procedure not duplicated elsewhere.

**Modifiers.** Occasionally a service or procedure needs to be modified. In that case, there are two-digit numerical modifiers that can be applied to the five-digit code. These modifiers can indicate unusual procedural services (-22), bilateral procedure (-50), multiple procedures (-51), two surgeons (-62), surgical team (-66), or repeat procedure by same physician (-76). When any of these or other modifiers are used and a full five-digit code for the modifier is desired, use 099 before the modifier code. Thus, they become 09922, 09950, 09962, and so on. The modifiers are delineated in the front of each section of the CPT to alert the coder to modifiers available for that section.

If more than one modifier is needed for a procedure, use (-99) before any other modifier. Thus, if a procedure required a modifier of -22 and -51, code -99 before the other modifiers. For instance, "33411 Replacement, aortic valve; with aortic annulus enlargement, noncoronary cusp," becomes 33411-99. This can also be written 33411 and 09999 indicating multiple modifiers.

**HCFA Common Procedure Coding System (HCPCS).** Medicare uses a supplement to the CPT codes. Level I of the HCPCS is the regular CPT system.

Level II is a coding system that uses a five-digit alphanumeric code to clarify procedures. The code begins with a letter from A to V followed by four numbers. An example might be A4550 Surgical trays, A4615 Nasal Cannula, or E0609 Blood Glucose Monitor with special features (voice synthesizers, automatic timers, and so on). Injections are listed under J codes. All of these codes can have an additional two-digit letter modifier. These modifiers can be simply LT for left, RT for right, or even CC to indicate a code change when resubmitting a claim that was previously denied by Medicare. The Level II codes were developed by Medicare for all procedures performed in the medical office in place of CPT codes which may not be specific. For instance, to bill a cyanocobalamin or Vitamin B$_{12}$ injection, the CPT code for an intramuscular injection is used (90782), but a Level II code for the medication (J3420) is also required.

Level III codes are similar to Level II but are assigned by the fiscal intermediary rather than the national administration. These codes use the letter codes W, X, Y, and Z.

## Diagnosis Coding

In addition to coding for procedures, a code is required for each diagnosis. Diagnosis codes are found in the current International Classification of Diseases, 9th Revision, Clinical Modification or ICD-9-CM, also referred to as ICD-9 or simply ICD. It is expected that in the future there will be a new way of coding diagnoses, known as ICD-10. This will be an alphanumeric code and will take the place of the current ICD-9 system. This is a collection of codes published by the World Health Organization for every disease, illness, condition, injury, and cause of injury known. The codes are found in three volumes, the first two of which depend upon each other for diagnosis coding.

Volumes I and II are used for coding diagnoses in ambulatory care centers and outpatient departments of hospitals; Volume III is used for inpatient procedures. The ICD-9-CM is usually now available in separate versions: one for physician offices and one for hospitals. The physician version has Volume I and II combined into one book, and the hospital version has all three volumes combined in one book.

Volume I, Tabular List, contains all the codes in numerical order. This volume is the second place that is referred to when coding a diagnosis.

Volume II, Alphabetic Index, contains all possible diagnoses, including symptoms, accidents and their causes, and concurrent diagnoses. This volume also contains a table of drugs and chemicals and a list of external causes for injuries. This volume is the first place that is referred to when coding a diagnosis.

Volume III, Procedures: Tabular List and Alphabetic Index, includes procedures used. The procedure codes of the CPT are more commonly used in the United States and are accepted by all the insurance companies. If you are unable to find a correct procedure code in the CPT, Volume III of the ICD-9-CM does contain helpful information. Often there is enough information in this volume to help identify a procedure in the CPT.

In the codes, initials such as NEC and NOS will be encountered. NEC means "not elsewhere classified" and is used only if there is not enough information to find a more specific code. NOS refers to "not otherwise specified." If a more specific diagnosis can be found, do not use a diagnosis with either of these references.

ICD-9-CM codes have a three-digit base with modifiers to that base added *after a decimal point*. For instance,

the code for cellulitis is 682. When looking back to Volume I, the code for 682 is broken down according to various areas of the body. Cellulitis of the leg is 682.6 and includes ankle, hip, knee, and thigh. Cellulitis of the foot is 682.7. Another example is pyelonephritis. Chronic pyelonephritis is 590.0 and acute pyelonephritis is 590.1.

The fifth digit defines the diagnosis even more specifically. In the preceding example, under 590.0 there are two choices: 590.00 without lesion of renal medullary necrosis, or 590.01 with lesion of renal medullary necrosis. If that specific information is known, code the fifth digit.

The fifth digit may also define a location more specifically. As in the example for cellulitis where the fourth digit identified a location, the fifth digit can also define a location. The diagnosis osteomyelitis is found in Volume II as

> Osteomyelitis (general) (infective) (localized) (neonatal) (purulent) (pyogenic) (septic) (staphylococcal) (streptococcal) (suppurative) (with periostitis) 730.2

When found in Volume I, 730.2 reads:

> Unspecified osteomyelitis, osteitis or osteomyelitis NOS, with or without mention of periostitis

There is also noted a requirement of a fifth digit to indicate the location of the disease. Thus, 730.27 is Unspecified osteomyelitis of the ankle or foot.

Some diagnosis codes cannot stand alone. For instance, in Volume II we find "Tuberculosis, kidney" as 016.0 [*590.81*]. These two codes when checked in Volume I read:

> 016.0 Tuberculosis of kidney
> Renal tuberculosis
> (Use additional code to identify manifestation, as:
> tuberculous: nephropathy (583.81)
> pyelitis (590.81)
> pyelonephritis (590.81).)

Looking up 590.81 we find:

> *Pyelitis or pyelonephritis in diseases classified elsewhere*
> *Code first underlying disease as:* tuberculosis (016.0).

The italics refer to manifestation codes and these must be shown after the underlying disease code. Thus, both codes 016.1 and 590.81 must be used when completing the claim form for this diagnosis.

Injury codes also cannot stand alone. If a patient comes in for treatment of a fractured arm, the first code to be found will be the diagnosis of the injury: 812.21 fracture of the humerus shaft. Upon referring to Volume I, 812.21 states this is a fracture of the shaft of humerus, closed. Since fractures are not usually a disease but rather the result of an injury, the cause of the injury must be coded as well. Again, refer to the back of Volume II under the appendix for E codes—Index to External Causes. For this exercise, Jaime Carrera fell from a ladder. Under "Fall, Ladder" the code E881.0 is given. Checking that code in Volume I, E881.0 states Fall from ladder. (E881.1 is fall from scaffold.) It is apparent that diagnosis codes are precise.

It is important to document all information related to an injury. Insurance carriers will often deny an injury claim until they have received information that there is no other insurance available to pay the medical charges. Often auto insurance, homeowner liability insurance, or workers' compensation insurance will pay the entire cost of treatment. These policies are primary and the medical insurance policies pay *after* the primary coverage is exhausted. In these situations, make sure the correct insurance company is billed first for the physician's services. If the medical insurance company pays the bill and later discovers there is accident coverage available, the medical insurance company will bring a claim against the accident policy to seek reimbursement of the monies it has paid out. This is called subrogation.

**Supplementary Health Factors.** V Codes are the last main section of Volumes I (numeric) and II (alphabetic). This section contains "Supplementary Classification of Factors Influencing Health Status and Contact with Health Services." These codes reflect exposure to diseases, such as "V01.1 Exposure to tuberculosis." They also reflect potential health hazards to the patient, such as "V16.1 Family history of malignant neoplasm in lung."

Well-child examinations, routine pregnancy examinations and delivery, screening for diseases, or conditions such as "V78.0 Iron deficiency anemia" are also found in this section. Again, just because the code is found in Volume II does not mean coding is complete. It must be checked in Volume I to make certain the code is accurate.

If the diagnosis is Weight gain, Volume II shows: "Weight gain (abnormal) (excessive) 783.1." When 783.1 is checked in Volume I, it reads:

Abnormal weight gain
*Excludes:* excessive weight gain in pregnancy (646.1)
        obesity (278.0).

When 278.0 is checked, it states

Obesity
*Excludes:* adiposogenital dystrophy (253.8)
obesity of endocrine origin NOS (259.9).

At this point, the patient's chart must be checked to determine whether the correct code is 278.0, 259.9, or 783.1.

**Coding Accuracy.** The more accurate the coding on the claim form, the less chance there is for error, the more quickly the physician is reimbursed, and the better chance that the physician's reimbursement will reflect the actual charge. Many insurance carriers keep a fee profile of each physician's charges. This profile reflects the amount of each charge for each service and can affect the physician's reimbursement for those services.

If an error is made in the coding, the insurance carrier will always downcode. That is, insurance will pay the lesser of the two amounts in question. For instance, Dr. Woo spent 45 minutes with an established patient for a complex medical problem, but instead of billing 99215, the medical assistant billed 99213 which reflects a time of 15 minutes and a problem of low complexity. Even though the diagnosis indicates a complex group of problems, the insurance company will pay according to the physician's fee profile for a 15-minute visit.

Do not guess when coding. The coding that is used becomes a permanent part of the patient's medical record with the insurance carrier. If an incorrect code is used, that coded diagnosis will stay with that patient. This can be a very difficult problem for insureds if they change insurance carriers or if other health problems occur.

Consider a patient with hip pain. She has a history of ovarian cancer for which she has had radiology treatments. The hip pain is thought to be possible metastases from the original cancer site. When ruling out this possibility, the physician indicates the following code for the claim form:

198.89  Secondary malignant neoplasm of other
        specified sites: hip.

When the pain is finally discovered to be arthritis and it is determined that the patient needs a hip replacement, the insurance carrier denies coverage for this operation. Reason: the patient's condition is terminal and the company does not want her to spend her last months having surgery and recovering from surgery when she is already in poor health. And, of course, there is the cost factor to consider in the eyes of the insurance carrier.

Incorrect coding can be a problem with ruling out a diagnosis. For instance, a patient presents many symptoms of peptic ulcer disease. Do not immediately code that patient as having that disease until the diagnosis is confirmed. Instead, code the symptoms. When the tests come back and a specific diagnosis of peptic ulcer can be made, then code the disease as

533.70 chronic  without mention of hemorrhage or
                perforation without mention of
                obstruction.

When coding:

● Be as precise as possible
● Do not guess
● Do not code what is not there

## CODING THE CLAIM FORM

In order for the insurance company to understand what is being billed, the claim form is completed by the medical assistant or billing clerk in the ambulatory care setting. The physician completes a charge slip at the time of the visit. This **charge slip** (see Figure 19-1), also known as an encounter form, includes the date of service, the visit or consult code, diagnoses for this visit, procedures done and lab tests ordered, and, if necessary, the date the patient is to return. This information is then translated onto the claim form. In some physician offices, charge slips are referred to as **superbills**.

The **HCFA-1500** is the claim form accepted by most insurance carriers. This form is prepared using words and CPT codes for procedures performed and ICD-9-CM codes for diagnoses. Keep in mind that the codes must correlate; for instance, if a person had an ICD-9-CM diagnosis code of earache, otitis media, or 382.9, and the CPT procedure code indicated was 69090, ear piercing, the insurance company would question the claim and reject it for payment. The person completing the claim form must be *as precise as possible*. If the coding is wrong, the claim will be denied and the physician will not receive pay-

ment. Coding must correlate with the physician's note in the chart; otherwise, fraud is committed.

Coding the claim form is a precise way to communicate with the insurance carrier. Coding indicates the complexity of the visit, the diagnosis for the visit, and the specific procedures performed during the visit. This results in very little confusion, and a minimum of communication is needed between the carrier and the physician's office because all information is contained in the codes.

For instance: Leo McKay, a regular patient, is seen for an extended visit to determine the cause of his abdominal pain. Symptoms include diarrhea, fever, nausea, and anorexia. An abdominal ultrasound is ordered as well as lab tests, and the results are unknown at the time of the insurance billing. The visit lasts 30 minutes and includes a full physical examination and a history of the present illness.

The CPT procedure coding for this visit is 99214, which reflects the examination and time spent with the patient, the history taken of this illness, and a medical decision of moderate complexity.

The ICD-9-CM diagnosis coding for abdominal pain is 789.0, for diarrhea 787.91, for nausea 787.02, and for anorexia 783.0. The claim form is submitted to the insurance carrier with these codes, and even though they are all symptoms, the claim will be paid because the visit and the tests ordered interrelate.

When the test results are known, they show a positive diagnosis of Giardia lamblia. The diagnosis code is changed to 007.1. Any further charges sent to the insurance carrier while Leo McKay is being treated for this problem are coded 007.1. The symptom codes from the first submission are dropped.

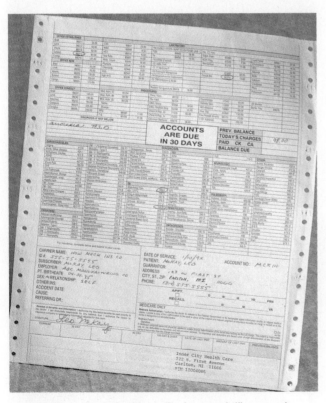

**Figure 19-1** Sample charge slip (or superbill), currently known as an encounter form. The physician marks the procedures performed (CPT codes) and the diagnosis (ICD-9-CM codes). There are a variety of charge slip formats available. Note this sample charge slip is different than the charge slips shown in Chapters 17 and 20.

## COMPLETING THE HCFA-1500 (12-90)

The HCFA-1500 (12-90) has been adopted by insurance carriers as the only acceptable form on which to submit insurance claims. However, each insurance carrier has its own thoughts on how the form should be completed and no two companies agree entirely on the information required, the boxes checked, and the rationale about what information goes in which boxes.

To illustrate the completion of a claim form, a fictitious insurance carrier will be used. (Insurance carriers change their rules and regulations for submitting claims constantly. One example is Medicare, which changes its requirements several times a year.) In order to avoid out-of-date material, this claim for payment is sent to How Much Insurance Company. Using the example given of Leo McKay in the coding section, the HCFA-1500 in Figure 19-2 shows the properly completed claim form:

**Example:**

Block 1.    X in "other."
Block 1a.   555-55-5555
Block 2.    McKay, Leo M
Block 3.    04 01 35 X in "M."
Block 4.    McKay, Leo M
Block 5.    123 West First Street
            Carlton, MI
            11666 (814) 983-2831
Block 6.    X in "self."
Block 7.    Same as insured.
Block 8.    X in "single"—no other boxes marked
            in this block for this claim.
Block 9.    Leave blank. (If the patient has other
            insurance, that information would go
            here.)
Block 10.   a.  X in "no."
            b.  X in "no."
            c.  X in "no."
Block 11.   1122334
            a.  Leave blank.
            b.  ABC Manufacturing Company
            c.  How Much Insurance Company
            d.  X in "no."
Block 12.   Needs date and "signature on file"
            typed in.
Block 13.   Needs "signature on file" typed in.
Block 14.   01 10 xx
Block 15.   In this example, Leo did not have previ-
            ous symptoms of similar nature, so this
            will be left blank.
Block 16.   Leave blank.
Block 17.   Leo is a regular patient of Dr. Woo so
            no referring physician name goes here.
            If he had been referred to Dr. Woo by
            another physician, the referring physi-
            cian's name would go here.
Block 18.   Leave blank.
Block 19.   Leave blank.
Block 20.   X in "yes" since outside labs were
            ordered in this example.
Block 21.   Use only ICD-9-CM codes here.
            1.  789.0
            2.  787.91
            3.  783.0
            4.  This can be left blank since there
                were only three diagnoses. A claim
                may be submitted using only one
                diagnosis code if it substantiates the
                charges.
Block 22.   Leave blank.
Block 23.   Leave blank.
Block 24.   A.  1/10/xx
            B.  3 (indicates office visit)
            C.  Leave blank.
            D.  99214
            E.  1,2,3
            F.  85.00

G.  1 (indicates one unit)
H.  Leave blank.
I.  Leave blank.
J.  Leave blank.
K.  Leave blank. (In Medicare, Medicaid,
    and Workers' Compensation claims,
    the medical provider's number is
    entered here.)

Line 2.     A.  1/10/xx
            B.  3
            C.  Leave blank.
            D.  82270
            E.  1,2
            F.  13.00
            G.  1
Block 25.   91-5555555 and X in "EIN."
Block 26.   MCK111
Block 27.   X in "no" unless physician accepts
            assignment for that plan.
Block 28.   98.00
Block 29.   -0-
Block 30.   98.00
Block 31.   Physician's name, telephone number,
            date claim sent in.
Block 32.   Leave blank since care provided at Dr.
            Woo's office
Block 33.   Inner City Health Care
            222 South First Avenue
            Carlton, MI 11666
            (PIN#) 10004086

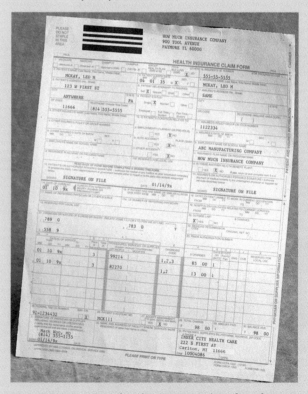

**Figure 19-2**    Completed HCFA-1500 claim form for
Leo McKay.

Remember, many insurance carriers will require some of the boxes to be filled in and others left blank. The billing person for the medical office will need to comply with the current requirements of the insurance carrier that is being billed. There is no right or wrong answer for every insurance carrier. If there is a question about billing, check with that carrier about their requirements.

Although the HCFA-1500 is the most common claim form in the ambulatory care setting, medical assistants who become claims processing specialists in different settings will need to be familiar with the UB92 (Figure 19-3). The **Uniform Bill 92 (UB92)** form was originally developed in the 1970s as a unique form for filing inpatient, home health care, hospice, and long-term

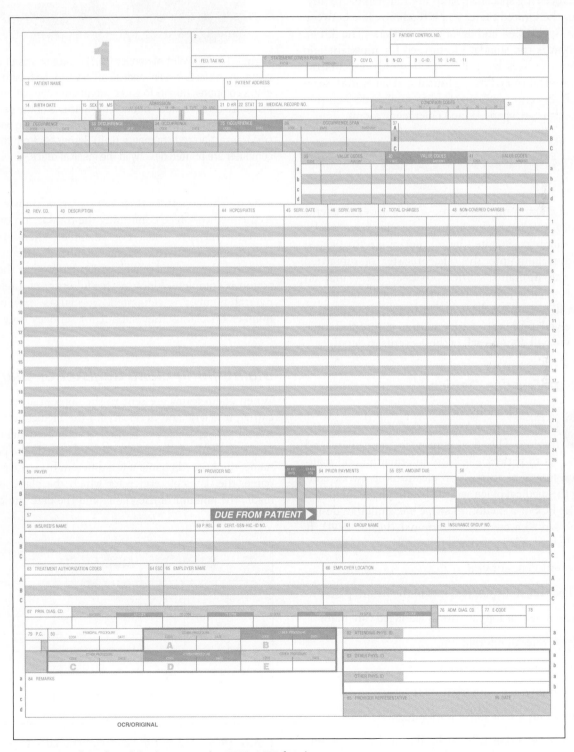

**Figure 19-3** UB92 claim form (also known as the HCFA-1450 form).

care benefits under a health plan. It is also known as the HCFA-1450 and may also be referred to as a summary bill.

Although medical assistants in ambulatory care facilities will not typically encounter hospital billing forms such as the UB92, many medical assistants are now finding opportunities as claims processing specialists in hospital, nursing facility, and clinic billing offices. As a claims processing specialist, skills are transferable to anywhere in the United States and interchangeable between provider specialties and insurance carriers. The UB92 claim form is the standard form used for inpatient and outpatient services by acute care hospitals, psychiatric, drug, and alcohol facilities, clinical and laboratory services, walk-in centers, nursing facilities, subacute facilities, home health care agencies, and emergency rooms.

## OVERSEEING THE CLAIMS PROCESS

Once the claim form has been coded, a series of events take place: the medical assistant, who may have used a referral number generated by a point-of-service device, enters the claim into the office register of submitted claims; the insurance carrier processes the claim; an explanation of benefits is sent to the insured; and, if necessary, follow-up procedures are instituted if payment is not received from the carrier within a specified time period. We will discuss each of these events in detail.

### Point-of-Service Device

A new electronic device now available to some health care providers is a **point-of-service (POS) device**. This device provides immediate and direct access to patient eligibility information and managed care functions through an electronic network connecting the medical office and the health plan's computer.

The POS is a small card-swipe box similar in design and function to a credit card terminal (Figure 19-4). It allows medical office personnel to:

- Record a patient visit
- Check eligibility for patients in the health plan
- Enter referrals for patients in managed care plans
- Verify referral information
- Check authorization status
- Enter inpatient authorization requests
- Enter outpatient authorization requests

After the information is input by the medical assistant, the POS communicates with the health plan's computer

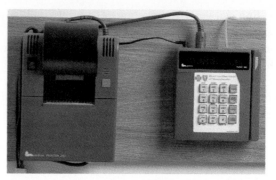

**Figure 19-4** Point-of-service (POS) device allows direct communication between medical offices and the health care plan's computer. (Right) To enter information, the patient's insurance card is swiped through the machine or the patient's identification number is entered on the keypad along with specific transaction code numbers. (Left) Responses from the plan's computer are printed directly in the medical office.

system. The computer then returns an acknowledgment to the medical office confirming the transaction or giving an error message code. For example, when visits are recorded accurately, a reference number is generated that is used as the medical office's confirmation that the transaction is complete. Upon successful entry of a referral, a referral number is generated. Specialists may use this number on claims they submit for services they render under the referral.

### Maintaining Claim Register or Diary

When claim forms are sent to the appropriate insurance carrier, it is wise and necessary for the medical office personnel to keep a diary or register of submitted claims (Figure 19-5). This **claim register** should include the patient's name, the insured's name if it is different from the patient's name, the dates of service for which the claim is being made, the amount of the claim, and the date the claim is

| Date | Patient Name | Insured Name | Insurance Company | Dates Billed | Total Charges | Amount Received |
|---|---|---|---|---|---|---|
| 1-18-_ _ | McKay, Leo | — | How Much Ins Co. | 1-10-_ _ | 98.00 | |
| | | | | | | |
| | | | | | | |
| | | | | | | |
| | | | | | | |
| | | | | | | |
| | | | | | | |
| | | | | | | |

**Figure 19-5** Example of claim register used to track insurance claims.

submitted. When payment is received, date of payment should be entered. When aging and reconciling accounts, the bookkeeper then can check the diary to note where the claim is in the process.

## The Insurance Carrier's Role

Upon receipt of the claim form, the claims processor at the insurance carrier checks the codes to make sure that the procedures and accompanying diagnoses agree. The processor then analyzes the information to make certain that:

1. The coverage was in force at the time of treatment
2. The physician has contracted with the insurance carrier
3. There are no exclusions or restrictions on the policy for payment of that diagnosis
4. There are no pre-existing condition restrictions
5. The diagnosis and procedures done are reasonable

The processor also checks to make sure that the billed amount falls within the usual, customary, and reasonable fee that the insurance carrier has developed for that specific procedure.

## Explanation of Benefits

Upon completion of the processing of the claim, the insurance company sends an **Explanation of Benefits (EOB)** to the insured. This form includes the dates, charges, amounts applied toward the deductible, amounts not covered either due to an exclusion or excess over the usual, customary, and reasonable charge, and the amount the company is paying for this claim. Some Explanation of Benefits forms even serve as a "bill" or "notice" in that they indicate the amount the insured must forward to the physician for payment in full of the account.

## Following Up on Claims

Occasionally, claims may be denied because the claim form was not properly coded. However, if there is no payment from the carrier and no other notification after a period of four to six weeks, it is necessary to follow up on the claim. The claim register will enable the office to keep track of the progress of claims.

To follow up, a toll-free number is provided by most carriers. The necessary information to have before making the call includes a copy of the claim form and the patient's name and insurance identification number. The carrier should be able to give the status of the claim. If payment is delayed, the carrier should be able to give the date when it can be expected. It is possible that payment was sent to the insured, in which case a statement should be sent to the patient. If there is a problem with the claim, the medical assistant may need to investigate the cause of the error and submit a revised claim.

For information on billing and collection procedures, see Chapter 20.

## THE COMPUTERIZED CLAIMS PROCESS

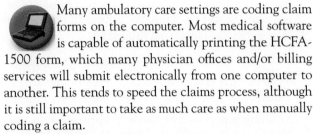

Many ambulatory care settings are coding claim forms on the computer. Most medical software is capable of automatically printing the HCFA-1500 form, which many physician offices and/or billing services will submit electronically from one computer to another. This tends to speed the claims process, although it is still important to take as much care as when manually coding a claim.

Typically, a computer program will receive instructions to print claims forms and to track the forms on a standard schedule. The information for each patient is keyed into the computer; once entered, the information is stored and can be utilized, with revisions as necessary, for future claim forms for that patient. This eliminates some of the tedious typewriting involved in filling out the claim form and ensures greater accuracy since much of the information only needs to be entered once.

## LEGAL AND ETHICAL ISSUES

A primary legal concern with medical insurance is a **breach of confidentiality** or the unauthorized release of confidential patient information to a third party. As patients check in at the office for an appointment, they should be given an Authorization for the Release of Medical Information Statement to sign *before* being seen by the physician or certainly *before* completing and submitting any insurance claim form. Many offices have a form unique to the specific provider's practice, which is signed annually and maintained in the patient's chart. The purpose of this form is to allow the provider to submit claim forms without the patient's signature each time a claim is submitted. The phrase "signature on file" must be keyed or stamped in Block 12 of each claim form filed for that patient.

Other types of legal issues related to medical insurance include fraud and insurance abuse. **Fraud** is defined as an intentional deception or misrepresentation that an individual makes, knowing it to be false, which could result in some unauthorized benefit. Examples of fraud in the medical office may include, but are not limited to:

- Using a higher level of service code in order to increase practice revenue
- Billing for services, equipment, or supplies that were not provided or required

● Misrepresenting a patient diagnosis to justify the level of services performed to increase practice revenue

**Insurance abuse** is defined as incidents or practices of providers, physicians, or suppliers of services and equipment that, while not considered fraudulent, are inconsistent with accepted sound medical, business, or fiscal practices. Examples of insurance abuse in the medical office may include, but are not limited to:

● Overcharging for services, equipment, or supplies

● Submitting claims for items or services that are not medically necessary to treat the patient's condition

● Billing practices that result in payment by a government program when the claim is the legal responsibility of another third-party payer

Coding errors pose another type of legal and ethical issue. The Omnibus Budget Reconciliation Acts of 1986 and 1987 state that physicians can be assessed civil penalties if they "know of or should know that claims filed with Medicare or Medicaid on their behalf are not true and accurate representations of the items or services actually provided." This means that physicians can be held responsible not only for negligent mistakes they make but also for mistakes made in their behalf by their medical assistants completing insurance claim forms. The penalties assessed are usually in the form of a monetary fine and may also involve exclusion from Medicare and Medicaid programs for a period of time.

## HEALTHCARE COMPLIANCE

The Office of Inspector General (OIG) issued compliance program guidelines in 2000 to assist physicians in solo or small group practices. These guidelines, consisting of seven steps, are not mandatory but focus on the development of meaningful voluntary compliance programs. They serve as a resource to be considered in addition to other OIG outreach efforts and other federal agency efforts to promote compliance.

### Seven Basic Elements of a Voluntary Compliance Program

1. Conduct periodic internal monitoring and auditing.
2. Implement compliance and practice standards by developing written standards and procedures.
3. Designate a compliance officer or contacts to monitor compliance efforts and enforce practice standards.
4. Conduct appropriate training and education on practice standards and procedures.

---

### SPOTLIGHT ON AAMA ESSENTIALS THROUGH CAAHEP

● Establishing a positive relationship with the patient during the first appointment assists the medical assistant in gathering important data and information necessary for coding and billing services at a later time.

● When following insurance and coding procedures, the medical assistant must always maintain a professional attitude and confidentiality when talking to patients regarding their care and treatment.

● The medical assistant responsible for coding procedures must prepare the billing and insurance forms with care and be understanding and positive when discussing the payment schedule with the patient.

---

5. Respond appropriately to detected violations by investigating allegations and disclosing incidents to appropriate government entities.
6. Develop open lines of communication, such as (1) discussions at staff meetings regarding how to avoid erroneous or fraudulent conduct and (2) community bulletin boards, to keep practice employees updated regarding compliance activities.
7. Enforce disciplinary standards through well-publicized guidelines.

Each practice is encouraged to undertake reasonable steps to implement the seven basic elements as best reflects their practice. Advantages of participating in a compliance program include:

● Helps prevent fraudulent or erroneous claims

● Demonstrates the practice is making a good faith effort to submit claims appropriately

● Considered analogous to practicing preventive medicine

Employees have an affirmative, ethical duty to come forward and report fraudulent or erroneous conduct so that it may be corrected. Individuals who fail to detect or report violations of the compliance program may be subject to discipline. Disciplinary actions could include verbal warnings, written reprimands, probation, demotion, temporary suspension, discharge of employment, restitution of damages, and referral for criminal prosecution. Including disciplinary guidelines in training and procedure manuals is sufficient to meet the well-publicized standard.

## DOCUMENTATION

An auditor should check claim forms, whether submitted electronically or by hard copy, to see that they are completed correctly. Include all pertinent dates and diagnostic and procedural coding information necessary for insurance payers to generate reimbursement. Auditors will look specifically for any indicators of insurance fraud and abuse.

**CASE STUDY 19-1**

Leo McKay, an established patient at Inner City Health Care, schedules a visit, complaining of nausea and severe abdominal pain. Dr. Mark Woo spends 30 minutes taking a history and doing an examination. He suspects an ulcer and orders lab tests (CBC complete, guaiac, lipid panel, and UA) to be done in the office and sends Mr. McKay for an upper GI series. Mr. McKay returns in 10 days to the test results which show a duodenal ulcer.

### CASE STUDY REVIEW

1. What would the proper diagnosis codes be for Mr. McKay?
2. What would the proper procedure codes be for Mr. McKay?
3. In coding the claim form for Mr. McKay's visit, what ethical principle and legal principle should guide the medical assistant?

## SUMMARY

Much material has been covered in this chapter. Remember, you can be the person to make the difference in insurance billing. By checking and double-checking your work, you make certain that the physician's time is being billed at the appropriate rate, that all procedures are billed with the proper diagnoses, and that the billing is sent to the correct insurance carrier. It takes much less time to double-check work once

and have it correct *before* it is sent out than to send it out with errors that cause difficulty in the future.

An understanding of medical insurance coverages and coding procedures is vital to a thriving ambulatory care setting. The astute medical assistant will perceive the challenges involved in proper coding techniques and understand their role in the management of the physician's office.

## REVIEW QUESTIONS

### Multiple Choice

1. CPT codes:
   a. are for diagnosis coding
   b. have five digits and may have two-digit modifiers
   c. have three-digit codes with a decimal point and one to two additional digits
   d. are updated semiannually
2. When coding a diagnosis, go first to:
   a. CPT
   b. Volume I of ICD-9-CM
   c. Volume II of ICD-9-CM
   d. E codes in ICD-9-CM

3. A plus symbol on a CPT code indicates:
   a. unusual procedural services
   b. bilateral procedures
   c. procedure is an add-on to a previously described procedure
   d. repeat procedure by the same physician
4. Level II of HCPCS:
   a. uses a five-digit alphanumeric code to clarify procedures
   b. is the same as the regular CPT system
   c. is assigned by the fiscal intermediary
   d. uses the letter codes W, X, Y, and Z

**ADMINISTRATIVE**

**Administrative Procedures**

- Understand and apply third-party guidelines
- Obtain reimbursement through accurate claims submission
- Monitor third-party reimbursement
- Understand and adhere to managed care policies and procedures

**Practice Finances**

- Document and maintain accounting and banking records
- Manage accounts receivable

**GENERAL (TRANSDISCIPLINARY)**

**Professionalism**

- Adhere to ethical principles

**Communication Skills**

- Use professional telephone technique
- Recognize and respond to verbal and nonverbal communications
- Receive, organize, prioritize, and transmit information

**Legal Concepts**

- Maintain confidentiality
- Document accurately
- Follow employer's established policies dealing with the health care contract
- Follow federal, state, and local legal guidelines

## SCENARIO

At Doctors Lewis & King, patient billing is typically done at time of service, and a charge slip noting date, description of charges, and fees is given to the patient upon leaving the office. Office policy states that, if possible, patients should pay their part of the fee, or their copay, at time of service. Marilyn Johnson, the office manager, has found that this is the most efficient way to ensure timely payment and eliminates the need to mail a separate statement. However, the office is flexible and, if the patient cannot pay all or part of the charge at the visit, Marilyn works out a payment schedule that is acceptable to both office and patient.

## INTRODUCTION

In the ambulatory care setting, patient billing is a critical administrative function that helps to maintain a healthy, viable practice. Timeliness is essential in billing, for the ambulatory care setting depends on its accounts receivable to pay its bills in a responsible manner. Billing need not be a complex activity, but it must be completely accurate. In offices still using pegboard accounting, billing and collection procedures are done manually, often using the patient's ledger card as the basis for the statement. If the office is computerized, patient bills and collection notices are typically computer generated.

While not all ambulatory care settings expect payment at the time of service, it is certainly common. The best method of patient billing and collections is a method that is customized to the practice and that regards the patient as a consumer who should be respected. Patients appreciate knowing in advance what charges and fees to expect. Many offices include these in their informational brochures or post them in a prominent place in the office.

## BILLING PROCEDURES

The ambulatory care setting's cash flow and collection process are dependent on accurate billing techniques. The financial status of the practice is reflected in monthly statements indicating unpaid patient balances, which, if they persist, are reviewed for appropriate action, including referral to a **collection agency**. Copies of all billing forms will be retained in the patient account record.

Timeliness and accuracy have a significant influence upon prompt payment and how soon collection of the patient account will be finalized. In other words, billing performance can be measured by the time it takes to generate and submit a complete statement, that is, a statement with full documentation. If an office is experiencing problems generating patient bills, a billing timeliness analysis worksheet can be constructed to identify internal delays that affect how quickly an account is billed and thus paid. By focusing on inefficiencies in the revenue cycle, processes may be identified that need to be streamlined. For example, the date of service and insurance verification, the date the bill was generated, and the date the bill was submitted to the patient or third party can determine the efficiency of the billing process.

A billing efficiency report is another instrument that may be used to monitor efficiency. This report lists the previous month's billing backlog, which is added to the number of new accounts. The number of processed accounts is then subtracted. The weekly number of accounts that were rebilled also is noted, and the amount of time billing personnel spent on billing accounts is recorded. Production efficiency is calculated from this data. Inherent to this system is the careful monitoring of follow-up bills: whether they were paid, if the insurance was paid, and assessing the patient's responsibility for payment.

## CREDIT AND COLLECTION POLICIES

Even uncomplicated patient billing should be done according to credit and collection policies established by the physician employers of the ambulatory care setting. Having a formalized policy makes decision making easier and gives the medical assistant responsible for billing and collections authority to act. For example, some questions the physicians and office manager may want to address include:

- When will payment be due from the patient?

- What kind of payment arrangements can be made if the patient does not pay at time of service?

- Will a collection agency be utilized? Who decides?

- At what point should a patient be reminded of an overdue bill?

- How is that reminder initially managed: by telephone or letter?

- At what point will a patient bill be considered delinquent?

- If exceptions to office policy are to be made, who makes these exceptions?

By answering these and other questions, a straightforward credit and collection policy can be devised that is a guide to both patients and the medical assistant in charge of billing.

### Patient Teaching Tip

Patients appreciate knowing their responsibility in terms of payment. Whoever schedules the first appointment with a new patient should diplomatically inform the patient of office policy on payment of fees. If the patient anticipates a problem in paying promptly, a schedule can be worked out that is agreeable to both parties.

## PAYMENT AT TIME OF SERVICE

Because the best opportunity for collection is at the time of service, many ambulatory care settings provide the patient with a bill and require payment at that time. This assures prompt collection, eliminates further bookkeeping work, and provides better cash flow for the practice. To accommodate the patient, most offices accept cash, personal checks, and possibly credit cards.

It is important to note that payment at time of service will be adjusted according to the patient's insurance and the terms of that policy. If the patient is a member of an HMO, and the ambulatory care center is a participating provider, it is bound to the terms of that agreement.

It is always helpful to discuss fees with patients when scheduling the first appointment, especially if payment is appreciated at time of service. See also Chapter 17 for a discussion of fees.

## TRUTH-IN-LENDING ACT

 In those situations where a payment schedule is arranged, it must be determined by the office whether or not interest will be charged. Ambulatory care settings may decide to charge interest for installment arrangements.

Medical assistants need to be aware of the conditions of the **Truth-in-Lending Act** (also called the Consumer Credit Protection Act of 1968) which was established to protect consumers by requiring that providers of installment credit state the charges clearly in writing and express the interest as an annual rate. When there is a bilateral agreement between the physician and patient to pay in more than four installments, the physician must disclose finance charges in writing. Even if no finance charges are made, the forms must still be completed.

## COMPONENTS OF A COMPLETE STATEMENT

Statements to patients must be professional looking, neat, accurate, and inclusive of all services and charges. If the statement is to be mailed, an enclosed self-addressed envelope is a convenience for many patients and may result in a faster turnaround of payment.

Charge slip (also known as superbill), statement, and insurance reporting information are often combined on one form (Figure 20-1). A well-prepared patient statement should contain not only information for the patient, but information needed to process medical insurance claims as well.

- Patient's name and address

- Patient's insurance identification number

- Insurance carrier

- Date of service

- Description of service

- Accurate procedure (CPT) and diagnosis (ICD-9-CM) codes for insurance processing (see also Chapters 18 and 19)

- Physician's signature

| DATE | PATIENT | SERVICE CODE | FEES CHARGE | PAID | ADJ. | BALANCE DUE | | PREVIOUS BALANCE | NAME | RECEIPT NO. |
|---|---|---|---|---|---|---|---|---|---|---|
| | | | | CREDITS | | | | | | |

THIS IS YOUR RECEIPT _____ ▲
AND/OR A STATEMENT OF YOUR ACCOUNT TO DATE _____ ▲

PATIENTS NAME                                      ☐ M ☐ F

ADDRESS

CITY                          STATE        ZIP

| OFFICE VISITS AND PROCEDURES | | | | | | | |
|---|---|---|---|---|---|---|---|
| 99211 | EST PT - MINIMAL OV | 1 | | | | HOSPITAL VISIT | 14 |
| 99212 | EST PT - BRIEF OV | 2 | | | | EMERGENCY | 15 |
| 99213 | EST PT - INTERMEDIATE OV | 3 | | | | CONSULTATION | 16 |
| 99214 | EST PT - EXTENDED OV | 4 | | 93000 | | EKG | 17 |
| 99215 | EST PT - COMPREHENSIVE OV | 5 | | 93224 | | ELECTROCARDIOGRAPHIC MONITORING | 18 |
| 99201 | NEW PT - BRIEF OV | 6 | | 93307 | | ECHOCARDIOGRAPHY | 19 |
| 99202 | NEW PT - INTERMEDIATE OV | 7 | | 85025 | | CBC | 20 |
| 99203 | NEW PT - EXTENDED OV | 8 | | 81000 | | URINALYSIS WITH MICROSCOPY | 21 |
| 99204 | NEW PT - COMPLEX OV | 9 | | 36415 | | ROUTINE VENIPUNCTURE | 22 |
| 99205 | NEW PT - COMPREHENSIVE OF | 10 | | 71020 | | RADIOLOGY EXAM-CHEST-2 VIEWS | 23 |
| 99238 | HOSPITAL DISCHARGE | 11 | | 30300 | | REMOVE FOR. BODY-INTRANASAL | 24 |
| 99025 | NEW PT - SURGERY PROC. PRIMARY | 12 | | | | | 25 |
| | NURSING HOME VISIT | 13 | | | | | 26 |

RELATIONSHIP                    BIRTHDATE

SUBSCRIBER OR POLICY HOLDER

☐ MEDICARE ☐ MEDICAID ☐ BLUE SHIELD ☐ 65-SP.

INSURANCE CARRIER

AGREEMENT #

GROUP #

**D - OTHER SERVICES**

**AUTHORIZATION TO RELEASE INFORMATION:** I HEREBY AUTHORIZE THE UNDERSIGNED PHYSICIAN TO RELEASE ANY INFORMATION ACQUIRED IN THE COURSE OF MY EXAMINATION OR TREATMENT.
SIGNED (PATIENT, OR PARENT IF MINOR)

NEXT APPOINTMENT         AT         AM PM

DATE _____

RETURN _____ DAYS _____ WEEKS _____ MONTHS

PLACE OF SERVICE    ☐ OFFICE  ☐ OTHER _____

DIAGNOSIS OR SYMPTOMS _____

**CAPITAL AREA HEALTH CARE**
839 SYCAMORE PARK
BOISE, ID 83725
(208) 863-4210

DOCTOR'S SIGNATURE _____

03626

**Figure 20-1**   Sample charge slip shown is a multipurpose form used to document information for insurance claims as well as to provide the patient with a receipt and documentation of procedures, diagnoses, and fees.

● Ambulatory care center name, address, telephone number, and possibly fax number

## Computerized Statements

If the ambulatory care setting uses a computer system of bookkeeping, then statements will be computer generated. Typically, the medical assistant issues instructions to search the patient database for outstanding balances and directs the computer to print statements.

During this process, the computer program will also "age" accounts (see Aging Accounts in this chapter) and print collection letters (already in the database) for overdue accounts.

# MONTHLY AND CYCLE BILLING

The billing schedule is often determined by the size of the medical practice. Monthly billing is a system in which all accounts are billed at the same time each month. In a smaller ambulatory care setting, monthly billing may be the most efficient method. Cycle billing staggers bills during the month and is a flexible system for larger practices.

## Monthly Billing

In a **monthly billing** system, one or two days are devoted to billing and mailing all statements. Typically, statements should leave the office on the 25th of the month to be received by the first of the month. The major disadvantage of monthly billing is that a medical assistant may neglect other activities during this time-consuming period. To avoid these problems, billing statements may be prepared intermittently over a one- or two-week period and stored until the mailing date. To avoid confusion caused by delays in mailing, a message to "Disregard if payment has already been made" should be printed on the form. Patients become annoyed and the practice appears disorganized if a statement arrives several days after payment has been made.

## Cycle Billing

In a **cycle billing** system, all accounts are divided alphabetically into groups, with each group billed at a different time. In this way, office personnel with numerous bills to process each month will be able to handle them in a more efficient manner. Statements are prepared on the same

To cycle bill patient accounts:

1. Divide the alphabet into four sections: A–F, G–L, M–R, S–Z.
2. Prepare statements for patients whose last names begin with A through F on Wednesday and mail them on Thursday of Week 1.
3. Prepare statements for patients whose last names begin with G through L on Wednesday and mail them on Thursday of Week 2.
4. Prepare statements for patients whose last names begin with M through R on Wednesday and mail them on Thursday of Week 3.
5. Prepare statements for patients whose last names begin with S through Z on Wednesday and mail them on Thursday of Week 4.

**Figure 20-2**    Typical schedule for cycle billing system.

schedule each month. They can be mailed as they are completed, or held and mailed at one time. A typical cycle billing schedule is shown in Figure 20-2. The system can be varied to suit the needs of the individual practice.

## PAST-DUE ACCOUNTS

As efficient and effective as the billing process may be, there will still be collections on some accounts. The most common reasons for past due accounts include:

- Inability to pay. People may have financial hardships from time to time.
- Negligence. People may forget to make a payment because they have been away or dealing with a family emergency.
- Unwillingness to pay. When a patient complains about a charge or refuses to pay, it may have nothing to do with finances. Often, they are dissatisfied with the care or treatment they have received. These patients should be referred to the physician or office manager for immediate attention.

## COLLECTION PROCESS

The process of collecting delinquent accounts begins with first establishing how much has been owed for how long.

Ideally, collection of accounts receivable should be prompt and conducted in a timely fashion. Management consultants recommend that fees should be collected at the time of service and that a collection ratio of at least 90 percent should be maintained. A collection ratio is a method used to gauge the effectiveness of the ambulatory care setting's billing practices. Typically, the collection

ratio is figured by dividing the total collections by the net charges (gross charges minus adjustments). This yields a percentage, which is the collection ratio.

Another important factor is the accounts receivable ratio, which measures the speed with which outstanding accounts are paid. The desirable ratio is less than two months for collection of accounts receivable. To figure the accounts receivable ratio, divide the current accounts receivable balance by the average monthly gross charges. This yields the typical turnaround for collecting accounts receivable. Also see Chapter 21 for more information on account receivable and collection ratios.

The longer an office puts off attempting to collect delinquent accounts, the less chance there is of receiving payment. Statistics show that the value of the dollar decreases rapidly in the collection process. The more time and energy you put into collections, the less value you receive in return. In other words, you may manage to collect the full amount due, but when you consider the time and expense involved, it may not have been worth the effort and expense. Therefore, the value of the debt to be received following successful collection must be considered when determining how aggressive to be in debt collections. It is evident that as time passes the value of outstanding accounts as well as the percentage that will be collected declines.

## AGING ACCOUNTS

**Account aging** is a method of identifying how long an account is overdue. This means that past due accounts are identified according to the length of time they have been unpaid. When using a pegboard bookkeeping system, color-coded strips are attached to the ledger cards to show the age of an account, or the cards can be stored behind a color-coded divider in a separate file labeled "Unpaid." For example, a red strip might be used for accounts one month overdue, a blue strip for accounts two months overdue, and other colors for additional months overdue. A written code such as "OD3/2/23" should be written on the ledger card to indicate when the overdue notice was mailed, meaning "Overdue notice No. 3 mailed on February 23."

Depending upon the type of patient served, different aging systems are used. In a computerized billing system, the accounts are automatically aged, and the aging schedule or process is shown on the computerized ledger card. A typical aging schedule for a private patient is shown in Figure 20-3.

### Computerized Aging

 Aging accounts using a computerized system is very simple. Before printing billing statements, the medical assistant keys the appropriate

Charge slip (Superbill) given to patient at time of visit.

1. Itemized statement mailed at end of first month.
2. Itemized statement with overdue notice mailed when account is past due two months.
3. Telephone call reminding patient of overdue account and offering to help arrange a payment schedule.
4. Letter stating, "We have not received payment for your account," when account is past due three months.
5. Letter or telephone call stating, "Your account will be turned over to a collector," if this is the policy of the facility.
6. Certified letter stating (if outside collectors are used), "Your account was turned over to a collection agency." No further telephone calls are necessary, as they might antagonize the patient and leave the medical assistant open to verbal abuse.

**Figure 20-3**    Sample aging process for a patient with private insurance.

commands to age the accounts. The program can age accounts according to several criteria: for example, by past due balance, zero balance, or credit balance accounts. Accounts can also be aged by government agency category or by insurance carrier. All Medicare or Medicaid accounts might be aged separately from other accounts.

The computer can also generate and print an accounts receivable report showing each overdue account, the balance overdue, and a breakdown showing how long the account is overdue. This breakdown is usually divided into accounts 0 to 30 days overdue, 31 to 60 days overdue, 61 to 90 days overdue, and 90 days or more overdue. Additional reports can be generated from the accounts receivable report. For example, the office staff may wish to reprint a report showing accounts that have been delinquent for more than 90 days or accounts that are delinquent by more than a certain dollar amount.

## COLLECTION TECHNIQUES

Ambulatory care settings use both telephone and written communications in their collection techniques. While both have some measure of effectiveness, some practices prefer to call the patient with a past due account before officially initiating collection proceedings. The patient may have misplaced the statement, forgotten a payment, or been away on an extended vacation; a quick telephone call can often resolve the situation without the time and expense involved in collections. Also, the patient appreciates the courtesy and personal approach.

## Correspondence to Insurance Carriers

Many patients have some form of medical insurance. Most claim departments of insurance carriers and government agencies employ large numbers of employees who have varying levels of experience. Payment can be delayed because of an overburdened claim department, a form that has been lost in transit, a misfiled form, an inexperienced employee, or numerous other reasons.

The medical assistant should maintain an up-to-date claims register (see Chapter 18) or tickler file and take firm control of the practice's collection procedures to ensure that claims are paid promptly. In offices where the medical assistant files claims for patients, a follow-up collection policy is important to maintain strong cash flow. When carriers do not pay in full or question or deny a claim, the medical assistant will have to determine the nature of the problem and notify the patients.

## Telephone Collections

The medical assistant is likely to use the telephone for collection procedures. Telephoning is often an effective measure, for a patient may remember a call more so than a bill received in the mail.

A successful telephone collection call is enhanced by keeping to the facts, being tactful, pleasant, and diplomatic. When making calls to patients regarding past due accounts, there are some things to keep in mind in order to maintain the desired relationship with patients. Always remain courteous and respectful. Do not treat patients with suspicion or threats. Remember, the health profession is dedicated to helping people; avoid antagonizing patients.

Most people do not let their bills become past due on purpose or out of spite. Keep this in mind when making calls. Work with patients to encourage and enable them to pay any fees they owe.

Certain legal rules and ethical guidelines govern telephone collections.

- When making collection calls, callers must identify themselves and ascertain that they are talking to the person who is responsible for the account.
- A collection call could be embarrassing to the patient; therefore it should not be made to the patient's place of employment.
- In most states, a debtor may be contacted only between 8 A.M. and 9 P.M.
- Do not threaten to turn the person over to collection agencies.

Violating these rules makes the caller vulnerable to charges of harassment under the **Fair Debt Collection Practice Act.**

When collecting by telephone, it is helpful to keep complete accurate records of who said what and how much was promised as payment. If, after two weeks nothing has been resolved as a result of the calls, then another course of action, such as retaining the services of a collection agency or **credit bureau**, may be the solution, especially for large sums of money owed.

## Collection Letters

Collection letters are sent to encourage patients and third-party carriers to pay overdue balances. After two statements are mailed to patients and the charge slip has brought no response, the ambulatory care setting begins sending collection letters.

Lack of payment from a patient is usually not considered serious until after 60 days. When the patient fails to respond to the charge slip, to the statement, or to a 60-day statement with an "Overdue" remark, a series of collection letters begins. One typical collection letter series is shown in Figure 20-4 A through C.

## USE OF AN OUTSIDE COLLECTION AGENCY

Occasionally, the ambulatory care setting may turn over highly delinquent accounts to an outside collection agency. Discretion is always advised here, however, for the expense of collection may not justify the fees to be collected. For unpaid accounts with large balances, however, this is often a viable solution.

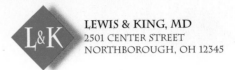

LEWIS & KING, MD
2501 CENTER STREET
NORTHBOROUGH, OH 12345

June 14, 20—

Mr. John O'Keefe
12 Gravers Lane
Northborough, OH 12345

Dear Mr. O'Keefe:

Your account with our office is three months past due, and you have not responded to our previous requests for payment. Please pay your balance of $852 at this time, or contact us with an explanation of why you cannot pay.

Please call me at 312-824-6925 if you have a question about your account. Otherwise, we expect your payment immediately.

Sincerely,

Marilyn Johnson
Office Manager

NORTHBOROUGH
FAMILY MEDICAL GROUP

(A)

**Figure 20-4**　Sample collection letters: (A) First letter.

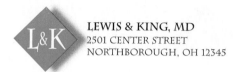

LEWIS & KING, MD
2501 CENTER STREET
NORTHBOROUGH, OH 12345

July 15, 20—

Mr. John O'Keefe
12 Gravers Lane
Northborough, OH 12345

Dear Mr. O'Keefe:

Your son, Chris, was seriously ill in March when he came to Dr. King for treatment. Dr. King was pleased to use her experience and education to treat Chris, and it was in this same spirit of cooperation that we expected you to pay your account within a reasonable amount of time.

Four months have passed and you have still not remitted the $852 outstanding balance on your account. We cannot continue to keep your unpaid account on our books. If you are experiencing financial difficulties, please call the office so we can arrange a payment schedule that is agreeable to both of us.

Sincerely,

Marilyn Johnson
Office Manager

NORTHBOROUGH
FAMILY MEDICAL GROUP

**(B)**

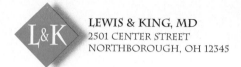

LEWIS & KING, MD
2501 CENTER STREET
NORTHBOROUGH, OH 12345

August 17, 20—

CERTIFIED MAIL

Mr. John O'Keefe
12 Gravers Lane
Northborough, OH 12345

Dear Mr. O'Keefe:

This is our final attempt to collect your account of $852, which is five months past due. You have ignored all our previous letters [or letters and phone calls], so we have no alternative but to turn over your account to a collection company.

Your account is being assigned to Ambler Medical Collection Service, which will pursue whatever legal means is necessary to collect this debt. If you contact me at 312-824-6925 within seven days, we will retrieve your account from the collection service to protect your credit rating.

Sincerely,

Marilyn Johnson
Office Manager

NORTHBOROUGH
FAMILY MEDICAL GR

**(C)**

**Figure 20-4**   *(continued)*  (B) Second letter. (C) Third letter.

One service of the collection agency is to provide an intercept letter. For a nominal fee, this may be sent from the agency as the last resort before the account is turned over to collection. This communication alerts patients to the fact that if a response is not received, their account will go to collection. This often is the only action needed for the patient to pay the outstanding bill. Another service of a credit bureau or collection agency is to provide credit ratings of patients at the physician's request. Physicians who pay for this service are able to monitor patients' ability to pay their bills, as well as to trace a "skip," someone who leaves with an outstanding bill and no forwarding address.

When selecting a collection agency, be certain to hire one that is compatible with the medical office's philosophy. Ask for referrals from other physicians, ambulatory care centers, and hospitals. Ask the agency about its approach to collections and request sample letters and reminder notices.

## USE OF SMALL CLAIMS COURT

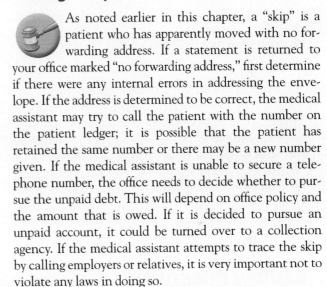

In certain circumstances, the ambulatory care center may consider bringing a case to small claims court. Typically, small claims courts handle cases that involve only limited amounts of debt (these vary from state to state), they do not permit representation by an attorney, and they are generally efficient and streamlined in their proceedings. Nonetheless, preparing for small claims courts and taking time to appear will require a certain investment of staff. It is also important to note that, if the court finds in the medical office's favor, the medical office still must collect the money from the defendant.

## SPECIAL COLLECTION SITUATIONS

In patient billing and collections, a number of special situations may arise.

### Bankruptcy

If a patient has declared bankruptcy, statements may no longer be sent nor any attempt be made to collect delinquent accounts. Because a physician's fee is an unsecured debt, it is one of the last to be paid. Bankruptcy laws are federal and are subject to the Federal Wage Garnishment Law of attaching property to satisfy debt.

### Estates

Collection of fees when a patient has died must be directed to the executor of the estate or the one responsible for overseeing the estate. Some general guidelines to follow include:

- Show courtesy by not sending a statement in the first week or so after a death.
- Address the statement to "Estate of (name of patient)" with the patient's last known address.
- If unsure of how to proceed, contact the office's attorney or the clerk of the probate court for advice.

### Tracing "Skips"

As noted earlier in this chapter, a "skip" is a patient who has apparently moved with no forwarding address. If a statement is returned to your office marked "no forwarding address," first determine if there were any internal errors in addressing the envelope. If the address is determined to be correct, the medical assistant may try to call the patient with the number on the patient ledger; it is possible that the patient has retained the same number or there may be a new number given. If the medical assistant is unable to secure a telephone number, the office needs to decide whether to pursue the unpaid debt. This will depend on office policy and the amount that is owed. If it is decided to pursue an unpaid account, it could be turned over to a collection agency. If the medical assistant attempts to trace the skip by calling employers or relatives, it is very important not to violate any laws in doing so.

## STATUTE OF LIMITATIONS

A statute of limitations is a statute that defines the period in which legal action may take place. When applying this concept to collections, the time period is usually defined by the class the account falls into. These include open book accounts, which may have periodic charges against them; written contracts; and single-entry accounts, which only have one charge against them. The time period in which legal action must take place against any of these accounts varies from state to state; if an unpaid account is more than three years old, it is wise to investigate the statute of limitations in your state before spending time and effort in collections.

**CASE STUDY**

**20-1**

For patient accounts more than 60 days overdue, the offices of Doctors Lewis & King begin a series of collection proceedings to attempt to collect the monies. Initially, they place a telephone call to the patient to determine whether a billing problem might be present that can be clarified over the telephone. If they cannot reach the patient, or the patient does not respond to the call, then collections begin. Marilyn has assigned this function of the billing process to Ellen Armstrong because Ellen has a warm telephone manner and is good with patients.

## CASE STUDY REVIEW

1. Why is Ellen's telephone manner of importance in the collection process?
2. In addition to telephone collections, what patient letters might Ellen send?
3. Ellen has come across an account that is delinquent and discovers that the patient has declared bankruptcy. What can Ellen do now?

## SUMMARY

Billing and collection activities in the ambulatory care setting are intricately linked to daily financial practices and claims processing, and the medical assistant responsible for billing should also be well aware of these other functions. Billing need not entail a complex or elaborate system, but whether accomplished by manual or computer methodology, it needs to be precise, professional, and comprehensive, as all communications with patients should be. If collections become necessary, courteous and straightforward letters and telephone exchanges are the most effective. The goal of all billing and collections is to maintain the relationship with the patient while ensuring good cash flow and payment of accounts receivable in the ambulatory care setting.

## REVIEW QUESTIONS

### Multiple Choice

1. The Consumer Credit Protection Act:
   a. is designed to place limits on the amount of debt consumers are liable for
   b. is also known as the statute of limitations
   c. is also known as the Truth-in-Lending Act
   d. does not apply to medical facilities
2. Cycle billing is a system of billing:
   a. completed every fourth month
   b. done by computer
   c. completed by the 25th of the month
   d. in which accounts are divided alphabetically for billing purposes
3. One of the most common reasons patient bills go unpaid is:
   a. inability to pay because of financial hardship
   b. patients consider the cost of medical care too high
   c. patients think their insurance should cover all medical bills
   d. patients think physicians make too much money

4. Aging accounts:
   a. is a process of identifying overdue patient accounts
   b. describes patients that have a long-term relationship with the ambulatory care center
   c. describes elderly patients
   d. applies to accounts considered inactive
5. If an unpaid account goes to small claims court:
   a. the medical office must engage an attorney representative
   b. the medical office is still responsible for collecting even if the court finds in its favor
   c. there is no need to show up at court
   d. a very large sum of money must be at issue
6. A credit bureau:
   a. provides information about a patient's credit history
   b. collects outstanding debts
   c. produces database software
   d. provides information about a patient's medical history

7. The Truth in Lending Act requires disclosing any finance charges:
   a. when the agreement is unilateral
   b. when payment is to be received in more than 4 payments
   c. and requires the interest be expressed as an annual rate
   d. b and c above

8. It will be most difficult to collect past-due accounts from:
   a. those who just forgot their bill
   b. those who are unwilling to pay
   c. those who are having financial hardships
   d. those who have no insurance

9. A "skip" is defined as:
   a. the time period when legal action cannot be taken
   b. an estate involved in probate
   c. one who moves without a forwarding address and leaves an unpaid bill
   d. one who has paid a portion of a debt

10. Lack of payment is usually not considered serious until after:
    a. 120 days
    b. 45 days
    c. 60 days
    d. 90 days

## Critical Thinking

1. Why is prompt and accurate billing important to the success of the ambulatory care setting and to the patient?

2. In establishing credit and collection policies, what issues should the ambulatory care center address?

3. Why is payment at time of service a good collection practice?

4. What information would you include in a complete statement?

5. What are the advantages and disadvantages of monthly billing? Cycle billing?

6. Describe a sample aging process for a patient with private insurance.

7. Write a series of collections letters, using the characters in this book.

8. With another student, role-play a telephone collections call. One student can be the medical assistant, one student, the patient.

9. Independently of one another, make notes on how the medical assistant handled the call in number 8. Then compare and discuss the observations.

10. Have a small group discussion on the ethics of collections. Each student can explain either a pro or a con position toward collections.

## WEB ACTIVITIES

Research the World Wide Web for information on debt collections. Consider key words such as *credit law, collections, debt recovery*. What sources of information are found that might be helpful to an ambulatory care facility?

## REFERENCES/BIBLIOGRAPHY

Andress, A. A. (1996). *Saunders manual of medical office management*. Philadelphia: W. B. Saunders.

Humphrey, D. D. (1996). *Contemporary medical office procedures* (2nd ed.). Albany, NY: Delmar.

Keir, L., Wise, B. A., & Krebs, C. (1998). *Medical assisting: Administrative and clinical competencies* (4th ed.). Albany, NY: Delmar.

Kinn, M. E., & Woods, M. A. (1999). *The medical assistant: Administrative and clinical* (8th ed.). Philadelphia: W. B. Saunders.

Murato, S. (1994, October 24). Practice management. *Medical Economics*. Montvale, NJ: Medical Economics Publication.

# 21

# ACCOUNTING PRACTICES

## KEY TERMS

Accounting
Accounts Payable
Accounts Receivable (A/R) Ratio
Assets
Balance Sheet
Collection Ratio
Cost Accounting
Cost Analysis
Cost Ratio
Financial Accounting
Fixed Cost
Income Statement
Liability
Managerial Accounting
Owner's Equity
Utilization Review (UR)
Variable Cost

## OUTLINE

**Bookkeeping and Accounting Systems**
Single-Entry
Pegboard
Double-Entry
Computerized Systems
Computer Service Bureaus
**The Accounting Function**
**Cost Analysis**
Fixed Costs
Variable Costs

**Financial Records**
Income Statement
Balance Sheet
**Useful Financial Ratios**
Accounts Receivable Ratio
Collection Ratio
Cost Ratio
**Expenses of the Ambulatory Care Setting**
Accounts Payable
Payroll

## OBJECTIVES

*The student should strive to meet the following performance objectives and demonstrate an understanding of the facts and principles presented in this chapter through written and oral communication.*

1. Define the key terms as presented in the glossary.
2. Understand the purpose and range of the accounting function in the ambulatory care setting.
3. Describe the four different types of bookkeeping and accounting systems.
4. Compare and contrast financial, managerial, and cost accounting.
5. Explain the use and validity of the income statement and the balance sheet.
6. Recall three useful financial ratios and explain.
7. Identify proper steps in accounts payable management.
8. Discuss the impact of utilization review on reimbursement.

**ADMINISTRATIVE**

**Practice Finances**

- Apply bookkeeping principles
- Document and maintain accounting and banking records
- Manage accounts receivable
- Manage accounts payable
- Process payroll

**GENERAL (TRANSDISCIPLINARY)**

**Legal Concepts**

- Document accurately

**Operational Functions**

- Apply computer techniques to support office operations

When James Whitney, one of the physician-owners at Inner City Health Care, and Jane O'Hara, CMA, the office manager, decided to add a new medical assistant to the staff, they first reviewed the financial records for the previous year. While the volume of work in the center generated the need for an additional employee, Whitney and O'Hara had to be sure it was financially feasible. In addition to past records, they also had to make some projections for the upcoming year; with certain new managed care fees, they had to be sure that anticipated revenues would be sufficient to sustain the salary of a new employee.

## INTRODUCTION

Medical financial management in the ambulatory care setting is most important in the daily functioning of the office business as it directly affects overall bookkeeping and accounting procedures. Accounting generates financial information for the ambulatory care setting and is defined as a system of monitoring the financial status of a facility and the specific results of its activities. It provides financial information for decision making.

Previous chapters have included the topic of proper daily financial practices (Chapter 17), the accurate coding and the specific processing of insurance forms (Chapter 18 and Chapter 19), and the efficient management of collecting on accounts (Chapter 20). All of this is essential to obtain maximum reimbursement and create profitability for the practice.

This chapter ties many of these elements together and creates a total picture of their interdependence. Each element is critical to the ambulatory care setting's accurate accounting practices.

## BOOKKEEPING AND ACCOUNTING SYSTEMS

Medical offices utilize a variety of ways to monitor their financial accounts and the total financial operations of the business. Some small offices still use the single-entry bookkeeping and pegboard systems, while others prefer double-entry or computerized systems, or a combination.

### Single-Entry

The single-entry system has been used in the physician's office for many years. This includes a daily journal or log, patients' statements, ledgers, checks, and disbursement (expenditure) records. Information is first recorded in the journal, which provides a chronological record of financial transactions. Information from the journal is then transferred to the ledger through the process of posting. All amounts entered in the journal must be posted to the accounts kept in the ledger to summarize the results. This system has been used extensively in ambulatory care settings because of its simplicity and inexpensive nature.

However, it is difficult to find errors, for there are no internal controls, which is a topic that will be further discussed in this chapter.

### Pegboard

As discussed in Chapter 17, the pegboard system is often called "one write" or "write-it-once" system. The pegboard system is easier to use than the single-entry system and has greater internal controls. The pegboard system provides control over collections, payments, and charges. It utilizes No Carbon Required (NCR©) forms that are layered or shingled on pegs on the left of the board so that both income and disbursement entries need to be written only once. Many pegboard plans include a charge slip, which simplifies third-party payment processing for both the medical office and the patients. The charge slip is used to record the input needed during the patient's visit, while serving as the patient's receipt for services performed and fees charged. An advantage of the pegboard system is its accuracy; since data are entered at the time of service and not recopied, few errors can creep in.

## Double-Entry

The double-entry system is based on the fact that each transaction has two aspects; that is, a dual effect on the accounting elements. This system is based on the accounting principle that assets equal liabilities and owner's equity. **Assets** are the properties owned by the business (supplies, equipment, accounts receivable, and so on). **Liabilities** include what is owed to creditors. **Owner's equity** is the amount by which the business assets exceed the business liabilities. Net worth, proprietorship, and capital are often used as synonyms for owner's equity.

The double-entry system requires that the two aspects involved in every transaction be recorded on each side of the equation and that the two sides always be in balance. Although this accounting system requires time and skill, it provides a comprehensive financial picture and has built-in accuracy controls. It is orderly, fairly simple, flexible, and accurate, making it impossible for certain types of errors to remain undetected for long. For example, if one aspect of a transaction is properly recorded but the other aspect is overlooked, the records are out of balance. This occurrence may be easily discovered and subsequently corrected.

## Computerized Systems

 The majority of medical offices is relying on accounting software packages to prepare financial records, such as ledgers and reports, and to retrieve patient information. A computerized accounting system is most likely to be based on the principles of either the pegboard, write-it-once, or a double-entry bookkeeping system, or a combination of both.

Just as the pegboard system is customized to the individual ambulatory care setting, a computer system can also be customized to meet the needs of the practice. Most large multi-speciality clinics have a computer system designed particularly for their needs. Medical office software packages have the capabilities of including the most common procedure (CPT) and diagnostic (ICD-9-CM) codes within a database to be recalled when completing insurance claim forms or printing other computer-generated reports.

Computers also have the flexibility of assigning codes in other categories to indicate whether a bill has been paid with cash, a check, or by a third-party payer. Codes may also be assigned to place and type of service and the professional performing the service. This facilitates the tracking of payments and also allows for the analysis of specific sources that generate income for the practice. Adjustments to reflect discounts or reduced fees may also be entered into the computer. The computer is used in the preparation of billing statements, insurance forms, collection letters, and a number of financial ratios

and statements to assist in monitoring the practice's financial stability.

**Computers and Managed Care.** Computerization of the medical facility has increased due to the emphasis placed on the importance of accurate documentation of medical records and the shift from fee-for-service contracts to managed care plans. As medical facilities realized they needed to monitor more information, an increasing number of offices opted for computerization.

## Computer Service Bureaus

An option for ambulatory care settings that cannot afford the purchase of their own computers and software is to use a computer service bureau. In this case, the ambulatory care setting provides the data and the bureau provides basic billing and accounting services, furnishing financial statements, completed insurance forms, payroll materials, and checks.

Service bureaus handle accounts from the medical facilities in one of three ways:

1. Through the office's own computer terminal, on-line sharing occurs where the office is tied directly to the bureau's mainframe computer
2. Through on-line servicing, where the office has its own terminal which allows direct communication with the service bureau's computer
3. Through off-line batch processing, where the medical assistant or bookkeeper sends daily batches of data to the bureau to process

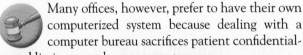 Many offices, however, prefer to have their own computerized system because dealing with a computer bureau sacrifices patient confidentiality and limits control over computer usage.

## THE ACCOUNTING FUNCTION

**Accounting** is a system of monitoring the financial status of a facility and the financial results of its activities. Accounting may be divided into two major categories: financial and managerial. **Financial accounting** provides information primarily for entities external to the organization such as the government. In contrast, **managerial accounting** generates financial information that can enable more efficient internal management. **Cost accounting** helps to determine what it costs the ambulatory care setting to perform particular services and is an integral part of managerial accounting. A hospital cost report for Medicare is essentially part of financial accounting, since the report is generated for an external user—the Health Care Financing Administration (HCFA), which administers the Medicare program. However, it is also a part of cost accounting because a cost report on Medicare will show what it costs to care for patients on Medicare.

## COST ANALYSIS

A very important aspect of the practice is the cost analysis. The purpose of the analysis is to determine the costs of each service. There are two factors to consider: fixed costs and variable costs.

### Fixed Costs

Fixed costs are costs that do not vary in total as the number of patients vary. For example, the annual depreciation cost of the equipment is fixed because it will remain the same regardless of the number of patients who use it.

### Variable Costs

Variable costs are those that vary in direct proportion to patient volume such as clinical supplies and laboratory procedures. Average costs to treat patients decline because of fixed costs not variable costs. The greater the volume, the more widely the fixed costs are spread and the less cost any one unit is responsible for.

Patient cost factors include administrative costs, such as the cost of billing and collections, personnel costs for office staff providing patient care, equipment costs, and costs for clinical supplies. The physician cost will include costs for interpreting tests, diagnosing illnesses, and the costs of professional liability insurance.

### COMPUTERIZING THE AMBULATORY CARE SETTING

If the ambulatory care setting is to be more computerized, whether through a service bureau or a complete on-site system, it is important to remember:

• Computerization will require more time than estimated.

• The paper-pencil bookkeeping system will have to be maintained concurrently for a period of time.

• A poorly managed paper-pencil system will not be made better by computerization.

• Adequate on-site computer training for all staff is essential.

• Notify patients of the move to a computer system and the changes that will occur.

For more information on computers in the ambulatory care setting, see Chapter 11.

### SPOTLIGHT ON AAMA ESSENTIALS THROUGH CAAHEP

● Maintaining the medical practice's financial profitability requires a medical assistant who is not only knowledgeable in this area, but who also maintains a high level of integrity and honesty.

● The medical assistant responsible for monitoring the accounts payable function of the office must be of high character, good moral standing, and above reproach in terms of handling money and other financial transactions.

● If required to perform any tasks related to employee salaries, the medical assistant needs to demonstrate a high degree of confidentiality and should never discuss topics related to specific employee salaries with anyone other than the employer-physician.

Calculating and reviewing costs provide the ambulatory care setting with data to set fees, market the practice, determine profit, and monitor the practice's performance.

## FINANCIAL RECORDS

Indicators of the financial status of the medical facility include financial statements that reflect the daily operations of the business. These records comprise an accounting information system that is maintained for numerous reasons, one of which is to provide source data for use in the preparation of various reports. Two financial statements common to the ambulatory care setting are the income/expense statement and the balance sheet.

### Income Statement

Figure 21-1 shows a sample income statement. The statement shows the cumulative profit and total expenses for the month. The statement is itemized to show operating expenses and employees' withholding taxes and retirement contributions. This statement enables the practice to monitor increases and decreases daily.

### Balance Sheet

Sometimes called the statement of financial condition or statement of financial position, the balance sheet is an

**INNER CITY HEALTH CARE**
**INCOME STATEMENT**

| | Month of ___, 20__ | Year-to-Date | Budget for Year | Overhead Percentages |
|---|---|---|---|---|
| A. Revenue: | | | | |
| 1. Office #1 | $ | $ | $ | |
| 2. Office #2 | $ | $ | $ | |
| | $ | $ | $ | 100% |
| B. Total Revenue: | | | | |
| C. Expenses: | | | | |
| 1. Non–doctor (staff) salaries—gross | $ | $ | $ | % |
| 2. Staff fringes | | | | |
| – Payroll taxes | $ | $ | $ | |
| – Empl. benefits | $ | $ | $ | |
| – Empl. seminars | $ | $ | $ | |
| – Uniforms | $ | $ | $ | |
| – Retirement plan | $ | $ | $ | |
| | $ | $ | $ | % |
| 3. Occupancy costs: | | | | |
| – Rent—Off. #1 | $ | $ | $ | |
| – Rent—Off. #2 | $ | $ | $ | |
| – Property taxes | $ | $ | $ | |
| – Insurance | $ | $ | $ | |
| – Utilities | $ | $ | $ | |
| – Janitor/Grounds | $ | $ | $ | |
| | $ | $ | $ | % |
| 4. Medical expenses: | | | | |
| – Medications | $ | $ | $ | |
| – Supplies | $ | $ | $ | |
| – Lab fees | $ | $ | $ | |
| | $ | $ | $ | % |
| 5. Office expenses: | | | | |
| – Office supplies | $ | $ | $ | |
| – Postage | $ | $ | $ | |
| – Telephone | $ | $ | $ | |
| | $ | $ | $ | % |
| 6. Malpractice ins. | $ | $ | $ | % |
| 7. Professional expenses: | | | | |
| – Auto expenses (Doctors') | $ | $ | $ | |
| – Dues/subscriptions | $ | $ | $ | |
| – Books and videos | $ | $ | $ | |
| – Dues/memberships | $ | $ | $ | |
| – Entertainment | $ | $ | $ | |
| – Professional development | $ | $ | $ | |
| – Travel | $ | $ | $ | |
| | $ | $ | $ | % |

*(continues)*

**Figure 21-1** A sample income statement that shows profit and expenses for one month.

itemized statement of the assets, liabilities, and owner's equity of a medical facility as of a specified date. Its purpose is to provide information regarding the status of these basic accounting elements.

The balance sheet is made possible through the double-entry system of accounting since every transaction is recorded by two sets of entries made in a ledger or journal. Increases in assets are recorded as debits; decreases are recorded as credits. Increases in liabilities and owner's equity are recorded as credits; decreases are recorded as debits.

Debit and credit entries to one or more accounts make up the system. In any recording, the total dollar amount of the debit entries must equal the total dollar

| | Month of ___ , 20__ | Year-to-Date | Budget for Year | Overhead Percentages |
|---|---|---|---|---|
| 8. Equipment costs: | | | | |
| – Depreciation/amortization | $ | $ | $ | |
| – Rent | $ | $ | $ | |
| – Service/maintenance | $ | $ | $ | |
| – Interest (if on equipment purchase loans) | $ | $ | $ | |
| | $ | $ | $ | % |
| 9. Marketing expenses | | | | |
| – Advertising | $ | $ | $ | |
| – Other fees | $ | $ | $ | |
| | $ | $ | $ | % |
| 10. Professional expenses: | | | | |
| – Accounting | $ | $ | $ | |
| – Legal | $ | $ | $ | |
| – Consulting | $ | $ | $ | |
| – Ret. Plan Admin. | $ | $ | $ | |
| | $ | $ | $ | % |
| 11. | | | | |
| 12. | | | | |
| 13. | | | | |
| 14. | | | | |
| D. Total Non–Doctor Expenses: | $ | $ | $ | % |
| E. Operating New Income Before Doctors' Costs (B minus C) | $ | $ | $ | % |
| F. Associate Physician's Costs: | | | | |
| – Salaries—gross: | $ | $ | $ | |
| – Benefits | $ | $ | $ | |
| – | $ | $ | $ | |
| – | $ | $ | $ | |
| G. Total Non–Owner Doctors' Costs | $ | $ | $ | % |
| H. New Income Available to Owner– Doctors (E minus G) | $ | $ | $ | % |
| I. Owner–Doctors' Costs: | | | | |
| 1. Salaries—gross: | | | | |
| –Dr. A | $ | $ | $ | |
| –Dr. B | $ | $ | $ | |
| 2. Bonuses—gross: | | | | |
| –Dr. A | $ | $ | $ | |
| –Dr. B | $ | $ | $ | |
| 3. Retirement contributions: | | | | |
| –Dr. A | $ | $ | $ | |
| –Dr. B | $ | $ | $ | |
| 4. "Semi-personal" expenses: | | | | |
| –Dr. A | $ | $ | $ | |
| –Dr. B | $ | $ | $ | |
| J. Total Owner–Doctors' Costs | $ | $ | $ | |
| K. Net Income (H minus J) | $ | $ | $ | |

**Figure 21-1**    (*continued*)

amount of the credit entries. Each ledger or journal entry should have the:

1. Date of transaction
2. Journal or ledger account names involved
3. Dollar amount of the charges
4. Brief explanation of the transaction

## USEFUL FINANCIAL RATIOS

There are a few financial ratios that can help evaluate how the practice is doing. Data from the current year and previous year's financial statements can be converted into ratios to highlight different financial characteristics.

Ratios should always be viewed in relationship to the total financial picture, however.

While two of these ratios were discussed in Chapter 20, some elaboration is in order in the context of this chapter.

## Accounts Receivable Ratio

The **accounts receivable (A/R) ratio** formula measures the speed in which outstanding accounts are paid. The accounts receivable ratio provides a picture of the state of collections and probable losses. The longer an account is past due, the less likelihood of successfully making the collection.

$$\frac{\text{Total Accounts Receivable}}{\text{Monthly Receipts}} = \text{Turnaround Time}$$

**Example:**

$$\frac{\$120,000}{\$60,000} = \begin{array}{l} \text{2 Months Turnaround Time} \\ \text{for Payment on an Account} \end{array}$$

The goal of an efficient billing and collecting policy should be a turnaround time of two months or less.

## Collection Ratio

The **collection ratio** shows the percentage of outstanding debt collected. The goal should be a 90 percent collection ratio. Total receipts divided by total charges give the unadjusted collection ratio, but adjustments may include federal and state insurance programs (Medicare and Medicaid, Workers' Compensation), managed care adjustments, and any other adjustments as directed by the physician.

| | |
|---|---|
| Total Receipts | = $40,000 |
| + Managed Care Adjustments | $3,000 |
| + Medicare Adjustments | $2,000 |
| TOTAL | $45,000 |
| Total Charges | $52,000 |

$$\frac{\text{Total Receipts } \$45,000}{\text{Total Charges } \$52,000} = \begin{array}{l} \text{86.5\% Collection Ratio} \\ \text{after Adjustments} \end{array}$$

## Cost Ratio

The **cost ratio** formula shows the cost of a procedure or service and can help in determining, for instance, the cost effectiveness of maintaining a laboratory in the ambulatory care setting. The ratio is:

$$\frac{\text{Total Expenses}}{\text{Total Number of Procedures for 1 Month}}$$

$$\frac{\text{Total Laboratory Expenses for September}}{\text{Total Number of Procedures Performed for September}}$$

$$\frac{\$48,000}{240} = \$200 \text{ per Procedure}$$

A conclusion might be reached that the lab is too costly because each procedure is not billed at $200.00.

# EXPENSES OF THE AMBULATORY CARE SETTING

While the ambulatory care setting is trying to maximize its income, it is also responsible for overhead costs, such as payroll and other accounts payable. Good financial management ensures that these costs are always met in a timely fashion.

## Accounts Payable

**Accounts payable** are an unwritten promise to pay a supplier for property or merchandise purchased on credit or for a service rendered. Accounts payable are the most common liability or financial obligation in a physician's office. These include expenses such as medical and office supplies, salaries, equipment, and services. Payments for these expenses are made by check to ensure complete, accurate records of all money received and disbursed. See Chapter 17 for information on writing checks.

The administrative medical assistant, the bookkeeper, or the office manager will monitor the accounts payable accounting functions. All bills received in the ambulatory care setting should be paid promptly. Some statements note that a discount of one or two percent is possible if paid within ten days of receipt of the bill. Such discounts should be noted and the bills paid within the time limit to warrant the discount.

The responsible person will check the accuracy of the statement, prepare the check, and mark on the statement date of payment, check number, and amount paid. The statements (noting payment) and checks are submitted for final approval and signature on the check by either the physician or office manager.

## Payroll

The administrative medical assistant is likely to be involved in making certain the W-4 form, the Employee's Withholding Allowance Certificate, is completed by all employees. However, salary calculations, withholding taxes, and social security calculations are the responsibility of the office manager. See Chapter 22.

## UTILIZATION REVIEW

In the present health care climate where there has been an increase in managed care plans with a corresponding decrease in the traditional indemnity fee-for-service contracts, more attention has been focused on how the billing and financial management process should proceed. Because of the influence of governmental mandates in the practice of medicine, and the growth of the utilization review industry, more accurate recordkeeping and documentation in all facets of the ambulatory care setting have become necessary. There are nearly 300 utilization review firms throughout the country. These companies aggressively sell their services to employers and to insurance carriers. Utilization review (UR) is actually a review of the service required before it may be performed. If the reviewer determines that the procedure or treatment is not needed, then it will not be approved or covered under the patient's insurance plan. Policies that once permitted medical decisions to be made solely by the physician are now made by other health professionals who are employed by UR firms. Some clinics may find it beneficial to have one medical assistant whose main responsibility is to present procedures to utilization review for acceptance or denial. Because of the increasing concern for quality of health care at low cost, more physicians also are realizing they need more documentation of both medical and financial information with more accessible means for retrieval.

**CASE STUDY 21-1**

Because the owners of Inner City Health Care need to make adequate income to pay all overhead and share in a profit, they are instituting new measures to reduce their costs of operating. However, they have fixed costs that they cannot change. So they plan to look at their variable costs to determine where they can reduce expenses without any reduction in quality of service.

### CASE STUDY REVIEW

1. What are some fixed costs that Inner City is likely to have?
2. What are some of the variable costs that should be considered when looking at profitability?
3. How may utilization review procedures affect the profitability of Inner City Health Care?

## SUMMARY

Medical financial management is crucial to the profitability of the ambulatory care setting. It is necessary for each medical facility to decide on which accounting system best serves the individual practice. Careful monitoring of billing procedures and aging accounts, and accurately documenting both the medical and financial record will help in providing a sound financial analysis and a strong financial foundation for the ambulatory care setting.

## REVIEW QUESTIONS

**Multiple Choice**

1. The "write-it-once" is a bookkeeping system also known as:
   a. single-entry
   b. pegboard
   c. double-entry
   d. disbursement

2. An example of a fixed cost is:
   a. salaries
   b. cost of supplies
   c. depreciation of equipment
   d. cost of treating patients

3. An itemized statement of financial position is the:
   a. income statement
   b. balance sheet

c. trial balance
d. collection ratio

4. The Employee's Withholding Allowance Certificate is the:
   a. W-2
   b. W-4
   c. FICA
   d. W-3

5. Utilization review:
   a. looks at the utility of all personnel
   b. examines how useful the ambulatory care center is to patients
   c. is a review of a procedure or treatment before it is performed to determine whether it is needed by the patient
   d. only affects hospitals

6. Assets include:
   a. equipment and supplies on hand
   b. building or property
   c. accounts receivable
   d. all the above

7. A computer service bureau:
   a. is the service you hire to care for the office computer system
   b. causes the office to sacrifice patient confidentiality
   c. can function through linkage of computers, on-line servicing or off-line batch processing.
   d. b and c above

8. In a medical facility where the total receipts including any adjustments are $83,500 and the total charges equal $97,750, the collection ratio:
   a. would be great at 94%
   b. would be quite good at 88%
   c. should be almost 85%
   d. shows a modest return at 75%

9. Money can be saved with accounts payable when:
   a. paid promptly
   b. discounts are realized
   c. realizing that buying in bulk is too expensive
   d. a and b above

## Critical Thinking

1. Why is medical financial management important?
2. List one advantage and one disadvantage of the single-entry bookkeeping system.
3. Discuss the pros and cons of an on-site complete computer system and a computer service bureau.
4. How may fixed and variable costs differ?
5. Review the importance of financial records and identify and state the differences between the two primary records.
6. Identify three useful ratios in calculating how a practice is doing.
7. Give examples of the preceding three ratios.
8. How does utilization review affect financial reimbursement in the ambulatory care setting?

## WEB ACTIVITIES

Using the World Wide Web, research companies producing and servicing medical software for use in the ambulatory care setting.

## REFERENCES/BIBLIOGRAPHY

Andress, A. A. (1996). *Manual of medical office management.* Philadelphia: W. B. Saunders Company.

Kinn, M. E., & Woods, M. A. (1999). *The medical assistant: Administrative and clinical* (8th ed.). Philadelphia: W. B. Saunders Company.

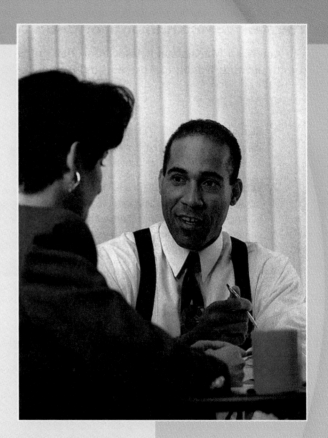

# PROFESSIONAL
# PROCEDURES

# OFFICE AND HUMAN RESOURCE MANAGEMENT

# Chapter 22

# THE MEDICAL ASSISTANT AS OFFICE MANAGER

## KEY TERMS

Agenda
Ancillary Services
Benchmark
Benefit
Bond
Brainstorming
Charisma
Embezzle
Emulate
Externship
Fringe Benefit
"Going Bare"
Hierarchy
Internet
Itinerary
Liability
Malpractice
Marketing
Minutes
Negligence
Paradigm
Practicum
Procedures Manual
Professional Liability Insurance
Profit Sharing
Risk Management
Search Engine
Self-actualization
Shadow
Subordinate
Teamwork
Web Site
Work Statement

## OUTLINE

The Medical Assistant as Manager
Qualities of a Manager
Management Styles
  People-oriented Personality
  Things-oriented Personality
  Idea-oriented Personality
  Other Management Styles
  Changing Styles for the Twenty-
    first Century
The Importance of Teamwork
  Getting the Team Started
  Using a Team to Solve a Problem
  Planning and Implementing a
    Solution
  Recognition
Supervising Personnel
  Staff Meetings
  Supporting Staff Members
Travel Arrangements
  Itinerary
Supervising Student Practicums
Time Management

Procedures Manual
  Organization of the Procedures
    Manual
  Updating and Reviewing the
    Procedures Manual
Marketing Functions
  Seminars
  Brochures
  Newsletters
  Press Releases
  Special Events
Record and Financial
  Management
  Payroll Processing
Facility and Equipment
  Management
  Inventories
  Equipment and Supplies
    Maintenance
Risk Management
Liability Coverage and Bonding

## OBJECTIVES

*The student should strive to meet the following performance objectives and demonstrate an understanding of the facts and principles presented in this chapter through written and oral communication.*

1. Define the key terms as presented in the glossary.
2. Describe the qualities of a manager.
3. Identify three types of personalities and their management styles.
4. Differentiate between authoritarian and democratic management styles.
5. Discuss characteristics of managers and leaders.

*(continues)*

6. Recall a minimum of four descriptions of managers/leaders for the new millennium.

7. List three benefits of a teamwork approach.

8. Discuss the importance of a meeting agenda.

9. List pieces of information that should be included in meeting minutes.

10. Identify the steps required to make travel arrangements.

11. Define the term itinerary and list important information the itinerary should contain.

12. List three methods of increasing productivity and efficient time management.

13. Describe the purpose of a procedures manual.

14. Describe the general concept of marketing and recall at least three marketing tools.

15. Describe the purpose and benefit of marketing.

16. Define records management, financial management, facility and equipment management, and risk management.

17. Describe the steps involved in payroll processing.

18. Describe liability coverage and what bonding means.

## ROLE DELINEATION COMPONENTS

### ADMINISTRATIVE
**Practice Finances**
- **Process Payroll**
- **Manage renewals of business and professional insurance policies (adv)**

### GENERAL (TRANSDISCIPLINARY)
**Professionalism**
- **Work as a team member**
- **Manage time effectively**
- **Prioritize and perform multiple tasks**
- **Facility planning (adv)**
- **Lead/motivate employees (adv)**
- **Plan and conduct staff meetings (adv)**
- **Train/orient employees (adv)**

(*continues*)

## SCENARIO

Marilyn Johnson has been employed by Doctors Lewis & King for the past eight years. Three years ago, she was promoted to the position of office manager when the facility added the second office for its associates in the next suburb. Marilyn has a baccalaureate degree in business administration. Her responsibilities at Doctors Lewis & King include various duties involving personnel, finances, and office efficiency.

## INTRODUCTION

The skills and growing complexity of medical specialization have broadened the scope of employment options for the medical assistant. Many ambulatory health care facilities are turning to managed care as a means of ensuring consumer use of the appropriate level of care and to facilitate cost containment. This approach has created opportunity for medical assistants to advance to the office manager (OM) position based on individual facility needs.

In general, the office manager should have a minimum of an associate's degree. Large corporate settings may employ an OM and a human resource (HR) person with some crossover of responsibilities depending on the needs and organizational structure of the facility. Most HR positions require a minimum of a bachelor's degree with validation that the person has been accepted to an accredited master's program. The role of the medical assistant as a human resources manager is covered in Chapter 23.

**Communication Skills**

- Promote the practice through positive public relations
- Serve as liaison (adv)

**Legal Concepts**

- Comply with established risk management and safety procedures
- Follow employer's established policies dealing with the health care contract
- Follow federal, state, and local legal guidelines
- Maintain awareness of federal and state health care legislation and regulations
- Participate in the development and maintenance of personnel, policy, and procedure manuals
- Develop and maintain personnel, policy, and procedure manuals (adv)

**Instruction**

- Locate community resources and disseminate information
- Develop educational materials (adv)

**Operational Functions**

- Maintain supply inventory
- Evaluate and recommend equipment and supplies
- Supervise personnel (adv)
- Negotiate leases and prices for equipment and supply contracts (adv)
- Negotiate managed care contracts (adv)
- Create spreadsheets and input data (adv)
- Create databases and input data (adv)
- Perform computer searches (adv)
- Transmit and receive data and messages by Internet, e-mail, and web site (adv)

# THE MEDICAL ASSISTANT AS MANAGER

The office manager of a medical office or ambulatory care facility is a role that can have vast and diverse responsibilities. In some offices, there may be one office manager and a separate human resources manager. In others, one person may be responsible for all duties that can fall under the role of office manager and human resources manager. This chapter covers the following office manager duties:

1. Create and update the office procedures manual
2. Supervise office personnel
3. Assist in improving work flow and office efficiencies (time management)
4. Prepare staff meeting agenda, conduct the meeting, and record minutes
5. Supervise the purchase, repair, and maintenance of office equipment
6. Supervise the purchase and storage of office supplies
7. Supervise the purchase and storage of controlled substances
8. Approve financial transactions and account disposition; generate financial reports as needed
9. Make travel arrangements and prepare an itinerary
10. Prepare patient education materials and arrange patient/community education workshops as needed
11. Arrange and maintain practice insurance and develop risk management strategies

## QUALITIES OF A MANAGER

Qualifications of the manager will vary from office to office, however, some general requirements are common to any office setting. Attributes needed to perform as a high quality manager include but are not limited to the following:

- *People Skills.* The office manager must like people in general and enjoy working with them. Building confidence and self-esteem in others and being interested in promoting constructive relationships are essential qualities of the office manager. The ability to function as an effective team leader provides a role model for other staff members to **emulate.**

- *Truthfulness.* Lead by example! If an honest mistake is made, be the first to admit to the error and seek the best solution for preventing it from happening again. Respond honestly to requests. For example, two staff members ask for the same day off. The office manager will make the decision that only one member may have the day off and will review the policy manual to determine the appropriate criteria for designating who will have the request granted.

- *Fairmindedness.* It is important to always be fair with co-workers. Decisions that impact one fellow employee create a ripple effect. That is, you may have to make the same decision for another employee at another time. Decisions should be based, as much as possible, on the assumption that what is granted to one employee will be granted to others in similar situations. This approach will decrease the risk of being accused of playing favorites or being unfair.

- *Effective Communication Skills.* Communication skills include written and oral methods. The manager must communicate clearly, diplomatically, tactfully, and with respect for the feelings of others.

● *Organizational Skills.* Being organized includes being able to prioritize tasks, working efficiently and methodically. Know when and be willing to delegate tasks when others have the expertise and time to complete the task within the time lines.

● *Objectivity.* The manager must be able to view challenges without bias or prejudice. For example, when promotions are made, the office manager must be able to focus on the job description criteria and individual qualifications without introducing personal preference.

● *Problem-solving Skills.* The office manager must be a problem solver. This may include being creative and doing away with old **paradigms** and traditional approaches to solving a problem. When difficult issues arise, focus on the situation, issue, or behavior, not on the person. A discussion about solving the problem without laying blame is much more productive. Positive solutions may be more readily attained when discussing what was observed rather than what was told by someone else.

● *Technical Expertise.* The office manager should have a working knowledge of each procedure performed in the office, although it is not necessary to be the acknowledged technical expert. A good office manager is continually learning and encourages **subordinates** to seek opportunities to continue their education and advance their technical skills.

## MANAGEMENT STYLES

There is a direct correlation between a person's personality and his or her management style. Three types of personalities and their management styles are discussed here (Institute for Management Excellence, 1998; Pyzdek, 1996).

### People-oriented Personality

A team-oriented management style is most often used by people-oriented personalities. This personality is comfortable teaching, coaching, helping, communicating, advising, motivating, guiding, leading, and inspiring others. People-oriented managers tend to use the participatory management style by establishing and communicating the purpose and direction of the task and soliciting the participation of employees. These managers are leaders who use actions and words to show the way and inspire employees. They tend to coach by evaluating and advising, motivating and guiding.

**SPOTLIGHT ON AAMA ESSENTIALS THROUGH CAAHEP**

● Creating a positive office atmosphere helps to ease the patient's fears and feelings of helplessness.

● Training and supporting staff members in cultural diversity issues establishes a precedent for meeting the widely diverse needs of all patients.

● Being able to accept and offer criticism and to implement change are required attributes of a successful office manager.

### Things-oriented Personality

Things-oriented personalities tend to have more process-oriented management styles. They are most comfortable with physical dexterity, building, constructing, modeling, remodeling, and working with tools or instruments. The autocratic management style is often used by this personality. Autocratic managers function on the premise that in most cases employees cannot make a contribution to their own work, and that even if they could, they wouldn't. Autocratic managers deal with this perception by using "carrots" and "sticks." The "carrot," in most cases, is a monetary incentive and the "stick" is docked pay for poor quality work.

### Idea-oriented Personality

The innovation-oriented management style is most often employed by idea-oriented personalities. These managers are most comfortable working with ideas and information. Management by wandering around (MBWA) is often used by them to collect information that can then be used to generate new ideas and approaches to doing the job. MBWA users are observant and ask questions to get at the problem. Once the problem has been clearly identified they enjoy research, data collection, and then brainstorming sessions to arrive at solutions.

### Other Management Styles

In some organizations the **hierarchy** is viewed as a "chain-of-command." The person in the topmost position on the organizational chart is the ultimate authority. This person may delegate authority to a subordinate who may, in turn, delegate authority to positions further down in the hierarchy. But these managers must possess complete knowledge of the work being done by their subordinates. This management style is often referred to as the authoritarian style. The manager holds all authority and responsibility and communicates from the top of the hierarchy down.

In the democratic management style, the person at the top of the organization holds final responsibility but also delegates authority to others by developing a shared vision of the goals and objectives of the organization. Communication is very active, flowing upward to higher authorities and downward to subordinates.

## Changing Styles for the Twenty-first Century

Today, managers are often seen as administrators rather than leaders. An administrator is one who executes, directs, or manages affairs. A leader, on the other hand, is a person who shows the way or guides. As we move into the twenty-first century, office managers will be called upon to be leaders and possess leadership qualities.

A good leader is one who can inspire others by example. In the medical office setting, a leader has the ability to inspire employees in a direction that benefits the entire facility. A leader excels in achieving goals and therefore influences others to be goal setters and achievers as well. Managers become leaders by demonstrating on a daily basis that they believe in their vision for the organization. Leaders have **charisma**, that is, they motivate others and inspire allegiance and devotion. Table 22-1 contrasts some management and leadership characteristics. Table 22-2 contains suggested management techniques and a brief description of the managers and leaders of the new millennium. Notice the importance of leadership characteristics as opposed to management characteristics in these descriptions.

| TABLE 22-1 | MANAGEMENT AND LEADERSHIP CHARACTERISTICS |
|---|---|
| **Management Characteristics** | **Leadership Characteristics** |
| Punishment | Reward |
| Demands respect | Invites speaking out |
| Drill sergeant | Motivator |
| Limits and defines | Empowers |
| Imposes discipline | Values creativity |
| Bottom line | Vision |
| Control | Change |
| Hierarchy | Network |
| Rigid | Flexible |
| Automatic annual raises | Pay for performance |
| Dominates | Facilitates |
| Issues orders | Acts as role model |
| Demands unquestioning obedience | Coaches and mentors others |
| Knows all the answers | Asks the right questions |
| Not interested in new answers | Seeks to learn and draw out new ideas |

*Source:* The Institute for Management Excellence. (1996, October). Managers vs. leaders. *Management vs. Leadership* [On-line]. Available: www.itstime.com/oct96b.htm.

## THE IMPORTANCE OF TEAMWORK

The use of **teamwork** to improve the efficiency of the office may at first seem incongruent to your desire to improve office efficiency, since it seems that several people are now involved in solving a problem that you the manager should solve and explain. Teamwork builds morale and actually results in getting more accomplished with the resources you have because the team members

| TABLE 22-2 | DESCRIPTIONS OF MANAGERS AND LEADERS |
|---|---|
| Management by Coaching and Development (MBCD) | Managers see themselves primarily as employee trainers. |
| Management by Competitive Edge (MBCE) | Individuals and groups within the organization compete against one another to see who can achieve the best results. |
| Management by Decision Models (MBDM) | Decisions are based on projections generated by artificially constructed situations. |
| Management by Exception (MBE) | Managers delegate as much responsibility and activity as possible to those below them, stepping in only when absolutely necessary. |
| Management by Performance (MBP) | Managers seek quality levels of performance through motivation and employee relations. |
| Management by Styles (MBS) | Managers adjust their approaches to meet situational needs. |
| Management by Walking Around (MBWA) | Managers walk around the company, getting a "feel" for people and operations; stopping to talk and to listen. |
| Management by Work Simplification (MBWS) | Managers constantly seek ways to simplify processes and reduce expenses. |

*Source:* The Institute for Management Excellence. (1996, October). Management styles. *Management vs. Leadership* [On-line]. Available: www.itstime.com/oct96.htm.

develop ownership of the solution to a problem and want to make it work. When it works, it flatters them and builds their esteem.

Efficiency of a team results from the collective working together to plan how to "work smarter" and how to dovetail tasks and support each other so that wasted effort is avoided. In order to achieve all of these things, a team must not only be given the responsibility and the authority to plan and execute their plan to solve a problem, but they must know your expectations for them. Sometimes this means that you, the office manager, must stick your neck out for them. They will reward you handsomely for doing so.

## Getting the Team Started

A successful teamwork approach is not a mysterious event that just happens, it is the result of clear vision, specific goals, and a well-planned strategy on the part of the team leader. For teamwork to be successful, individual team members must understand and support the specifics of the problem they are being asked to solve. This is probably the most significant task of the team leader or the office manager. It is helpful in taking this important step to let the team develop its own work statement, for in this way they assume ownership of the goals and objectives you want them to achieve. The work statement frequently outlines specific tasks and their sequential order of accomplishment. Its purpose is to ensure that everyone is working toward the team goals and objectives.

A major pitfall at this stage may be diverse opinions which can lead to a work statement that does not meet the manager's goals and objectives for the team. It is your job as office manager to try to direct the team back to what you want them to work on without undermining their team spirit. Take care at this stage not to begin making assignments or to let team members start solving the problem until the work statement is complete. Under some circumstances it may be necessary for you, the office manager, to exercise your authority in defining the work statement, but be careful, as this approach could harm the team's collective spirit.

The next step in team development is to establish a timetable for achieving results and identifying the standards that must be maintained. Without a timetable a team feels no sense of urgency and tends to lose direction. You also have to paint a clear picture of the standards that must be maintained as you attempt to solve the problem. You should let the team develop both the standards as well as the timetable, but with your leadership and support.

## Using a Team to Solve a Problem

Problem solution is the next step in team development. Some people call this stage brainstorming a solution.

Brainstorming is fun, but unless it is controlled by the leader, it will bog down into needless arguments and hurt feelings. In a successful brainstorming session everyone should feel free to contribute solutions to the problem without any consideration for practicality or flaws in the proposal. Only after everyone has had a chance to speak are the solutions looked at in terms of practicality and for technical correctness. At this point the team should not look at what is wrong with the solution, but what needs to be done to make it a workable solution.

Prioritization of the solutions comes next. In order to do this it is helpful to assign scores for impact on solving the problem and for changeability, or the difficulty in implementing a particular solution in your office environment. The result will be a list of solutions to the problem in descending order from the greatest impact on the problem with the least cost or difficulty in implementation. Do a needs assessment, remove oneself from the issue, and look at it from a different perspective. Benchmark (compare) your facility to other facilities and organizations to see how they accomplish tasks, compensate employees, and so on.

## Planning and Implementing a Solution

The team should work out a detailed plan for implementation of the solution selected, including a schedule. Assignments should be made, resources of equipment and funds available to the team should be defined, and any remaining problems assigned to subteams that will function just as the primary team did in solving them. The team should continue to meet to discuss progress and to resolve additional problems that may occur.

## Recognition

A successful team should not be disbanded until it is acknowledged for its efforts and physical recognition is given in the case of an important problem that was solved. In some cases, a dinner or luncheon is in order. This is the most important phase of team development, as it is responsible for developing a team spirit or sense of self-actualization within the organization. Once this spirit is implanted into an organization, it becomes infectious.

## SUPERVISING PERSONNEL

Creating an atmosphere in which open and honest communication can take place is critical to supervising personnel. This type of communication may be encouraged through the establishment of regular staff meetings, with each staff member sharing ideas for improvement and areas of concern. Eliciting the help of others in problem-solving strategies will promote harmony (Figure 22-1).

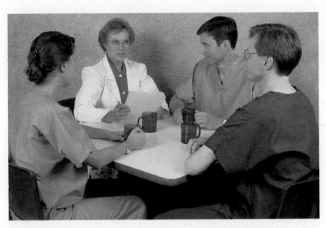

**Figure 22-1** Consistently scheduled staff meetings can help office managers understand staff concerns as well as allow managers to communicate with the staff. This personal communication can help promote harmony among the health care team.

## Staff Meetings

The office manager usually initiates the staff meeting idea and should officiate at such meetings. Failure of the office manager to be present may convey a message that the meeting is an event not worthy of attention. It is important that the office manager be familiar with basic parliamentary procedures. The purchase of books such as *Robert's Rules of Order* or *Parliamentary Procedure at a Glance* is an excellent investment.

Successful staff meetings are announced well in advance or on established time lines to enable the majority of the office personnel to attend. An **agenda** identifying the subjects to be covered during a given meeting should be issued prior to the meeting so that each attendee arrives prepared with input and/or questions relevant to the topics. Procedure 22-1 outlines the procedural steps for creating a meeting agenda. Figure 22-2 is a sample agenda. Each meeting should end with opportunity for nonagenda items to be discussed or suggested for inclusion in the next meeting. The meeting should have a fixed time to end.

A written record in the form of **minutes** should be maintained and sent to all team members regardless of whether they attended the meeting. This policy will keep all members informed about policy changes and decisions that impact the office operations. The minutes also trigger a reminder for any new procedures or revisions to be made in the procedures manual. See Chapter 15 for additional information related to agendas and minutes.

The first paragraph of the minutes should contain the following pieces of information:

- Kind of meeting (scheduled staff meeting, special meeting)

---

**AGENDA**

STAFF MEETING Wednesday, February 16, 2002
2:00 PM — Conference Room

1. Read and approve minutes of last meeting

2. Reports
   A. Satellite facility — Marilyn Johnson
   B. Patient flow — Joe Guerrero
   C.

3. Discussion of new telephone system

4. Unfinished Business
   A. Review new procedure manual pages
   B.

5. New Business
   A. Appoint committee for design of new marketing brochure
   B.

6. Open discussion and/or topics for next meeting's agenda

7. Set next meeting time

8. Adjourn

**Figure 22-2** Sample meeting agenda.

- Name of the organization (Doctors Lewis & King)
- Date, time, and place of the meeting
- Names of those attending and who was the chair of the meeting
- Approval of previous minutes

The following paragraphs should address each of the agenda topics and include a brief summary of discussions, actions taken, name of person making any motions, the exact wording of the motion, and whether the motion was approved.

In addition to recording action plans under each agenda topic, it is desirable to summarize all action items agreed to in the meeting in one section of the minutes. This will facilitate easy access to information at a later date should it be required.

The last paragraph should include the date, time, and place of the next meeting and the hour of adjournment for this meeting. The person preparing the minutes should always sign them. A copy of the minutes should always be maintained in a book for easy reference.

## Supporting Staff Members

The office manager may also be responsible for the following roles related to supporting staff employees. In large offices or clinics some of these responsibilities may be delegated to the human resources manager and are more fully covered in Chapter 23.

- Interview, hire, and terminate employees as delegated by the physician(s)/employer.

- Supervise or personally train employees. These responsibilities apply to new staff members as well as to updating current staff.

- Make weekly work schedules, vacation schedules, and determine how sick days will be covered effectively.

- Provide adequate staffing for employee absences.

- Establish probation periods within the legal boundaries of the employer and conduct performance evaluations as delegated by the physician(s)/employer.

- Establish increases and changes in the benefit package. These responsibilities should always be discussed with the physician(s)/employer first to be sure that the office manager is acting within the guidelines and scope of tasks delegated to that position.

## TRAVEL ARRANGEMENTS

The office manager may be asked to make travel arrangements for physicians going on vacation or to conventions, symposiums, or out-of-town seminars and continuing medical education (CME) courses. If the physicians do a fair amount of travel or if they live in a metropolitan area, they may utilize the services of a travel agent. Attention to detail is extremely important in preventing travel disruptions.

Read carefully the instructions for completing registration forms, complete them, and mail them as quickly as possible to secure reservations to conventions, etc. Next make hotel and travel arrangements. General information regarding the physician's travel preferences should be maintained in a file folder and be referred to when making travel arrangements. Helpful information to maintain in this file includes:

- Name of travel agents used in the past (ranked by reputation and recommendation)

- Physician's or office credit card numbers

- Car rental preference

- Preferred airline, class of travel, seating choice

- Hotel/motel accommodations (bed size, suite, studio, connecting rooms, price range, amenities)

- Shuttle service

Next, contact the travel agent and identify the destination, date and time for departure and return, number traveling in party, and seating preference. A travel agent can also assist with rental car and hotel accommodations if needed. Take your time and pay attention to detail. When tickets are received, always check to see that all departure and arrival times match what is needed and that a confirmation number has been provided for car rentals and hotel arrangements. Procedure 22-2 outlines the procedural steps involved in making travel arrangements through a travel agent.

The Internet may be used to search for the lowest cost air, auto, and lodging reservations. The procedures do not require extensive knowledge of travel and airline reservation protocols. Searching for information on the **Internet** requires the use of a search engine if you do not already have a list of favorite travel **web sites**. A **search engine** is a special computer program available through your Internet service provider. With a search engine, you enter only the subject of your search and the engine will provide a list of web sites related to your subject. For example, if you are making travel arrangements you might access a search engine such as Lycos and key in the subject "air fares." The engine will return either a list of web sites or ask you to further refine your subject with suggestions such as cheap air fares, international travel, etc. Once you have refined your search, you may have choices such as Only-Travel.com, Expedia.com, or Priceline.com. Select the appropriate web site and follow its instructions.

Priceline.com and similar web sites are services that allow you to name the price you want to pay; Priceline finds a major airline willing to release seats on flights where they have unsold space. You need to have a reasonable idea of the price of the service you are trying to purchase; unreasonably low bids will just waste your time and effort. Procedure 22-3 outlines the steps for making travel arrangements via the Internet.

## Itinerary

If you have utilized a travel agent in making the travel arrangements the agency will most likely provide several copies of the **itinerary**. An itinerary is a detailed plan for a proposed trip. The office should maintain one copy of the itinerary in case the physician must be reached for emergencies. The physician should have one copy to carry with him or her and a copy to leave with family members.

---

## TRAVEL ITINERARY

**James Whitney, MD**
**Inner City Health Care**
**400 Inner City Way**
**Seattle, WA 98400**

Sept 15, 20--        INVOICE: 880133795

**29 Sept 20-Friday**

| | | | |
|---|---|---|---|
| USAIR | 6:30 | Coach Class | Equip-Boeing 757 Jet |
| LV: Seattle | | 11:55P | Nonstop    Miles-2125    Confirmed |
| AR: Pittsburgh | | 7:23A | Elapsed time-4:28    Arrival Date-30Sept |
| | | | Seat-31C |

**30 Sept-Saturday**

Alamo                    1 Compact 2/4 DR    Drop-101CT    Confirmed
Pickup-Pittsburgh              Pittsburgh Airport    Chg-USD .00
Rate-        59.98    Baserate              Guaranteed        Extra Hr 10.00-UN
Phone-412-472-5060

Confirmation-1870649

**01 Oct 20-Sunday**

| | | | |
|---|---|---|---|
| USAIR | 1419 Coach Class | | Equip-Boeing 737 Jet |
| LV: Pittsburgh | 3:05P | | Nonstop    Miles-2125    Confirmed |
| AR: Seattle | 5:27P | | Elapsed time-5:22 |
| Lunch | | | Seat-20A |

Ticket Number/s:
Whitney/James        35709334923        BA Card            461.00
    Air Transportation    416.36        Tax    44.64    TOTAL    461.00
                                Sub Total            461.00
                                Credit Card Payment    461.00-
                                Amount Due            0.00

TICKET IS NON REFUNDABLE. TRIP INSURANCE IS AVAILABLE. RECONFIRM ALL FLTS 24 HRS PRIOR TO DEPARTURE

**Figure 22-3**   Sample travel itinerary.

You may need to develop the itinerary if you have made the travel arrangements via computer. Figure 22-3 shows a sample travel itinerary.

Important information to be included on any itinerary includes:

- Air travel: departure and arrival date and time, meals, airline name and telephone number, airport
- Car rental: name of provider, telephone number, confirmation number
- Hotel/motel: name, confirmation number, dates, telephone number
- Meeting location: name, address, room number, telephone number

## SUPERVISING STUDENT PRACTICUMS

The student **practicum** is a transitional stage that provides opportunity for the student to apply theory learned in the classroom to a health care setting through practical, hands-on experience. Institutions accredited by the Committee on Accreditation of Allied Health Education Programs (CAAHEP) call this period **externship**. Some institutions may use the term *internship* and still others may operate through a co-operative education program. The number of hours for the practicum are predetermined along with criteria for site selection and tasks performed by the student.

The office manager should schedule an information interview with the extern student before the practicum begins. During this time a discussion of the expectations of the office manager and the extern may be established. A tour of the facility and introductions to key personnel aids the extern in feeling more comfortable the first day of "work."

Since the extern will be writing in medical records where correct spelling is mandatory or may be scheduling appointments and must write telephone numbers without transposition, some pretesting may be offered. By giving a spelling test of ten commonly used medical terms or verbally stating five telephone numbers for the extern to write down, an immediate evaluation is attained.

The office manager should directly supervise or identify someone else to supervise the extern. During the first few days of the practicum, the extern may simply shadow the supervisor, learning the routine, physician preference, and protocols for that particular office. As the extern begins to feel comfortable in the new environment, minimal tasks should be assigned. Based on the extern's ability to follow directions and perform tasks, increased skill-level tasks may be added.

The supervisor will supervise and evaluate the extern's progress; schedule activities that will provide experience in all aspects of medical assisting, including administrative, clinical, and laboratory procedures; maintain accurate records of attendance and hours "worked"; and communicate the extern's progress to the medical assisting supervisor from the educational institution. Procedure 22-4 provides steps for supervising a student practicum.

When working with externs, it is important to remember that they still have much to learn. When you take time to explain each step and to provide the rationale for each, students will learn more quickly. Demonstrating new and/or different techniques and approaches helps students by providing them with options that they may find more comfortable.

Remember that this type of learning is very stressful. The extern is not yet accustomed to communication with a "real" patient, let alone working with a physician. Your role as office manager is to reduce as much stress as possible for everyone concerned. Introduce the extern to the patient and ask the patient's permission to allow the student to perform a procedure. Many patients will be very tolerant when they realize the circumstances and will be quite cooperative.

## TIME MANAGEMENT

Because medical office managers are responsible for numerous tasks and may experience many interruptions during the course of the day, it is important that they become disciplined and work well independently as well as with others. By focusing and pinpointing specific goals, which in turn may be translated into tasks to be completed during the workday, much can be accomplished.

Many office managers find it helpful to develop a "To Do" list on which tasks to be accomplished are listed. These tasks may be prioritized or simply listed as they come to mind or occur during the day. As each task is completed, it is crossed off. At the end of the day a sense of accomplishment is the reward for a clean list. Any tasks not yet completed may be prioritized and transferred to the next day's "To Do" list.

As much as possible, try to handle a paper only once. Read it, decide what action needs to be taken, and complete it. When responding to telephone calls, try also to bring closure to the call so that it is not necessary to make another call.

Do not procrastinate. Complete tasks as they arise whenever possible. Sometimes it takes longer to list a task on the "To Do" list and then have to rethink the solution than to just do it.

## PROCEDURES MANUAL

The procedures manual provides detailed information relative to the performance of tasks within the facility in which one is employed. Each procedures manual should be designed for that specific office setting and should satisfy its requirements.

The procedures manual serves as a guide to the employee assigned a specific task and may also be useful in evaluating the employee's performance. If a temporary employee is assigned the task, the procedures manual will be invaluable in assuring that each procedure is completed as outlined.

The physician(s) and the office manager should have copies of the procedures manual and it should also be accessible to all employees. Copies of individual sections may be given to the employee responsible for the task; the employee should be instructed to follow these guidelines and told that they may be used as employee evaluation tools.

### Organization of the Procedures Manual

It is best to use a loose-leaf binder with separator pages denoting each procedure. Many office managers find it helpful to divide the binder into administrative and clini-

| Administrative Section | Clinical Section |
|---|---|
| Personnel Management | Physical Examinations |
| Communication | Infection Control |
| (oral and written) | Collecting Specimens |
| Patient Scheduling | Laboratory Procedures |
| Records Management | Surgical Asepsis |
| Financial Management | Emergencies |
| Facility and Equipment | |
| Management | |

**Figure 22-4** Many offices find that dividing the procedures manual into tabbed sections helps organize the material. A table of contents for the manual can also help locate information easily.

cal sections with subdivisions for each primary task performed (Figure 22-4).

To facilitate using the procedures manual, a consistent format should be developed and used throughout the manual. Each procedure should be a step-by-step outline or list of steps to be taken to complete a task as desired in that facility. Providing the rationale for a step, when appropriate, enhances the learning process, especially for new staff members. Procedure 22-5 provides steps for developing and maintaining a procedures manual.

## Updating and Reviewing the Procedures Manual

When new procedures are added to the office routine, a new procedure page should be developed immediately. The new page is then useful as an educational tool or job aid while team members are learning new techniques.

An annual page-by-page review should be done to ascertain if each procedure is still being used and assure that each page is correct in each detail and satisfies all criteria established by the staff personnel. This contributes to an efficient office and gives all employees a sense of pride and satisfaction that they are performing within the scope of their training and to their greatest potential. The procedures manual should be reviewed by personnel performing the various tasks and their suggestions should be evaluated and incorporated into the revisions when appropriate. All new procedure pages and revisions should be dated (Rev. 02/15/02).

## MARKETING FUNCTIONS

Effective communication skills are essential in the management of the ambulatory care setting. These skills are used by the office manager inside the ambulatory care setting to establish friendly, professional relationships with colleagues and patients. Communication is just as critical when relating to external audiences: other organizations, potential new patients, and community members. Developing relationships outside the office is often called marketing, a concept that office managers may utilize to enhance the image and visibility of an ambulatory care setting while also providing benefits to patients, potential patients, and the neighboring community.

In its broadest sense, **marketing** can be defined as the process by which the provider of services makes the consumer aware of the scope and quality of these services. While marketing is a tool traditionally used by for-profit organizations to promote and sell products and services, it has become increasingly acceptable among health care organizations, whether they are for- or not-for-profit.

Marketing functions and materials are diverse and can include seminars and workshops, patient education brochures, brochures that describe the ambulatory care setting and its scope of services, newsletters, press releases, and special events such as open houses or participation in community health care events. Depending on the size and resources of the medical office, the manager may choose to use all or some of these tools (Figure 22-5).

 When producing written material and organizing events, it is essential that ethical guidelines be respected at all times. Marketing tools should be appropriate, in good taste, and designed to quietly enhance the reputation of the office. Cultural issues should always be considered. For example, patient education brochures for a practice with many Spanish-speaking patients should be produced in bilingual editions, with English on one side and Spanish on the other. Legal issues are important as well; when presenting material of a medical nature, it is extremely important that information be accurate and up-to-date.

Effective marketing is a valuable tool for the office manager, especially as managed care calls on all health care professionals to become more competitive in order to survive. Marketing can increase visibility and credibility. The effective manager will enlist the talents and skills of the entire team in developing a marketing plan.

## Seminars

As consumers become increasingly aware of lifestyle choices, they look to health care professionals for information and guidance. Seminars and workshops are useful vehicles for presenting health-related information; while expert advice can be given, there is also the opportunity for patients and health care professionals to interact.

| Marketing Tool | Potential Uses and Value |
|---|---|
| Seminars | Can educate patients and provide good will in the community. All staff—administrative and clinical—can work as a team to organize, publicize, and deliver the seminars. |
| Brochures | Brochures are typically of two types: patient education brochures and brochures on office services. Can be simple 8 1/2" x 11" fact sheets, with text only, or more elaborate brochures folded to 4" x 9" that incorporate both text and graphics or photos. Both types of brochures are informative for patients and present a professional image of the ambulatory care setting. |
| Newsletters | Newsletters can be produced on a biannual or quarterly basis and can form the nucleus of a marketing program. Because they are versatile tools, they can include a wide range of information from health-related articles to staff introductions to insurance updates. They should be sent to individuals on the office's mailing list and be available in the reception area. |
| Press Releases | Periodic press releases on new equipment, new staff, and expanded or remodeled office space can be a vital link to the local community. |
| Special Events | Special events are an effective way to join with other community organizations to promote wellness. They can include participation in health fairs, cosponsorship of a charity event, or an open house on the premises to acquaint the community with new services or equipment. |

**Figure 22-5** Marketing tools and their use in a medical environment.

Seminars can be organized to meet patient and community needs. Some popular seminar topics include hypertension, diabetes, eating disorders, and exercise and weight management programs.

No matter what the topic area, the content should be oriented to the lay person's level of understanding, with a focused message and a delivery designed to maintain attention. Interactive seminars, which encourage audience participation, can be productive and enjoyable. Audiovisuals, such as projected slides, will provide visual reinforcement. Handouts, either from professional organizations or those produced by office staff, can elaborate on seminar content and help the participant review and remember what was said.

## Brochures

Despite the promise of a paperless society, brochures continue to be valuable sources of information. In the health care setting, patients welcome a rack of brochures as a source of current, accurate background on medical issues. New patients also find that a brochure on office services will answer many questions about the practice, its philosophy, and its scope of services, and provide physician profiles.

Today, it is possible to produce a professional-looking brochure in the office using one of the computer programs that integrate text and graphics. If a brochure is produced in-house, it is important to consider writing, design, and production. Writing should be clear, to the point, and grammatically correct. Always proofread carefully before printing. Design should be kept simple; while computer programs offer sophisticated options, these are best left to experienced designers. Avoid the use of too many typefaces; choose a typeface and size for readability, and, if using artwork or photography, consider its reproduction qualities. Typically, brochures will be printed in one or two colors. Black or another dark ink is best for readability.

Often, a local printer will be able to advise the office manager on how to prepare a brochure or handout for printing. The simplest handouts can be quick-copied (a high-speed photocopy) on a white or lightly colored or textured stock. After printing, brochures should be made accessible to patients and other visitors in a rack or neatly arranged in piles (Figure 22-6). Occasionally, a brochure will be mailed; one that folds to 4" × 9" will fit into a standard #10 business envelope.

**Patient Education Brochures.** Like seminars, patient education brochures can address a variety of topics, including hypertension, diabetes, eating disorders, and exercise and weight management programs. When writing these brochures, always research material carefully, request permission for copyrighted materials, and present the information in a manner that is accessible to your patient population.

**Office Brochures.** A brochure on the practice can provide a wide range of information and will orient the new patient to the practice. One way to determine what information to include is to develop a list of frequently asked patient questions. Once this list is compiled, it can serve as the beginning of the brochure outline. Issues to consider might include:

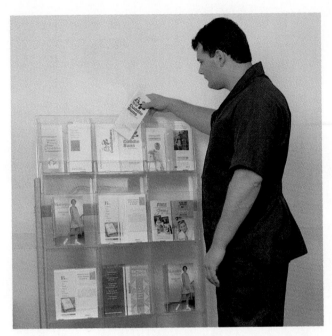

**Figure 22-6** Brochures and handouts should be accessible and inviting to patients and office visitors.

- Brief history of the practice
- Brief resumes or credentials of physicians
- Philosophy of the practice
- Scope of services
- How to reach the practice in case of emergency
- Insurances accepted
- Rights of patients
- Policies regarding the release of information
- Scheduling information: How to schedule an appointment, cancellation policies
- Amenities on the premises such as parking, pharmacy, lab
- Location, map if necessary, and location of satellite offices

## Newsletters

Newsletters are effective communication tools because they encourage regular contact with patients and other readers. Newsletters are a versatile medium, too; they can contain patient education articles, updates on staff changes, awards, information on insurance carriers, calendars of events, even recipes that are consistent with a healthful lifestyle.

Most newsletters can be written and produced in the office. Like brochures, they should be simple in design and format. An additional factor in newsletter production is mailing; an up-to-date database must be maintained, postal regulations must be followed, and the costs of mailing considered.

## Press Releases

Press releases are simple, inexpensive marketing tools. Use them to announce new staff, promote a new service, or publicize a series of seminars. If a professional, courteous relationship is developed with the local press, most will be happy to receive and publish releases. When writing releases, always follow proper format, which includes a date of release, a contact person's name and telephone number, and a short headline. Releases are best kept to one double-spaced typed page. At the end of the release, type "30" or a number sign (#). Maintain an active list of local newspapers and editors' names so that you can mail or fax the release to the appropriate editor.

## Special Events

While they can be time-consuming to organize and participate in, special events are rewarding, for they present an opportunity to interact with the community. They have high visibility, for often a group of community organizations will collaborate to cosponsor an event such as a walk-a-thon, blood pressure clinic, health fair for seniors, or wellness day for children and families. Sponsorship can be as simple as a donation to the cause; other times, staffing a booth or offering a service such as blood pressure checks is appropriate.

Like all marketing efforts, special events require organizational skills and teamwork, but they often result in heightened communication with the community and provide an educational service to patients and their families.

## RECORD AND FINANCIAL MANAGEMENT

Physicians entrust a great deal of responsibility to their medical office managers. The daily payments received through the mail and office visits must be processed and prepared for banking. Office expenses must be processed and paid in a timely fashion to capitalize on any discounts available. Employee requirements and records such as Social Security records, Withholding Allowance Certificates (W-4 forms) (Figure 22-7) indicating the number of exemptions claimed, and Employment Eligibility Verification Forms (I-9) ensuring that all persons employed are either United States citizens, lawfully admitted aliens, or aliens authorized to work in the United States must be completed and filed with the appropriate federal agencies. Also, state and local tax records must be filed and maintained for each employee.

Page 2

Form W-4 (2000)

**Deductions and Adjustments Worksheet**

Note: Use this worksheet only if you plan to itemize deductions or claim adjustments to income on your 2000 tax return.

1 Enter an estimate of your 2000 itemized deductions. These include qualifying home mortgage interest, charitable contributions, state and local taxes, medical expenses in excess of 7.5% of your income, and miscellaneous deductions. (For 2000, you may have to reduce your itemized deductions if your income is over $128,950 ($64,475 if married filing separately). See Worksheet 3 in Pub. 919 for details.) ... 1 $

2 Enter: $7,350 if married filing jointly or qualifying widow(er)
$6,450 if head of household
$4,400 if single
$3,675 if married filing separately ... 2 $

3 Subtract line 2 from line 1. If line 2 is greater than line 1, enter -0- ... 3 $
4 Enter an estimate of your 2000 adjustments to income, including alimony, deductible IRA contributions, and student loan interest ... 4 $
5 Add lines 3 and 4 and enter the total. (Include any amount for credits from Worksheet 7 in Pub. 919) ... 5 $
6 Enter an estimate of your 2000 nonwage income (such as dividends or interest) ... 6 $
7 Subtract line 6 from line 5. Enter the result, but not less than -0- ... 7 $
8 Divide the amount on line 7 by $3,000 and enter the result here. Drop any fraction ... 8
9 Enter the number from the Personal Allowances Worksheet, line H, page 1 ... 9
10 Add lines 8 and 9 and enter the total here. If you plan to use the Two-Earner/Two-Job Worksheet, also enter this total on line 1 below. Otherwise, stop here and enter this total on Form W-4, line 5, page 1 ... 10

**Two-Earner/Two-Job Worksheet**

Note: Use this worksheet only if the instructions under line H on page 1 direct you here.

1 Enter the number from line H, page 1 (or from line 10 above if you used the Deductions and Adjustments Worksheet) ... 1
2 Find the number in Table 1 below that applies to the LOWEST paying job and enter it here ... 2
3 If line 1 is MORE THAN OR EQUAL TO line 2, subtract line 2 from line 1. Enter the result here (if zero, enter -0-) and on Form W-4, line 5, page 1. Do not use the rest of this worksheet ... 3

Note: If line 1 is LESS THAN line 2, enter -0- on Form W-4, line 5, page 1. Complete lines 4-9 below to calculate the additional withholding amount necessary to avoid a year end tax bill.

4 Enter the number from line 2 of this worksheet ... 4
5 Enter the number from line 1 of this worksheet ... 5
6 Subtract line 5 from line 4 ... 6
7 Find the amount in Table 2 below that applies to the HIGHEST paying job and enter it here ... 7 $
8 Multiply line 7 by line 6 and enter the result here. This is the additional annual withholding needed ... 8 $
9 Divide line 8 by the number of pay periods remaining in 2000. For example, divide by 26 if you are paid every other week and you complete this form in December 1999. Enter the result here and on Form W-4, line 6, page 1. This is the additional amount to be withheld from each paycheck ... 9 $

**Table 1: Two-Earner/Two-Job Worksheet**

| Married Filing Jointly | | | All Others | | |
|---|---|---|---|---|---|
| If wages from LOWEST paying job are— | Enter on line 2 above | | If wages from LOWEST paying job are— | Enter on line 2 above | |
| $0 - 4,000 | 0 | | $0 - $5,000 | 0 | |
| 4,001 - 7,000 | 1 | | 5,001 - 11,000 | 1 | |
| 7,001 - 13,000 | 2 | | 11,001 - 17,000 | 2 | |
| 13,001 - 19,000 | 3 | | 17,001 - 22,000 | 3 | |
| 19,001 - 25,000 | 4 | | 22,001 - 27,000 | 4 | |
| 25,001 - 31,000 | 5 | | 27,001 - 40,000 | 5 | |
| 31,001 - 37,000 | 6 | | 40,001 - 50,000 | 6 | |
| 37,001 - 41,000 | 7 | | 50,001 - 65,000 | 7 | |
| 41,001 - 45,000 | 8 | | 65,001 - 80,000 | 8 | |
| 45,001 - 55,000 | 9 | | 80,001 - 100,000 | 9 | |
| 55,001 - 63,000 | 10 | | 100,001 and over | 10 | |
| 63,001 - 70,000 | 11 | | | | |
| 70,001 - 85,000 | 12 | | | | |
| 85,001 - 100,000 | 13 | | | | |
| 100,001 - 110,000 | 14 | | | | |
| 110,001 and over | 15 | | | | |

**Table 2: Two-Earner/Two-Job Worksheet**

| Married Filing Jointly | | All Others | |
|---|---|---|---|
| If wages from HIGHEST paying job are— | Enter on line 7 above | If wages from HIGHEST paying job are— | Enter on line 7 above |
| $0 - $50,000 | $420 | $0 - $30,000 | $420 |
| 50,001 - 100,000 | 780 | 30,001 - 60,000 | 780 |
| 100,001 - 130,000 | 870 | 60,001 - 120,000 | 870 |
| 130,001 - 250,000 | 1,000 | 120,001 - 270,000 | 1,000 |
| 250,001 and over | 1,100 | 270,001 and over | 1,100 |

Form W-4 (2000)

**Purpose.** Complete Form W-4 so your employer can withhold the correct Federal income tax from your pay. Because your tax situation may change, you may want to refigure your withholding each year.

**Exemption from withholding.** If you are exempt, complete only lines 1, 2, 3, 4, and 7 and sign the form to validate it. Your exemption for 2000 expires February 16, 2001.

**Note:** You cannot claim exemption from withholding if (1) your income exceeds $700 and includes more than $250 of unearned income (e.g., interest and dividends) and (2) another person can claim you as a dependent on their tax return.

**Basic instructions.** If you are not exempt, complete the Personal Allowances Worksheet below. The worksheets on page 2 adjust your withholding allowances based on itemized deductions, adjustments to income, or two-earner/two-job situations. Complete all worksheets that apply. They will help you figure the number of withholding allowances you are entitled to claim. However, you may claim fewer (or zero) allowances.

**Child tax and higher education credits.** For details on adjusting withholding for these and other credits, see Pub. 919, How Do I Adjust My Tax Withholding?

**Head of household.** Generally, you may claim head of household filing status on your tax return only if you are unmarried and pay more than 50% of the costs of keeping up a home for yourself and your dependent(s) or other qualifying individuals. See line E below.

**Nonwage income.** If you have a large amount of nonwage income, such as interest or dividends, you should consider making estimated tax payments using Form 1040-ES, Estimated Tax for Individuals. Otherwise, you may owe additional tax.

**Two earners/two jobs.** If you have a working spouse or more than one job, figure the total number of allowances you are entitled to claim on all jobs using worksheets from only one Form W-4. Your withholding usually will be most accurate when all allowances are claimed on the Form W-4 prepared for the highest paying job and zero allowances are claimed on the others.

**Recent name change?** If your name differs from that shown on your social security card, call 1-800-772-1213 for a new social security card.

**Personal Allowances Worksheet** (Keep for your records.)

A Enter "1" for yourself if no one else can claim you as a dependent ... A

B Enter "1" if:
• You are single and have only one job; or
• You are married, have only one job, and your spouse does not work; or ... B
• Your wages from a second job or your spouse's wages (or the total of both) are $1,000 or less.

C Enter "1" for your spouse. But, you may choose to enter -0- if you are married and have either a working spouse or more than one job. (Entering -0- may help you avoid having too little tax withheld.) ... C

D Enter number of dependents (other than your spouse or yourself) you will claim on your tax return ... D

E Enter "1" if you will file as head of household on your tax return (see conditions under Head of household above) ... E

F Enter "1" if you have at least $1,500 of child or dependent care expenses for which you plan to claim a credit ... F

G **Child Tax Credit:**
• If your total income will be between $18,000 and $50,000 ($23,000 and $63,000 if married), enter "1" for each eligible child.
• If your total income will be between $50,000 and $80,000 ($63,000 and $115,000 if married), enter "1" if you have two eligible children, enter "2" if you have three or four eligible children, or enter "3" if you have five or more eligible children ... G

H Add lines A through G and enter total here. Note: This may be different from the number of exemptions you claim on your tax return. ▶ ... H

For accuracy, complete all worksheets that apply.
• If you plan to itemize or claim adjustments to income and want to reduce your withholding, see the Deductions and Adjustments Worksheet on page 2.
• If you are single, have more than one job and your combined earnings from all jobs exceed $34,000, OR if you are married and have a working spouse or more than one job, and the combined earnings from all jobs exceed $60,000, see the Two-Earner/Two-Job Worksheet on page 2 to avoid having too little tax withheld.
• If neither of the above situations applies, stop here and enter the number from line H on line 5 of Form W-4 below.

- - - - - - - - Cut here and give Form W-4 to your employer. Keep the top part for your records. - - - - - - - -

| Form **W-4** Department of the Treasury Internal Revenue Service | **Employee's Withholding Allowance Certificate** ▶ For Privacy Act and Paperwork Reduction Act Notice, see page 2. | OMB No. 1545-0010 **2000** |
|---|---|---|

1 Type or print your first name and middle initial / Last name / 2 Your social security number

Home address (number and street or rural route)

3 ☐ Single ☐ Married ☐ Married, but withhold at higher Single rate
Note: If married, but legally separated, or spouse is a nonresident alien, check the Single box.

City or town, state, and ZIP code

4 If your last name differs from that on your social security card, check here. You must call 1-800-772-1213 for a new card. ▶ ☐

5 Total number of allowances you are claiming (from line H above OR from the applicable worksheet on page 2) ... 5
6 Additional amount, if any, you want withheld from each paycheck ... 6 $
7 I claim exemption from withholding for 2000, and I certify that I meet BOTH of the following conditions for exemption:
• Last year I had a right to a refund of ALL Federal income tax withheld because I had NO tax liability AND
• This year I expect a refund of ALL Federal income tax withheld because I expect to have NO tax liability.
If you meet both conditions, write "EXEMPT" here ... 7

Under penalties of perjury, I certify that I am entitled to the number of withholding allowances claimed on this certificate, or I am entitled to claim exempt status.

Employee's signature (Form is not valid unless you sign it) ▶ _____ Date ▶ _____

8 Employer's name and address (Employer: Complete lines 8 and 10 only if sending to the IRS.) / 9 Office code (optional) / 10 Employer identification number

Cat. No. 10220Q

**Figure 22-7** The Form W-4 indicates the number of exemptions claimed by the employee for income tax purposes.

## Payroll Processing

In some cases it is the office manager's responsibility to prepare payroll checks for each employee and record all deductions withheld. A W-2 form (Figure 22-8) summarizing all earnings and deductions for the year must be prepared for each employee by January 31 of each year. The Social Security Administration must receive a report of W-2 forms each year.

To comply with all governmental regulations, federal, state, and local, it is important that the office manager who processes payroll maintain complete, up-to-date records on every employee. This information should be gathered from new employees and updated every year and upon any change in employee status. Every employee file should contain social security number, number of exemptions claimed on the W-4 Form, the employee's gross salary, and all deductions withheld for all taxes including Social Security, federal, state, local, plus unemployment tax (where applicable), and disability insurance (where applicable).

In order to process payroll, the physician's office must have a federal tax reporting number, obtained from the Internal Revenue Service. In some states, a state employer number also is needed.

**Preparing Payroll Checks.** When preparing payroll checks, it is important to keep a record of all tax and insurance amounts deducted from an employee's earnings. Many ambulatory care settings that operate on a manual bookkeeping system find that the write-it-once system is the most efficient way to accurately maintain these records. Payroll records should include:

- Employee name, address, and telephone number
- Social security number
- Date of employment

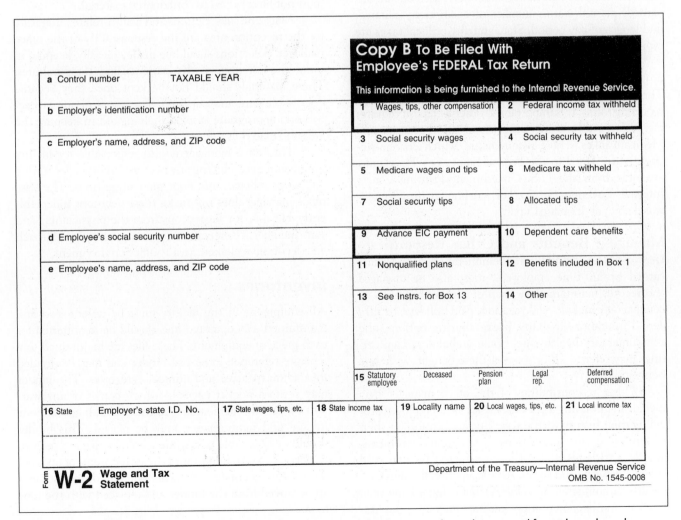

**Figure 22-8** The Form W-2 summarizes all earnings and deductions for the year and must be prepared for each employee by January 31.

Each paycheck stub should contain:

- Number of hours worked, including regular and overtime (if hourly)
- Date of pay periods
- Date of check
- Gross salary
- Itemized deductions for federal income tax, social security (FICA) tax, state taxes, city or local taxes
- Itemized deductions for health insurance, disability insurance
- Other deductions such as uniforms, loan payments, and so on
- Net salary (gross earnings minus taxes and deductions)

**Figuring Taxes.** When figuring federal income taxes and social security taxes, use the charts provided by the Internal Revenue Service. Federal tax is based on amount earned, marital status, number of exemptions claimed, and length of pay period. State and city or local taxes are typically a percentage of the gross earnings.

All federal and state taxes withheld must be paid on a quarterly basis to the appropriate government offices. These monies should be accompanied by the required reporting forms. It is important to observe deposit requirements for withheld income tax and social security and Medicare taxes. These requirements, which change frequently, are listed in the Federal Employer's Tax Guide, available from the U.S. Government Printing Office, Internal Revenue Service, or on-line at ftp://ftp.fedworld.gov/pub/irs-pdf/p15.pdf.

**Managing Benefits and Other Responsibilities.** Benefits, or additional remuneration to the salary earned by full-time employees, must also be managed and records maintained for each employee. Examples of benefits may include paid vacation, paid holidays, health/dental insurance, disability, profit-sharing options, and complimentary health care. Some ambulatory care settings may refer to all or some of these benefits as fringe benefits.

Other responsibilities of the office manager may include maintaining a personal file for each employee providing their history with the facility, application for their current position, evaluations, promotions, problems, awards, entitlements, legal forms required by state and federal agencies, and so on. All Occupational Safety and Health Administration (OSHA) data, hazard material training and documentation, cardiopulmonary resuscita-

tion (CPR) certifications, and continued education units (CEUs) must be recorded and maintained.

## FACILITY AND EQUIPMENT MANAGEMENT

The physical plant or building must be observed and maintained with safety being a key ingredient. It should be the responsibility of each staff member to report to the office manager any facility repairs that require attention and suggest replacement or recommend new pieces of equipment as required by the practice to support the health care needs of its population.

The office manager is usually responsible for the maintenance of the office and may hire ancillary services to provide janitorial and laundry services, dispose of hazardous materials, and maintain aquariums or plants that may enhance the environment of the facility. The office manager must stress the importance of patient confidentiality at the close of each day. Ancillary services must not have access to confidential material.

Magazine subscriptions and health-related literature for the reception area are the responsibility of the office manager. Selections should be made carefully, keeping in mind the interests of the patients and their cultures. These materials should not be kept once they become dog-eared, torn, and outdated. The use of plastic protectors and appropriate storage shelving aid in keeping the area and materials tidy.

The office manager is also responsible for facility improvements including any necessary repairs, decorating and color scheme, and floor plan suggestions. The wise office manager does not make these decisions independently, but asks for suggestions from the physician(s) and staff members. Remember, the team-building approach adds a cohesive element to any office environment.

### Inventories

All equipment in the facility must be inventoried and maintained. Documented files should be maintained for each piece of equipment. These files are maintained in a separate reference loose-leaf binder and may be divided into administrative and clinical categories. The binder may contain pocket pages in which copies of any warranties, service agreements/contracts, and instructions for use and maintenance may be placed. This binder should be accessible to anyone who may need to refer to its pages. It is also important that as new items or updated service agreements/contracts are purchased, the old ones are removed from the binder and replaced with the new items.

## *Equipment and Supplies Maintenance*

The office storage areas should be well maintained, and each item should always be put back in its place with lids replaced properly to prevent any accidents. Medication storage requires special attention. Many medications must be stored at certain temperatures, kept dry, or stored in dark, airtight containers. Narcotics should always be stored in a locked cabinet. Require two individuals to sign off when narcotic supplies are used and maintain a daily inventory.

Laboratory equipment must be maintained and quality control measures utilized. Calibration checks are required for a number of pieces of equipment: sphygmomanometers and centrifuges to name two. Microscopes and various types of scopes used during physical examinations and specialty procedures contain light sources that must be checked before each use. A replacement supply of bulbs should be available.

## RISK MANAGEMENT

The office manager must practice **risk management**. The risk management process includes the identification, analysis, and treatment of risks within the medical office. The office manager should evaluate the practice to determine when potential risks are present and act to eliminate the risks or to prevent injuries from the risks.

 A comprehensive safety program is essential to risk management. This safety program is responsible for meeting the basic safety needs of patients, employees, and visitors. The manager will make sure that all safety guidelines and practices are followed throughout the office and that all staff members work within the scope of their training and qualifications.

The primary principle behind the risk management role is loss prevention. With the increased number of legal actions occurring in the health care field, the risk management program is even more vital for the protection of the facility's assets. Maintenance of practice liability coverage is essential to protect the facility from risk that cannot be avoided.

## LIABILITY COVERAGE AND BONDING

**Negligence** is performing an act that a reasonable and prudent physician would not perform or failure to perform an act that a reasonable and prudent physician would perform. The common term used to describe professional **liability**, or legal responsibility, today is **malpractice**, a term that has negative connotations. It is much easier to prevent malpractice than to defend it in litigation so every effort should be taken to prevent negligence.

Insurance policies specifically designed to protect the physician's assets in the event a liability claim is filed and awarded in the patient's favor are available. Any physician not carrying such insurance is said to be **"going bare"** and would personally be responsible for any court costs, damages, and attorney fees if a malpractice suit were lost.

Practicing medical assistants should carry **professional liability insurance** for protection. Medical assistants who are members of the American Association of Medical Assistants (AAMA) have the option of purchasing personal and professional insurance through the organization at corporate rates.

Some physicians will carry the names of their employees on their policies. If this is the case, always ask to see the policy and verify that your name is printed on the policy—no name indicates no coverage. The manager may need to see that professional liability insurance has been purchased, all appropriate names are listed, and the premiums are paid in a timely fashion.

Professional liability insurance is important if the physician/employer is sued. In this event, the physician and the medical assistant could be named in the suit. If the case were lost, both the physician and the medical assistant could be liable.

Individuals who are responsible for handling financial records and money in the medical office may be bonded. A **bond** is purchased for a cash value in an employee's name which insures that the physician will recover the amount of loss in the event that an employee **embezzles** funds. It is the office manager or the human resources manager's responsibility to ask prospective employees if they are bondable. Individuals who are not bondable may not be the best candidates for the position.

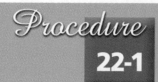

## 22-1  Preparing a Meeting Agenda

**PURPOSE:**
To prepare a meeting agenda, a list of specific items to be discussed and/or acted upon, in order to maintain the focus of the group and allow business to be transacted in a timely fashion.

**EQUIPMENT/SUPPLIES:**
List of participants
Order of business
Names of individuals giving reports
Names of any guest speakers
Computer and paper to print agendas

**PROCEDURE STEPS:**
1. Reserve proposed date, time, and place of meeting. RATIONALE: Ensure that the facilities are available for the meeting.

2. Collect information for meeting agenda by previewing the previous meeting's minutes for old business items, checking with others for report items, determining any new business items. RATIONALE: Ensure that all old and new business items have been identified.

3. Prepare a hard copy of the agenda and have it approved by chair of the meeting. RATIONALE: Confirmation by the chair of the agenda content ensures that agenda is correct and complete.

4. Send agenda to meeting participants two weeks in advance of the meeting. RATIONALE: Permits participants to prepare for the meeting by completing any tasks required and preparing any necessary documentation.

## 22-2  Making Travel Arrangements

**PURPOSE:**
To make travel arrangements for the physician.

**EQUIPMENT/SUPPLIES:**
Travel plan
Telephone and telephone directory
Computer
Physician's or office credit card to pay for reservations

**PROCEDURE STEPS:**
1. Confirm the details of the planned trip: dates, time, and place for departure and arrival; preferred mode of transportation (plane, train, bus, car); number of travelers; preferred lodging type and price range; and whether travelers checks are required. RATIONALE: Confirming pertinent travel details ensure that correct arrangements will be made.

2. Make travel and lodging reservations by calling travel agent or using the computer for on-line ticket services. RATIONALE: Ensure that space for physician is reserved at desired times.

3. Pick up tickets or arrange for their delivery.

4. Check to see that ticket arrangements are accurate (dates, times, places).

5. Check to see that car rental and lodging accommodations are accurate and confirmed. RATIONALE: Avoid inaccuracies and confusion with schedule.

6. Make additional copies of the itinerary or create the itinerary if making arrangements via computer. The itinerary should list date and time of departures and arrivals, including flight numbers and seat assignments. Note mode of transportation to lodging (shuttle, bus, car, taxi). Include name, address, and telephone number of lodgings and meeting places.

7. Maintain one copy of the itinerary in the office file.

8. Give several copies of the itinerary to the physician. RATIONALE: Ensure that a copy is on file with the office and that there are sufficient copies for the traveler(s) and their families.

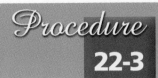

# Making Travel Arrangements Via Internet

**PURPOSE:**
To make travel arrangements for the physician using the Internet.

**EQUIPMENT/SUPPLIES:**
Travel plan
Computer
Physician's or office credit card to pay for reservations.

**PROCEDURE STEPS:**
1. Confirm the details of the planned trip: dates, time, and place for departure and arrival; preferred mode of transportation (plane, train, bus, car); number of travelers; preferred lodging type and price range; and whether travelers checks are required. RATIONALE: Confirming pertinent travel details ensures that correct arrangements will be made.
2. Go to the computer and access the Internet.
3. Select a search engine to locate web pages under the subject "air fares." Web pages may provide links to air fares, auto reservations, and hotel/ motel reservations. Follow web page instructions for making arrangements. Review and copy confirmation of your transaction. RATIONALE: The Internet can be a time saver and cost-effective way of securing travel arrangements.
4. Pick up tickets or arrange for their delivery, if necessary. Tickets purchased on the Internet may be mailed or picked up at an airport, or they may be electronic tickets.
5. Make additional copies of the itinerary or create the itinerary. The itinerary should list date and time of departures and arrivals, including flight numbers and seat assignments. Note the mode of transportation to lodging (shuttle, bus, car, taxi). Include name, address, and telephone number of lodgings and meeting places.
6. Maintain one copy of the itinerary in the office file.
7. Give several copies of the itinerary to the physician. RATIONALE: Ensure that a copy is on file with the office and that there are sufficient copies for the traveler(s) and their families.

# Supervising a Student Practicum

**PURPOSE:**
To prepare a training path for a student extern being assigned to the office. To make the involved office personnel aware of their responsibilities. To preplan which jobs the student extern performs and in what sequence they will be assigned. To make the externship successful by providing as much supervision and assistance as necessary.

**EQUIPMENT/SUPPLIES:**
None needed

**PROCEDURE STEPS:**
1. Review the clinical externship contract or agreement between your agency and the educational institution. RATIONALE: Guidelines and procedures are reviewed and refreshed in your mind.
2. Determine the amount of supervision the extern will require. RATIONALE: Prepares you to speak with the student and site supervisor regarding supervision.
3. Identify the supervisor who will be immediately responsible for the extern. RATIONALE: Establishes a person who knows he or she is to supervise the student and be responsible for the externship procedures.
4. Plan what tasks the extern will be allowed or encouraged to perform. RATIONALE: The office may or may not permit the student to perform

*(continues)*

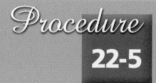

## Procedure 22-4 *(continued)*

invasive procedures. Determining tasks the student can and can not perform beforehand promotes a better relationship.

5. Create a schedule outlining the time the extern will be assigned to each unit. RATIONALE: Establishing a schedule keeps everyone appraised of what is happening and when.

6. Begin orientation for the extern as soon as he or she arrives at the office. Include a tour of the office and introduction to the staff. RATIONALE: Orients student and staff to each other and establishes guidelines for procedures.

7. Give the extern a copy of the Office Policy Manual and the work schedule for the entire externship. Answer any questions the extern might have. RATIONALE: Orients student and staff to each other and establishes guidelines for procedures.

8. Maintain an accurate record of the hours the extern works. Also log the date and reason for any missed days, late arrivals, or early dismissals. RATIONALE: Provides necessary documentation for the hours completed by the student.

9. Check with the extern frequently to be sure the extern is receiving meaningful training from the work experience. RATIONALE: Verifies that necessary training is being provided.

10. Consult physicians and staff members with whom the extern has worked for their opinion of the student's capabilities. Follow up on any problems that might be identified. RATIONALE: Verifies that necessary training is being provided.

11. Report the extern's progress to the medical assisting supervisor from the educational institution. This person usually visits once or twice each rotation. RATIONALE: Verifies that necessary training is being provided.

12. Prepare the student extern evaluation report from comments provided by the supervisor assigned and each employee who worked with the extern. RATIONALE: Provides necessary documentation for the externship experience.

## Procedure 22-5  Developing and Maintaining a Procedures Manual

**PURPOSE:**

To develop and maintain a comprehensive, up-to-date procedures manual covering each medical, technical, and administrative procedure in the office, with step-by-step directions and rationale for performing each task.

**EQUIPMENT/SUPPLIES:**

Computer or electronic typewriter (electronic storage allows changes and revisions to be made easily)
Binder, such as a three-ring binder
Paper
Standard procedures manual format

**PROCEDURE STEPS:**

1. Write detailed, step-by-step procedures and rationales for each medical, technical, and administrative function. Each procedure is written by experienced employees close to the function and then reviewed by a supervisor and/or office manager. Rationales help employees understand *why* something is done. RATIONALE: Establishes consistent guidelines to be followed.

2. Collect the procedures into the Office Procedures Manual. RATIONALE: Provides a reference

*(continues)*

## *Procedure* 22-5 *(continued)*

guide with step-by-step instruction and examples where appropriate.

3. Store one complete manual in a common library area. Provide a completed copy to the physician/employer and the office manager. Distribute appropriate sections to the various departments. RATIONALE: Provides a reference guide with

step-by-step instruction and examples where appropriate.

4. Review the procedures manual annually and add any new procedures, delete or modify as necessary, and indicate the revision date (Rev. 10/12/02). RATIONALE: Maintains current office protocols.

---

**22-1**

Dr. Lewis and Dr. King have requested sigmoidoscopy procedures to be scheduled for two different patients. The patients are scheduled. Both patients are put on a strict diet and pretest protocol for several days to prepare for the procedures. The day of the appointments, it is discovered that the two sigmoidoscopy procedures have been scheduled at the same time. The problem is that the office has only one sigmoidoscope available.

### CASE STUDY REVIEW

1. Divide the class into two groups to discuss problem-solving solutions. Assume that rescheduling a patient is not an acceptable solution because of the patient's pretest protocol. The patients would be very upset if the procedure could not be performed due to a scheduling problem.
2. How could this problem have been avoided?
3. Both patients have been told about the scheduling problem and one is very upset and argumentative. What role should the office manager assume in this predicament?

---

**22-2**

The office manager for Doctors Lewis and King has many leadership qualities and utilizes them effectively in her management style. She sets realistic goals and becomes a role model for subordinates to emulate. She empowers her subordinates and encourages creativity.

### CASE STUDY REVIEW

1. Divide the class into small groups and ask them to brainstorm the pros and cons of this management style.
2. Discuss with your small group other management styles and your comfort level working under these management styles.
3. Within your group, develop a set of questions that might be asked at an interview to determine the management style of this manager prior to accepting employment.

## SUMMARY

The office manager is the glue that holds the office together and keeps it running smoothly. When the manager sets a positive example for others, is considerate and aware of the diversity of others, a positive environment is created for teamwork. A teamwork approach enables the entire office to be more productive, provide the best health care, and foster an enjoyable work relationship.

The role of office manager varies greatly depending upon the size of the medical practice, the physician's trust in the manager's competency level, and the physician's comfort in delegating authority to others. An effective office manager is a tremendous asset to physicians. The personal and financial rewards are worthwhile to the medical assistant who desires a new dimension to explore and enjoys a challenge.

## REVIEW QUESTIONS

### Multiple Choice

1. The office manager should have a minimum of a (an):
   a. associate's degree
   b. bachelor's degree
   c. master's degree
   d. doctoral degree
2. When the office manager is too busy to perform a task, he or she should:
   a. refuse to do it
   b. delegate the task to someone who is knowledgeable
   c. put it off and do it when there is time later
   d. hope that no one will notice it did not get done
3. For teamwork to be successful, individual team members must:
   a. do as they are told by the office manager
   b. not ask why they are doing something a certain way
   c. understand and support the task
   d. think independently and solve the problem on their own
4. People-oriented personalities:
   a. are most comfortable with physical dexterity, building, construction, and working with tools or instruments
   b. are most comfortable working with ideas, information, and data
   c. are most comfortable teaching, coaching, helping, leading, and inspiring others
   d. use "carrots" and "sticks"
5. Meeting minutes:
   a. should address each agenda topic and include a brief summary of discussions, actions taken, name of each person making a motion, the exact wording of motions, and motion approval or defeat
   b. are a detailed plan for a proposed trip
   c. include information regarding mode of transportation and lodging reservations
   d. must follow parliamentary procedures

6. When working with externs, it is important to remember that:
   a. they should have expert knowledge about their field
   b. they do not need supervision when working with a patient
   c. they are very experienced with working on real patients
   d. they have much to learn
7. The procedures manual:
   a. is a detailed plan for a proposed trip
   b. provides detailed information regarding mode of transportation and lodging reservations
   c. provides detailed information relative to the performance of tasks within the health care facility
   d. summarizes action details of staff meetings
8. Which of the following statements is *not* correct regarding a student practicum?
   a. It is a transitional stage that provides opportunity for students to apply theory learned in the classroom to a health care setting through hands-on experience.
   b. It assumes that the student is an employee who does not need to be introduced to patients.
   c. It may require the student to shadow another medical assistant for a few days.
   d. It involves an evaluation of the student's progress.
9. Developing relationships outside the office is often called:
   a. marketing
   b. benchmarking
   c. advertising
   d. sales
10. Record and financial management involves all of the following *except:*
    a. payroll processing
    b. preparing payroll checks
    c. figuring taxes
    d. equipment and supplies maintenance

## Critical Thinking

1. How would you, as the office manager, handle someone who is spreading a harmful rumor about another employee in the office?
2. Discuss teamwork and the benefits of the teamwork approach.
3. How can the office manager promote open and honest communication?
4. This chapter identifies various management styles. Under which management style would you feel most comfortable working and why? Does this management style promote a teamwork atmosphere? Why or why not?
5. The student practicum can be a very stressful time for the extern. As an office manager, how can you help the extern feel more at ease the first day of "work"?
6. This chapter describes various tactics you can use to keep yourself organized, such as making a "To Do" list, handling a paper only once, and avoiding procrastination. Describe things that you do to keep yourself organized.
7. Describe how a procedures manual for a single-physician practice would differ from a procedures manual for a multi-physician practice.
8. Describe how a procedures manual could become outdated and need revision.
9. In what cases would a press release be used?
10. Explain why the primary principle behind the risk management role is loss prevention.

## WEB ACTIVITIES

Use the web sites described in the text, or alternative sites you know about, to plan a trip between two cities within the United States. Compare the fares for Sunday departure and Friday return dates with the fares for low volume days as obtained from the Priceline.com site. Also compare fares on flights purchased within one week of departure with fares on flights purchased a month prior to departure. Follow the instructor's instructions on completing and turning in your results.

## REFERENCES/BIBLIOGRAPHY

Colbert, B. J. (2000). *Workplace readiness for health occupations.* Albany, NY: Delmar.

Frew, M. A., Lane, K., & Frew, D. R. (1995). *Comprehensive medical assisting: Competencies for administrative and clinical practice* (3rd ed.). Philadelphia: F. A. Davis.

Institute for Management Excellence (June 1998). Linking personality with management style. [On-line]. Available: http://itstime.com/jun98.htm.

Lewis, M. A., & Tamparo, C. D. (1998). *Medical law, ethics, and bioethics for ambulatory care* (4th ed.). Philadelphia: F. A. Davis.

McConnell, C. R. (1998). *Case studies in health care supervision.* Gaithersburg, MD: Aspen Publishers.

Pyzdek, T. (1996). Management styles: Participatory management style. [On-line]. Available: http://www.qualityamerica.com/knowledgecente/articles/CQMStyle2.html.

*Chapter*

**23**

# THE MEDICAL ASSISTANT AS HUMAN RESOURCES MANAGER

## KEY TERMS

Conflict Resolution
Educational History
Evaluation
Exit Interview
Involuntary Dismissal
Job Description
Letter of Reference
Letter of Resignation
Mentor
Networking
Overtime
Probation
Resumes
Salary Review
Work History

## OUTLINE

**Tasks Performed by the Human Resources Manager**
**The Office Policy Manual**
**Recruiting and Hiring Office Personnel**
  Job Descriptions
  Recruiting
  Preparing to Interview Applicants
  The Interview
  Selecting the Finalists
**Orienting and Training New Personnel**
**Evaluating Employees and Planning Salary Review**
  Performance Evaluation
  Salary Review

**Dismissing Employees**
  Involuntary Dismissal
  Voluntary Dismissal
  Exit Interview
**Maintaining Personnel Records**
**Complying with Personnel Laws**
**Special Policy Considerations**
  Temporary Employees
  Smoking Policy
  Discrimination
  Employees with Chemical Dependencies or Emotional Problems
**Providing/Planning Employee Training and Education**
**Conflict Resolution**

## OBJECTIVES

*The student should strive to meet the following performance objectives and demonstrate an understanding of the facts and principles presented in this chapter through written and oral communication.*

1.  Define the key terms as presented in the glossary.
2.  Describe the role of the human resources manager.
3.  Explain the function of the office policy manual.
4.  Identify methods of recruiting employees for a medical practice.
5.  Discuss the interview process.
6.  Describe appropriate evaluation tools for employees.
7.  Recall procedures to follow when dismissing employees.
8.  Identify items to keep in an employee's personnel record.
9.  List and define a minimum of four laws related to personnel management.
10. Recall effective methods of resolving conflicts.

## ADMINISTRATIVE

**Practice Finances**

- Manage personnel benefits and maintain records (adv)

## GENERAL
## (TRANSDISCIPLINARY)

**Legal Concepts**

- Follow federal, state and local legal guidelines
- Participate in the development and maintenance of personnel, policy and procedure manuals
- Develop and maintain personnel, policy and procedures manuals (adv)

**Instruction**

- Train and orient personnel (adv)
- Conduct continuing education activities (adv)

**Operational Functions**

- Supervise personnel (adv)
- Interview and recommend job applicants (adv)

Jane O'Hara, CMA, is the officer manager at Inner City Health Care. She also functions in the role of the human resources manager. Part of her responsibilities includes recruiting, hiring, training, and dismissing employees.

In one day Jane may meet with Dr. Rice to update the policy manual, place an advertisement in the local newspaper for a new medical assistant, welcome a new physician to the practice, being sure she completes all of the necessary forms, and meet with Karen Ritter to evaluate her salary.

## INTRODUCTION

The medical assistant, while performing the tasks and assuming the responsibility of an office manager, also may function in the role of the human resources manager.

The title human resources manager is often reserved for an individual who manages a human resources department in a large, corporate setting. Many of the duties performed by this individual, however, may be performed in a sole proprietor's medical practice with only one or two employees.

## TASKS PERFORMED BY THE HUMAN RESOURCES MANAGER

Tasks usually assigned to the human resources manager include determining job descriptions, hiring, training, and dismissing employees, and maintaining employee personnel records. But with today's quest for greater office efficiency and the tremendous increase in federal and state regulatory requirements, the skills required of a human resources manager have greatly broadened. Former responsibilities have been expanded to include writing the policy manual, planning employee evaluation, preventing and investigating discrimination

and harassment claims, and complying with regulatory agencies. The human resources manager also assists in providing training and educational opportunities for employees so they are up to date in all aspects of quality patient care.

Increasingly, human resource managers are expected to be able to support the organization's efforts that focus on productivity, service, and quality. In a climate in which there are too few persons for the positions to be filled, and the delivery methods for health care are changing almost daily, productivity, service, and quality are essential to a successful practice. It becomes the responsibility of the human resource manager to see that every employee's productivity level is high, that the service is A+, and that quality is at the highest level. Today's customers, the patients, will often choose their health care provider on the basis of service and quality.

The position of human resources manager now requires a higher level of education and experience to better grasp the legal and regulatory aspects of personnel management. The human resources manager also must have excellent people skills, a strong sense of fairness, and the ability to resolve conflicts. None of this is accomplished in a vacuum. It requires working in close cooperation with the office manager and the physician-employer(s).

This chapter discusses these responsibilities in groups of eight separate but overlapping functions:

1. Creating and updating the office policy manual
2. Recruiting and hiring office personnel
3. Orienting and training new personnel
4. Evaluating and planning salary review
5. Dismissing employees

6. Maintaining personnel records
7. Complying with all state and federal regulations regarding personnel
8. Planning/providing employee training and education

## THE OFFICE POLICY MANUAL

The procedures manual described in Chapter 22 identifies specific methods of performing tasks. The policy manual provides more general guidelines for office practices.

---

**Possible content of policy and procedure manual**

| Policy Manual | Procedure Manual |
|---|---|
| General practices and policies of an office | Daily guide; step-by-step instructions for procedures |

---

The policy manual will identify clear guidelines and directions required of all employees as well as define appropriate expectations and boundaries of the employment relationship. Having written policies means not having to determine a policy on a case-by-case basis. Policy manuals will vary by the size of the practice or problems to be addressed, but some topics include the mission statement of the practice, biographical data on each physician, employment policies, wage and salary policies, benefits to be awarded, and employee conduct expectations.

Establishing and stating the mission of the practice clearly identifies for employees the goals and objectives to be sought by each employee. Having biographical data of each physician helps employees to respond to queries from patients about a physician's training, education, and interests.

Employment policies might include statements on equal employment opportunity, job requirements for particular positions and to whom the person reports, recruitment and selection procedures, orientation of new employees, probation, and dismissal. Wage and salary policies should be in writing. How are employees classified, what are the working hours, how is overtime compensated, how are salary increases determined, what benefits (medical, retirement, vacation, holidays, sick leave) does the practice have? The answers to such questions are part of the policy manual. Employee conduct is another piece of the policy manual. Guidelines should be established about uniforms and appearance. Can an employee hold a second job outside the practice? Is smoking allowed? Are staff members responsible for housekeeping duties? A statement regarding the confidentiality of all information received in the practice is essential in this area of the policy manual.

Having a policy manual with clearly written directives helps employees understand the expectations and boundaries of the employment relationship. The policy manual should be reviewed with each new employee and updated on a regular basis. See Procedure 23-1 for details on developing and maintaining a policy manual.

## RECRUITING AND HIRING OFFICE PERSONNEL

Before recruiting and hiring personnel to fill positions within the medical office, the human resources manager and physician-employer must know exactly what the role and responsibilities of the position are by having a job description for the position and follow a recruiting policy that is effective, fair, and observes all appropriate laws and regulations.

### Job Descriptions

Before any position is filled, a **job description** must be in place. This is done cooperatively with the office manager and the physician-employer. Once the job qualifications are defined, the human resources manager can begin efforts to fill the position.

In daily operations most job descriptions are on file, but if the situation involves a new or greatly expanded office, a complete set of job descriptions is needed before recruiting can begin. Even when a written description is on file, it should be reviewed when a new employee is to be hired. The person who is leaving the position is often an excellent resource for the accuracy of the current job description and any changes that should be made.

The job description must include basic qualifications for the position and have enough information to provide both the supervisor and the employee with a clear outline of what the job entails (Figure 23-1). Necessary work experience, skills, education, and any special certification or licensure that is expected is to be identified in the job description. See Procedure 23-2 for details on preparing job descriptions.

Another important point with respect to the job description is that a review and update of the description should be done every year. Most jobs change constantly whether from a minor shifting of duties or the addition

### JOB DESCRIPTION FORMAT

**JOB TITLE:**
Describes the job in one to three words; should be a title an employee can identify with and be proud of.

**REPORTS TO:**
Identifies position or person to whom the employee reports.

**PURPOSE/OBJECTIVE:**
A short statement outlining the purpose or mission of the job, explaining basically why this job exists; should make the person feel like an integral part of the whole organization.

**RESPONSIBILITIES AND DUTIES:**
*Duties* are statements that outline a particular function or task and identify what is being done; all statements are related to the work to be performed. Duties should identify the most predominant and significant tasks and convey a measure of frequency of occurrence. *Responsibilities* are simply names or titles for types of work areas. Duties are subsets of responsibilities.

**WORK RELATIONSHIPS AND AUTHORITY BOUNDARIES:**
When significant to the job, a statement describing the relationships and degree of interface of the job with internal and external groups.

**POSITION REQUIREMENTS:**
Education and experience that are required for the person to function in this capacity.

**Figure 23-1** This sample format describes the main features of a job description with definitions for each feature. (From *Personnel Management Handbook*, 2nd ed., by Maryann Ricardo, The McGraw-Hill Companies, Inc. Copyright 1992. Reprinted with permission.)

of some new technical procedure or device. Without updating a job description, the wrong person may be recruited to fill a vacancy.

## Recruiting

A major challenge facing the human resource manager today is recruitment. Medical assistants are listed in the top ten occupations with the fastest employment growth through 2006 according to the U.S. Department of Labor, Bureau of Labor Statistics. One reason for this demand is the aging of the U.S. population. It is estimated that over 80% of jobs are in the service industry, and all health care positions fit into that category. When physician-employers have been unsuccessful in recruiting qualified medical assistants, they have turned to contracting out some work, such as transcription and billing.

The human resources manager begins the recruitment process. Often a process called networking is a highly effective method of finding employees. **Networking** is a process in which people of similar interests exchange information in social, business, or professional relationships. For instance, the human resources manager may network with members of the American Association of Medical Assistants and express an interest in a new employee for a position that is open. Current employees are often an excellent resource because they may know of a qualified person who is looking for a position.

Checking with nearby universities, community, and technical colleges' medical assistant departments is another good resource. Employing a private or state placement agency is another possibility. While newspaper advertisements may generate many **resumes**, they are only marginally effective as a search tool. It is often far too time consuming to review the large volume of applications generated by this approach.

## Preparing to Interview Applicants

Once several applicants have expressed interest in the position, preparation for the interview begins. The human resources manager should have a number of resumes to consider. Some may have already filled out a job application when they dropped off a resume. The resumes and applications can be reviewed together. Some important points to remember in reading resumes and applications follow.

Under **educational history**, look beyond the degree earned. Look for a good performance record at school and the kinds of supplemental education achieved. Does attendance at seminars and short-course training programs relate to your position needs? When reading a person's **work history**, make note of unexplained gaps in employment. You may want to ask specific questions in the interview. Has advancement been gained in each new position? Are the responsibilities and duties of the applicant's positions explained or will questions need to be asked of the prospective employee?

Look for information that indicates if this candidate really enjoys the kind of work setting you have. Is the applicant comfortable serving the infirm? Can you truly identify the level of skill from the descriptions or are the skills vague? The cover letter, if one is included, should address the specifics required of your position. Does the person display a negative or a positive attitude? Do not excuse any errors or unprofessional appearance in the job application or the resume. Each should be letter perfect. An individual who is careless in this respect is likely to be careless on the job.

Some applications will be set aside after using the preceding guidelines. With the remaining candidates, determine who is to be interviewed and make telephone calls to establish interviews. You may make note of the quality of speaking skills, especially if this person will be using the telephone on the job. Make an interview appointment date with only those who seem truly interested in the position during your telephone conversation.

## The Interview

The interview is usually conducted by only one person if second interviews are anticipated. The physician-employer, office manager, or another employee may be present in either the first or the second interview, however. This is a decision made by the human resources manager and the physician-employer (Figure 23-2). The interviewer(s) will want to review the application and resume prior to the interview for particular points to ask the candidate. An interview worksheet is an excellent tool to use to make certain that you are fair and equitable with each candidate. The worksheet should provide enough room for notes taken during the interview.

Suggested items for the interview worksheet are:

- Applicant's name
- Telephone number
- Education and training
- Work experience
- Special skills
- Professional demeanor
- Voice and mannerisms specific to position
- Responses to questions
- Ability to problem solve when given a scenario
- Any health-related or work-related problems applicant discloses
- Interviewer's personal impressions and recommendations

Conduct interviews in a quiet and private setting. Do not schedule interviews back to back without time to collect your thoughts or to allow you to compare notes with others participating in the interview. Ask job-related questions such as Describe your last job. What did you like best about it? What did you like least? What is most important to you about a job? Describe your administrative and clinical skills. Figure 23-3 shows some sample questions. Let the applicant do the most of the talking.

Any questions related to age, sex, race, religion, or national origin are inappropriate. Inquiries about medical

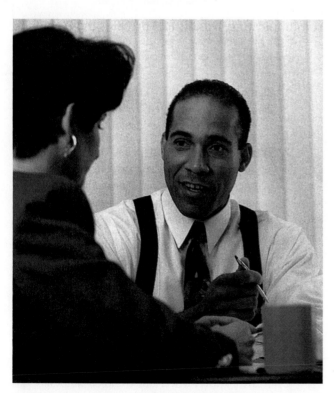

**Figure 23-2** The interview can be conducted on a one-to-one basis with only the applicant and one staff member or with several staff members meeting with the applicant at once.

---

**General Questions**
- What are your strengths and weaknesses?
- Why did you leave your last job?
- Identify what is most important to you in a job.

**Questions Related to Work Relationships**
- Describe an individual you have enjoyed working with.
- Explain how a conflict with a coworker was resolved.
- How would a coworker describe you?

**Questions Related to Problem Solving**
- Describe a work-related decision that made you very proud.
- Identify a task/procedure/assignment you could not do, and explain why.
- How do you approach a task when it seems mundane or boring?

**Questions Related to Integrity**
- If asked to do something illegal or unethical, what would you do?
- Tell us about a time when you broke a confidence.
- If you saw a coworker put a patient at risk, what would you do?

**Figure 23-3** Common interview questions.

history, drug use, or arrest records may not be made. Keep your questions related to performance on the job. If you may want to bond this employee, you may ask candidates if they have been bonded before or are willing to be bonded. It may be best to leave salary discussions for a second interview, but it can also be helpful to determine if applicants' salary expectations are in line with what you can offer. A question such as What salary are you expecting? is appropriate. Do not make a job offer until all the candidates selected for interview have been interviewed, and do not prejudge someone on appearance or any other physical factor during or following the interview. Only the person's qualifications are to be considered.

At the close of the interview, let the applicant know when a decision will be made or whether a second interview will be conducted. A tour of the facility and introduction to key staff members may be offered, but are not necessary at the time of the first interview. Finally, thank the applicant for participating in the interview and being interested in the position.

## Selecting the Finalists

Shortly after the final interview is complete, the human resources manager should compare notes with all the others involved in the interview to select the top candidates. This is done by comparing notes and impressions from the interviews and by taking into consideration the ability of a candidate to work with patients and colleagues having a variety of problems and cultural backgrounds. The next step is to check references of former employers, supervisors, coworkers, and teachers. A large corporate medical practice may even have a consent form each candidate is asked to sign that gives permission to check references and call former employers. You may need to recognize, however, that even with a release from a potential new hire, many organizations and businesses restrict the release of reference information to only name, dates of employment, and title of position served. Telephone checks for references are an excellent strategy since you receive an immediate response. If you stress confidentiality when you make the contact, it will be easier for the person to respond to your questions. Always check with more than one reference and former employer to get an accurate assessment of the candidate. A sample telephone reference check form is shown in Figure 23-4.

A checklist of questions to ask might include:

1. What were the dates of employment of (name of applicant) in your firm?
2. Describe the job performed.
3. Reason for leaving the job?
4. Strong points of the employee?
5. Limitations of the employee?

**TELEPHONE REFERENCE CHECK FORM**

Name of Applicant _____

Person Contacted _____

Position _____

Telephone Number _____

Relation to Applicant _____

1. I would like to verify some information given to us by (applicant's name) who is applying for a position with our organization. What are the dates of his employment with you?
   _____, 20___ to _____, 20___
2. What was the nature of his job?
3. What did you think of his work?
4. How did he get along with the other employees?
5. Did you see any difference in his job performance during the employment period?
6. What was his salary?
7. Why did he leave the job?
8. What are his strong points?
9. What are his limitations?
10. Please describe his attitude.
11. What degree of supervision did he need?
12. Could you comment on his attendance and dependability?
13. Were there any personal difficulties that you know of that may have interfered with his work?
14. Given the right opportunity, would you rehire him?
15. Is there anything else that we should know?

Reference call made by _____ Date _____

**Figure 23-4** A telephone reference check form such as this one can help the interviewer ask consistent questions of several references. (From *Personnel Management Handbook*, 2nd ed., by Maryann Ricardo, The McGraw-Hill Companies, Inc. Copyright 1992. Reprinted with permission.)

6. Can you comment on attendance and dependability?
7. Any personal difficulties you were aware of that interfered with the work?
8. Would you rehire?
9. Anything else we should know about this candidate?

Offer the position when a first-choice candidate has been determined and indicate when a response is needed. Be prepared with a second-choice candidate should the preferred candidate respond negatively. At the time of the offer, the candidate should understand the salary offered, the starting date, the practice policies, and the benefits. When a candidate has accepted the position, a confirmation letter should be written that clearly spells out details discussed earlier. Give specific instructions on when and where the new employee should report the first day on the job. If practical, the employee should be given the policy and procedures manuals to read.

For the unsuccessful applicants, send a letter explaining that they are no longer being considered for the position and thank them for applying. Copies of these letters as well as the interview checklists should be kept for a minimum of six months should any questions arise regarding your choice of candidates. See Procedure 23-3 for details on interviewing.

## ORIENTING AND TRAINING NEW PERSONNEL

Orienting and training new employees is the responsibility of both the human resources manager and the office manager who is most likely to work the closest with the new employee. It is common for a new employee to be placed on probation for sixty to ninety days during which time both the employee as well as supervisory personnel may determine if the environment and the position are satisfactory for the employee. Procedure 23-4 outlines how to orient and train personnel.

Important elements to orientation include the introduction of the new employee to other staff members, assigning a mentor who can respond to questions, and making the employee aware of the procedures to be performed in this new position. If the procedure's manual is detailed and accurate, this manual now becomes the daily "guide" for the new employee. Sometimes the individual leaving a position may still be present and is asked to assist in the orientation process. This is especially beneficial if there is a good working relationship between the employee who is leaving and the management of the practice. Depending upon the responsibilities of the new employee, a supervisor may be asked to monitor all procedures for a period of time for accuracy, safety, and patient protection. During the probation period, the employee should be officially evaluated by the human resources manager (see sample form in Figure 23-5). This evaluation becomes part of the employee's personnel record.

## EVALUATING EMPLOYEES AND PLANNING SALARY REVIEW

It is very important that all employees know whether they are performing their job as expected and know how they can improve their performance if necessary.

### PROBATIONARY EMPLOYEE EVALUATION FORM

Name_____

Hire Date _____

Job Title _____

Pay Rate_____ Supervisor _____

Do you recommend the employee continue in employment?
_____ Yes _____ No

Please state your reasons for whatever action you recommend. Use the guidelines below to make your decision.

1. Has the employee required more training than is normally needed for the job?

2. Has the employee grasped this job with very little training?

3. Is the employee performing at, above, or below (circle one) the standard for this job?

4. If below, when do you expect the employee to reach the standard?

5. Does the employee get along well with all staff members?

6. Has the employee maintained a good attendance record and a good work attitude?

7. Has the employee expressed any dissatisfactions?

_____    _____

Supervisor's Signature                          Date

**Figure 23-5** Sample probationary employee evaluation form. (From *Personnel Management Handbook,* 2nd ed., by Maryann Ricardo, The McGraw-Hill Companies, Inc. Copyright 1992. Reprinted with permission.)

## *Performance Evaluation*

Not only is evaluation of employees necessary during the probation period, it is necessary for current employees as well. Evaluations should be performed no less than once a year on the anniversary of the hire date. Some human resources managers may wish to evaluate an employee more often, especially if a problem has surfaced in an evaluation.

The evaluation may take many forms; it can be formal or informal; it may involve more than one person. The results of the evaluation, however, must be a part of the employee's personnel record. For that reason, a formal evaluation is preferred. Many practices use a written evaluation that requires that the employee evaluate himself prior to meeting with the human resources manager (Figure 23-6). The human resources manager uses the same form for evaluation. During the meeting, notes are compared as the evaluation is conducted.

# PERFORMANCE REVIEW FORM

_____          _____
          Employee Name                              Title

_____          _____
          Supervisor                              Department

TYPE OF REVIEW (Check One)
_____ Quarterly
_____ Annual
_____ Probation
_____ Other _____

Review Period Covered _____ to _____

PERFORMANCE DEFINITIONS

| | |
|---|---|
| 5 = Outstanding | Performance that is clearly superior, beyond the call of duty, or substantially above standard level. Seldom attained level of performance but achievable. |
| 4 = Above Standard | Very commendable performance; exceeds the norm for the job. |
| 3 = Standard | Competent and consistent performance; expected level of activity and performance for the job. Most often rating received. |
| 2 = Below Standard | Performance needs improvement. This level of performance is unacceptable; needs improvement to meet the standards for the job.<br>**Employee new to the job:** Performance might receive below standard rating due to lack of job knowledge and is expected to improve with experience.<br>**Experienced Employee:** Performance is below acceptable level and requires direction and/or counsel. |
| 1 = Unsatisfactory | Performance is unacceptable. Job activity is clearly and substantially lacking in quality, quantity, or timeliness. May also not be meeting cost or budget constraints. Needs much improvement to meet the standards for the job. |

| (office use only)<br><br>EVALUATION SUMMARY<br>Total I _____<br>+ Total II _____ | FINAL RATING: CHECK ONE (office use only)<br><br>_____ Merit Increase Recommended<br>_____ No Merit Increase—Satisfactory Performance/No Growth<br>_____ No Merit Increase (Probationary/Special Evaluation)<br>_____ No Merit Increase (Performance Probation)<br>    Re-evaluate in 90 Days for Unsatisfactory or in 180 Days for Needed Improvement |
|---|---|

**GENERAL PERFORMANCE RATING (PART I)**

| *General Criteria* | *Rating* | *Comments Supporting Rating* |
|---|---|---|
| 1. **Patient Relations:** How well does the employee communicate a "we care" image to the patients, visitors, physicians, and fellow employees? | | |
| 2. **Work Responsibilities:** What is the quality of the employee's work relative to quality, quantity, and timeliness? | | |
| 3. **Teamwork:** Does the employee have a team spirit? Does the employee interact well with co-workers/supervisor/manager? | | *(continues)* |

**Figure 23-6**    Sample performance review form. (Adapted from *Personnel Management Handbook*, 2nd ed., by Maryann Ricardo, The McGraw-Hill Companies, Inc. Copyright 1992. Reprinted with permission.)

| General Criteria | Rating | Comments Supporting Rating |
|---|---|---|
| 4. **Adaptability:** Is the employee open to change and new ideas? Does the employee remain flexible to changes in routine, work-load, and assignments? | | |
| 5. **Personal Appearance:** How well does the employee maintain appropriate personal appearance, including proper attire, hygiene? | | |
| 6. **Communication:** Does the employee communicate well? Is information given and received clearly? Does he/she have good verbal and written skills? | | |
| 7. **Dependability:** Can the employee be relied upon for good attendance? Does the employee perform and follow through on work without supervisory intervention or assistance? | | |

Subtotal I _____ ÷ 7  General Criteria = _____

**JOB-SPECIFIC CRITERIA RATING (PART II)**  (To be used with Job Description attached)

| Responsibility and Standard | Rating | Comments Supporting Rating |
|---|---|---|
| Complete a section for each responsibility listed on the employee's job description. | | |

Subtotal II _____ ÷ _____ = _____
# job duties

Contributions made since last review:

_____

_____

_____

Education or training received since last review:

_____

_____

_____

Action to be taken based on performance:

_____

_____

_____

Comments:

_____

_____

_____

| | | |
|---|---|---|
| _____ | | _____ |
| Employee Signature | | Date |
| _____ | | _____ |
| Supervisor Signature | | Date |
| _____ | | _____ |
| Physician Signature | | Date |

**Figure 23-6**  *(continued)*

The climate of the performance evaluation should be comfortable and provide privacy (Figure 23-7). The meeting should be friendly, but the employee must sense the importance of the evaluation. Do not allow any disagreements to escalate into arguments during the evaluation. Without reading the employee's self-evaluation, ask the employee to tell about the self-assessment. Acknowledge the employee's point of view and identify when you agree or differ from the self-assessment. Be prepared to describe specific examples of positive performance and/or negative performance.

When negative performance is identified, ask the employee for possible solutions. Then a plan can be determined to alter the negative performance. In this way, a trusting atmosphere is established in that both of you are working together for a solution that will benefit the medical practice. Always look for and seek a win-win situation whenever possible. The action plan determined should then be evaluated at the next performance evaluation.

At the close of the evaluation, always express your confidence in the individual to make any changes necessary, offer assistance where needed, and thank the employee for participating. End any evaluation with a positive statement about some portion of the employee's performance.

There are occasions when reviews are performed more frequently than annually. A review would occur two to three months after a significant promotion to measure how things are progressing. Reviews occur more often when general performance falls well short of past efforts or a serious error in judgment has been made. This type of review may end with a reprimand, a warning to correct the problem by a given date, or possibly, immediate dismissal. Document any steps to be taken to correct a problem and any reason that is cause for dismissal.

## Salary Reveiw

Although the practice is common in some areas, it may be better not to tie salary increases or bonuses with the annual performance evaluation. Conduct the **salary review** at the beginning of the new year separate from performance evaluations.

Salary review is important. Unfortunately, in smaller medical offices and ambulatory care settings, the review of salary may have to be raised by the employee. Physician-employers tend to forget that their employees have been with them for over a year without a raise or a discussion of financial reimbursement. If such is the case, it is perfectly acceptable for the employee to raise the issue on a yearly basis. However, the best approach is for the human resources manager to conduct salary reviews at the beginning or end of each calendar year.

Data should be collected prior to a salary review. The human resources manager should network with other

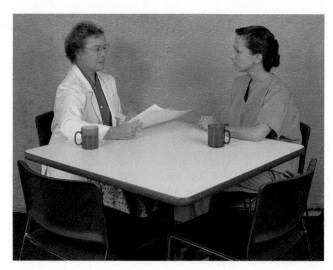

**Figure 23-7**    A comfortable, private setting encourages discussion during an employee evaluation.

human resources managers to determine wages and salaries for comparable individuals with comparable skills. Remember, also, that it is far more cost-effective to reward good employees with a salary increase than it is to train a new employee who commands a lesser salary than current employees. Reward employees well and provide benefits that encourage them to stay with the practice. Employees who stay with the practice for a long time not only fully understand how best to serve their physician-employers, they have established a relationship with patients that is very beneficial.

How much of a raise is to be awarded at the time of salary review is difficult to determine and will depend upon many factors which might include the profits of the year, the patient load, the workload, and the current cost of living.

The critical shortage of health care employees today is reflected in the shortage of medical assistants across the country. Newspapers advertising for individuals to work in the ambulatory care setting tell the story. A consideration worth mentioning is that often the salary does not match the education, experience, and special training required of someone working in the health care field. Educators often hear, "Why would I spend a year or more in education to be paid what I would make working in a fast food restaurant?" Because it is costly in time and resources to replace employees, it is best to invest that cost into a fair and just salary increase for valued employees.

## DISMISSING EMPLOYEES

Most human resources managers do not enjoy rating the performance of other employees particularly when difficult topics are involved and it may be necessary to dismiss an employee. However, the written performance evaluation actually establishes the format for such a dismissal when necessary and is more likely to remove the emotion from the situation. Involuntary dismissal is still difficult when it is necessary.

## Involuntary Dismissal

Involuntary dismissal results from two primary causes: poor performance or serious violation of office policies or job descriptions. When it becomes apparent to the human resources manager that the effectiveness of an employee is dropping well below expectations, it will be known in the review or a performance review may be called. The review allows the employee to be informed of the shortcomings, to explain any reasons for the present situation, and to determine a plan to alleviate the problem. If the problem is a serious one, probation is usually invoked and any lack of significant improvement in the time provided results in immediate dismissal.

When the problem is a violation of either office policy or procedures, both a verbal and a written warning are given to the employee. Involuntary dismissal follows if the situation persists. Dismissal may be immediate if the action is a serious violation of policy. Serious violations will depend upon the office practice, but some causes for immediate dismissal include theft, making fraudulent claims against insurance, placing the patient in jeopardy by not practicing safe techniques, and breach of patient confidentiality.

Some key points to keep in mind when dismissal is necessary are:

1. The dismissal should be made in privacy.
2. Take no longer than 10 minutes for the dismissal.
3. Be direct, firm, and to the point in identifying reasons.
4. Do not engage in an in-depth discussion of performance.
5. Explain terms of dismissal (keys, clearing out area, final paperwork).
6. Listen to employee's opinion and emotions; it is not necessary to agree.
7. Accompany the employee to their desk to pack their belongings.
8. Escort the employee out of the facility; do not allow to finish the work of the day.

## Voluntary Dismissal

Other reasons for dismissal may be more pleasant. Changes in personnel occur for many good reasons and people voluntarily leave their jobs. They may relocate, seek advancement in another facility, or simply have personal reasons for leaving. These employees will give their manager proper notice and be able to turn their current projects and duties over to their replacements. They have time to say good-bye to their friends and leave with a good feeling about their employment.

## Exit Interview

An exit interview is an excellent opportunity for the employee who voluntarily leaves a practice and the human resources manager to discuss the positive and negative aspects of the job and what changes might be made for a new person coming into the facility. A sample exit interview form is shown in Figure 23-8. It also allows the opportunity for the employee to ask for a letter of reference or to view the personnel file before leaving. In a voluntary dismissal, request a letter of resignation for the personnel file.

Any dismissal process, voluntary or involuntary, must include a statement in the personnel file. For involuntary dismissal, be certain that the reasons for the dismissal are well documented. Be honest, nonjudgmental, and do not allow emotions to escalate into hostility and anger. State only the facts in the personnel file; do not

---

### EXIT INTERVIEW FORM

1. What did you like and dislike about the work you have been doing?
   (Including: support on the job; opportunity for personal growth; recognition and rewards)

2. What kind of people have you found the doctors, your immediate supervisor, and co-workers to be?
   (Including: attitude; fairness; scheduling and assignment of work; work expectations; technical competence; assistance and guidance available; team spirit)

3. What is your view of our management practices and policies?
   (Including: clarity and fairness of practice policies; communications; management and staff)

4. How have you felt about performance appraisals, your salary and benefits?
   (Including: adequacy of salary; regularity and fairness of appraisals)

5. What are your principal reasons for leaving the practice?
   (Including: primary dissatisfactions; job or personal changes)

6. In what areas do you feel we need to improve?

Interviewer signature: _____ Date _____

Employee signature: _____ Date _____

**Figure 23-8** Sample exit interview form. (From *Personnel Management Handbook*, 2nd ed., by Maryann Ricardo, The McGraw-Hill Companies, Inc. Copyright 1992. Reprinted with permission.)

state opinion. Remember that employees have the right to view their personnel file at any time.

The physician-employer should always be informed of any dismissal as quickly as possible. Some will be involved in the actual dismissal process. A physician-employer is most likely going to be concerned about ongoing assistance in the practice and that a break not occur in quality care given to patients.

## MAINTAINING PERSONNEL RECORDS

An important aspect of the responsibilities of the human resources manager is maintaining personnel records. All documentation and correspondence related to each employee from application to dismissal, from awards to reprimands including the formal reviews, must be kept in the confidential personnel file. Access to this file is limited to certain management personnel and the employee. Not all of these people are allowed to see the entire file. These files are usually kept for a period of three to five years.

This file also includes the kind of information normally maintained for payroll and business practices. That information includes name, address, and sex of employee. The position title, date of beginning employment, rate of pay (hourly or otherwise), total overtime pay, deductions or additions to wages, wages paid each pay period, and date of dismissal.

## COMPLYING WITH PERSONNEL LAWS

This text is not meant to be a legal guide for a human resources manager. The practice attorney should always be contacted if there is any question regarding personnel laws which may vary in some states depending upon the size of the practice. Only a brief introduction of the laws related to the ambulatory care setting are given.

**Overtime** must be addressed in each practice. Who is reimbursed for overtime and how is that reimbursement determined? Typically, medical receptionists and secretaries, insurance billers, medical transcriptionists, and medical assistants are likely to be paid overtime. Overtime pay at a rate of not less than one and one-half times the regular rate of pay after a forty-hour work week is standard. Each week stands alone and one week cannot compensate for another. If the practice does not want to be involved in overtime situations, require that any overtime be preauthorized in advance.

The Equal Pay Act of 1963 prevents wage discrimination for jobs that require equal skill, effort, and responsibility. The Civil Rights Act of 1964 prevents employers from discriminating against individuals on the basis of race, color, religion, sex, age, or national origin.

Sexual harassment violates Title VII of the Civil Rights Act. Steps must be taken to ensure that all employees are working in an atmosphere that is not hostile, where sexual gestures, the presence of pornographic or offensive materials, or obscene language are not allowed.

Employees have a right to expect safe working conditions. The Occupational Safety and Health Act (OSHA) was established to prevent injuries and illnesses resulting from unsafe or unhealthy working conditions. Compliance with this law requires that each employee be aware of possible risks associated with chemical hazards and bloodborne pathogens and be aware of how to protect themselves. Since there are many of these hazards in a medical practice, compliance and protection for employees are extremely important, and training sessions should be held in this area.

The Immigration Reform Act requires employers to verify the right of employees to work in the United States. Documentation acceptable for verification is a Social Security card or birth certificate. The United States Department of Justice Immigration and Naturalization Service will provide instructions and a form for employees and employers to complete (Figure 23-9).

Employers cannot discriminate or condemn any full-time employee for jury duty. While the employer does not have to continue pay during jury duty, the employee cannot lose seniority, insurance, or other benefits. Many employers continue an employee's full pay during the time of service on a jury since the reimbursement for jury service is so small. This is a way to benefit your employees and encourage good citizenship.

This list is by no means comprehensive, but does include personnel regulations most likely to affect the medical practice. Any concerns should be directed to the practice's attorney.

## SPECIAL POLICY CONSIDERATIONS

There are several other managerial issues that may arise in a medical office for which the office manager will have to plan. These can include policies for temporary employees, smoking, avoiding discrimination, and having a support system in place for employees who need physical or emotional help.

### Temporary Employees

Temporary employees who may be employed for ninety days or less include students who are serving an internship

**U.S. Department of Justice**
Immigration and Naturalization Service

OMB No. 1115-0136
**Employment Eligibility Verification**

**Please read instructions carefully before completing this form. The instructions must be available during completion of this form. ANTI-DISCRIMINATION NOTICE. It is illegal to discriminate against work eligible individuals. Employers CANNOT specify which document(s) they will accept from an employee. The refusal to hire an individual because of a future expiration date may also constitute illegal discrimination.**

**Section 1. Employee Information and Verification.** To be completed and signed by employee at the time employment begins.

| Print Name:     Last | First | Middle Initial | Maiden Name |
|---|---|---|---|

| Address (Street Name and Number) | Apt. # | Date of Birth (month/day/year) |
|---|---|---|

| City | State | Zip Code | Social Security # |
|---|---|---|---|

| I am aware that federal law provides for imprisonment and/or fines for false statements or use of false documents in connection with the completion of this form. | I attest, under penalty of perjury, that I am (check one of the following):<br>☐ A citizen or national of the United States<br>☐ A Lawful Permanent Resident (Alien # A_____)<br>☐ An alien authorized to work until ___/___/___<br>(Alien # or Admission # _____) |
|---|---|

| Employee's Signature | Date (month/day/year) |
|---|---|

**Preparer and/or Translator Certification.** *(To be completed and signed if Section 1 is prepared by a person other than the employee.) I attest, under penalty of perjury, that I have assisted in the completion of this form and that to the best of my knowledge the information is true and correct.*

| Preparer's/Translator's Signature | Print Name |
|---|---|

| Address (Street Name and Number, City, State, Zip Code) | Date (month/day/year) |
|---|---|

**Section 2. Employer Review and Verification.** To be completed and signed by employer. Examine one document from List A OR examine one document from List B **and** one from List C as listed on the reverse of this form and record the title, number and expiration date, if any, of the document(s)

| List A | OR | List B | AND | List C |
|---|---|---|---|---|

Document title: _____

Issuing authority: _____

Document #: _____

Expiration Date (if any): ___/___/___

Document #: _____

Expiration Date (if any): ___/___/___

**CERTIFICATION - I attest, under penalty of perjury, that I have examined the document(s) presented by the above-named employee, that the above-listed document(s) appear to be genuine and to relate to the employee named, that the employee began employment on** *(month/day/year)* ___/___/___ **and that to the best of my knowledge the employee is eligible to work in the United States. (State employment agencies may omit the date the employee began employment).**

| Signature of Employer or Authorized Representative | Print Name | Title |
|---|---|---|

| Business or Organization Name | Address (Street Name and Number, City, State, Zip Code) | Date (month/day/year) |
|---|---|---|

**Section 3. Updating and Reverification.** To be completed and signed by employer

| A. New Name (if applicable) | B. Date of rehire (month/day/year) (if applicable) |
|---|---|

C. If employee's previous grant of work authorization has expired, provide the information below for the document that establishes current employment eligibility.

Document Title:_____ Document #:_____ Expiration Date (if any):___/___/___

**I attest, under penalty of perjury, that to the best of my knowledge, this employee is eligible to work in the United States, and if the employee presented document(s), the document(s) I have examined appear to be genuine and to relate to the individual.**

| Signature of Employer or Authorized Representative | Date (month/day/year) |
|---|---|

Form I-9 (Rev. 11-21-91) N

**Figure 23-9** Employment Eligibility Verification, Form I-9.

from a local college practicing their skills for when they will be on the job. They should be reviewed every two to three weeks in cooperation with their college supervisor. Give them as much actual hands-on experience as possible; they are your future employees and the employees of your colleagues.

## Smoking Policy

Smoking on the premises has become a greater concern in the past ten years. Many places of employment do not allow smoking at all. Some states and cities have laws that may govern this issue for you. When a policy is established, it should cover everyone—employers, employees, and patients. The objective is to have a policy that is workable and enforceable, promotes health, encourages employee morale and productivity, and sets examples for patients. A designated place for smoking may be necessary.

## Discrimination

The Americans with Disabilities Act (ADA) establishes guidelines prohibiting discrimination against a "qualified individual with a disability" in regard to employment. Someone with a disability who satisfies the skills necessary for the job, has the experience, education, and any other job requirements, and who, with reasonable accommodation, can perform the job cannot be discriminated against. Employers often find that persons with disabilities are their finest employees. Of particular note for medical personnel is that persons with AIDS are included in the guidelines set forth by the ADA. Persons with AIDS cannot be discriminated against. It can be assumed that if you are providing a safe working environment and all employees follow the rules for standard precautions, that reasonable accommodation has been made for the person with AIDS.

## Employees with Chemical Dependencies or Emotional Problems

Employees with chemical dependency or emotional problems are ill and are to be treated as such. The situation should be approached constructively rather than punitively. Make a commitment to the employee to assure that the employee is fit for and capable of quality patient care. The human resources manager and physician-employer must be able to recognize the problem when it exists and deal openly and honestly with the issue. If drug or alcohol treatment becomes necessary and an employee is temporarily suspended from employment, do not allow the employee to return unless it is made certain the employee will not endanger herself or anyone else.

## PROVIDING/PLANNING EMPLOYEE TRAINING AND EDUCATION

Health care changes daily; new procedures are established, a better technique is discovered for performing a particular task. Major changes regularly occur in medical insurance. Computer systems are updated or new software is added. A more sophisticated telephone system is installed to make certain patients are responded to promptly. New state or federal regulations demand additional training or compliance to safety regulations not previously necessary. New medications become available which physicians may prescribe and employees must understand. All this demands that employees receive a continuing and constant update in their area of employment.

Training and education may be done within the practice or outside the practice. When an employee is a member of a professional organization such as the American Association of Medical Assistants or the American Association of Medical Transcriptionists, many monthly meetings will include continuing education opportunities. Numerous seminars and conferences held throughout the country may be beneficial to employees. Local hospitals often have continuing education opportunities that might be beneficial. The human resources manager will keep abreast of these opportunities and encourage employees to attend. Any continuing education opportunity that may benefit the employee on the job and the medical practice itself should ideally be paid for by the physician-employer(s).

It is often best to provide training and education within the facility when the training necessary is very specific to the medical practice. For instance, training on new computer software is apt to be very specific to the particular setting. When sophisticated new equipment is purchased, companies often provide in-house training for the individuals who will be using the equipment. Take advantage of as many of those opportunities as are available and for as many of your employees as possible. When the training is quite expensive or time consuming, make certain one person receives the training. Then have that individual train others. Whenever possible, provide training outside of regular hours when patients are not being seen—before or after the office closes or during a lunch period. Always pay employees for any time served over their regular working hours.

Careful attention to continuing education and training for employees will pay for itself many times over

## SPOTLIGHT ON AAMA ESSENTIALS THROUGH CAAHEP

- Conducting an exit interview with an employee who voluntarily leaves his or her position provides an atmosphere where the positive and the negative aspects of the position can be discussed. It can also identify what changes might be necessary when a new person fills the position.

- Part of being a good human resources manager is being able to solve conflicts between other employees, coworkers, supervisors, and physician-employers.

- Being able to acknowledge what stresses employees on the job will help to generate new ways or tasks to decrease or prevent stress.

again. The more confident and secure employees feel in the skills they are expected to perform, the more satisfied the practice's patients will be.

## CONFLICT RESOLUTION

A good human resources manager will be a master at **conflict resolution**, solving problems between any two parties. The most difficult task is to prevent or solve conflicts that occur between employees or between employees and supervisors or physician-employers. Most conflict occurs because of poor communication or a misunderstanding, so effective communication is a goal for any manager.

Volumes of materials have been written about successful conflict management. One can probably never get enough material on the subject. Some guidelines that may be helpful in preventing and resolving conflicts follow:

- Listen to your employees. What do they say? What do they communicate nonverbally?

- Be prepared to temporarily assist an employee having a difficult time.

- Create a safe environment for an employee to admit a mistake.

- Manage by walking around and talking to your employees.

- Acknowledge the stressors of the job and compensate employees.

- Give ample verbal positive comments and pats on the back.

- Be honest with employees at all times.

- Provide office staff meetings in which employees can express their concerns.

- Treat employees fairly.

- Do not tolerate negative comments or actions among employees.

- Remember birthdays and special occasions with cards or small gifts.

- Provide small rewards when possible.

- Expect to work longer and harder than any employee.

- Have the physician-employer host a social lunch every 60 days.

- Keep employees informed of changes impacting them.

- Encourage an open door policy for concerns and complaints.

- Be a role model for all employees.

- Keep confidences.

- Encourage continuing education through workshops and seminars.

There is no end to such a list. A human resources manager who cares about each employee, who "carries water for the workers in the trenches," who administers fairly and honestly creates an environment where conflict will be at a minimum.

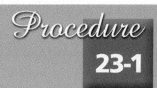

## 23-1 Develop and Maintain a Policy Manual

**PURPOSE:**
To develop and maintain a comprehensive, up-to-date policy manual of all office policies relating to employee practices, benefits, office conduct, and so on.

**EQUIPMENT/SUPPLIES:**
Computer
Binder, such as a three-ring binder
Paper
Standard policy manual format

**PROCEDURE STEPS:**
1. Following office format, develop precise, written office policies detailing all necessary information pertaining to the staff and their positions. The information should include benefits, vacation, sick leave, hours, dress codes, evaluations, rules of conduct, and grounds for dismissal. RATIONALE: Well-defined policies clearly outlined for each employee are necessary for efficient and effective staff operations.
2. Identify procedures for reimbursing overtime, preventing discrimination and harassment, creating a safe working environment, and allowing for jury duty.
3. Include a policy statement related to smoking.
4. Identify steps to follow should an employee become disabled during employment.
5. Determine what employee opportunities for continuing education, if any, will be reimbursed; include requirements for recertification or licensure.
6. Provide a copy of the policy manual for each employee.
7. Review and update the policy manual regularly. Add or delete items as necessary, dating each revised page.

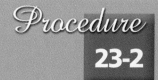

## 23-2 Preparing a Job Description

**PURPOSE:**
To provide a precise definition of the tasks assigned to a job, to determine the expectations and level of competency required, and to specify the experience, training, and education needed to perform the job for purposes of recruiting and performance evaluation.

**EQUIPMENT/SUPPLIES:**
Computer
Paper
Standard job description format

**PROCEDURE STEPS:**
1. Detail each task that creates the job. RATIONALE: A detailed job description identifies clear expectations for each employee.
2. List special medical, technical, or clerical skills required.
3. Determine the level of education, training, and experience required for the position.
4. Determine where the job fits in the overall structure of the office.
5. Specify any unusual working conditions (hours, locations, and so on) that may apply.
6. Describe career path opportunities.

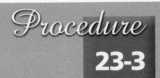

## 23-3    Interviewing

**PURPOSE:**
To screen applicants for training, experience, and characteristics to select the best candidate to fill the position vacancy.

**PROCEDURE STEPS:**

1. Review resumes and applications received.
2. Select candidates who most closely match the education and experience being sought.
3. Create an interview worksheet for each candidate listing points to cover.
4. Select an interview team; this team should always include the human resources or office manager and the immediate supervisor to whom the candidate will report.
5. Call personally to schedule interviews; this allows you to judge the applicant's telephone manners and voice.
6. Remind the interviewers of various legal restrictions concerning questions to be asked.
7. Conduct interviews in a private, quiet setting. RATIONALE: Careful interviewing of potential employees is an important step in hiring the best candidate for the position.
8. Put the applicant at ease by beginning with an overview about the practice and staff, briefly describing the job, and answering preliminary questions.
9. Ask questions about the applicant's work experience and educational background using the resume and interview worksheet as a guide.
10. Provide the most promising applicants additional information on benefits and a tour of the office if practical.
11. Applicant's general salary requirements may be discussed, but avoid discussion of a specific salary until a formal offer is tendered.
12. Inform the applicants when a decision will be made and thank each for participating in the interview.
13. Do not make a job offer until all the candidates have been interviewed.
14. Check references of all prospective employees.
15. Establish a second interview between the physician-employer(s) and the qualified candidate if necessary.
16. Confirm accepted job offers in writing, specifying details of the offer and acceptance.
17. Notify all unsuccessful applicants by letter when the position has been filled.

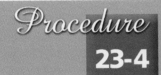

## 23-4    Orient and Train Personnel

**PURPOSE:**
To acquaint new employees with office policies, staff, what the job encompasses, procedures to be performed, and job performance expectations.

**PROCEDURE STEPS:**

1. Tour the facilities and introduce the office staff.
2. Complete employee-related documents and explain their purpose.
3. Explain the benefits programs.
4. Present the office policy manual and discuss its key elements.
5. Review federal and state regulatory precautions for medical facilities.
6. Review the job description.
7. Explain and demonstrate procedures to be performed and the use of procedure manuals supporting these procedures.
8. Demonstrate the use of any specialized equipment.
9. Assign a mentor from the staff to help with the orientation. RATIONALE: Without proper orientation and training, the best new employee can fail.

**CASE STUDY 23-1**

Bruce Goldman, CMA, has been with Inner City Health Care for one year. It is time for his first annual evaluation. The office manager, Jane O'Hara, gives Bruce a performance review form to complete before the formal evaluation. The following day, Bruce has an appointment to meet with Jane to discuss the evaluation. During the meeting, they discover they agree on most points.

### CASE STUDY REVIEW

1. How should Jane handle discussing Bruce's frequent long lunches that extend beyond his scheduled lunch break time?
2. Would it be appropriate for Jane to ask a fellow CMA who works with Bruce to sit in to help her to evaluate him?
3. How should Jane end the formal evaluation?

## SUMMARY

As you have seen from this discussion, human resources management is a challenge. It is, however, a rewarding one. While physician-employers are responsible for patients' physical care, the human resources manager is responsible for the employees in the organization. The human resources manager who is successful will manage these employees in a way that enables and encourages them to give the very best patient care possible. The medical assistant who has good communication skills and acquires additional training in human resources management will always have variety on the job and will have the satisfaction of watching a health care team run smoothly and efficiently.

## REVIEW QUESTIONS

### Multiple Choice

1. Human resources managers:
   a. need no special training for the job
   b. are responsible for hiring, training, and managing personnel
   c. usually work harder and longer hours than employees
   d. both b and c
2. The following questions may be asked in an interview:
   a. How old are you?
   b. Have you ever been arrested?
   c. Can you supply a birth certificate or a Social Security card?
   d. Do you plan to start a family soon?
3. Causes for immediate dismissal of an employee include:
   a. being late for work three times within a month
   b. theft, making fraudulent insurance claims
   c. placing a patient in jeopardy and breaching confidentiality
   d. both b and c

4. The most difficult tasks of the human resources manager may be:
   a. resolving conflicts between personnel and dismissing an employee
   b. evaluating employees and planning salary review
   c. planning for continuing education
   d. communicating with the physician-employer
5. The human resources manager will work closely with:
   a. the physician-employer
   b. the office manager
   c. all employees
   d. all the above
6. OSHA:
   a. requires employers to verify an employee's right to work in the United States
   b. protects employees who have disabilities from employment discrimination
   c. protects employees with chemical dependencies or emotional problems
   d. protects employees from unsafe or unhealthy working conditions

7. Conflict between employees:
    a. usually is the result of personality differences
    b. results when the manager is dictatorial
    c. usually is the result of poor communication or a misunderstanding
    d. is better ignored to allow employees to work it out
8. Employees receiving training or education necessary to the job:
    a. will seek that training after hours and not expect reimbursement
    b. will be continuous and constant in the health care field
    c. should always be paid for any time served over regular working hours
    d. both b and c
9. Personnel records:
    a. are usually kept for three to five years and may include payroll data
    b. are not available for everyone to view and must be kept confidential
    c. include all papers related to employment and personal data
    d. all the above
10. Dismissal:
    a. may be voluntary or involuntary
    b. should always be documented
    c. is a good time for an exit interview
    d. all the above

## Critical Thinking

1. Discuss the importance of having employees participate in providing input to the job description.
2. How are references checked for prospective employees?
3. Discuss the advantages of having established policies and procedures for performance reviews.
4. How and when might physician-employers be directly involved in personnel matters?
5. You have an employee who gossips about other employees and is negative to everyone. She is otherwise an excellent employee. Plan a strategy to correct the situation.
6. You have just accepted a position to work in a larger more specialized clinic where you will be able to use skills you are not currently able to exercise. Identify two or three main points for a letter of resignation you will prepare.

7. An employee approaches you, the human resource manager, identifying that he/she has just become responsible for the care of an aging parent that may require occasional time away from work. You have no policy about how this absence should be treated. What kind of policy might be helpful? Where would you look for suggestions?
8. An exit interview form has been introduced in this chapter. Another simple form for an exit interview is to use the ABCs. A stands for "awesome." What do we do that is really good? B stands for "better." What could we do better in our organization? C stands for "change." What would you recommend we change? Discuss the merits of both forms for an exit interview.
9. Do a simple comparison of salaries in your community. Compare the hourly wages of a secretary, a medical assistant, a plumber, your automobile mechanic, and a person working in a fast-food restaurant. What conclusions can you make, if any?
10. What might physician-employers and human resource managers do to make certain they keep valued employees? Is salary really the most important issue?

## WEB ACTIVITIES

Research the World Wide Web for information about how to hire individuals. Consider http://www.ruf.rice.edu/~humres/Training/HowToHire as one resource for your search. Are there any differences in hiring for the medical profession as opposed to other types of businesses? What tips do you *not* find mentioned in the text?

## REFERENCES/BIBLIOGRAPHY

Andress, A. A. (1996). *Manual of medical office management.* Philadelphia: W. B. Saunders Company.

Kinn, M. E., & Woods, M. A. (1999). *The medical assistant: Administrative and clinical* (8th ed.). Philadelphia: W. B. Saunders Co.

Mathis, R. L., & Jackson, J. H. (2000). *Human resource management* (9th ed.). Cincinnati, OH: South-Western College Publishing.

Ricardo, M. (1992). *Personnel management handbook* (2nd ed.). New York: McGraw-Hill, Inc.

Sullivan, D. (1992). *Effective management in nursing.* New York: Addison-Wesley.

## SCENARIO

Dr. Ray Reynolds currently is the senior physician at Inner City Health Care, a multi-physician urgent care center. When he began his practice thirty-two years ago, however, he had a private practice and employed one full-time and two part-time medical assistants. Dr. Reynolds felt the office ran smoothly, except when an assistant had to be replaced. Retraining a new person consumed a great deal of valuable time. Even if the new employee came with experience from another medical office, the procedures still required retraining.

Dr. Reynolds finds that when he needs to replace a medical assistant now, he looks at the applicants' resumes and interviews only those candidates who are certified medical assistants (CMAs) or registered medical assistants (RMAs). The office is too busy to spend time training and retraining new people.

## INTRODUCTION

Thirty years ago medical assistants were trained on the job by the practitioner for whom they were employed. Quality control of training varied since there were no established criteria for evaluating such training.

Hence, the certification examination was developed by AAMA and the RMA examination was developed by the AMT. Both examinations, along with methods of continuing education and recertification, or revalidation, establish criteria for evaluating training.

## PURPOSE OF CERTIFICATION

Certification is intended to set a consistent minimum standard for evaluating an individual's professional competence as a medical assistant. The **certification examination** is offered by the **American Association of Medical Assistants (AAMA)**. Hiring physicians view the credential as professional and an indication of entry-level skills. Maintaining the credential demonstrates a lifelong commitment to continuing education. The graduate medical assistant has a goal and challenge to which to aspire, first by earning the credential, and second by maintaining the credential through recertification.

Formal medical assistant education programs are offered throughout the country in vocation-technical high schools and colleges, proprietary schools, postsecondary vocational schools, community and junior colleges, and four-year colleges and universities. Medical assistants may be trained on the job; however, physicians recognize that their offices operate more efficiently with professionally educated personnel.

## PREPARING FOR THE EXAMINATION

Preparation for the examination requires forethought, scheduling, and discipline. It is important to plan well in advance to ensure confidence and a positive test result, earning your credential. If you are sitting for the examination immediately upon graduation, your preparation time for the examination may only require two to three months. If you have been out of school for some time or your work experience has been very specialized, you may need six to eight months to prepare for the examination.

During the forethought stage, determine the date you want to sit for the examination. Check with the appropriate Web site or make a telephone call to the examination department to obtain the current application form. The application form will contain information such as dates, times, and locations of test sites, policies regarding deadlines, incomplete applications, examination verification information, and information regarding study guides.

It is also important to consider looking for a study group or partner. The right study environment can be invaluable to your success for several reasons. First, it is important to select a study partner or group who shares your commitment to a successful outcome and who plans to sit for the examination near the same date you have selected. A study partner can also give you some accountability for keeping to the planned schedule.

Once it has been determined when and where you will sit for the examination and who your study partner, if any, will be, a meeting should be scheduled to discuss the review/study approach. It may be that your group will decide to review/study each subject provided in the Curriculum Content Outline accompanying the application. Other groups review/study only those areas in which they feel less confident. A plan that meets the needs of each group member and that all can agree to works best.

Meeting once or twice a week helps the group stay focused and on task. Independent study should be done throughout the week. During the independent study time, each group member may be asked to write 10 multiple choice questions relevant to the weeks' study topic. Answers to these questions should be on a separate page. Some find it helpful to also provide the rationale or textbook page number that supports their answer. When the group meets, a discussion of the study topic could take place and copies of the questions distributed for answering. The questions could then be corrected and discussion of any questionable or missed answers could take place.

Once a schedule has been established and agreed upon, discipline is required. It is critical that each group member spend time individually preparing for the next group meeting. Someone should be put in charge of each group meeting to keep the event from turning into a social time. To help with this, it is a good idea to set a specific time limit for the study/review session. If individuals want to visit after the session, they are free to do that without disrupting the purpose of the session. All members should be committed to being prepared and attending each scheduled review/study session.

## REGISTERED MEDICAL ASSISTANT (RMA)

The American Medical Technologists (AMT), a national certifying body for health professionals, established the **Registered Medical Assistant (RMA)** credential in 1972. The RMA/AMT has its own bylaws, officers, local, state, and national organizations. Applicants for the RMA examination are graduates of schools accredited by the **Accrediting Bureau of Health Education Schools (ABHES)**, a regional accrediting commission, or other acceptable agency. Currently, there are over 52,000 RMAs certified by AMT. Registered medical assistants

### SPOTLIGHT ON AAMA ESSENTIALS THROUGH CAAHEP

● Joining professional organizations, such as AAMA and AMT, and participating in the activities they afford, such as becoming certified or registered, helps a medical assistant to grow both personally and professionally.

● Obtaining certification or registration as a medical assistant requires a professional attitude, a high degree of understanding of medical assistant skills, and a positive approach to working with all types of patients and coworkers.

● A skilled and credentialed medical assistant should possess the ability to see beyond the complaining patient who may not be feeling well, and project a positive and professional caring attitude toward that patient.

and members of the AMT Registry are entitled to wear the RMA insignia.

AMT certification examinations are intended to evaluate the competence of entry-level practitioners. Content areas defined and validated by subject-matter experts, educators, and individuals working in their respective fields make up the test. Registration is granted in conjunction with other indicators of training and experience, since the tests provide only one source of information regarding examinee competence.

## Examination Format and Content

The AMT registration examination consists of 200 to 210 multiple-choice questions. Examinees are required to select the single best answer; multiple answers for a single item are scored as incorrect. Test questions may require examinees to recall facts, interpret graphic illustrations, interpret information presented in case studies, analyze situations, or solve problems. The approximate percentages of questions in content areas are as follows:

1. General Medical Assisting Knowledge—42.5%
   • anatomy and physiology
   • medical terminology
   • medical law
   • medical ethics
   • human relations
   • patient education

2. Administrative Medical Assisting—22.5%
   - insurance
   - financial bookkeeping
   - medical secretarial-receptionist

3. Clinical Medical Assisting—35.0%
   - asepsis
   - sterilization
   - instruments
   - vital signs
   - physical examinations
   - clinical pharmacology
   - minor surgery
   - therapeutic modalities
   - laboratory procedures
   - electrocardiography
   - first aid

## Application Process

The following criteria have been established for applicants sitting for the RMA Examination:

1. Applicant shall be of good moral character.
2. Applicant shall be a graduate of an accredited high school or acceptable equivalent.
3. Applicant must meet one of the following requirements:
   A. Applicant shall be a graduate of a
      - medical assistant program or institution accredited by an organization approved by the United States Department of Education
      - medical assistant program accredited by a Regional Accrediting Commission or by a national accrediting organization approved by the United States Department of Education
      - formal medical services training program of the United States Armed Forces
   B. Applicant shall have been employed in the profession of medical assisting for a minimum of five years, no more than two years of which may have been as an instructor in a postsecondary medical assistant program.
4. All applicants taking the AMT examination must pass to receive the Registered Medical Assistant (RMA) credential.

## Application Completion and Test Administration Scheduling

The candidate should allow ample time for documentation to be completed before considering the scheduling of a test when submitting an application. It is the candidate's responsibility to keep abreast of the progress of the application and to aid in the timely response of references and employers. Tests may be scheduled *only* after applications are completed.

Examinations are administered throughout the year at testing center locations. Although most centers offer tests every week of the year, several locations administer tests only on specific days of the year. A complete and up-to-date list of sites will be forwarded when the candidate's application is approved. Most examinations may be scheduled within three days of application completion.

## CERTIFIED MEDICAL ASSISTANT (CMA)

The American Association of Medical Assistants (AAMA) offers the certification examination. After successfully passing the certification examination, the **Certified Medical Assistant (CMA)** credential is awarded by the Certifying Board of the AAMA. The credential appears after your name and distinguishes you as a professional signifying achievement in a demanding career field.

CMAs are recognized by peers for their commitment to continued professional development. Survey results indicate that employers recognize the value of the credential by paying higher salaries and offering more benefits to CMAs. Broader career advancement opportunities and enhanced job security represent other benefits of certification. The CMA credential is a national credential and therefore is valid wherever the practitioner is employed within the United States.

## Examination Format and Content

The CMA certification examination is a comprehensive test of the knowledge actually utilized in today's medical office. The content is drawn from an in-depth analysis of the numerous tasks medical assistants perform on a daily basis. The consultant for the examination is the **National Board of Medical Examiners (NBME)**, the same organization that develops licensure and specialty board examinations for physicians nationwide.

Examination questions are formulated by the Certifying Board's **Task Force for Test Construction**. This group is comprised of practicing medical assistants, physicians, and medical assisting educators from across the United States. Working with NBME, the Task Force updates the CMA examination annually to reflect changes in medical assistants' day-to-day responsibilities, as well as the latest developments in medical knowledge and technology.

The three major areas tested include:

1. *General medical knowledge:* terminology, anatomy, physiology, professionalism, communication, medicolegal guidelines/requirements
2. *Administrative knowledge:* typing and data entry, equipment, records management, screening and processing mail, scheduling and monitoring appointments, resource information/community services, managing physician's professional schedule and travel, managing the office, office policies and procedures, managing practice finances
3. *Clinical knowledge:* principles of infection control, treatment area, patient preparation and assisting the physician, patient history interview, collecting and processing specimens, preparing and administering medications, emergencies, first aid

Students must enroll as an AAMA member before their graduation date to be eligible for the reduced student rate. Once they are a student member they may stay at the student rate for one year after graduation if they don't choose to be an active or associate member and pay the higher dues amount. The additional year of membership at the reduced rate helps the recent graduate maintain membership while finding a job and getting established in a career.

## Application Process

Candidates will want to read all instructions carefully before completing the application form. Incomplete or incorrect applications will not be processed and will be returned to the candidate. Postmark deadlines for applications, cancellations, and examination location changes are strictly enforced.

The examination is offered at over 250 test sites nationwide. A complete listing of the locations is included in the application. Applications are available from the AAMA Certification Department, 20 North Wacker Drive, Suite 1575, Chicago, IL 60606-2903 or telephone 312-424-3100 or e-Mail: certification@aama.ntl.org.

The appropriate application form must be completed and postmarked by October 1 for the January exam and by March 1 for the June exam.

The certification examination is scheduled from 9:00 AM to 1:00 PM the last Friday of January and the last Saturday in June.

It is recommended that the application be sent by certified mail, return receipt requested to verify delivery. The application must be typewritten or printed using black ink only. Be sure the application is signed and dated properly and the eligibility category section is completed appropriately.

Tear off the application page from the instruction pamphlet. Do not mail the instructions back with the application. Keep this information for future reference along with a copy of everything submitted, including a copy of your completed payment check or money order. If you are paying by VISA or MasterCard, provide the requested information at the top of the application.

A guide for the certification examination entitled *A Candidate's Guide to the AAMA Certification Examination* provides explanations of how to approach the types of questions used on the examination and tips on how to study for the content that will be tested. A sample 120-question examination is included.

## Eligibility Categories and Requirements

You must fulfill one of the four eligibility categories to apply for the CMA examination. Figure 24-1 describes these requirements.

## Grounds for Denial of Eligibillity

The following are grounds for denial of eligibility for the Certified Medical Assistant (CMA) credential, or for discipline of Certified Medical Assistants (CMAs):

- obtaining or attempting to obtain certification, or recertification of the CMA credential, by fraud or deception

- knowingly assisting another to obtain or attempt to obtain certification or recertification by fraud or deception

- misstatement of material fact or failure to make a statement of material fact in application for certification or recertification

- falsifying information required for admission to the CMA examination, inpersonating another examinee, or falsifying education or credentials

- copying answers, permitting another to copy answers, or providing or receiving unauthorized advice about examination content during the CMA examination

- unauthorized possession or distribution of examination materials, including copying and reproducing examination questions and problems.

Individuals who have been found guilty of a felon, or pleaded guilty to a felon, are not eligible to take the CMA Exam. However, the Certifying Board may grant a waiver based upon mitigating circumstances, which may include, but need not be limited to the following:

## CATEGORY 1—CAAHEP GRADUATING STUDENT OR RECENT GRADUATE

*Graduating students* must have completed, by January 31 for the January test and by June 30 for the June test, formal training, including an externship, in a medical assisting program accredited by CAAHEP. If the student fails to complete the program by the required date, the exam will be considered invalid. Scores will not be released, and refunds will not be provided.

*Requirement:* Applications must be signed by the program director and an official transcript must accompany the application.

*Recent graduates* must take the exam within 12 months of graduation to qualify for the discounted fee.

*Requirement:* An official transcript must accompany the application to verify graduation from the program.

## CATEGORY 2—CAAHEP GRADUATE

The candidate must be a graduate of a medical assisting program accredited by CAAHEP.

*Requirement:* An official transcript must accompany the application to verify graduation from the program.

## CATEGORY 3—ABHES GRADUATE

The candidate must have graduated from an ABHES accredited medical assisting program that was ABHES accredited at the time of graduation.

*Requirements:* An official transcript must accompany the application to verify graduation from the program.

## CATEGORY 4—RECERTIFICANT

The candidate must be a Certified Medical Assistant applying for the CMA Examination to recertify his or her credential.

*Requirement:* A copy of the candidate's CMA certificate should accompany the application. (Contact the AAMA Certification Department if you are unable to locate your certificate. The month and year that you passed the CMA Examination will be required to research your records.)

**Figure 24-1** CMA Eligibility Categories and Requirements through June 2002. (Source: *AAMA's CMA Examination.* AAMA Certification Department, Dept. 79-7999, Chicago, IL 60678-7999.)

- the age at which the crime was committed
- the circumstances surrounding the crime
- the nature of the crime committed
- the length of time since the conviction
- the individual's criminal history since the conviction
- the individual's current employment references
- the individual's character references
- other evidence demonstrating the ability of the individual to perform the professional responsibilities competently, and evidence that the individual does not pose a threat to the health or safety of patients

## How to Recertify

Recertification of the CMA credential may be achieved by either reexamination or by the continuing education method. Recertification credits are evaluated on supportive documentation, and on their relevancy to medical assisting as defined by the AAMA Medical Assistant Role Delineation Study or the Content Outline for the Certification/Recertification Examination.

A total of 60 points is necessary to recertify the CMA credential. At least 20 points must be from AAMA continuing education units (CEUs). The remaining 40 points may be any formal credit (e.g., non-AAMA CEUs, contact hours, college credit) that has relevancy to medical assisting as defined by the AAMA Medical Assistant Role Delineation Study (shown in the appendices) or the Content Outline for the Certification/Recertification Examination. All 60 points may be from AAMA CEUs, but 20 *must be* from AAMA CEUs.

Continuing education courses are offered by local, state, and national AAMA groups. Guided study programs are also available through AAMA's "Quest for Excellence" program. *The Professional Medical Assistant,* the official bimonthly publication of AAMA, provides articles designated for continuing education units.

The CMA credentials must be recertified every five years. Certificates are current through December 31 of the fifth year following certification or recertification. For example, if you certified or recertified in 1996, your credential would hold current status through December 31, 2001. Failure to recertify will result in a **not current status**.

A CMA need not be a member of the AAMA, nor currently employed, in order to recertify. Figure 24-2 illustrates the Continuing Education Verification Form used to submit CEUs to AAMA for recertification. The entire recertification by continuing education instructions and application can be downloaded from AAMA's website (www.aama-ntl.org). Review of recertification applications can take up to 90 days. If all criteria are met, recertification is granted. The date that the application is

postmarked to the AAMA Executive Office will be the date of recertification.

Upon meeting recertification requirements, the applicant receives a seal to affix to the original certificate. A Recertification Certificate is also available for purchase. AMT promotes continued education and **revalidation** of the RMA credential. Revalidation is processed through the American Medical Technologists Institute for Education (AMTIE) and is required on a five-year cycle. *Vital Signs,* a quarterly publication by AMT, is designed for registered medical assistants and students of ABHES schools.

The American Medical Technologists Institute for Education (AMTIE) offers STEP, a continuing education home-study program for healthcare practitioners. STEP is published in AMT's *Journal of Continuing Education Topics & Issues*. Health care practitioners may earn continuing education credit for reading articles, answering self-study questions, and returning answer sheets to the AMT office for scoring. AMT records credit earned and issues annual reports of STEP activities to program participants.

### AAMA's CMA Recertification by Continuing Education
### Continuing Education Verification Form

**Name:** Jane Doe  **Social Security Number:** 000-00-0000  **Page Number:** 1

Read the application instructions before completing this sheet. If additional space is needed, this form may be photocopied. You may use computer-formatted facsimiles of any part of this application. TYPE or neatly PRINT the information. This form is also available in a Word or WordPerfect format. You may call the AAMA to request it be sent to you by email or on disk. On each page you use, enter your name, Social Security number, and the page number above. To convert credits to points, see How to Convert Credit to Recertification Points in the instructions. For information on how to determine the content category, refer to the section Content Areas Defined. Supportive documents must be attached to this form. Also attach a photocopy of your original certificate. Do *not* send your original certificate.

| 1 | 2 | 3 | 4 | 5 | 6 | 7 | 8 | 9 |
|---|---|---|---|---|---|---|---|---|
| Date of activity (m/d/y) | Sponsor (group or organization issuing the credit for the continuing education activity) | Program title | Amount and type of credit earned (eg, CEU, CME, contact hour or college credit) | Recertification points — AAMA CEUs | Other credit | Points per content area — Gen. | Adm. | Clin. |
| If using more than one page, copy the cumulative total for each column (5–9) from the previous page ☜ |||||||||
| 7/3/00 | AAMA 10259 | Managing the Medical Office | .4 CEU | 4 | | | 4 | |
| 8/24/00 | Trident Chapter of Medical Assistants | Medical Nutritional Needs | .6 CEU | 6 | | 6 | | |
| 9/2/98 | Eli Lily Co. | Aspects of Diabetes | .2 CEU | | 2 | | | 2 |
| 10/11/00 | Tri-City Chapter of Medical Assistants | Improving Your Coding Skills | .4 CEU | 4 | | | 4 | |
| 11/17/00 | 28784 | Quality Urinalysis Testing | .2 CEU | 2 | | | | 2 |
| 1/9/01 | Administrative Seminars Inc. | Personnel Management | .8 CEU | | 8 | | 8 | |
| 3/19/01 | Riverside Hospital | Hepatitis In-service | 1 Contact Hr. | | 1 | | | 1 |
| 4/24/99 | South Carolina AAMA St. Soc. | Child Abuse | .4 CEU | 4 | | 2 | 1 | 1 |
| 6/21/01 | U. of South Carolina | AIDS Awareness | 2 Semester Hrs. | | 30 | 15 | | 15 |
| 9/8/01 | American Heart Association | CPR | 4 Contact Hrs. | | 4 | 1 | | 3 |
| | | | | | | | | |
| | | | | | | | | |
| **Total points in each column (5–9):** (If using more than one page, copy the cumulative total for each column (5–9) to the top of the next page.) |||| 20 | 45 | 24 | 17 | 24 |

**Figure 24-2**  Sample Continuing Education Verification Form for AAMA. (Source: *AAMA's CMA Examination*. AAMA Certification Department, Dept. 79-7999, Chicago, IL 60678-7999.)

It is February, and Juan Estaban is beginning to research the procedures and requirements for taking the medical assisting certification examination. Juan is enrolled in a CAAHEP-accredited program.

**24-1**

## CASE STUDY REVIEW

1. If Juan wants to take the examination in June, what is the procedure for applying?
2. Juan is setting up a study schedule. He plans to review course textbooks and tests, purchase a certification review study guide, and set up a study group. Set up a sample study schedule.
3. What criteria should Juan use when asking people to join his study group?

It is May, and Nancy McFarland, who graduated from an ABHES-accredited program four and a half years ago, is beginning to research the procedures and requirements for taking the medical assistant examination. Nancy completed her internship at Inner City Health Care and was hired to work there full-time (35 hours per week) when she graduated.

**24-2**

## CASE STUDY REVIEW

1. If Nancy wants to take the exam in January, what is the procedure for applying?
2. Nancy is setting up a study schedule. She plans to review course textbooks and tests, purchase a study guide, and set up a study group. Develop a simple study schedule.
3. What criteria should Nancy use when asking people to join her study group?

## SUMMARY

Many advantages for certification/recertification and registration have been discussed in this chapter. Although certification examinations are not legally required for practicing medical assistants, it is the goal of CAAHEP-accredited and ABHES-accredited institutions to encourage graduates to sit for and maintain their credentials.

Membership in the AAMA or in the AMT is also encouraged. In addition to the previously mentioned advantages of AAMA, other benefits such as receiving quarterly newsletters, *The Professional Medical Assistant* journal, credit card privileges, group insurance plans, legal advice, a loan program, and a discounted car rental program are available.

With nearly 400 local AAMA chapters and 51 affiliate state societies, there is the benefit of networking with others in the profession. As an information source for both professional and association issues, the executive staff at the AAMA's national headquarters is available to answer questions at a toll-free number (1-800-228-2262).

AMT currently has 37 chapters which meet regularly and allow networking with other Registered Medical Assistants plus other allied health professionals registered through the AMT, including phlebotomists, medical laboratory technicians, and dental assistants.

## REVIEW QUESTIONS

### Multiple Choice

1. The goal and challenge of each graduating medical assistant should be to:
   a. find employment
   b. have a good benefit package
   c. possess entry-level skills
   d. earn the CMA credential and maintain it

2. The certification examination is:
   a. a comprehensive test based on tasks medical assistants perform daily
   b. all true/false questions
   c. developed by the AMTIE
   d. developed by the NBME

3. Benefits from membership in a professional organization such as AAMA or AMT include all of the following *except:*
   a. discounted rates on legal representation
   b. legal advice
   c. nationwide networking opportunities
   d. professional journal publications
4. Recertification of the CMA credential options include:
   a. submit work experience
   b. reexamination or CEU method
   c. submit on-the-job training
   d. submit military training
5. Applications for the CMA exam must be postmarked by:
   a. October 1 for January exam and March 1 for June exam
   b. October 31 for January exam and March 31 for June exam
   c. September 30 for January exam and April 30 for June exam
   d. September 1 for January exam and April 1 for June exam
6. The RMA was established by the:
   a. ABHES
   b. CAAHEP
   c. AMT
   d. AAMA
7. Candidates who graduate from a medical assisting program that is not CAAHEP-accredited on the date of graduation, but is accredited by CAAHEP within 36 months of that date, are eligible to apply for the CMA exam under which category(ies)?
   a. Category 1
   b. Category 4
   c. Categories 3 or 4
   d. Categories 1 or 2
8. RMA examinations:
   a. are offered at Cogent testing center locations
   b. are offered twice a year
   c. are offered three times a year
   d. are offered six times a year

## Critical Thinking

1. Describe the purpose and benefits of certification.
2. Identify the necessary qualifications for maintaining current CMA status
3. Identify the necessary qualifications for the certification examination as an RMA.

4. Differentiate between the methods of recertification for the CMA.
5. Identify several approaches to collecting CEUs.
6. List advantages of membership in a professional organization for medical assistants.

## WEB ACTIVITIES

 Using the World Wide Web, search your local and state AAMA or AMT web sites. Print and turn in to your instructor the location, meeting schedules, and any upcoming events planned for your state.

## DOCUMENTATION

Upon successfully passing the Certification Examination and earning the CMA credential, one should begin to document all CEUs earned. Copies of the form illustrated in Figure 24-2 may be obtained from the AAMA for this purpose. It is important to have the following information for CEU documentation:

- complete date of the activity
- sponsor (group or organization issuing the credit for the CE activity)
- program title
- amount and type of credit earned (e.g., CEU, CME, contact hour or college credit)
- recertification points (AAMA CEUs or other credit)
- points per content area (general, administrative, clinical)

## REFERENCES/BIBLIOGRAPHY

AAMA. (1997–1998). AAMA *certification/recertification examination for medical assistants;* January and June 2000 Application Instructions. Chicago: AAMA.

American Medical Technologists. [On-line]. Available: http://www.amt1.com.

Frew, M. A., Lane, K., & Frew, D. R. (1995). *Comprehensive medical assisting: Competencies for administrative and clinical practice.* Philadelphia: F. A. Davis Company.

# Chapter 25

# EMPLOYMENT STRATEGIES

## KEY TERMS

Accomplishment Statements
Application/Cover Letter
Application Form
Bullet Point
Career Objective
Chronological Resume
Contact Tracker
Functional Resume
Interview
Power Verbs
References
Resume
Targeted Resume

## OUTLINE

**Developing a Strategy**
  Self-Assessment
**Job Analysis and Research**
**Budgetary Needs Analysis**
**Resume Preparation**
  Resume Specifications
  Clear and Concise Resumes
  Accomplishments
  References
  Accuracy
  Resume Styles
  Vital Resume Information

**Application/Cover Letters**
**Completing the Application Form**
**The Look of Success**
  Personal and Professional Poise
**The Interview Process**
  Preparing for the Interview
  The Actual Interview
  Closing the Interview
**Interview Follow-Up**
  Follow-Up Letter
  Follow Up by Telephone

## OBJECTIVES

*The student should strive to meet the following performance objectives and demonstrate an understanding of the facts and principles presented in this chapter through written and oral communication.*

1. Define the key terms as presented in the glossary.
2. List the steps involved in job analysis and research.
3. Describe a contact tracker and its usefulness.
4. Give three examples of accomplishment statements.
5. Differentiate chronological, functional, and targeted resumes.
6. Identify the purpose and content of a cover letter.
7. Demonstrate effective ways to anticipate and respond to an interviewer's questions.
8. Describe appropriate overall appearance and dress for an interview.
9. Identify the benefits of writing a follow-up letter.

**GENERAL (TRANSDISCIPLINARY)**

**Professionalism**

- Project a professional manner and image
- Demonstrate initiative and responsibility
- Adhere to ethical principles

**Communication Skills**

- Use effective and correct verbal and written communications
- Recognize and respond to verbal and nonverbal communications

## SCENARIO

Eun Mee Soo is a graduate of a CAAHEP-accredited medical assisting program and recently passed the certification examination. She is now preparing her resume and beginning her job search. Eun Mee plans to move out of state (she always dreamed of moving north), so she will also be looking for a new apartment. All of these changes are a bit unsettling for Eun Mee. She is beginning to wonder if she should not relocate at this time but stay close to home until she feels more secure.

## INTRODUCTION

So you are about to graduate from the medical assistant program! This time is often unsettling since many changes are occurring; the loss of security the classroom environment provided, loss of contact with fellow classmates, and loss of a structured schedule are just a few changes. Questions such as: Am I ready for my first job? How do I find a job? What do I say at the interview? begin to surface.

The focus on employment may represent apprehension and doubt or be sparked with anticipation and a sense of fulfillment. This chapter has been included to provide direction and to help answer some of the questions related to the job search.

## DEVELOPING A STRATEGY

Positive thinking is one of the primary keys to success in planning your career and job search. Positive thinking leads to positive attitudes, positive feelings about yourself and others, and positive words and actions.

There is a job out there for you! Those individuals who are successful at finding that first job devote a minimum of forty hours per week at job strategy tactics. In other words, finding their first job is their first job. These individuals do not become discouraged by rejection, rather they learn from it and work harder for the next opportunity.

### Self-Assessment

Perhaps the first place to begin the job campaign is with a self-assessment exercise. This exercise should stimulate your thought process related to the type of employment upon which you want to focus. Take a moment now to complete the exercise, Self-Evaluation Work Sheet (Figure 25-1).

## JOB ANALYSIS AND RESEARCH

Begin to compile a list of potential employers in your immediate area or the geographical area in which you want to work. This may be accomplished by looking through the yellow pages of the telephone directory and/or the business listings. Select facilities that are within your geographic boundaries, provide the work setting and/or specialty you have selected, and appear to offer the basic guidelines you have established.

Now begin your research. Many offices have brochures available that describe their services, appointment scheduling, telephone policy, fees and insurance protocol, confidentiality issues, after-hours medical coverage, and mission statement or philosophy of practice criteria. Most of the larger medical centers offer community education series and prepare a calendar of events publication. Also found in these publications are articles on wellness issues, safety precautions, financial reports, and introductions of new procedures, equipment, and staff members. These documents are an excellent resource tool for learning more about a particular facility and should be studied carefully.

The computer can be of great value in your job search. There are multitudes of employment sites on the Internet and it is possible to search newspaper want ads for almost any large city you desire. The yellow pages are also on-line for most cities, permitting you to easily search for medical facilities that are in line with your goals and objectives.

It may also be helpful to develop your own list of "Hot Line" telephone numbers. Television and radio sta-

---

## SELF-EVALUATION WORK SHEET

Respond to the following questions honestly and sincerely. They are meant to assist you in self-assessment.

1. List your three strongest attributes as related to people, data, or things.
   i.e.; Interpersonal skills related to people
   Accuracy related to data
   Mechanical ability related to things

   _____ related to _____
   _____ related to _____
   _____ related to _____

2. List your three weakest attributes as related to people, data, or things.
   _____ related to _____
   _____ related to _____
   _____ related to _____

3. How do you express yourself? excellent, good, fair, poor
   Orally _____ In writing _____

4. Do you work well as a leader of a group or team? Yes _____ No _____

5. Do you prefer to work alone and on your own? Yes _____ No _____

6. Can you work under stress/pressure? Yes _____ No _____

7. Do you enjoy new ideas and situations? Yes _____ No _____

8. Are you comfortable with routines/schedules? Yes _____ No _____

9. Which work setting do you prefer?
   Single-physician setting _____ Multiple-physician setting _____
   Small clinic setting _____ Large clinic setting _____
   Single specialty setting _____ Multi-specialty setting _____

10. Are you willing to relocate? _____ Willing to travel? _____

**Figure 25-1**  Self-evaluation work sheets can help determine a person's strengths, weaknesses, and preferences before the job search begins.

---

tions often share these numbers. By compiling these numbers into a list, you can efficiently make calls to determine if positions are open and the correct name and spelling of the person to whom the application should be addressed. A visit to your local employment agency may also provide additional resources. Remember to check for job openings on bulletin boards in laundromats, churches, health clubs, and any variety of locations. The Chamber of Commerce in your community may be another resource to consider. Journals and publications such as *The Professional Medical Assistant* (PMA) and your local AAMA chapter will be valuable resources to utilize. Network with professionals at every opportunity. Employers will often report employment opportunities to the Job Placement Center in the college campus or to your medical assistant instructors.

Competition in today's employment arena is very keen. Solicit all help possible as you search for that first job. Friends, relatives, and acquaintances provide the most successful leads to potential employment opportunities. Tell everyone you are looking for a job, the type of position, and the setting in which you would most like to work. Do not forget to tell your personal physician, ophthalmologist, and dentist about your employment goals. They have contact with other professionals who may need help and want to hire a medical assistant.

Direct contact with employers is the second most successful means of finding employment. It takes a lot of nerve and self-confidence to call on prospective employers unannounced or to pick up the telephone to call and ask if they are likely to be hiring medical assistants in the near future. This is an effective approach, however.

The third most effective way to gain employment is a combination of the methods previously discussed. For example, you are visiting the physician's office for an allergy injection. The medical assistant administering the injection asks how your classes are progressing and you share that you are about to graduate and are looking for an entry-level position. The medical assistant tells you that the office next door has a position open. After the injection, if you are dressed appropriately, you could stop in to inquire about the position and ask for an application form.

Don't overlook your externship facility if you participated in an externship program. Very frequently new MAs entering the job market are hired by the site where they did their externship. The site has had time to come to know them, their work ethic, and their knowledge. In addition the site has already invested time in some training so former externs are knowledgeable of the policies and procedures of the facility. Even if the site decides to advertise for the position and interview candidates, you will have an advantage over the other applicants provided your performance was good during your work there.

Review the reasons for employers not hiring shown in Figure 25-2. This figure lists the qualities employers want and do not want in an employee.

When you are serious about the job search and are giving forty hours per week to the process, you will contact numerous individuals. By devising some means of recording these contacts, their responses, and your action, you will not become confused or forget valuable information. A **contact tracker** such as the one suggested in Figure 25-3 may be helpful.

## BUDGETARY NEEDS ANALYSIS

It is critical that you know just how much income is required to meet your living expenses. To accomplish this, begin to keep a diary of all purchases and payments. By

### REASONS FOR EMPLOYERS NOT HIRING

Employers in business were asked to list reasons for not hiring a job seeker. Given in rank order (from most unwanted to least unwanted), the 15 biggest gripes are as follows:

1. Poor appearance (not dressed properly, poorly groomed).
2. Acting like a know-it-all.
3. Cannot express self clearly; poor voice, diction, grammar.
4. Lack of planning for work—no purpose or goals.
5. Lack of confidence or poise.
6. No interest in or enthusiasm for the job.
7. Not active in school extracurricular programs.
8. Interested only in the best dollar offer.
9. Poor school record (academic, attendance).
10. Unwilling to start at the bottom.
11. Making excuses, hedges on unfavorable record.
12. No tact.
13. Not mature.
14. No curiosity about the job.
15. Critical of past employers.

**Figure 25-2** Reasons for employers not hiring. (Courtesy of Highline Community College, Counseling/Career Center, Des Moines, WA)

reviewing your checkbook register you should be able to itemize basic expenditures; i.e., rent, utilities, payments (car, credit card), food, clothing, insurance, taxes, and so on. Once a monthly expenditure record is established, an estimate of the money required to live on may be calculated.

## CONTACT TRACKER

| | Company Name/Address | Telephone Number | Contact's Name | Resume Sent | Application/ Cover Letter | Application Form Sent | Follow-Up Phone | Follow-Up Letter | Result |
|---|---|---|---|---|---|---|---|---|---|
| 1. | | | | | | | | | |
| 2. | | | | | | | | | |
| 3. | | | | | | | | | |
| 4. | | | | | | | | | |
| 5. | | | | | | | | | |
| 6. | | | | | | | | | |

**Figure 25-3** A simple contact tracker such as this can help organize all communication you may have with potential employers.

# RESUME PREPARATION

A **resume** is a summary data sheet or a brief account of your qualifications and progress in the career you have chosen. It is a useful tool for selling yourself and provides opportunity to describe your education, what you have done, and what you can do, and lists those who can vouch for your integrity and experience. A resume that is well thought out and written in such a way as to create interest in what you have to contribute to the employer may reward you with many interviews. During the interview your resume serves as a reference from which the interviewer may be prompted to ask questions.

## Resume Specifications

The resume should be limited to one page in length. Keep a 1 to 1½ inch margin on all four sides of the page to create a picture-like frame. Capitalize major headings and single space between lines. Double space between sections. The use of **bullet point** lists instead of paragraphs aids the interviewer in gleaning key points quickly.

Select a high-quality bond stationery that is standard 8½ × 11 inches with a weight of between 16 and 25 pounds. This paper weight provides aesthetic benefit and will also accept the ink better resulting in a clean, sharp print resolution. Buff or ivory paper with matching envelope has the greatest eye appeal and distinguishes your resume from others.

Use a computer or word processor to produce your resume. It allows you the freedom to experiment with placement to create a picture-perfect resume or to individualize the resume for a particular position or facility.

## Clear and Concise Resumes

Your resume must be short and easy to read and understand. Use statements that are positive and reflect confidence and portray you as a problem solver. Be sure that any information given within your resume or application form is not misleading or exaggerated. Leave out the word *I* when writing your resume. This is your personal resume and it is understood that you are referring to yourself.

## Accomplishments

Use **accomplishment statements** if you have them from your externship or work experience. Accomplishment statements begin with **power verbs**, give a brief description of what you did, and the demonstrable results that were produced. Figure 25-4 provides a list of sample power verbs. Some accomplishment statement examples are: "Utilized computer skills to schedule and reschedule patient appointments" and "Demonstrated skills in setting up sterile trays and assisting with sterile procedures."

| | | | | | |
|---|---|---|---|---|---|
| Accompanied | Billed | Computed | Demonstrated | Enumerated | Graded |
| Accumulated | Bought | Conducted | Deposited | Established | Graphed |
| Achieved | Budgeted | Conferred | Described | Estimated | Greeted |
| Acquired | Built | Constructed | Detailed | Evaluated | Headed |
| Administered | Calculated | Consulted | Determined | Examined | Hired |
| Admitted | Cashed | Contacted | Developed | Exchanged | Identified |
| Advised | Catalogued | Contracted | Devised | Exhibited | Implemented |
| Allowed | Changed | Contrasted | Diagnosed | Expanded | Improved |
| Analyzed | Charged | Contributed | Directed | Expedited | Improvised |
| Answered | Charted | Controlled | Discovered | Experienced | Increased |
| Applied | Classified | Converted | Dismantled | Fabricated | Indexed |
| Appointed | Cleaned | Convinced | Dispatched | Facilitated | Indicated |
| Appraised | Cleared | Coordinated | Distributed | Figured | Influenced |
| Arranged | Closed | Copied | Documented | Filled | Informed |
| Assembled | Coded | Corrected | Drew | Financed | Initiated |
| Assessed | Collated | Corresponded | Drove | Finished | Inspected |
| Assigned | Collected | Counseled | Earned | Fitted | Installed |
| Attached | Commanded | Created | Educated | Fixed | Instructed |
| Attained | Communicated | Debated | Employed | Formalized | Insured |
| Attended | Compiled | Decided | Encouraged | Formulated | Integrated |
| Authorized | Completed | Delegated | Engineered | Fulfilled | |
| Balanced | Composed | Delivered | Entertained | Generated | *(continues)* |

**Figure 25-4** These sample power verbs may help you define your previous job responsibilities.

| | | | | | |
|---|---|---|---|---|---|
| Interpreted | Maintained | Overcame | Prompted | Related | Showed |
| Interviewed | Managed | Packaged | Proofread | Relayed | Sold |
| Introduced | Manufactured | Packed | Proposed | Renewed | Solicited |
| Inspected | Marked | Paid | Proved | Reorganized | Sorted |
| Inventoried | Marketed | Participated | Provided | Repaired | Stocked |
| Investigated | Measured | Patrolled | Published | Replaced | Stored |
| Invoiced | Met | Perfected | Purchased | Reported | Straightened |
| Issued | Modified | Piloted | Ran | Requested | Summarized |
| Judged | Monitored | Placed | Rated | Researched | Supervised |
| Justified | Motivated | Planned | Read | Responsible for | Supplied |
| Kept | Negotiated | Posted | Rearranged | Retrieved | Taught |
| Learned | Nominated | Prepared | Rebuilt | Revised | Telephoned |
| Lectured | Noted | Prescribed | Recalled | Routed | Tested |
| Led | Notified | Presented | Received | Scheduled | Trained |
| Licensed | Observed | Priced | Recommended | Secured | Transferred |
| Listed | Obtained | Printed | Reconciled | Selected | Transported |
| Listened | Opened | Processed | Recorded | Sent | Typed |
| Loaded | Operated | Procured | Reduced | Separated | Verified |
| Located | Ordered | Produced | Referred | Served as | |
| Logged | Organized | Programmed | Registered | Serviced | |
| Mailed | Outlined | Promoted | Regulated | Set up | |

**Figure 25-4**    *(continued)*

## References

Select a variety of **references** to be included on or with your resume. References may be listed on a separate sheet of paper that matches your resume. An individual who knows you or has worked with you long enough to make an honest assessment and recommendation regarding your background history is an excellent reference person. Use only nonrelated persons as references unless the work relationship has been formalized.

Choose references who are well-respected and are clear speakers and writers. No matter how much someone likes you and your work, it can hurt you if they cannot convey the information in a business-like manner. Professional references such as a former instructor, physician, externship supervisor, or fellow coworkers are excellent reference choices.

Always ask permission to use someone as a reference *before* the name is printed on the resume or reference list. You will want to verify the correct spelling of the reference's name, title, place of employment and position, and telephone number for prospective employers.

Help your references aid you in obtaining an interview and employment. A personal visit or telephone call to discuss your career objectives and how you plan to conduct your job search will be helpful. Ask for any suggestions they may have to offer. Provide them with a copy of your resume and cover letter. This helps them visualize the position for which you are applying and picture how you may benefit that employer.

Keep in touch with references. Check back to see who has called and how things went. Knowing what employers ask may produce some valuable pointers for your next letter, resume, or interview.

Finally, thank your references. They will appreciate knowing how you are doing and that you value their assistance.

Leave out "References Upon Request" if necessary to shorten your resume to save space. Employers know they can ask for references at a later date.

## Accuracy

Proofread, proofread, and proofread your resume. Ask someone who is a good speller or your references to edit your resume. Then proofread it again yourself. Do not rely on your computer spell check; it does not differentiate between words such as to, too, two or here and hear. Eliminate repetition of information such as task descriptions. Summarize employment prior to ten years ago or leave it off if not relevant to the position you are seeking.

## Resume Styles

Various resume styles have been developed, each having specific advantages and disadvantages. You will want to choose the style or combination of styles that best describes your strengths and ability to do the job. It may be to your advantage to check with the human resources department of the facility to which you are applying to see if there is a resume style preference.

**Chronological Resume.** The **chronological resume** is used by individuals who have job experience. The job history begins with the most recent experience first and concludes with the earliest experience at the bottom.

The chronological resume is advantageous when:

- The position is in a highly traditional field, such as teaching, law, or health care, where specific employers are of paramount interest

- You are staying in the same field as prior jobs

- Job history shows real growth and development

- Prior titles are impressive

The chronological resume is *not* advantageous when:

- Your work history is spotty

- You are changing career goals

- You have been in the same job for many years

- You are looking for your first job

Figure 25-5 is an illustration of a chronological resume.

---

**Ashley Jackson**
2031 Craig Street
Renton, Washington 98055
(206) 255-1365

---

**WORK EXPERIENCE**

September, 1996–Present    GROUP HEALTH COOPERATIVE
 Direct support for a dermatology/surgery practice.
 Patient preparation.
 Medical and surgical asepsis.
 Assist with sterile procedures.
 Patient follow-up.

June, 1994–August, 1996    VALLEY INTERNAL MEDICINE
 Clinical responsibilities.
 Assisted with surgeries in ambulatory care setting.
 Patient preparation.
 Medical and surgical asepsis.
 Assisted with sterile procedures.

March, 1994–June, 1994    VALLEY INTERNAL MEDICINE
 Medical Assistant Externship
 Administrative duties and clinical responsibilities utilizing
 all medical assisting skills, including patient induction,
 chief complaint, vital signs, patient preparation, EKGs,
 medical and surgical asepsis, and sterile procedures.

**EDUCATION/CERTIFICATION**

Associate in Applied Science degree, June, 1994, Highline
Community College, Des Moines, Washington, 98198-9800.

Certified Medical Assistant, June, 1994.

**Figure 25-5**    Sample chronological resume.

**Functional Resume.** The functional resume highlights specialty areas of accomplishment and strengths. It allows you to organize these in an order that supports your work objective.

The functional resume is advantageous when:

- Your experience can be sorted into areas of function; i.e., administrative, clinical, supervisory
- You are changing careers
- You are reentering the job market after an absence
- Your career path or growth is not clear from a chronological listing
- You have had a variety of different, apparently unconnected work experiences

- Much of your work has been volunteer, freelance, or temporary
- You want to eliminate repetition of descriptions of job duties
- You have extensive specialized experience

The functional resume is *not* advantageous when:

- You want to emphasize a management growth pattern
- Your most recent employers have been highly prestigious and the specific employers are of paramount interest

A sample of a functional resume for a person reentering the job market is shown in Figure 25-6.

---

**Joan Bishop**
4320 Spraig Street
Renton, Washington 98055
(206) 255-2620

---

**TEACHING:**

Instructed community groups on issues related to child abuse.

Taught volunteers how to set up community program for victims of domestic violence.

Ran workshops for parents of abused children.

Instructed public school teachers on signs and symptoms of potential and actual child abuse.

**COUNSELING:**

Consulted with parents for probable child abuse and suggested courses of action.

Worked with social workers on individual cases, in both urban and suburban settings.

Counseled single parents on appropriate coping behaviors.

Handled pre-take interviewing of many individual abused children.

**ORGANIZATION/COORDINATION:**

Coordinated transition of children between original home and foster home.

Served as liaison between community health agencies and schools.

Wrote proposal to state for county funds to educate single parents and teachers.

**WORK HISTORY:**

1986–1990   Community Mental Health Center, Tacoma, Washington
            Volunteer Coordinator—Child Abuse Program
1990–1994   C.A.R.E.—Child-Abuse Rescue-Education, Trenton, New Jersey
            County Representative

**EDUCATION:**

1970   B.S. Sociology, Douglass College, New Brunswick, New Jersey

**Figure 25-6**   Sample functional resume; this style is useful for a person reentering the job market.

**Targeted Resume.** The targeted resume is best for focusing on a clear, specific job target. It should contain a career objective, and list your skills, capabilities, and any supporting accomplishments related to that objective. Graduating students will find this resume style enables them to list classes related to their career objective, grade point average, student awards, and achievements. This information adds substance to a resume when work experience is minimal and should be at the beginning of the resume since it is your most significant asset.

The targeted resume is advantageous when:

- You are very clear about your job target
- You have had a variety of experiences that appear unrelated to each other, but that include skills that you can use in a skills list related to your job target

- You can go in several directions and want a different resume for each
- You are just starting your career and have little experience, but know what you want and are clear about your capabilities
- You are able to keep your resume on a computer disk

The targeted resume is *not* advantageous when:

- You want to use one resume for several different applications
- You are not clear about your abilities and accomplishments

Figure 25-7 provides a sample of a targeted resume.

---

**Ashley Jackson**
2031 Craig Street
Renton, Washington 98055
(206) 255-1365

---

**CAREER OBJECTIVE:** To obtain a challenging position as a medical assistant
in an ambulatory care/surgery facility.

**ACHIEVEMENTS:**
Certified Medical Assistant.
Graduate of an Accredited Medical Assistant Program.
Experienced in providing assistance with surgeries in an ambulatory care setting.
Excellent communication and interpersonal skills.

**SKILLS AND CAPABILITIES:**
Post-surgery patient follow-up.
Patient induction.
Vital signs.
Patient preparation.
EKGs.
Medical and surgical asepsis.
Sterile procedures.

**WORK HISTORY:**
September, 1996–Present    Group Health Cooperative, Seattle, WA,
                           Surgical Medical Assistant.
June, 1994–August, 1996    Valley Internal Medicine, Renton, WA,
                           Clinical Medical Assistant.
March, 1994–June, 1994     Valley Internal Medicine, Renton, WA,
                           Externship Student/Trainee.

**EDUCATION/CERTIFICATION:**
Associate in Applied Science Degree, Highline Community College.
Certified Medical Assistant.

**AFFILIATIONS:**
American Association of Medical Assistants

**Figure 25-7**    Sample targeted resume; this style is useful when focusing on a specific job target.

## *Vital Resume Information*

All resume styles must contain certain vital information about the job applicant. Essential information includes:

- Your full name, address including street number, city, state, and zip code.

- Your telephone number or a number where a message may be left. Always include the area code with the number.

- Your education. Begin with the most recent school attended and include the name, address, and graduation date with the diploma, certificate, or degree earned.

- Work experience. List company name and address. Do not underestimate the value of any job; relate transferable skills to your career objective.

## APPLICATION/COVER LETTERS

The **application/cover letter** is a means of introducing yourself and submitting your resume to a potential employer with the goal of obtaining an interview. A well-written cover letter will highlight your qualifications and experience for employment and will enhance the information contained within your resume. The letter should follow a standard business style and should never be more than one page in length. It should be printed on the same paper as the resume.

Since this may be your first contact with a potential employer, the letter should sell you and describe your intentions regarding employment, display your personality, and create an interest in reading your enclosed resume.

Some guidelines to follow in writing the application/cover letter include:

1. Address your letter to a specific individual whenever possible. You may need to make a telephone call to obtain the name and correct spelling.
2. Keep the letter short, use correct grammar and spelling, and follow standard business letter format.
3. The first paragraph should state your reason for writing and focus the reader's attention.
4. The second paragraph should identify how your education, experience, and qualifications relate to the job and refer to the enclosed resume.
5. The last paragraph should close with a request for an interview.
6. Do not reproduce cover letters. An original letter should be sent to each individual.
7. The cover letter and resume should be mailed in a business size envelope that matches its contents or in an 8½ × 11 manila envelope containing your return address.

A sample of an application/cover letter is shown in Figure 25-8A.

An alternate example of an application/cover letter using Information Mapping® to highlight and draw attention to specific information in your letter is shown in Figure 25-8B. This format is considered easier to read because the focus is on specific blocks of information. In addition, its uniqueness draws attention to your letter and resume and may result in your being selected when competition is keen.

## COMPLETING THE APPLICATION FORM

Sooner or later during the job search you will be asked to complete an **application form**. How well you complete this task may be a key factor in obtaining an interview and/or that first job.

Reading through the application form questions, you may be tempted to write in "See resume" rather than repeat pertinent information already contained within your resume. Do not fall into this pitfall. Answer every item completely. Read all the directions carefully. Look for seemingly insignificant directions placed at the top or bottom of the page that state "Print Carefully," "Complete in Your Own Handwriting," or "Please Type." Employers may use this to assess your ability to read and follow directions.

If the application is to be handwritten, use black ink to complete the form. Black ink is considered legal and often is an indelible (permanent) ink and is more legible if the form must be duplicated. Concentrate when completing the form and be sure to print clearly and make no errors.

The current trend is toward on-line application forms. These forms are prepared by keying information into the appropriate spaces or blocks by using a computer. The completed forms may then be printed and mailed to the perspective employer or sent electronically. Sending electronically is increasingly the preferred method. All of the concerns relative to care in following instructions, providing complete and accurate information, and proofing the application for any errors before sending are applicable.

If you are asked to list experience but the application does not specify "paid experience," be sure to list any volunteer or externship experience that relates to the position you are seeking. Part-time employment can be important as an indicator of your willingness to work, your ability to serve the public, and your organizational skills.

You may be asked to complete the application form "on the spot." Plan ahead for this event and carry a completed copy of your resume, reference list, and

2031 Craig Street
Renton, Washington 98055
August 22, 20____

Sarah Molles, Manager
Seattle Group Health Cooperative
304 Fourth Avenue
Seattle, Washington 98124-1716

Dear Ms. Molles:

I read your advertisement in the *Seattle Times* for a medical assistant to assist in a dermatology surgery practice. I meet the qualifications listed and would like to be considered for the position.

I am currently a certified medical assistant graduated from a two-year accredited program. I have experience as a clinical assistant in an internal medicine clinic and have excellent communication and interpersonal skills.

I would like to request an interview to discuss how I could be of value to your organization in the subject position.

Yours truly,

*Ashley Jackson*

Ashley Jackson

Enclosure, Resume

**Figure 25-8(A)** Sample application/cover letter.

---

2031 Craig Street
Renton, Washington 98055
August 22, 20____

Sarah Molles, Manager
Seattle Group Health Cooperative
304 Fourth Avenue
Seattle, Washington 98124-1716

SUBJECT: SURGICAL MEDICAL ASSISTANT POSITION

| | |
|---|---|
| **Background** | I read your advertisement in the *Seattle Times* for a medical assistant to assist in a dermatology surgery practice. I meet the qualifications listed and would like to be considered for the position. |
| **Qualifications** | I am a certified medical assistant graduated from a two-year accredited program. I have experience as a clinical assistant in an internal medicine clinic and have excellent communication and interpersonal skills. |
| **Requested Action** | I would like to request an interview to discuss how I could be of value to your organization in the subject position. |

Yours truly,

*Ashley Jackson*

Ashley Jackson

Enclosure, Resume

**Figure 25-8(B)** Sample information mapped letter.

application/cover letter with you. Information not included in your resume, such as which years you attended high school and your salary history, should also be carried with you. These documents should provide all the information needed to complete the application form and may be submitted with the application form. This demonstrates to the potential employer your seriousness and preparedness for finding a job.

## THE LOOK OF SUCCESS

The look of success begins with the outward appearance. First impressions are lasting, so strive for a favorable, professional look from head to toe.

Hair should be clean, shiny, and healthy looking, and worn in an appropriate style for the ambulatory care setting. Long hair should be worn off the collar in perhaps a French braid or twist. Long hair that is worn on the shoulders or down the back has the potential for being caught in equipment. It also serves as a host for many airborne pathogens.

The skin should have a healthy glow. Consultation with a cosmetician may prove helpful in solving skin problems or provide opportunity for trying new products. A basic understanding of your personal skin type and selection of cosmetics that complement your skin tone aid in the presentation of a professional appearance. The natural look is most appropriate for the medical office.

Daily bathing, whether by soaking in a tub and using a loofah sponge or using a pulsating shower, cleanse and relax the body. If your skin tends to be dry, apply lotion or emollient cream to replace the natural oils depleted by the water. Many lotions, talcum powders, and deodorants are scented. Remember to use caution where perfumes and scents are concerned since many magnify when the body is under stress and the scent may be offensive or cause allergic reactions in others.

Bathe the feet, carefully washing between each toe, and take care to dry the feet completely. This aids in the prevention of fungal growth. To prevent ingrown toenails, trim the nails straight across rather than rounding the nails as you do the fingernails.

Fingernails should be manicured on a weekly basis. Nails should be short and oval shaped or have rounded corners. Cuticles should be softened by soaking the fingertips in warm water. Gently use an orange stick or a cotton-tipped swab and push the cuticle back. To prevent hangnails, apply cuticle oil as you gently push the cuticle back. Only clear nail polish should be worn in the ambulatory care setting. Nail polish that is chipped or cracked must be removed or replaced immediately as it creates crevices in which pathogens may hide, multiply, and be spread.

First impressions are lasting so make yours professional in all respects. Conservative business attire is appropriate. A tailored suit or a classic dress are effective in portraying a professional image. Pay attention to details such as your jewelry and shoe selection. Shoes should be polished and in good repair. They should fit properly and be comfortable and easy to walk in (Figure 25-9).

## *Personal and Professional Poise*

When you feel well and know that you look good, you project a confident and professional appearance. In other words, you are professionally poised. Webster's dictionary defines poise as balance and stability; ease and dignity of manner. Personal poise combines all of the previously mentioned body appearances plus smoothness of movement and physical flexibility.

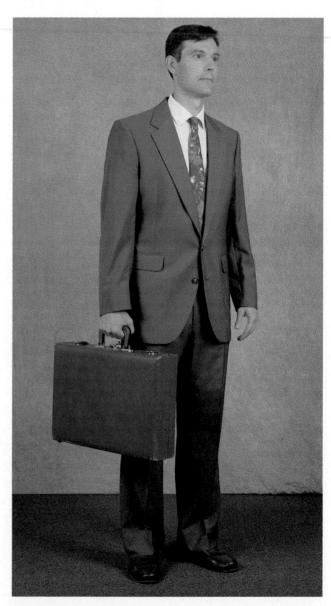

**Figure 25-9**    Medical assistant appropriately dressed and prepared for the interview.

SPOTLIGHT ON AAMA
ESSENTIALS THROUGH CAAHEP

- Positive thinking is one of the primary keys to success in planning a career and conducting a job search.

- A person's outward appearance and first impression are lasting; they can make the difference between a positive and a negative job interview.

- Feeling well and dressing in an appropriate manner will help you to project the image of a confident and poised professional member of the health care team.

## THE INTERVIEW PROCESS

If your application/cover letter and resume have made a favorable impression with the organization, you may be invited for an interview. An interview is a meeting in which you and the interviewer discuss the employment opportunities within that particular organization. It will be the interviewer's responsibility to determine if you have the personality, education, and skills to perform the job. You, on the other hand, will be selling your qualifications and assessing if this is an organization in which you want to be employed.

Being well prepared for the interview will increase your self-confidence and ability to focus during the actual interview. Knowing that your application/cover letter, resume, and references all support your career goal and objectives allows you time to concentrate on interview preparation and presentation.

### Preparing for the Interview

Before the interview takes place, you will want to study carefully the organization for which you are interviewing. Be prepared to relate your skills and interests to the needs of this organization. In other words, what can you contribute and why should they hire you? The interview is your opportunity to sell yourself and identify ways in which you can benefit the employer.

A copy of your resume and cover letter should be brought along to the interview just in case the interviewer can not locate the original or wants another copy. You should also have copies of letters of recommendation, a list of references, a copy of your transcript from the schools you attended, and copies of any certificates such as

AIDS training, First Aid, and CPR. These items should not be presented unless dictated by events that take place during the interview. You might also have with you the name of the interviewer and a copy of any questions you plan to ask the interviewer. A last minute review will refocus your thoughts before you go into the interview. You could also keep your list available for quick reference in the event that your mind goes blank when you are asked if you have questions.

In order to arrive five to ten minutes early, you may need to check a map for directions or make a trip the day before your interview. Try to travel about the same time as you would for the interview so you have an idea of the time it takes, traffic flow, construction areas encountered, and parking availability.

Introduce yourself confidently to the receptionist and identify by name the person you wish to see and the time of your appointment. Always arrive alone. The employer wants to see you and sense your self-reliance and responsibility. While you wait, try to relax and observe the office setting, other employees, what they are wearing, and their manner of conducting business. This may be helpful to you during the interview and in making a decision to work here.

### The Actual Interview

When you enter an interviewer's office, think of yourself as a guest and take your cues from him or her. Most interviewers will introduce themselves and extend their hand. A firm handshake, responding by introducing yourself and smiling confidently convey a positive professional image. Remain standing until you are invited to be seated. Keep your personal items on your lap or place them on the floor near your chair. Do not invade the interviewer's territory by placing your things on the desk.

Sit erect in the chair with your feet flat on the floor or crossing only your ankles. Avoid nervous mannerisms while you speak and maintain good eye contact. Be natural and positive about the position, organization, and yourself. Present a professional image by using medical terminology when responding to questions or providing information. Observe the interviewer carefully for cues. Respond to questions completely, trying not to repeat yourself or give more information than was requested.

Be prepared for the kinds of questions that may be asked during the interview process. Ask yourself, "If I were the employer, what would I want to know about the applicant?" Figure 25-10 contains examples of standard questions asked by most employers. Consider how you would respond to each question.

Remember that the interviewer is asking questions to determine if you are qualified for the position and if you are the kind of person that will fit into the organization.

## TYPICAL QUESTIONS ASKED DURING AN INTERVIEW

1. I see from your resume you graduated from _____ college. What did that college have to offer that others didn't?

2. What subjects did you enjoy the most and why?

3. What do you see yourself doing five years from now?

4. Tell me about yourself.

5. What do you consider to be your greatest strengths and weaknesses?

6. How do you think a friend or professor who knows you well would describe you?

7. What qualifications do you have that make you think you would be successful in this position?

8. In what ways do you think you can make a contribution to our organization?

9. What two or three accomplishments have given you the most satisfaction?

10. How well do you work under pressure?

11. Will you be able to work overtime occasionally?

12. Do you have any questions you would like to ask?

**Figure 25-10** Knowing how you would answer some of these typical questions can prepare you for your interview.

*Think* before answering questions; try to provide the information requested in a positive and professional manner. *Listen* carefully so that you understand what information the question is requesting. *Ask* for clarification if you are uncertain. This demonstrates your ability to be open enough to ask questions when in doubt.

### Closing the Interview

By observing the interviewer and listening carefully, you will be able to determine when the interviewer feels he or she has enough information about you to make a decision. Usually during the closing the interviewer will ask if you have any additional questions. This is your opportunity to collect information helpful in making a decision to accept or decline an offer. Your questions provide another opportunity to sell yourself, show that you have done your homework about the organization, and have listened carefully during the interview. Select three or four questions that will help you the most.

Questions about the organization are excellent choices. Examples might be:

- "What are the opportunities for advancement with this organization?"

- "I read that your organization has educational benefits. Could you explain briefly how that program works?"

- "You mentioned in-house training programs for employees. Could you give one or two examples?"

You may also have some questions about the job itself. Examples of these types of questions are:

- "Is this a newly created position? If so, what results are you hoping to see?"

- "Was the last person in this position promoted? What contributed to their advancement?"

- "What do you consider the most difficult task on this job?"

- "What are the lines of authority for this position?"

Do not use this question time to ask about salary, sick leave, vacations, or retirement benefits. At this point, your focus should be on the value and skills you can contribute to the organization. These questions may be asked during a second interview or when a position is offered.

Before you leave, thank the interviewer for taking time to discuss the position with you. If you definitely are interested in the position, ask to be considered as a candidate for the position. If follow-up procedures have not been explained, now is the time to ask when the final selection will be made and how you will be notified. A firm handshake as you leave, a pleasant smile, and confidence as you exit will leave a professional picture in the interviewer's mind.

## INTERVIEW FOLLOW-UP

Following up after the interview is essential. This is the time to telephone your references to let them know the name of the organization and the person's name with whom you interviewed, something about the position, and your qualifications. Share any information that will help your references support you in obtaining the position.

### Follow-Up Letter

Take time to write a follow-up letter to the interviewer a day or two after your interview. The letter should be written in standard business format and printed on the same paper as your application/cover letter and resume. Be sure that all spelling and grammar are correct.

The follow-up letter provides another opportunity to express your interest in the organization and the position. You can briefly emphasize the experience and skills you have to offer and again request being considered a candidate for the position.

Record the mailing date on your contact tracker and keep a copy of the letter in a file with other information about the organization. Figure 25-11 is a sample follow-up letter.

## Follow Up by Telephone

Allow a few days for your follow-up letter to reach the interviewer. If you do not hear from the interviewer within a week or by the designated time established during the interview, you may telephone to ask if you are still being considered for the position or if a decision has been made.

Speak directly into the mouthpiece of the telephone using good diction and voice volume. Identify yourself and provide some information to aid the interviewer in recalling who you are. Perhaps mentioning the date you interviewed will suffice. Be polite and professional and remember to thank the individual for speaking with you. At the end of the conversation say good-bye and wait until they hang up before you break the connection. Log the telephone call and its response on your contact tracker for future reference.

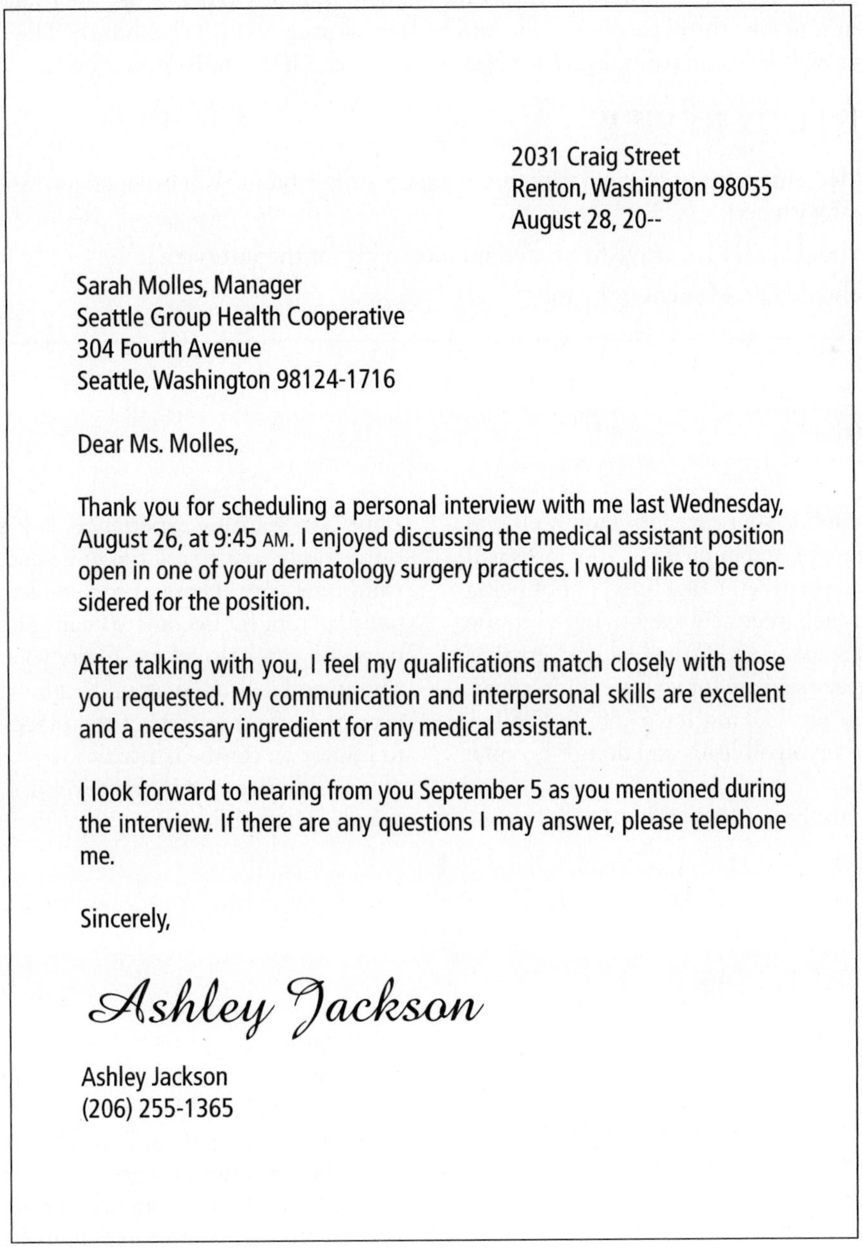

2031 Craig Street
Renton, Washington 98055
August 28, 20--

Sarah Molles, Manager
Seattle Group Health Cooperative
304 Fourth Avenue
Seattle, Washington 98124-1716

Dear Ms. Molles,

Thank you for scheduling a personal interview with me last Wednesday, August 26, at 9:45 AM. I enjoyed discussing the medical assistant position open in one of your dermatology surgery practices. I would like to be considered for the position.

After talking with you, I feel my qualifications match closely with those you requested. My communication and interpersonal skills are excellent and a necessary ingredient for any medical assistant.

I look forward to hearing from you September 5 as you mentioned during the interview. If there are any questions I may answer, please telephone me.

Sincerely,

*Ashley Jackson*

Ashley Jackson
(206) 255-1365

**Figure 25-11** Sample follow-up letter.

Eun Mee Soo is a recent graduate of an accredited medical assisting program and has no medical work experience except her externship at Inner City Health Care. Eun Mee has been employed part-time as a sales representative (clerk) in one of the city's prestigious clothing stores while she attended school.

## 25·1 CASE STUDY REVIEW

1. Which resume style would represent Eun Mee best and why?
2. What information should Eun Mee provide in the vital information section of the resume?
3. What is the purpose of an accomplishment statement? Provide an example of one that Eun Mee might use.

Doctors Lewis and King maintain a two-doctor family physicians' office. They are in need of a new medical assistant to take the place of one who will be leaving at the end of the month. They have established interviews with five applicants. Eun Mee Soo is the first candidate to be interviewed.

## 25·2 CASE STUDY REVIEW

1. Eun Mee enters the interview with some papers in her hand. What paperwork should she have brought with her?
2. Why should Eun Mee arrive five to ten minutes early for the interview?
3. How should Eun Mee enter the room?

## SUMMARY

Finding your first job is your first job. How well you research, plan, prepare, and implement your tasks will make the difference between being hired or not being hired. Learn from each interview session. Listen to the questions that were asked and formulate answers that you feel would be appropriate for your next interview. Tell everyone you are looking for a job and solicit their help. Follow up on all leads and do not become discouraged.

Once you have been hired at that first job, continue your learning experience. Ask appropriate questions and try not to ask the same question a second or third time. Pay attention to details and learn individual preferences. Become a team player and look for ways you can help others. Carry your share of responsibility and do not be afraid to admit you are unfamiliar with certain aspects of the office. Employers need to know you can be trusted to work within the scope of your education and not beyond. Practice being an asset to your employer.

## REVIEW QUESTIONS

### Multiple Choice

1. The resume:
   a. is a summary data sheet or brief account of your qualifications and progress in your career
   b. is also known as a contact tracker
   c. always includes references
   d. is used to introduce yourself and identify qualifications

2. References:
   a. must always be listed on the resume
   b. should be a relative
   c. should be someone who likes you and your work but may not be a good communicator
   d. should be someone who knows you or has worked with you long enough to make an honest assessment of your capabilities and integrity

3. The targeted resume is advantageous:
   a. when prior titles are impressive
   b. when reentering the job market after an absence
   c. when you are just starting your career and have little experience
   d. when you have extensive specialized experience
4. The application/cover letter is:
   a. a detailed data sheet describing your vital information, education, and experience
   b. introduces you to a prospective employer and captures their interest in you as a candidate for the position
   c. lists individuals who can vouch for you
   d. should be lengthy and detailed
5. The interview:
   a. does not require much thought or preparation
   b. requires you to think before answering questions, listen carefully, and ask for clarification if uncertain of the question
   c. provides time to ask questions about salary, vacation, and benefits
   d. does not require any follow-up
6. Preparing for the interview:
   a. bathe yourself, groom your hair and fingernails, and wear clean and pressed conservative business attire
   b. allow adequate time to get to the interview
   c. prepare a packet to give the interviewer containing certificates, letters of recommendation, a list of references, and your list of questions
   d. a, b, and c
7. Job analysis should include:
   a. compiling a list of potential employers
   b. gathering information about employers in whom you have interest
   c. preparing a budgetary needs analysis
   d. all of the above
8. The best source for job search data is:
   a. the Internet
   b. friends and acquaintances
   c. the yellow pages and classified ads
   d. all the above
9. A frequently overlooked potential employer is:
   a. your personal health care provider
   b. your externship site
   c. the local hospital
   d. all of the above

10. You can impress the interviewer by:
    a. acting like you know it all
    b. having poise and good appearance
    c. showing flexibility by having no specific goals
    d. all of the above

## Critical Thinking

1. Discuss the various resume styles and determine which style would be most suitable for you.
2. Discuss methods of researching a prospective employer.
3. Review Figure 25-2 and discuss the rationale behind each reason for employers not hiring.
4. Prepare a budget and discuss it with a classmate.
5. Collect and review numerous application forms.

## WEB ACTIVITIES

Select a location in the United States and use the Internet to research potential openings for medical assistants. Go to the Internet site Yahoo! [http://www.yahoo.com/] and research positions available at the location you have selected. Then research salaries for medical assistants in that area. If you have trouble working through the menu, select the site careers.yahoo.com and use the sections on job search and researching salaries to obtain the information. After you have completed these tasks, prepare an information packet on one of the facilities with a job opening for medical assistant. Include address, phone number, person to contact, and type of procedures performed at the location. You may need to do further Internet research to obtain some of this information. Follow the instructor's instructions on completing and turning in your results.

## DOCUMENTATION

Copy or design your own contact tracker form and document all pertinent information regarding your job search contacts.

## REFERENCES/BIBLIOGRAPHY

Yate, M. (1994). *Knock 'em dead the ultimate job seeker's handbook.* Holbrook, MA: Bob Adams, Inc.

Yate, M. (1993). *Resumes that knock 'em dead.* Holbrook, MA: Bob Adams, Inc.

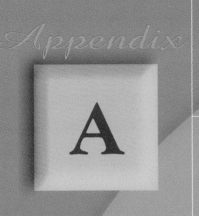

# COMMON MEDICAL ABBREVIATIONS AND SYMBOLS

| | |
|---|---|
| a̅a̅ | of each |
| AAMA | American Association of Medical Assistants |
| AAMT | American Association of Medical Transcription |
| ab | abortion |
| abd | abdomen |
| ABE | acute bacterial endocarditis |
| ABG | arterial blood gases |
| ABHS | Accrediting Bureau of Health Education Schools |
| ABO | blood groups |
| abs | absent |
| ac | before meals (ante cibum) |
| ac | acute |
| ACTH | adrenocorticotropic hormone |
| AD | right ear (auris dexter) |
| ADA | Americans with Disabilities Act |
| ADL | activities of daily living |
| ad lib | as desired |
| adm | admission |
| AFP | alpha fetal protein |
| AHD | arteriosclerotic heart disease |
| | atherosclerotic heart disease |
| AIDS | acquired immunodeficiency syndrome |
| AL | left ear (auris laevus) |
| alb | albumin |
| AM | before noon (ante meridiem) |
| AMA | against medical advice |
| | American Medical Association |
| AMI | acute myocardial infarction |
| amt | amount |
| ant | anterior |
| ante | before |
| A&P | anterior and posterior |
| | auscultation and palpation |
| | auscultation and percussion |

| | |
|---|---|
| aq | water |
| A/R | accounts receivable |
| ARU | automated routing unit |
| AS | left ear (auris sinistra) |
| ASA | acetylsalicylic acid |
| ASAP | as soon as possible |
| ASCAD | arteriosclerotic coronary artery disease |
| ASCVD | arteriosclerotic cardiovascular disease |
| | atherosclerotic cardiovascular disease |
| AU | each ear (aures unitas) |
| A&W | alive and well |
| Ba | barium |
| BaE | barium enema |
| BBB | bundle branch block |
| BC | birth control |
| BC/BS | Blue Cross/Blue Shield |
| BE | bacterial endocarditis |
| | barium enema |
| bid | twice a day |
| bil | bilateral |
| BM | basal metabolism |
| | bowel movement |
| BMR | basal metabolism rate |
| BP | blood pressure |
| BPH | benign prostatic hypertrophy |
| BS | blood sugar |
| | bowel sounds |
| | breath sounds |
| BSA | body surface area |
| BSI | body substance isolation |
| BSL | blood sugar level |
| BSN | bowel sounds normal |
| BSO | bilateral salpingo-oophorectomy |
| BSR | blood sedimentation rate |
| BUN | blood urea nitrogen |

| | |
|---|---|
| BW | below waist |
| | birth weight |
| | body weight |
| Bx | biopsy |
| C | Celsius |
| | centigrade |
| c̄ | with |
| C1 | first cervical vertebra |
| CA | cancer |
| | carcinoma |
| Ca | calcium |
| CAAHEP | Commission on Accreditation of Allied Health Education Programs |
| CAD | coronary artery disease |
| CAHD | coronary arteriosclerotic heart disease |
| caps | capsules |
| CAT | computerized axial tomography |
| CBC | complete blood count |
| CC | chief complaint |
| cc | cubic centimeter |
| CCU | coronary care unit |
| C&D | cystoscopy and dilation |
| CDC | U.S. Centers for Disease Control and Prevention |
| CE | continuing education |
| cerv | cervical |
| | cervix |
| CEU | continuing education unit |
| CHAMPUS | Civilian Health and Medical Program of the Uniformed Services |
| CHAMPVA | Civilian Health and Medical Program of the Veterans Administration |
| CHD | childhood disease |
| | congenital heart disease |

| | | | | | | |
|---|---|---|---|---|---|
| CHD | congestive heart disease | DOB | date of birth | fl | fluid |
| | coronary heart disease | DOD | date of death | fl dr | fluid dram |
| CHF | congestive heart failure | DOE | dyspnea on exertion | fl oz | fluid ounce |
| CHO | carbohydrate | dos | dosage | FMP | first menstrual period |
| CIN | cervical intraepithelial | DPM | doctor of podiatric medicine | FP | family practice |
| | neoplasia | DPT | diphtheria, pertussis, and | freq | frequent |
| ck | check | | tetanus | FSH | follicle-stimulating hormone |
| Cl | chlorine | DR | delivery room | ft | foot |
| cldy | cloudy | Dr | doctor | FTP | file transfer protocol |
| CLIA | Clinical Laboratory | dr | dram | fx | fracture |
| | Improvement | DRGs | diagnosis-related groups | | |
| | Amendments | DSD | dry sterile dressing | G | gravida |
| cm | centimeter | dsg | dressing | g | gram |
| CMA | certified medical assistant | DT | delirium tremens | GB | gallbladder |
| CME | continuing medical education | DTR | deep tendon reflex | GC | gonococcus |
| CNS | central nervous system | D&V | diarrhea and vomiting | | gonorrhea |
| C/O | complains of | DW | distilled water | GI | gastrointestinal |
| $CO_2$ | carbon dioxide | D/W | dextrose in water | gm | gram |
| COB | coordination of benefits | dx | diagnosis | GP | general practice |
| COPD | chronic obstructive | | | gr | grain |
| | pulmonary disease | ea | each | grav | pregnancy |
| CPR | cardiopulmonary resuscitation | EBV | Epstein-Barr virus | GTH | gonadotropic hormone |
| CPT | Current Procedural Code | ECG | electrocardiogram | GTT | glucose tolerance test |
| CPU | central processing unit | Echo | echocardiogram | gtt(s) | drop (drops) |
| crit | hematocrit | | echoencephalogram | GU | genitourinary |
| CS | cerebrospinal | E. coli | *Escherichia coli* | GYN | gynecology |
| CS | cesarean section | ECT | electroconvulsive therapy | | |
| C&S | culture and sensitivity | EDC | estimated date of confinement | h | hour |
| CSF | cerebrospinal fluid | | or expected date of | HBP | high blood pressure |
| CSR | continuous speech | | confinement | HCFA | U.S. Health Care Financing |
| | recognition | EDD | estimated date of delivery or | | Administration |
| CT | computerized tomography | | expected date of delivery | hCG | human chorionic |
| CVA | cerebrovascular accident | EEG | electroencephalogram | | gonadotropin |
| CVP | central venous pressure | EENT | eyes, ears, nose, and throat | HCL | hydrochloric acid |
| CVS | chorionic villus sampling | eg | for example | HCPCS | HCFA Common Procedure |
| cx | cervix | EKG | electrocardiogram | | Coding System |
| CXR | chest x-ray | elix | elixir | Hct | hematocrit |
| cysto | cystoscopic examination | EMG | electromyography | HCVD | hypertensive cardiovascular |
| | cystoscopy | EMS | emergency medical service | | disease |
| | | ENT | ear, nose, and throat | HEENT | head, eyes, ears, nose, and |
| DACUM | developing a curriculum | EOB | explanation of benefits | | throat |
| DC | doctor of chiropracty | eos | eosinophil | Hgb | hemoglobin |
| D&C | dilation and curettage | EPO | exclusive provider | H&H | hemoglobin and hematocrit |
| DDS | doctor of dentistry | | organization | HHS | U.S. Department of Health |
| DEA | U.S. Drug Enforcement | eq | equivalent | | and Human Services |
| | Agency | ER | emergency room | HMO | health maintenance |
| dec | decrease | ERT | estrogen replacement therapy | | organization |
| del | delivery | ESR | erythrocyte sedimentation rate | H/O | history of |
| diab | diabetic | EST | electroshock therapy | $H_2O$ | water |
| diag | diagnosis | exam | examination | H&P | history and physical |
| diff | differential white blood cell | ext | extract | HPI | history of present illness |
| | count | | | HPV | human papilloma virus |
| dil | dilute | F | Fahrenheit | HR | human resource |
| disc | discontinue | | female | hs | at bedtime |
| disp | dispense | fax | facsimile | | hour of sleep |
| DM | diabetes mellitus | FBS | fasting blood sugar | ht | height |
| DNA | deoxyribonucleic acid | FDA | U.S. Food and Drug | hx | history |
| | does not apply | | Administration | Hz | hertz |
| DNR | do not resuscitate | FH | family history | | |
| DO | doctor of osteopathy | FHR | fetal heart rate | ICCU | intensive coronary care unit |
| DOA | dead on arrival | FHS | fetal heart sound | ICD | International Classification of |
| | | | | | Diseases, Adapted |

| | | | | | | |
|---|---|---|---|---|---|
| ICD-9-CM | International Classification of Diseases, 9th revision, Clinical Modification | MBCE | management by competitive edge | noct | at night |
| ICU | intensive care unit | MBDM | management by decision models | non rep | do not repeat |
| ID | intradermal | MBP | management by performance | NOS | not otherwise specified |
| I&D | incision and drainage | MBS | management by styles | NPO | nothing by mouth |
| IM | internal medicine | MBWA | management by wandering around | NR | nonreactive |
| | intramuscular | | | | no refill |
| imp | impression | MBWS | management by work simplification | | normal range |
| inf | infusion | MCHC | mean corpuscular hemoglobin and red cell indices | NS | nonspecific |
| inj | injection | | | | normal saline |
| I&O | intake and output | MCO | managed care organization | | not significant |
| IPPB | intermittent positive pressure breathing | MCV | mean corpuscular volume and red cell indices | | not sufficient |
| | | | | N&T | nose and throat |
| IUD | intrauterine device | MD | muscular dystrophy | N&V | nausea and vomiting |
| IV | intravenous | | doctor of medicine | NVD | nausea, vomiting, and diarrhea |
| IVP | intravenous pyelogram | MDR | minimum daily requirement | | |
| | | med | medicine | O | oral |
| JAAMT | *Journal of the American Association for Medical Transcription* | mEq/L | milliequivalents per liter | | oxygen |
| | | mg | miligram | | pint |
| JAMA | *Journal of the American Medical Association* | MH | marital history | O₂ | oxygen |
| | | | medical history | OB | obstetrics |
| JCAHO | Joint Commission on Accreditation of Healthcare Organizations | | menstrual history | OB-GYN | obstetrics-gynecology |
| | | MHx | medical history | OC | office call |
| | | MI | maturation index | | on call |
| jt | joint | | myocardial infarction | | oral contraceptive |
| | | ml | milliliter | occ | occasionally |
| K | potassium | mm | millimeter | OD | drug overdose |
| kg | kilogram | mm³ | cubic millimeter | | right eye (oculus dexter) |
| KOH | potassium hydroxide | mmHg | millimeters of mercury | | doctor of optometry |
| KUB | kidney, ureter, and bladder | MMR | measles, mumps, and rubella | OGTT | oral glucose tolerance test |
| KV | kilovolt | MOM | milk of magnesia | OM | office manager |
| | | mono | mononucleosis | OOB | out of bed |
| L | liter | MP | menstrual period | OP | outpatient |
| | left | MRI | magnetic resonance imaging | O&P | ova and parasites |
| l | length | | | OPIM | other potentially infected material |
| LA | left atrium | MS | mitral stenosis | | |
| | lactic acid | | morphine sulfate | OPV | oral poliovaccine |
| L&A | light and accommodation | | multiple sclerosis | OR | operating room |
| lab | laboratory | MT | medical technologist | ortho | orthopedics |
| lac | laceration | | medical transcriptionist | OS | left eye (oculus sinister) |
| lap | laparotomy | MTCP | Medical Transcriptionist Certification Program | os | mouth |
| lat | lateral | | | OSHA | U.S. Occupational Safety and Health Administration |
| lb | pound | multip | multipara | | |
| LBBB | left bundle branch block | MVP | mitral valve prolapse | OT | occupational therapist |
| LDL | low-density lipoprotein | | | | occupational therapy |
| LE | lupus erythematosus | NA | not applicable | OTC | over the counter |
| liq | liquid | NaCl | sodium chloride | OU | both eyes (oculus unitas) |
| LLQ | lower left quadrant | narc | narcotic | OURQ | outer upper right quadrant |
| LMP | last menstrual period | NB | newborn | OV | office visit |
| LP | lumbar puncture | NBME | National Board of Medical Examiners | oz | ounce |
| LRQ | lower right quadrant | | | | |
| LUQ | left upper quadrant | N/C | no complaints | P | phosphorus |
| L&W | living and well | ND | doctor of naturopathy | | pulse |
| lymphs | lymphocytes | NEC | not elsewhere classified | PA | posteroanterior |
| | | neg | negative | P&A | percussion and auscultation |
| M | male | NG | nasogastric | PA | physician's assistant |
| m | meter | NGU | nongonococcal urethritis | PAC | phenacetin, aspirin, and codeine |
| ℳ | minim | NL | normal limits | | |
| MBCD | management by coaching and development | NMP | normal menstrual period | Pap | Papanicolaou (smear, test) |
| | | | | para | number of pregnancies |

| | | | | | |
|---|---|---|---|---|---|
| **para I** | primipara | **pro-time** | prothrombin time | **sed rate** | sedimentation rate |
| **PAT** | paroxysmal atrial tachycardia | **PSA** | prostate-specific antigen | **segs** | segmented neutrophils |
| **path** | pathology | **PSRO** | Professional Standards Review Organization | **seq** | sequela |
| **PBI** | protein-bound iodine | | | **SF** | scarlet fever |
| **pc** | after meals | **PT** | physical therapy | | spinal fluid |
| **PCC** | Poison Control Center | | prothrombin time | **SG** | specific gravity |
| **PCN** | penicillin | **pt** | patient | **SH** | social history |
| **PCP** | primary care physician | **PTA** | prior to admission | **SIDS** | sudden infant death syndrome |
| **PCV** | packed cell volume | **pulv** | powder | **sig** | instructions, directions |
| **PDR** | *Physician's Desk Reference* | **PVC** | premature ventricular concentration | **sigmoid** | sigmoidoscopy |
| **PE** | physical examination | | | **SMA 12/60** | Sequential Multiple Analyzer (12-test serum profile) |
| **peds** | pediatrics | **px** | physical examination | | |
| **PEG** | pneumoencephalography | | prognosis | **SOAP** | subjective data, objective data, assessment, and plan |
| **PERRLA** | pupils equal, round, regular, react to light, and accommodation | **q** | each; every | | |
| | | **q AM** | every morning | **SOB** | shortness of breath |
| **PET** | positron emission transmission or tomography | **QA** | quality assurance | **sol** | solution |
| | | **qd** | every day | **solv** | solvent |
| **PH** | past history | **qh** | every hour | **SOP** | standard operating procedure |
| | personal history | **q (2, 3, 4)h** | every 2, 3, or 4 hours | **SOS** | if necessary |
| | public health | **qid** | four times a day | **spec** | specimen |
| **pH** | hydrogen in concentration | **qn** | every night | **sp gr** | secific gravity |
| **PHO** | physician-hospital organization | **qns** | quantity not sufficient | **spont ab** | spontaneous abortion |
| | | **qod** | every other day | **SR** | sedimentation rate |
| **PI** | present illness | **qs** | of sufficient quantity | **SS** | signs and symptoms |
| | pulmonary infarction | **qt** | quart | **s̄s̄** | one-half |
| **PID** | pelvic inflammatory disease | **R** | registration | **Staph** | Staphylococcus |
| **PKU** | phenylketonuria | | right | **stat** | immediately |
| **PM** | after noon (post meridiem) | **RBC** | red blood cell | **STD** | sexually transmitted disease |
| | post mortem (after death) | **RBC/hpf** | red blood cells per high power field | **Strep** | Streptococcus |
| **PMN** | polymorphonuclear neutrophils | | | **subcut** | subcutaneous |
| | | **RBCM** | red blood cell mass | **supp** | suppository |
| **PMP** | past menstrual period | **RBCV** | red blood cell volume | **surg** | surgery |
| **PMS** | premenstrual syndrome | **RBRVS** | Resource-Based Relation Value Scale | **sx** | signs |
| **PNC** | penicillin | | | | symptoms |
| **PO** | postoperative | **REM** | rapid eye movement | **sym** | symptoms |
| **po** | by mouth | **resp** | respiration | **syr** | syrup |
| **POB** | place of birth | **Rh** | rhesus (factor) | | |
| **POMR** | problem-oriented medical record | **Rh-** | rhesus negative | **T** | temperature |
| | | **Rh+** | rhesus positive | **T$_3$** | tri-iodothyronine |
| **POS** | point-of-service plan | **RHD** | rheumatic heart disease | **T$_4$** | thyroxine |
| **pos** | positive | **RLQ** | right lower quadrant | **T&A** | tonsillectomy and adenoidectomy |
| **poss** | possible | **RMA** | registered medical assistant | | |
| **postop** | postoperative | **RNA** | ribonucleic acid | **tab** | tablet |
| **PP** | postprandial | **R/O** | rule out | **TB** | tuberculin |
| **PPB** | positive pressure breathing | **ROA** | received on account | **tbs** | tablespoon |
| **PPBS** | postprandial blood sugar | **ROM** | range of motion | | tuberculosis |
| **PPD** | purified protein derivative | | read-only memory | **TC** | throat culture |
| **PPO** | preferred provider organization | **ROS** | review of systems | | tissue culture |
| | | **RT** | radiation therapy | | total capacity |
| **PPT** | partial prothrombin time | **RUQ** | right upper quadrant | | total cholesterol |
| **preop** | preoperative | **Rx** | prescription | **ther** | therapy |
| **PRERLA** | pupils round, equal, react to light and accommodation | **S** | subjective data (POMR) | **therap** | therapeutic |
| | | **s̄** | without | **TIA** | transient ischemic attack |
| **primip** | woman bearing first child | **SA** | sinoatrial | **tid** | three times a day |
| **prn** | as the occasion arises, as necessary | **S&A** | sugar and acetone (urine) | **tinct** | tincture |
| | | **SBE** | shortness of breath on exertion | **TLC** | tender loving care |
| **procto** | proctoscopy | | | **TMJ** | temporomandibular joint |
| **prog** | prognosis | | subacute bacterial endocarditis | **top** | topically |
| **PROM** | premature rupture of membranes | **SC** | subcutaneous | **TOPV** | trivalent oral poliovirus vaccine |
| | | **SE** | standard error | | |

| | | | | | | |
|---|---|---|---|---|---|
| **TP** | total protein | **URI** | upper respiratory infection | **WBC** | white blood cell |
| **TPR** | temperature, pulse, and respiration | **urol** | urology | **WC** | white cell |
| | | **URQ** | upper right quadrant | **WDWN** | well developed, well nourished |
| **tr** | tincture | **URT** | upper respiratory tract | | |
| **trig** | triglycerides | **URTI** | upper respiratory tract infection | **WHO** | World Health Organization |
| **TSH** | thyroid stimulating hormone | | | **WN** | well nourished |
| **tsp** | teaspoon | **USP** | United States Pharmacopoeia | **WNF** | well-nourished female |
| **TUR** | transurethral resection of the bladder | **UT** | urinary tract | **WNL** | within normal limits |
| | | **UTI** | urinary tract infection | **WNM** | well-nourished male |
| **tus** | cough | **UV** | ultraviolet | **WO** | written order |
| **T&X** | type and crossmatch | | | **w/o** | without |
| | | **vac** | vaccine | **wt** | weight |
| **U** | unit | **vag** | vagina | | |
| **UA** | urinalysis | | vaginal | **x** | multiply by |
| **UB-92** | Uniform Bill-92 | **VD** | venereal disease | **XR** | x-ray |
| **UCG** | urinary chorionic gonadotropin | **VDRL** | Venereal Disease Research Library | | |
| **UCHD** | usual childhood diseases | | | **YOB** | year of birth |
| **ULQ** | upper left quadrant | **vit** | vitamin | **yr** | year |
| **ung** | ointment | **vit cap** | vital capacity | | |
| **URC** | usual, reasonable, customary | **vol** | volume | | |
| **urg** | urgent | **VS** | vital signs | | |

## Symbols

| | |
|---|---|
| * | birth |
| † | death |
| ♂ | male |
| ♀ | female |
| + | positive |
| − | negative |
| ± | positive or negative, indefinite |
| ÷ | divide by |
| = | equal to |
| > | greater than |
| < | less than |
| × | multiply by |
| # | number, pound |
| ' | foot, minute |
| " | inch, second |
| ℳ | minum |
| ʒ | dram |
| ℥ | ounce |
| μ | micron |
| ○ | pint |
| @ | at |

# TOP 200 DRUGS BY RETAIL SALES IN 2000

**B**

Courtesy of Source Prescription Audit, Scott-Levin, Newtown, PA 12/2000. "Top 200 drugs by retail sales in 2000." *Drug Topics* 2001; 6:18. Copyright © 2001 and published by Medical Economics Company at Montvale, NJ 07645-1742. All rights reserved.

## Top 200 Brand-Name Drugs by Retail Sales in 2000

| Rank | Product | Total retail dollars (000) | Rank | Product | Total retail dollars (000) | Rank | Product | Total retail dollars (000) |
|---|---|---|---|---|---|---|---|---|
| 1 | Prilosec | $4,102,195 | 36 | Synthroid | $649,256 | 71 | Relafen | $351,595 |
| 2 | Lipitor | 3,692,657 | 37 | Flovent | 647,980 | 72 | Serzone | 349,127 |
| 3 | Prevacid | 2,832,602 | 38 | Accutane | 636,246 | 73 | Cardura | 344,406 |
| 4 | Prozac | 2,567,107 | 39 | Flonase | 618,714 | 74 | Xalatan | 340,492 |
| 5 | Zocor | 2,207,042 | 40 | Avandia | 617,629 | 75 | Glucotrol XL | 321,631 |
| 6 | Celebrex | 2,015,508 | 41 | Ortho Tri-Cyclen | 616,997 | 76 | Detrol | 319,193 |
| 7 | Zoloft | 1,890,416 | 42 | Ultram | 601,465 | 77 | Seroquel | 318,844 |
| 8 | Paxil | 1,807,955 | 43 | Plavix | 599,512 | 78 | Humulin N | 317,017 |
| 9 | Claritin | 1,667,347 | 44 | Biaxin | 588,366 | 79 | Lotensin | 316,922 |
| 10 | Glucophage | 1,629,157 | 45 | Vasotec | 584,418 | 80 | Viracept | 315,510 |
| 11 | Norvasc | 1,597,091 | 46 | Pepcid | 568,684 | 81 | Avonex | 313,114 |
| 12 | Augmentin | 1,584,397 | 47 | Actos | 550,674 | 82 | Valtrex | 311,102 |
| 13 | Vioxx | 1,517,993 | 48 | Accupril | 500,796 | 83 | Allegra-D | 310,369 |
| 14 | Zyprexa | 1,418,411 | 49 | Enbrel | 500,363 | 84 | Adderall | 307,423 |
| 15 | Pravachol | 1,203,474 | 50 | Claritin D 24HR | 493,420 | 85 | Procrit | 298,764 |
| 16 | Premarin Tabs | 1,146,808 | 51 | Lamisil Oral | 487,920 | 86 | Claritin RediTabs | 298,253 |
| 17 | Neurontin | 1,131,678 | 52 | Ceftin | 455,965 | 87 | Cardizem CD | 283,968 |
| 18 | Oxycontin | 1,052,771 | 53 | Combivir | 452,844 | 88 | K-Dur 20 | 276,161 |
| 19 | Cipro | 1,023,657 | 54 | Serevent | 448,923 | 89 | Diovan | 270,144 |
| 20 | Zithromax Z-Pak | 961,579 | 55 | BuSpar Dividose | 434,023 | 90 | Remeron | 266,707 |
| 21 | Risperdal | 959,707 | 56 | Prinivil | 431,342 | 91 | BuSpar | 265,349 |
| 22 | Wellbutrin SR | 850,934 | 57 | Coumadin Tabs | 407,565 | 92 | Zerit | 264,738 |
| 23 | Zestril | 833,359 | 58 | Claritin D 12HR | 403,071 | 93 | Hyzaar | 264,128 |
| 24 | Effexor XR | 815,816 | 59 | Evista | 398,590 | 94 | Ziac | 258,299 |
| 25 | Allegra | 810,001 | 60 | Cozaar | 395,292 | 95 | Zithromax Susp | 252,501 |
| 26 | Viagra | 809,377 | 61 | Nasonex | 391,973 | 96 | Miacalcin Nasal | 245,241 |
| 27 | Ambien | 798,858 | 62 | Diflucan | 386,846 | 97 | Sporanox | 244,434 |
| 28 | Depakote | 758,329 | 63 | Aricept | 384,059 | 98 | Lotrisone | 243,440 |
| 29 | Levaquin | 753,711 | 64 | Procardia XL | 383,822 | 99 | Lescol | 238,343 |
| 30 | Imitrex | 747,631 | 65 | Cefzil | 382,250 | 100 | Xenical | 237,004 |
| 31 | Zyrtec | 739,543 | 66 | Adalat CC | 376,992 | 101 | Betaseron | 236,503 |
| 32 | Celexa | 737,487 | 67 | Aciphex | 372,138 | 102 | Asacol | 235,117 |
| 33 | Prempro | 711,798 | 68 | Lotrel | 353,784 | 103 | Monopril | 233,969 |
| 34 | Fosamax | 704,289 | 69 | Toprol XL | 353,725 | 104 | Humulin 70/30 | 229,600 |
| 35 | Singulair | 676,515 | 70 | Duragesic | 352,934 | 105 | Combivent | 229,550 |

| Rank | Product | Total retail dollars (000) | Rank | Product | Total retail dollars (000) | Rank | Product | Total retail dollars (000) |
|---|---|---|---|---|---|---|---|---|
| 106 | Flomax | $226,845 | 138 | Plendil | $169,716 | 170 | MS Contin | $125,606 |
| 107 | Zofran | 225,673 | 139 | Proscar | 166,868 | 171 | Effexor | 125,468 |
| 108 | Axid | 225,365 | 140 | Levoxyl | 164,919 | 172 | Pulmicort Turbuhaler | 122,785 |
| 109 | Lamictal | 221,847 | 141 | Bactroban | 163,939 | 173 | Proventil HFA | 121,417 |
| 110 | Baycol | 221,383 | 142 | Daypro | 163,783 | 174 | Serostim | 121,096 |
| 111 | Topamax | 219,865 | 143 | Lanoxin | 163,625 | 175 | Clozaril | 119,152 |
| 112 | Mevacor | 216,661 | 144 | Alphagan | 159,631 | 176 | Gonal-F | 119,096 |
| 113 | Neoral | 214,475 | 145 | Diovan HCT | 159,351 | 177 | Arava | 118,902 |
| 114 | Neupogen | 212,997 | 146 | Amaryl | 158,976 | 178 | Lupron Depot | 117,045 |
| 115 | Famvir | 205,223 | 147 | Tricor | 158,741 | 179 | Vicoprofen Non-Inj | 115,382 |
| 116 | Epivir | 205,172 | 148 | Ortho-Cyclen | 157,366 | 180 | Covera-HS | 115,239 |
| 117 | Ortho-Novum 7/7/7 | 203,989 | 149 | Humalog | 157,153 | 181 | Loestrin Fe 1/20 | 113,408 |
| 118 | Azmacort | 203,389 | 150 | Arthrotec | 152,530 | 182 | Elocon | 113,324 |
| 119 | Luvox | 199,293 | 151 | Patanol | 152,199 | 183 | Skelaxin | 113,307 |
| 120 | Coreg | 199,166 | 152 | Vancenase AQ DS | 150,883 | 184 | Meridia | 113,231 |
| 121 | Zestoretic | 198,956 | 153 | Accolat | 150,536 | 185 | Nasacort AQ | 112,518 |
| 122 | Tiazac | 198,727 | 154 | Cellcept | 150,193 | 186 | Dovonex | 110,975 |
| 123 | Avapro | 197,428 | 155 | Copaxone | 148,844 | 187 | Catapres-TTS | 109,703 |
| 124 | Benzamycin | 196,795 | 156 | Zithromax | 146,759 | 188 | Zyrtec Syrup | 109,389 |
| 125 | Triphasil | 196,589 | 157 | Hytrin | 145,267 | 189 | Propulsid | 107,279 |
| 126 | Zomig | 190,231 | 158 | Casodex | 143,906 | 190 | Tequin | 107,197 |
| 127 | Rebetron 1200 Pen | 189,843 | 159 | Xanax | 141,572 | 191 | Rezulin | 106,720 |
| 128 | Imitrex Statdose | 184,548 | 160 | Tobradex | 137,765 | 192 | Rebetron 1000 Pen | 106,624 |
| 129 | Sustiva | 183,008 | 161 | Prograf | 137,743 | 193 | Stadol NS | 105,637 |
| 130 | Amoxil | 176,847 | 162 | Crixivan | 137,645 | 194 | Prevpac | 105,011 |
| 131 | Lovenox | 175,402 | 163 | Lo/Ovral 28 | 137,138 | 195 | Loestrin Fe 1.5/30 | 103,323 |
| 132 | Ditropan XL | 174,058 | 164 | Differin | 136,023 | 196 | Phenergan Supp | 102,421 |
| 133 | Atrovent Inh | 174,018 | 165 | DDAVP | 133,016 | 197 | Viramune | 102,348 |
| 134 | Zantac | 172,662 | 166 | Macrobid | 131,419 | 198 | Cosopt | 102,212 |
| 135 | Altace | 172,308 | 167 | Betapace | 130,263 | 199 | Estratest Tabs | 101,697 |
| 136 | Alesse-28 | 171,698 | 168 | Ziagen | 127,284 | 200 | Prandin | 100,310 |
| 137 | Dilantin Kapseals | 171,374 | 169 | Zyban | 126,122 | | | |

## Top 200 Generic Drugs by Retail Sales in 2000

| Rank | Product | Total retail dollars (000) | Rank | Product | Total retail dollars (000) | Rank | Product | Total retail dollars (000) |
|---|---|---|---|---|---|---|---|---|
| 1 | Hydrocodone/APAP | $935,093 | 16 | Naproxen | $287,162 | 31 | Methylphenidate | $172,863 |
| 2 | Ranitidine HCl | 690,854 | 17 | Isosorbide Mononitrt | 286,576 | 32 | Amitriptyline | 168,586 |
| 3 | Atenolol | 532,836 | 18 | Carisoprodol | 286,430 | 33 | Trimethoprim/Sulfa | 168,446 |
| 4 | Lorazepam | 530,084 | 19 | Terazosin | 286,378 | 34 | Nifedipine ER | 157,299 |
| 5 | Albuterol Aerosol | 501,115 | 20 | Minocycline | 278,055 | 35 | Cimetidine | 156,799 |
| 6 | Alprazolam | 489,753 | 21 | Amoxicillin | 252,789 | 36 | Ipratropium Bromide | 154,735 |
| 7 | Propoxyphene-N/APAP | 457,763 | 22 | Ibuprofen | 248,035 | 37 | Hydrochlorothiazide | 148,603 |
| 8 | Cephalexin | 399,055 | 23 | Metoprolol Tartrate | 230,657 | 38 | Gemfibrozil | 148,226 |
| 9 | Tamoxifen | 393,067 | 24 | Furosemide Oral | 227,718 | 39 | Prednisone Oral | 141,904 |
| 10 | Clonazepam | 351,304 | 25 | Acetaminophen w/Cod | 216,379 | 40 | Methotrexate | 132,550 |
| 11 | Glyburide | 333,348 | 26 | Trimox | 214,918 | 41 | Captopril | 129,457 |
| 12 | Cartia XT | 331,837 | 27 | Acyclovir Systemic | 209,307 | 42 | Diclofenac Sodium | 123,457 |
| 13 | Albuterol Neb Soln | 325,017 | 28 | Cyclobenzaprine | 192,847 | 43 | Potassium Chloride | 121,779 |
| 14 | Verapamil SR | 301,604 | 29 | Warfarin | 178,317 | 44 | Clorazepate Dipot | 117,470 |
| 15 | Triamterene w/HCTZ | 292,778 | 30 | Trazodone HCl | 173,623 | 45 | Medrxyprgsterone Tab | 113,414 |

| Rank | Product | Total retail dollars (000) | Rank | Product | Total retail dollars (000) | Rank | Product | Total retail dollars (000) |
|---|---|---|---|---|---|---|---|---|
| 46 | Spironolactone | $113,240 | 98 | Dicyclomine HCl | $48,747 | 150 | Doxazosin | $28,189 |
| 47 | Clindamycin Systemic | 111,649 | 99 | Indapamide | 48,395 | 151 | Diltia XT | 27,569 |
| 48 | Doxycycline | 110,567 | 100 | Prednisolone Oral | 48,313 | 152 | Ketoconazole Topical | 26,558 |
| 49 | Diltiazem CD | 109,812 | 101 | Octicair | 47,988 | 153 | Levothyroxine | 26,415 |
| 50 | Estradiol Oral | 109,688 | 102 | Hydroxyzine | 47,063 | 154 | Dexamethasone Oral | 26,304 |
| 51 | Amiodarone | 108,066 | 103 | Bupropion | 46,855 | 155 | Chlorhexidine Glucon | 26,272 |
| 52 | Enalapril | 107,435 | 104 | Nystatin Systemic | 46,135 | 156 | Desoximetasone | 26,201 |
| 53 | Hydroxychloroquine | 105,895 | 105 | Triamcinln Acet Top | 45,627 | 157 | Bromocriptine | 26,133 |
| 54 | Methylprednis Tabs | 101,298 | 106 | Baclofen | 45,586 | 158 | Enulose | 26,002 |
| 55 | Diazepam | 100,210 | 107 | Ketoprofen | 45,484 | 159 | Indomethacin SR | 25,979 |
| 56 | Cefaclor | 99,915 | 108 | Sucralfate | 45,451 | 160 | Haloperidol | 25,865 |
| 57 | Propranolol LA | 98,875 | 109 | Theophylline SR | 44,118 | 161 | Valproic Acid | 25,856 |
| 58 | Nitroglycerin | 97,650 | 110 | Ticlopidine | 43,870 | 162 | Phenobarbital | 25,548 |
| 59 | Clonidine | 95,919 | 111 | Phenytoin Sodium Ext | 43,299 | 163 | Selegiline | 25,384 |
| 60 | Pentoxifylline | 95,402 | 112 | Clozapine | 43,091 | 164 | Megestrol Tabs | 24,555 |
| 61 | Glipizide | 93,619 | 113 | Atenolol Chlorthal | 43,068 | 165 | Quinine Sulfate | 24,441 |
| 62 | Temazepam | 93,513 | 114 | Guaif/Phenylprop | 43,027 | 166 | Clotrimazole Top | 24,320 |
| 63 | Nortriptyline | 91,972 | 115 | Lithium Carbonate | 42,933 | 167 | Hydroxyurea | 24,282 |
| 64 | Etodolac | 90,898 | 116 | Diphenoxylate w/Atro | 42,844 | 168 | Naproxen EC | 24,185 |
| 65 | Allopurinol | 89,571 | 117 | Nitrofurantoin Mcroc | 42,269 | 169 | Lindane | 24,164 |
| 66 | Diltiazem SR | 89,489 | 118 | Penicillin VK | 41,679 | 170 | Lonox | 24,056 |
| 67 | Glyburide Micronized | 79,195 | 119 | Oxybutynin Chloride | 41,307 | 171 | Nitroquick | 24,030 |
| 68 | Cefadroxil | 76,442 | 120 | Butalbital Cmpd w/Cd | 40,364 | 172 | Sulfasalazine | 23,899 |
| 69 | Clobetasol | 76,034 | 121 | Hydrocortsn Valerate | 39,458 | 173 | Cholestyramine | 23,516 |
| 70 | Morphine Sul Non Inj | 74,084 | 122 | Ery-Tab | 39,313 | 174 | Digoxin | 23,466 |
| 71 | Carbidopa/Levodopa | 73,230 | 123 | Carbidopa/Levdpa ER | 39,286 | 175 | Triazolam | 23,453 |
| 72 | Orphenadrine Citrate | 70,339 | 124 | Diclofenac Potassium | 38,006 | 176 | Acebutolol | 23,093 |
| 73 | Naproxen Sodium | 70,150 | 125 | Prednisolne Acet Oph | 37,289 | 177 | Clomipramine HCl | 22,853 |
| 74 | Nadolol | 69,757 | 126 | Promethazine/Codeine | 37,253 | 178 | Lactulose | 22,593 |
| 75 | Oxycodone w/APAP | 69,492 | 127 | Guanfacine HCl | 36,569 | 179 | Ibuprofen Liquid | 21,880 |
| 76 | Benzonatate | 68,749 | 128 | Clomiphene Citrate | 36,467 | 180 | Erythromycin Topical | 21,769 |
| 77 | Phentermine | 68,626 | 129 | Timolol Maleate XE | 36,124 | 181 | Colchicine | 21,372 |
| 78 | Carbamazepine | 67,842 | 130 | Indomethacin | 35,849 | 182 | Tobramycin Ophth | 21,259 |
| 79 | Methylphenidate SR | 67,025 | 131 | Timolol Maleate Oph | 35,258 | 183 | Hydroxyzine Pamoate | 20,798 |
| 80 | Labetalol | 66,498 | 132 | Sotalol | 35,134 | 184 | Ketorolac Oral | 20,523 |
| 81 | Butalbital/APAP/Caf | 65,896 | 133 | Desmopressin Acetate | 34,621 | 185 | Isosorbide Dinitrate | 20,205 |
| 82 | Azathioprine | 64,242 | 134 | Estropipate | 34,373 | 186 | Benztropine | 20,203 |
| 83 | Prochlorperaz Mal | 63,598 | 135 | Folic Acid | 33,673 | 187 | Diclofenac Sodium SR | 19,969 |
| 84 | Propranolol HCl | 62,698 | 136 | Sulindac | 33,369 | 188 | Diflorasone | 19,534 |
| 85 | Imipramine HCl | 61,106 | 137 | Bumetanide Non-Inj | 33,250 | 189 | Gentamicin Ophth | 18,966 |
| 86 | Methocarbamol | 59,187 | 138 | Hydrocortison Top Rx | 33,080 | 190 | Diltiazem | 18,792 |
| 87 | Metronidazole Tabs | 58,338 | 139 | Polymyxin B/Trimeth | 33,017 | 191 | Pentazocine/Naloxone | 18,783 |
| 88 | Hyoscyamine | 58,107 | 140 | Albuterol Oral Liq | 32,386 | 192 | Naproxen Delayed Rel | 18,730 |
| 89 | Neomycin/Polymx/HC | 57,961 | 141 | Oxazepam | 32,333 | 193 | Dipyridamole | 18,696 |
| 90 | Metoclopramide | 55,692 | 142 | Clindamycin Topical | 31,721 | 194 | Tetracycline | 18,627 |
| 91 | Doxepin | 53,206 | 143 | Guaifenesin/Pseudoep | 31,040 | 195 | Probenecid | 18,305 |
| 92 | Cromolyn Sod Neb Sln | 51,925 | 144 | Phenazopyridine HCl | 30,966 | 196 | Methyldopa | 18,283 |
| 93 | Tretinoin | 51,616 | 145 | Ketoconazole Syst | 30,812 | 197 | Benzoyl Peroxd Acne | 18,182 |
| 94 | Fluocinonide | 51,573 | 146 | Bisoprolol/HCTZ | 29,235 | 198 | Nystatin/Triamcinoln | 17,761 |
| 95 | Meclizine HCl | 51,400 | 147 | Promethazine Tabs | 29,058 | 199 | Erythromycin Ethylsc | 17,383 |
| 96 | Piroxicam | 51,077 | 148 | Thioridazine HCl | 28,833 | 200 | Methadone HCl Non-In | 17,188 |
| 97 | Adipex-P | 49,545 | 149 | Guaifenesin Rx | 28,595 | | | |

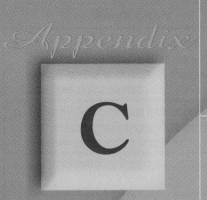

# MEDICAL ASSISTANT ROLE DELINEATION CHART

Reprinted with permission of the American Association of Medical Assistants.

*Asterisk denotes advanced skill

## ADMINISTRATIVE

### Administrative Procedures

- Perform basic clerical functions
- Schedule, coordinate and monitor appointments
- Schedule inpatient/outpatient admissions and procedures
- Understand and apply third-party guidelines
- Obtain reimbursement through accurate claims submission
- Monitor third-party reimbursement
- Perform medical transcription
- Understand and adhere to managed care policies and procedures
- * Negotiate managed care contracts (advanced)

### Practice Finances

- Perform procedural and diagnostic coding
- Apply bookkeeping principles
- Document and maintain accounting and banking records
- Manage accounts receivable
- Manage accounts payable
- Process payroll
- * Develop and maintain fee schedules (advanced)
- * Manage renewals of business and professional insurance policies (advanced)
- * Manage personnel benefits and maintain records (advanced)

## CLINICAL

### Fundamental Principles

- Apply principles of aseptic technique and infection control
- Comply with quality assurance practices
- Screen and follow up patient test results

### Diagnostic Orders

- Collect and process specimens
- Perform diagnostic tests

### Patient Care

- Adhere to established triage procedures
- Obtain patient history and vital signs
- Prepare and maintain examination and treatment areas
- Prepare patient for examinations, procedures, and treatments
- Assist with examinations, procedures and treatments
- Prepare and administer medications and immunizations
- Maintain medication and immunization records
- Recognize and respond to emergencies
- Coordinate patient care information with other health care providers

# GENERAL (TRANSDISCIPLINARY)

## Professionalism

- Project a professional manner and image
- Adhere to ethical principles
- Demonstrate initiative and responsibility
- Work as a team member
- Manage time effectively
- Prioritize and perform multiple tasks
- Adapt to change
- Promote the CMA credential
- Enhance skills through continuing education

## Communication Skills

- Treat all patients with compassion and empathy
- Recognize and respect cultural diversity
- Adapt communications to individual's ability to understand
- Use professional telephone technique
- Use effective and correct verbal and written communications
- Recognize and respond to verbal and nonverbal communications
- Use medical terminology appropriately
- Receive, organize, prioritize and transmit information
- Serve as liaison
- Promote the practice through positive public relations

## Legal Concepts

- Maintain confidentiality
- Practice within the scope of education, training, and personal capabilities
- Prepare and maintain medical records
- Document accurately

- Use appropriate guidelines when releasing information
- Follow employer's established policies dealing with the health care contract
- Follow federal, state and local legal guidelines
- Maintain awareness of federal and state health care legislation and regulations
- Maintain and dispose of regulated substances in compliance with government guidelines
- Comply with established risk management and safety procedures
- Recognize professional credentialing criteria
- Participate in the development and maintenance of personnel, policy and procedure manuals
- *  Develop and maintain personnel, policy and procedure manuals (advanced)*

## Instruction

- Instruct individuals according to their needs
- Explain office policies and procedures
- Teach methods of health promotion and disease prevention
- Locate community resouces and disseminate information
- *  Orient and train personnel (advanced)*
- *  Develop educational materials (advanced)*
- *  Conduct continuing education activities (advanced)*

## Operational Functions

- Maintain supply inventory
- Evaluate and recommend equipment and supplies
- Apply computer techniques to support office operations
- *  Supervise personnel (advanced)*
- *  Interview and recommend job applicants (advanced)*
- *  Negotiate leases and prices for equipment and supply contracts (advanced)*

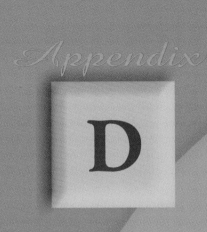

## Chapter 5   Coping Skills for the Medical Assistant

**Case Study 5-1**

1.  By being responsible, taking charge of the work environment, and being an inner-directed person, Ellen is more able to achieve her long-term goal of being an office manager. Certainly, she will learn by working closely with and observing Marilyn; there are also specific long-term, skill-building goals Ellen should set to give herself direction. If she gave herself three years to move into the office manager position, Ellen could set one long-term goal for each year. These might include (1) the first year, become proficient in all back-office clinical skills; (2) the second year, add front-office administrative tasks and skills; (3) the third year, begin to focus on office management.

2.  Short-term goals break down long-term goals into smaller, more manageable time segments and will help Ellen more easily evaluate her progress. Short-term goals also provide a sense of periodic reward necessary to sustain motivation toward a long-range goal.

    Ellen should review her three long-term goals and determine what short-term goals they include. For example, the first year, Ellen wants to become proficient in all back-office clinical skills; short-term goals may include practicing accuracy when performing clinical duties and understanding which supplies are needed for which procedures. For her second-year goal of developing front-office administrative tasks and skills, Ellen may become proficient on the computer and learn the intricacies of scheduling patients. For the third-year goal that focuses on office management, Ellen can learn team-building skills and develop a procedures manual.

3.  Ellen should take an active interest in her profession; she could attend seminars; speak with other medical assistants who are now office managers; read professional journals; and participate in professional organizations. This variety of exposure will enlarge Ellen's perspective and broaden her scope of information.

**Case Study 5-2**

1.  Ellen is demonstrating the classic signs and symptoms of burnout, which include:
    a.  she is a perfectionist
    b.  she has a decreased sense of humor
    c.  she displays frustration and irritability
    d.  she is critical of herself and others
    e.  she is physically and emotionally exhausted, yet continues to push herself
    f.  her work has become a chore
    g.  she feels like a failure if everything is not completed at the end of the day to her satisfaction

2.  Ellen needs to take time for self-analysis by asking herself some hard questions. These questions must be answered truthfully and completely.

3.  Ellen needs to institute some changes.
    a.  List negative words or phrases often used, and then substitute neutral replacements.
    b.  Create job diversity: Take a different route to work for a change; enter the office through a different door; change work routine where appropriate; investigate the possibility of a different work schedule.
    c.  Become creative: Change work area décor by adding a new calendar; change family photo on desk, add a foliage or silk plant to the area.
    d.  Revisit short- and long-term goals, and make adjustments where necessary; be sure all goals are realistic and attainable.
    e.  Pay more attention to personal habits: Change eating habits; exercise more; get more rest and sleep; renew old friendships; go to lunch with coworkers.

f. Implement time management techniques.

g. Delegate responsibility to others who are capable.

## Chapter 6 The Therapeutic Approach to the Patient with Life-Threatening Illness

### Case Study 6-1

1. These questions are intended to help. In this culture, the family is deeply involved.

2. Having such a document would make it easier for everyone involved to know how much information should and can be shared with another.

3. Most all of this concern is related to the culture.

4. Have an honest discussion with everyone involved so it is clear to the staff how the patient would like to have information handled.

### Case Study 6-2

1. Bruce should know that the human immunodeficiency virus (HIV) is transmitted between persons through sexual practices (sexual intimacy where body fluids might be exchanged); through direct blood-to-blood contact as in transfusions or needlestick injuries; and through intrauterine transmission. It is not transmitted through touching or other casual contact; AIDS is not an easily contracted disease.

2. AIDS patients and patients with the HIV virus often suffer extreme distress. Certainly, as a health care professional, Bruce needs to be sensitive to their needs and remember they may be both anxious and depressed. He should avoid being fearful and judgmental, but rather should be respectful toward patients with AIDS; while he should practice standard precautions, Bruce should also replace his fear with knowledge based on medical fact. He could be of assistance to HIV-infected or AIDS patients by referring them to support groups, social workers, legal advisors, and by helping the patient build coping skills.

3. Dealing with a large number of AIDS patients can be psychologically exhausting. While Bruce needs to combat his own prejudices, he also needs to be self-nurturing, not by withdrawing from AIDS patients but by giving himself a respite from time to time. If he routinely deals with AIDS patients, Bruce may benefit from a support group of his own that will help him build coping abilities.

## Chapter 7 Legal Considerations

### Case Study 7-1

1. It is critical that medical charts be kept current at all times. If the physician and medical assistant have maintained an accurate and up-to-date record of patient Boris Bolski's care, Joe can rely on the information in the chart to help him answer any questions. He should study the chart carefully.

Note: At all times, the patient's confidentiality must be respected. Typically, if the patient's attorney has issued the subpoena, the attorney will have the patient sign a release form. If the physician is subpoenaed by someone other than the patient's representative, the physician must be very careful about release of information and should proceed on a case-by-case basis. Certain records, because of their sensitive nature, may require a court order before being released.

2. Information in the chart should contain actual care rendered, dates that it was rendered, and charges made. Joe should note whether any comments were made on the chart that reflect patient input. Joe should also gather and review other material such as consent forms, insurance claim forms, and other documents related to patient care.

3. An expert witness is one who has the knowledge and experience to testify as to a reasonable and expected standard of care. Judges and jurors rely on the testimony of expert witnesses to understand the nature of medical information. Joe should answer questions in a factual way and in terms understood by the lay person.

## Chapter 8 Ethical Considerations

### Case Study 8-1

1. In most states, physicians and their employees are mandated to report all cases of suspected child abuse. Liz and Dr. Esposito must report the suspected abuse of Henry to the appropriate child protective agency.

2. and 3. Once the suspected abuse is reported, the responsible agency will respond to Henry's needs. However, in the meantime, Liz should take measures to protect and care for Henry, providing a safe environment if possible. While it may be difficult to do so, Liz should also view Juanita Hansen as a victim and seek treatment for her as well as for her son.

## Chapter 9 Emergency Procedures and First Aid

### Case Study 9-1

1. Wanda must first ascertain whether Annette is having trouble breathing. If she is, Wanda must direct her—and if necessary assist Annette—to receive immediate medical attention at the nearest hospital. If Annette says she is not having any breathing difficulty, Wanda should ask:

- What are your symptoms?

- Have you ever experienced an allergic reaction to an insect (specifically yellowjacket) sting before?

- Do you have hives?

- Are you experiencing any lightheadedness?
- Do you have any itching either at the site of the sting or in other body locations?

From these questions, Wanda needs to determine whether Annette is having a localized reaction, which can result in swelling, itching, and tenderness at the site of the sting, or a generalized reaction, which can be frightening for the patient and dangerous if it involves impairment of breathing functions.

2. If patients are allergic to an insect sting, it is possible that anaphylactic shock may ensue, which can lead to death. The patient must be directed to receive emergency care immediately, which will usually consist of the administration of epinephrine. If Annette must wait for EMS personnel, Wanda should stay with her over the telephone and calm her until EMS personnel arrive. For individuals who present at the ambulatory care setting with an apparent allergic reaction to a sting, the physician will prescribe epinephrine. Attempt to allay patient apprehension and monitor vital signs while waiting for EMS personnel to arrive.

3. Once Annette has received emergency treatment, Wanda can advise her to take certain precautions should she have another, and possibly more severe, reaction to an insect sting. For individuals with a known allergic reaction, the physician will prescribe epinephrine. These individuals should carry the epinephrine with them and self-inject, should they not be able to get immediate emergency care. The patient should then seek immediate emergency treatment. Advise all patients with known allergic reactions to be particularly careful when working or playing outdoors. Insects are not usually aggressive until their nests are approached; however, often these nests are not easy to detect and an individual may approach one without being aware of its presence. Patients with allergies to insects should always wear shoes out-of-doors, wear light-colored clothing, preferably with long sleeves and pant legs, look before taking a sip from a beverage when outdoors, and inspect lawn areas, shrubbery, and building walls periodically for evidence of nests of stinging insects.

## Case Study 9-2

1. Because of the possibility that Mrs. Johnson is experiencing a myocardial infarction, Bruce should get a wheelchair and immediately take Mrs. Johnson into an examination room and notify Dr. Lewis. Bruce should help Mrs. Johnson onto the examination table, place her in semi-Fowler's position, loosen tight clothing, and take her blood pressure, pulse, and respirations. Bruce should activate EMS if Dr. Lewis directed him to. Because Mrs. Johnson is extremely anxious, Bruce must attend to her psychological needs.

2. The equipment, supplies, and medications that Dr. Lewis may want and need to be available for Mrs. Johnson are

oxygen tank and mask, electrocardiograph, sphygmomanometer and stethoscope, and nitroglycerine, verapamil, and cardizem from the emergency cart.

3. Once the patient has been stabilized and Dr. Lewis has determined that Mrs. Johnson's symptoms are typical of angina pectoris, Bruce should continue to monitor Mrs. Johnson's vital signs and provide emotional support. He should notify the patient's family and remain with her until family members arrive to take Mrs. Johnson home.

4. Bruce can teach Mrs. Johnson and her family about the importance of using the prescribed form of nitroglycerin (sublingual tablets, transdermal patches) for angina attacks and the need to call Dr. Lewis if the nitroglycerin does not relieve symptoms. He can reinforce the need for regular exercise, a low-fat diet, stress reduction techniques, and no smoking.

## Chapter 10   Creating the Facility Environment

### Case Study 10-1

1. Audrey should greet the patient in a warm responsive manner and then assist Abigail Johnson to the extent she wants or needs assistance. In the examination room, privacy is especially important to patients. Space should be provided for patients to hang their clothes and undergarments. Mirrors are useful when dressing. Rooms should be soundproof so that conversations are not overheard. Audrey can ask Ms. Johnson if she would like help disrobing. Staff should always knock before entering a room.

2. Environments that give patients as much control as possible are preferable. These empower patients and make them feel comfortable with the circumstances. Harmonious surroundings can be created with color, type of lighting, fresh, clean odors, and avoidance of unnecessary clutter and equipment.

3. Because Audrey is obviously sensitive to Ms. Johnson, this patient is likely to feel less nervous about her physical exam. Audrey's warm yet unobtrusive manner should put Ms. Johnson at ease and, in the end, create the circumstances in which patient and physician can honestly and openly communicate.

## Chapter 11   Computers in the Ambulatory Care Setting

### Case Study 11-1

1. To minimize injury from excessive computer use, computer equipment needs to be chosen, set up, and used properly. Walter should consider using alternative keyboards to reduce wrist strain, using screen glare protectors to deflect monitor glare, positioning monitors for

individual comfort, and using chairs that offer lower back support.

The student should sketch out a diagram indicating positioning of chair, monitor, and keyboard. Annotate the sketch to explain why elements are positioned a certain way. See Figure 11-8 for general guidelines.

2. Walter should give staff who use computers frequently a general set of guidelines to ensure quality work and worker safety. They should take frequent short breaks away from the computer screen; they should change their posture from time to time and develop a variety of comfortable postures; they should look away from the monitor when printing, etc.; they should pay attention to any pain and take corrective action at once. Table 11-1 provides more detail on ensuring staff safety.

3. The inexperienced medical assistant can more easily overcome computer timidity if encouraged to build skills gradually. Walter needs to seek a fine line between setting firm goals for staff computer literacy but not setting expectations too high too quickly. A series of training courses either on or off the job will help build familiarity both with the hardware and the capabilities of the software. Staff should concentrate on learning one program at a time. Training after hours is preferable so center operations are not disrupted. When inexperienced users apply their skills in the workplace, they should have a "resource person" they can turn to as questions arise during computer use.

## Case Study 11-2

1. Confidentiality is most likely to be jeopardized with the use of fax machines, computer-based medical records, electronic transfer of medical records, invasion by hackers, and inappropriate discussion of patient records.

2. *Fax machines*—Establish written protocols to ensure confidentiality is maintained. To do this, locate fax machines in restricted access areas under the supervision of someone with the authority to access sensitive data. Personnel should first sign a confidentiality statement and be trained in sending a fax correctly to ensure the proper recipient receives the fax. Protocols should also include guidelines on what to do if a fax is received by an unintended recipient.

*Computer-based medical records*—The use of passwords is successful in controlling access to computer files and in providing an authentication mechanism. Development of a firewall to allow outside computers to access your computer while restricting access to your databases is essentially impossible. The office should not allow outside computers access to database computers and to communicate to an outside network or Internet while using a dedicated computer. Computer security protocols should be written, training should be provided to employees, and confidentiality statements should be signed by all

personnel having exposure to computer-based medical records before access is granted.

*Electronic transfer of medical records*—Follow the same procedures as computer-based medical records.

*Hackers*—Medical records sent over the Internet to an external location can be intercepted by hackers and posted on the Web for all to read. Encryption programs may be employed when sensitive medical records must be transmitted via electronic means.

*Inappropriate discussion*—All medical office employees should sign a confidentiality statement. During staff meetings, discuss the importance and ramifications of discussing confidential medical records via electronic methods.

3. Answers will vary.

# Chapter 12    *Telephone Techniques*

## Case Study 12-1

1. Triage is the act of evaluating the urgency of a medical situation. Because the young man is concerned about his mother's breathing, Audrey will automatically classify this call as a potential emergency. To gain additional information that will determine her actions, Audrey should ask the caller:

- The patient's name and age
- What happened to cause the situation
- Briefly, the patient's medical background that may shed light on the current breathing problem
- Whether the patient takes any regular medication
- If there are any other symptoms

Any breathing problems require emergency measures; after taking initial screening information, Audrey should inform Dr. Lewis, who will probably instruct Audrey to call 911 or the local emergency service to assist the patient as quickly as possible. Audrey will then follow up with the caller, and try to reassure him that help will be there as soon as possible. Once she has taken care of all urgent matters, Audrey should schedule a follow-up appointment for the patient with Dr. Lewis so he can ascertain the condition of the patient and determine the cause of the breathing difficulty.

2. Even though Audrey is not at the site, her Red Cross first aid and CPR training will give her the confidence to make difficult decisions under the pressure of time.

3. Audrey must be very careful not to give medical advice over the telephone, but only to triage the situation and help the caller assist the patient by making an appointment or by directing them to seek emergency assistance. In triaging, Audrey must always respect office procedures for handling emergency calls and act within the bounds of her training and expertise.

## Case Study 12-2

1. Wanda will need to know the caller's name and telephone and ask if she can return a call once she has collected the requested information.

2. The purpose of the call-back verification procedure is to verify that the person requesting the medical information is, in fact, employed by Claussen-Mason Laboratories.

3. After the verification has been established and permission by Dr. King has been given, Wanda may release the required information and then document the call appropriately in the telephone log book.

## Chapter 13   Patient Scheduling

### Case Study 13-1

1. Any ambulatory care center must institute cancellation procedures in order to assure quality patient care; free up care time for other patients; and protect physicians from potential legal complications.

2. In order to treat a patient, the patient's cooperation is necessary. A regular pattern of cancellations or no-shows may indicate that the patient is not committed to assisting in treatment. Sometimes, a physician may decide to terminate treatment, in which case a letter terminating services and discontinuing care would be sent to the patient by certified mail. Because Rhoda Au is a long-term patient, the physician may try to speak to her personally to discover if there is a reason for the repeated cancellations.

3. Whether using a manual or computer method, a system must be developed so it is evident to staff making appointments that, due to cancellations, time is now available to schedule other appointments.

   *In the manual system:* Note changes on the appointment sheet of all appointments that were changed, canceled, or failed to show using the steps in Procedure 13-3.

   *In the computer system:* Software programs differ, but cancellations are typically performed by deleting the patient's name from the time slot; that time then reopens for other appointments.

   Whether using a computer or manual system, be certain to keep a record of all canceled appointments including patient name, date, and time. Also record canceled appointments on the patient chart.

## Chapter 14   Medical Records Management

### Case Study 14-1

1. Karen should first instruct Liz in the principles of the numeric filing system used by Inner City Health Care. In addition to instructing Liz in filing methodology, Karen also needs to impress upon her the importance of maintaining up-to-date, easily accessible files. From a patient and physician point of view, good records enhance quality of care. Accurate files and documentation also are important should any litigation arise.

2. When filing any piece of documentation, Liz should follow these steps, which will enable her to efficiently process all written material.

   - Inspect
   - Index
   - Code
   - Sort
   - File

3. If all active and inactive patient files are to be computerized, Karen and Liz will need to be familiar with computer use and then investigate medical software that meets the needs of Inner City Health Care. They should expect the transition to be a gradual one and should set a series of intermediate goals, such as: first, scan all inactive files for archival storage; second, scan or input active client files; third, develop a system for efficiently transferring chart data from manual notation to computer input; fourth, gradually computerize other records such as correspondence.

## Chapter 15   Written Communications

### Case Study 15-1

1. While style manuals vary in content, certain elements are critical. Also, Marilyn wants it to be as comprehensive as possible, so her outline of major headings might include:

   - Introduction to the style manual
   - The Lewis & King letter format
   - A sample letter, noting standard elements that go into every letter
   - Procedures for all outgoing correspondence
   - Procedures for all incoming correspondence
   - Commonly used medical terms
   - Proofreading hints
   - Writing tips
   - Sample of form letters used by Lewis & King
   - Summary of mail classes and services
   - Summary of do's and don'ts in written communications

2. Marilyn can have medical assistants read a reference book on composition to educate them about usage and style; she can encourage them to enroll in a business

writing class; and she can help them build skills by giving manageable assignments that require an increasing level of ability.

3. After selecting the office letter style, Marilyn can identify standard components of any letter that leaves the offices of Lewis & King. These typically include:

- Date line
- Inside address of recipient
- Salutation
- Subject line
- Body of letter
- Complimentary closing
- Keyed signature and personal signature
- Reference initials, when applicable
- Enclosure notation, when applicable
- Carbon copy notation, when applicable
- Postscripts, when applicable
- Continuation page heading when the letter is more than one page

## Chapter 16    Transcription

### Case Study 16-1

Hospitals, multispecialty clinics, and solo physician practices offer competitive salaries and benefit packages. They may pay for professional memberships and registration fees for CE opportunities and an allowance for reference materials. The dictation from these settings encompasses a wide range of specialties, complexities, styles, and dialects. State-of-the-art equipment is often available so that new skills may be learned. There often are QA personnel to ask questions of and to obtain feedback on progress in document preparation.

Transcription services and home-based positions offer competitive pay rates and dictation from a wide range of specialties, complexities, styles, and dialects. There may be a more flexible work schedule available, with compensation based on production. There may or may not be QA personnel available.

Freelance MTs are in business for themselves. This environment offers the MT a sense of accomplishment and independence and the opportunity to work flexible hours. There may or may not be someone available to QA their work or answer questions when they get stuck. The freelance MT's earnings can be excellent if they are highly productive, transcribe accurately, and remain focused on building the business. At times there may be more work than can be readily handled and there may be slack periods with little to transcribe. Freelance MTs must maintain bookkeeping records and manage the business themselves or pay to have someone else handle the books.

### Case Study 16-2

1. The physician dictated *upper lip* in the first sentence and *lower lip* in the last sentence. The MT does not know which is correct.

2. To verify which lip is correct, the MT will need to pull the patient's chart and read through the documentation or flag the document asking the physician to acknowledge which is correct. The physician would also have to check the chart, so it is probably best if the MT does this.

3. If the information can be verified before the document is printed, the correction can be made before printing the document. If the document has been flagged, the physician will verify the correct site. To make the correction, simply draw a single line through the error and write the correction above or below the error while preserving legibility of the error. The correction notation should also include the initials of the person entering the correction, the date, and reference to the lab report as a cross-reference.

## Chapter 17    Daily Financial Practices

### Case Study 17-1

1. Selecting an appropriate bookkeeping method, taking responsibility for banking, managing the purchase of supplies, and establishing a petty cash system are all topics that Joann should become familiar with. Marilyn will review with Joann all the daily financial practices as reviewed in this chapter, including:

- Discussion and determination of patient fees
- Credit arrangements
- Managing patient accounts using either a manual or computerized bookkeeping method
- Taking care of all banking procedures, including understanding different accounts, types of checks, making deposits, accepting checks for payment, writing checks, and reconciling a bank statement
- The activities involved in purchasing, including preparing the purchase order
- Establishing a petty cash fund

2. If Marilyn wants to institute computerized bookkeeping methods at Doctors Lewis & King, it may be helpful to have Joann begin the process of computerization while Marilyn continues to maintain accounts with the manual method. The computerization process is a gradual one and often the two systems must run side-by-side until the computer method is up and running and all personnel are familiar and comfortable with using the new system. As Joann is setting up the system, Marilyn can work side by side with her, teaching Joann about how accounts have been maintained manually; she will acquaint Joann both with the specifics of the office's daily financial practices

and give her an understanding of the pegboard accounting method. At the same time, Marilyn will learn about the computer method by assisting Joann.

3. Part of daily financial practices includes accounts payable, or writing checks to pay bills, refund overpayments, and replenish petty cash. Joann must be careful about how she writes checks, making sure that they are legible, properly dated, include the name of the payee, the amount of payment in figures and words, and that the memo line is completed referencing the purpose of the check. The check stub must also be recorded to maintain an accurate record of payments made from the account. Before checks are sent, Joann should follow these rules:

- Check that numerical and written amounts agree.

- Check that everything is spelled correctly.

- Follow office procedure for having physicians or office manager approve and/or sign all checks.

- Determine that the check is made payable to correct payee, that the correct amount is paid, and that the current date is used.

## Chapter 18    *Medical Insurance*

### Case Study 18-1

|  | Total Charges | Allowed Charges |
| --- | --- | --- |
| Office visit | $85.00 | $80.00 |
| Return visit | +65.00 | +55.00 |
| **Total Charges** | $150.00 | $135.00 |
| Less deductible | −100.00 | −100.00 |
| Subtotal | $50.00 | $35.00 |
| Apply 80% coinsurance | × 80% | × 80% |
| **Insurance Payment** | $40.00 | $28.00 |
| **Patient Owes** | $10.00 | $7.00* |

*(or $22.00 if physician does not accept assignment; $7.00 plus $15.00 disallowed by Medicare)

## Chapter 19    *Medical Insurance Coding*

### Case Study 19-1

Note: Students will need to look these codes up in ICD-9-CM and CPT code books. Answers here are based on 2000 code books.

1. The proper ICD-9-CM diagnosis codes for Mr. McKay are:

787.0    nausea

789.0    abdominal pain

2. The proper CPT procedure codes for Mr. McKay are:

99204    new patient, extended office visit

85031    CBC, complete

82270    guaiac

80061    lipid panel

81000    urinalysis

3. When coding any claim form it is important that the medical assistant be as precise as possible, not guess, and not code what is not there. Coding must always correlate with the physician's notes in the chart; otherwise, fraud is committed and an ethical and legal principle violated.

## Chapter 20    *Billing and Collections*

### Case Study 20-1

1. Often, a quick telephone call may solve a collections problem, for the patient may have forgotten or misplaced the bill. No matter what the situation, a friendly tone is important. It is also critical to keep to the facts and remain tactful and pleasant. More is gained by remaining courteous than by assuming a threatening manner. In addition, legal rules and regulations apply to collection calls. A collection call should never be made in a way that is accusatory or that embarrasses the patient, for instance, by calling at the workplace.

2. If telephone collections are not effective, Ellen might send a series of letters once the account is 2 to 3 months past due. The first would ask the patient to pay the balance; the second, sent a month later, would again ask for immediate payment of the balance; the third would inform the client that the account is being assigned to a collection agency.

The student should draft three letters and then compare them with the collections letters in Chapter 20.

3. If a patient has declared bankruptcy, Ellen may not send any statements nor make any attempt to collect delinquent accounts. In a bankruptcy, a physician's fee is likely to be one of the last to be paid because it is unsecured.

## Chapter 21    *Accounting Practices*

### Case Study 21-1

1. In reviewing fixed costs, the owners of Inner City Health Care would consider items that do not vary in total according to the number of patients. For example, these might include rent and/or mortgage, utilities, and the annual depreciation cost of equipment.

2. Variable costs will vary in direct proportion to patient volume. Variable costs will include items such as clinical supplies, laboratory fees, professional liability insurance, and the costs of billing and collections.

3. Utilization review, which is a review of service before it is performed, demands more accurate recordkeeping and documentation than ever before. Utilization review companies sell their services to employers and insurance

carriers; these reviewers determine whether or not procedures or treatments are needed or will improve a patient's condition prior to the patient receiving medical services. If they decide a procedure or treatment is not needed, those services will not be covered by the insurance carrier. Thus, utilization review may affect the number of clinical procedures Inner City Health Care may perform and consequently its ultimate profitability. Also, if proper preauthorizations are not requested, Inner City may perform clinical procedures that the carrier may refuse to pay.

## Chapter 22    The Medical Assistant as Office Manager

### Case Study 22-1

1. Answers will vary, but the groups should discuss and incorporate the teamwork approach to plan and implement a solution.

2. The team previously should have identified the resources available and met to brainstorm possible problems that could occur and what their solutions might be.

3. The office manager should remain calm and try to keep the argument from escalating. Other patients may be present as well; they should not be disturbed. One of the duties of the office manager is to supervise personnel, so she would want to be supportive of the staff while being understanding of the patients' feelings.

### Case Study 22-2

1. Answers will vary, but pros may include that this management style communicates purpose and direction of tasks, solicits participation of others, inspires subordinates, encourages open communication, empowers others, serves as a role model, and is a continuous learner. Cons may include that she may be thought of as one who tattles to higher authorities.

2. Answers will vary.

3. Answers will vary.

## Chapter 23    The Medical Assistant as Human Resources Manager

### Case Study 23-1

1. Jane should be up-front with Bruce and state that it has been noticed that he frequently takes longer lunches than he is allotted. The two should work on an action plan to correct this situation, and a re-evaluation should be scheduled.

2. Although evaluations may involve more than the office manager or human resource manager and the employee, it probably would not be appropriate to involve the

employee's peer or fellow worker. It may affect work relationships and cause hard feelings.

3. Jane should end the formal evaluation on a positive note by stating her confidence in the individual to make any changes necessary, offering assistance where needed, and thanking the employee for participating. End with a positive statement about some portion of the employee's performance.

## Chapter 24    Preparing for Medical Assisting Credentials

### Case Study 24-1

1. Juan must request the application from the AAMA Certification Department or the Program Coordinator and be sure to complete the correct application. Juan should read all the instructions carefully before completing the application form. The application must be free from errors and each item must be completed in full. The application must be postmarked by March 1 for him to be allowed to take the June examination.

2. Answers will vary, but here is one sample schedule:

   March—Form study group. Contact people to see if they are interested. Set up a regular meeting time at least one time per week. Purchase study guides.

   April—Increase study group meetings to two times per week. Begin to review course textbooks and tests.

   May—Increase study group meetings to three times per week. Study independently two or three times per week also.

3. Juan should be careful to approach people he knows will take the examination seriously. He does not necessarily have to ask only those who are his friends.

### Case Study 24-2

1. Nancy must be of good moral character and have graduated from an accredited high school or acceptable equivalent. Nancy must determine the appropriate requirement she satisfies and have been employed in the profession of medical assisting for a minimum of five years, no more than two years of which may have been as an instructor in a postsecondary medical assistant program.

2. Since most examinations may be scheduled within three days of application completion, Nancy should begin her study schedule several months prior to January to allow plenty of time to study each of the categories covered on the test.

3. Nancy should begin early to find a study partner(s). The study partner(s) should take the examination seriously and have a similar date in mind for sitting for the exam. The partner(s) should also agree to and be committed to

the study schedule. Meeting once or twice a week helps keep the group focused. Independent study should be done throughout the week. During the independent study time, each group member could write 25 questions relevant to the weeks' study topic. When the group meets, a discussion of the study topic could take place and then copies of the questions distributed for answering. The questions could be corrected and discussion of any questionable or missed answers could take place.

## Chapter 25　Employment Strategies

### Case Study 25-1

1. The functional resume is probably the best resume style for Eun Mee to follow. The advantages of the functional style are that it allows areas of experience to be sorted into areas of function. This is useful when reentering the job market after an absence, when you have a variety of different, apparently unconnected work experiences, and when you have volunteer work experience.

2. Vital information should include full name, address including street number, city, state, and zip code, and telephone number including area code.

3. Accomplishment statements simply state your accomplishments and what you have done in previous employment settings. They are a way of tooting your own horn to help prospective employers realize your capabilities. Accomplishment statements should begin with power verbs and give a brief description of what you did and the demonstrable results that were produced. An example would be "During my experience as a sales representative, I serviced numerous customers who, as a result of my responsiveness to their needs, asked for me personally when they returned to the store for purchases."

### Case Study 25-2

1. The candidate should bring an extra application, cover letter, resume, and reference sheet.

2. Arriving early will give Eun Mee time to collect her thoughts and become composed. It will also demonstrate good work habits to the employer: punctuality.

3. The candidate should wait patiently until the employer calls her in and wait for the employer's cues. The candidate should return a firm handshake and wait to be offered a seat.

# GLOSSARY OF TERMS

**accessibility** making facilities or equipment available for use by any individual (Ch. 10).

**accession record (numeric system)** logbook used to assign numbers to correspondence or patients (Ch. 14).

**accomplishment statements** statements that begin with a power verb and give a brief description of what you did, and the demonstrable results that were produced (Ch. 25).

**account aging** process by which accounts are determined to be overdue (Ch. 20).

**accounting** system of monitoring the financial status of a facility and the financial results of its activities, providing information for decision making (Ch. 21).

**accounts payable** sum owed by a business for services or goods received (Ch. 17); also unwritten promise to pay a supplier for property or merchandise purchased on credit or for a service rendered (Ch. 21).

**accounts receivable** amount owed to a business for services or goods supplied (Ch. 17).

**accounts receivable (A/R) ratio assets** outstanding accounts receivable divided by the average monthly gross income for the past twelve months (Ch. 21).

**accreditation** process whereby recognition is granted to an educational program for maintaining standards that qualify its graduates for professional practice; to provide with credentials (Ch. 1).

**accredited** recognized as being outstanding (Ch. 4).

**Accrediting Bureau of Health Education Schools (ABHES)** entity accrediting institutions for the American Medical Technologists (Ch. 24).

**acquired immunodeficiency syndrome (AIDS)** disorder of the immune system caused by a human immunodeficiency virus (HIV), a retrovirus that destroys the body's ability to fight infection. As the disease progresses, the individual becomes overcome by disorders, including cancers and opportunistic infections. There is no known cure for AIDS (Ch. 6).

**active listening** received message is paraphrased back to the sender to verify the correct message was decoded (Ch. 4).

**acupuncture** treatment to relieve pain and disease by puncturing the skin with thin needles at specific points (Ch. 2, 3).

**adjustments** increases or decreases to patient accounts not due to charges incurred or payments received (Ch. 17).

**agenda** printed list of topics to be discussed during a meeting, sometimes giving time allocation (Ch. 15, 22).

**agent** person representing another (Ch. 7).

**algorithm** a special method for solving a specific kind of problem (Ch. 11).

**allied health professionals** health care providers with a range of educational backgrounds and skills who support, complement, or assist physicians and who are a critical part of the health care team (Ch. 2).

**allopathic** method of treating disease with remedies that produce effects different from those caused by the disease itself. Most traditional physicians today are considered allopathic physicians (Ch. 3).

**ambulatory care setting** health care environment where services are provided on an outpatient basis. Ambulatory is from the Latin and means "capable of walking." Examples include the solo-physician's office, the group practice, the urgent care center, and the health maintenance organization (Ch. 1, 2).

**American Association for Medical Transcription (AAMT)** nonprofit organization founded by medical transcriptionists to promote the profession (Ch. 16).

**American Association of Medical Assistants (AAMA)** premier organization dedicated to serving the interests of certified medical assistants (Ch. 24).

**Americans with Disabilities Act (ADA)** congressional act passed in 1990 to end discrimination against individuals with disabilities (Ch. 10).

**ancillary services** professional occupational companies hired to complete a specific job (Ch. 22).

**answering services** services employed to answer the calls of an ambulatory care setting after hours; unlike an answering machine, a live operator answers the call and forwards it appropriately (Ch. 12).

**antivirus program** software program that identifies the signature of a computer virus and works to eliminate it from the computer system. Antivirus programs are useful only if updated by frequently downloading from the program supplier updates on new viruses. Antivirus programs are usually incapable of detecting a new type of virus (Ch. 11).

**application/cover letter**   letter used to introduce yourself and your resume to a prospective employer with the goal of obtaining an interview (Ch. 25).

**application form**   form devised by a prospective employer to collect information relative to qualifications, education, and experience in employment (Ch. 25).

**applications software**   software that performs a specific data processing function (Ch. 11).

**articulating**   expressing oneself clearly and distinctly (Ch. 12).

**asepsis**   protecting against infection caused by pathogenic microorganisms (Ch. 3).

**assets**   properties of value that are owned by a business entity (Ch. 21).

**assignment of benefits**   signing over of benefits by the beneficiary to another party (Ch. 18).

**attribute**   inherent characteristic (Ch. 1).

**automated routing unit (ARU)**   telephone system that answers a call and uses a recorded voice to identify departments or services (Ch. 12).

**baccalaureate**   degree of bachelor conferred by colleges and universities (Ch. 1).

**balance**   amount owed (N); to verify posting accuracy (V) (Ch. 17).

**balance sheet**   itemized statement of assets, liabilities, and equity; a statement of financial condition (Ch. 21).

**bar code**   black bars that are read by an optical scanner. The bar code option on the HCFA-1500 insurance claim form permits the physician name and address to be coded on the top right corner (Ch. 18).

**basic insurance**   medical insurance that covers most physician fees, hospital expenses, and surgical fees according to the terms of the policy. The patient is usually responsible for a deductible (Ch. 18).

**benchmark**   making a comparison among different organizations relative to how they accomplish tasks, such as office computerization, organizing file systems, and employee remuneration (Ch. 11).

**beneficiary**   person under a policy eligible to receive benefits (Ch. 18).

**benefit**   remuneration that is in addition to the salary (Ch. 22).

**bias**   slant toward a particular belief (Ch. 4).

**bioethics**   branch of medical ethics concerned with moral issues resulting from high technology and sophisticated medical research. Social issues such as genetic engineering, abortion, and fetal tissue research raise important bioethical questions (Ch. 8).

**birthday rule**   method to determine which of two or more policies covering a dependent child will be primary; that parent with the birthday falling first in the calendar year has the primary policy (Ch. 18).

**bit**   smallest unit of data a computer can process; eight bits make up a byte (Ch. 11).

**blind copy**   protects the privacy of e-mail. Other recipients cannot identify who else may have received the transmitted message (Ch. 15).

**body language**   nonverbal communication that includes unconscious body movements, gestures, and facial expressions that accompany verbal messages (Ch. 4).

**bond**   binding agreement with an employee ensuring recovery of financial loss should funds be stolen or embezzled (Ch. 22).

**bond paper**   durable, strong paper usually used for correspondence (Ch. 15).

**brainstorming**   process of developing ideas through a synergistic interaction among participants in an environment free of criticism (Ch. 22).

**breach of confidentiality**   unauthorized release of confidential information (Ch. 16, 19).

**bubonic plague**   infectious disease with a high fatality rate transmitted to humans from infected rats and ground squirrels by the bite of the rat flea (Ch. 3).

**buffer words**   expendable words used while answering the telephone (Ch. 4, 12).

**bullet points**   asterisk or dot followed by a descriptive phrase; helps the reader identify important points easily (Ch. 25).

**burnout**   a state of fatigue or frustration brought about by a devotion to a cause, a way of life, or a relationship that failed to produce the expected reward (Ch. 5).

**byte**   amount of memory needed to store one character (such as a letter or number). Computer memory and disk space are measured in kilobytes, megabytes, and gigabytes (Ch. 11).

**candida**   a species of yeast (Ch. 19).

**capitation**   use of the number of members enrolled in a plan to determine salary of the physician; the physician is paid a fixed fee for each member no matter how many times that member is seen by the physician (Ch. 18, 19).

**caption**   method of designation used on file guides (Ch. 14).

**cardiopulmonary resuscitation (CPR)**   combination of rescue breathing and chest compressions performed by a trained individual on a patient experiencing cardiac arrest (Ch. 9).

**career objective**   expresses your career goal and the position for which you are applying (Ch. 25).

**cashier's check**   bank's own check drawn against the bank's account (Ch. 17).

**catchment**   40-mile radius of a military base where medical care is available to military dependents (Ch. 18).

**cellular telephones**   battery-operated portable telephones that are typically found in automobiles and other unfixed locations. One can receive and send messages from cellular phones (Ch. 12).

**central processing unit (CPU)**   brain of the computer that performs instructions defined by software (Ch. 11).

**certification**   guarantees as being true or as represented by or as meeting a standard (Ch. 1, 24).

**certification examination**   standardized means of evaluating medical assistant competency (Ch. 24).

**certified check**   depositor's own check that the bank has indicated with a date and signature to be good for the amount written (Ch. 17).

**certified medical assistant (CMA)**   a medical assistant who has successfully completed the AAMA's national certification examination and earned the status of being certified (Ch. 1, 24).

**certified medical transcriptionist (CMT)** recognized professional credential obtained through successful completion of both parts of the core certification examination administered by the MTCC at AAMT (Ch. 16).

**charge out-follow up** system of processing requests for health information to ensure proper return of the information (Ch. 15).

**charges** fee for services rendered; increases balance due (Ch. 17).

**charge slip** form used to record services supplied and charges and payments for those services; functions as billing form for insurance reimbursement. Also known as an encounter form. See also **superbill** (Ch. 19).

**charisma** personality and appearance characteristics that influence people to support the person possessing it; magnetism (Ch. 22).

**chart notes** (also called progress notes) physician's formal or informal notes about presenting problem, physical findings, and plan for treatment for a patient examined in the office, clinic, acute care center, or emergency department (Ch. 16).

**chief complaint (CC)** specific symptom or problem for which the patient is seeing the physician today (Ch. 16).

**chronological resume** resume format used when you have employment experience (Ch. 25).

**civil law** law related to actions between individuals (Ch. 7).

**claim** demand for payment; in this case it is a demand by the beneficiary to the insurance company for payment of medical expenses incurred during the effective dates of the medical policy (Ch. 18, 19).

**claim register** diary or register of claims submitted to each insurance carrier. When payment is received, the date and amount of payment is entered in the register (Ch. 19).

**clinical e-mail** electronic messages sent to or by the physician's office regarding medical questions or advice (Ch. 15).

**closed questions** questions answered with a yes or no (Ch. 4).

**clustering** grouping together of nonverbal messages into statements or conclusions (Ch. 4); also, scheduling system where patients with similar complaints are seen for consecutive appointments, e.g., ear infections at 9:00, 9:30, and 10:00 A.M. with physical examinations at 1:00, 2:00, and 3:00 P.M. (Ch. 13).

**coding** process of marking data to indicate how information is to be filed (Ch. 14).

**coinsurance** that percentage paid by the company or that paid by the insured (Ch. 18).

**collection agency** outside establishment that collects outstanding debts (Ch. 20).

**collection ratio** gross income divided by the amount that could have been collected less disallowances (Ch. 21).

**color coding** method of filing utilizing colors to ensure quick filing and retrieval of records. Three common methods are Tab Alpha Code System, Alpha-Z System, and color-coded file folders (Ch. 14).

**communication cycle** involves sending and receiving messages even when unconsciously aware of them (Ch. 4).

**compensation** overemphasizing of characteristics to make up for a real or imagined failure or handicap (Ch. 4).

**competency** legally qualified or adequate (Ch. 1).

**compliance** to act in accordance with conditions laid down (Ch. 1).

**confidentiality** ethical and legal rules in regard to patient privacy (Ch. 12, 16).

**confidentiality agreement** when signed, the agreement signifies that the medical transcriptionist is committed to keep all patient information confidential (Ch. 16).

**conflict resolution** solving problems between coworkers or any two parties (Ch. 23).

**congruency** the verbal message and the nonverbal message must agree (Ch. 4).

**consecutive or serial filing** numeric filing method where numbers are considered in ascending order using the entire set of figures (Ch. 14).

**consultation report** document that reports the findings and/or advice of another physician requested to see a patient by the attending physician (Ch. 16).

**contact tracker** form used to keep track of employment contact information such as name of employer, name of contact person, address and telephone number, date of first contact, resume sent, interview date, follow-up information, and dates (Ch. 25).

**continuing education (CE)** method of recertification of the certified medical transcriptionist credential (Ch. 16).

**continuing education units (CEU)** method for earning points toward recertification (Ch. 24).

**continuous speech recognition (CSR)** the process of direct conversion of spoken documentation into a written text, e.g., electronic version using a computer equipped with voice recognition software (Ch. 16).

**coordination of benefits (COB)** the provision of an insurance contract that limits benefits to 100 percent of the cost (Ch. 18).

**copayment** payment required when seen by the physician (Ch. 18).

**cost accounting** determines what it costs for a practice to perform particular services (Ch. 21).

**cost allocation** process of taking costs from one area and allocating them to others (Ch. 20).

**cost analysis** procedure that determines the costs of each service (Ch. 21).

**cost ratio** formula that shows the cost of a procedure or service and helps determine the financial value of maintaining certain services (Ch. 21).

**crash tray or cart** tray or portable cart that contains medications and supplies needed for emergency and first aid procedures (Ch. 9).

**credentialed** testimonials showing that a person is entitled to credit or has a right to exercise official power (Ch. 1).

**credit** decreases balance due (Ch. 17).

**credit bureau** outside agency that provides information about a patient's credit history (Ch. 20).

**crepitation** grating sound heard on movement of ends of a broken bone (Ch. 9).

**criminal law** law related to wrongs committed against the welfare and safety of society as a whole (Ch. 7).

**cross-reference** notation in a file to direct the reader to a specific record that may be filed under more than one name/subject, e.g., married name/maiden name or foreign names, where the surname is not easily recognizable (Ch. 14).

**culture** social behavior patterns and beliefs (Ch. 6).

**currency** paper money (Ch. 17).

**Current Procedural Terminology (CPT)** standard codes for procedures and services. Used by most ambulatory care settings in encoding the claim form and recognized by most insurance carriers (Ch. 18, 19).

**cut** placement of the tab on file folders (Ch. 14).

**cycle billing** method of spreading billing over the whole month instead of sending all bills at the end of the month (Ch. 20).

**database management software** computer applications software designed for the manipulation of data within a database. This software allows for creation and editing capabilities, sorting capabilities, and comparing and summarizing activities (Ch. 11).

**data input device** any device capapble of converting hard copy, motion, temperature, position, or other analog signals into digital input for use by a computer (Ch. 11).

**data output device** device that converts digital data from a computer into hardcopy, motion, position, or other analog signals (Ch. 11).

**data storage device** device capable of permanently or temporarily storing digital data (Ch. 11).

**data storage memory** permanent memory not part of the motherboard. Utilizes any suitable data storage device. Can be read-only or read-write type of memory (Ch. 11).

**day sheet** form used with pegboard system to record daily patient transactions (Ch. 17).

**decode** to translate into language that is easily understood; to interpret (Ch. 4).

**deductible** that amount of incurred medical expenses that must be met before the insurance policy will begin to pay (Ch. 18).

**defendant** person who defends action brought in litigation (Ch. 7).

**defense mechanism** behavior that protects the psyche from guilt, anxiety, or shame (Ch. 4).

**dementia** impairment of intellectual function that is progressive and interferes with normal activities (Ch. 6).

**denial** rejection of or refusal to acknowledge (Ch. 4).

**diagnosis code** numerical designation for a specific illness, injury, or disease; codes found in ICD-9-CM code book (Ch. 18, 19).

**diagnosis-related groups (DRGs)** classification of patients into categories based on primary diagnosis, procedure, and discharge status (Ch. 18).

**diaphragm** membrane separating the abdominal and thoracic cavities; functions in respiration (Ch. 12).

**digital dictation** dictation recorded directly into computers and managed by computers (Ch. 16).

**direct payment** payment made directly to the physician by the insurance company (Ch. 18).

**disbursement** to assign general ledger account information (account name or number) to a financial transaction (Ch. 17).

**displacement** displacing negative feelings onto something or someone else with no significance to the situation (Ch. 4).

**disposition** temperament, character, personality (Ch. 1).

**doctrine** principle of law established through past decisions (Ch. 7).

**documentation** written material that accompanies purchased software containing the information necessary for using the software appropriately; sometimes known as the manual (Ch. 11).

**double booking** scheduling system where multiple patients are given an assigned appointment time, e.g., 9:30 A.M., to be seen by different office personnel at that time (Ch. 13).

**durable power of attorney for health care** legal form that allows a designated person to act on another's behalf in regard to health care choices (Ch. 6, 7).

**E codes** ICD-9-CM codes for the external causes of injury, poisoning, or other adverse reactions that explain how the injury occurred (Ch. 19).

**editing** the process of manipulating text to avoid inaccuracies and inconsistencies within a document (Ch. 16).

**elective procedures** those procedures not necessary for the health of the patient (Ch. 18).

**electronic mail (e-mail)** communications that are sent, received, stored, and forwarded on-line from computer to computer by means of a modem (Ch. 12, 15).

**emancipated minor** persons under age 18 who are financially responsible for themselves and free of parental care (Ch. 7).

**Emergency Medical Services (EMS)** Emergency Medical Services (EMS) system is a local network of police, fire, and medical personnel trained to respond to emergency situations. In many communities the system is activated by calling 911 (Ch. 9).

**empathy** ability to be objectively aware of and have insight into another's feelings, emotions, and behaviors, and to be aware of the significance and meaning of these to the other person (Ch. 1, 12).

**emulate** imitate a characteristic of an individual in order to equal or surpass the original (Ch. 22).

**encode (encoding)** creating a message to be sent (Ch. 4).

**enunciation** speaking clearly; articulating (Ch. 12).

**envoy** an electronic data exchange system that allows you to access patient eligibility information via modem (Ch. 18).

**ergonomics** scientific study of work and space, including factors that influence worker productivity and that affect workers' health (Ch. 11).

**established patient** patient who has been seen previously in the office, with a pertinent history and medical information readily accessible in the chart (Ch. 13).

**ethical** conforming to accepted principles of right and wrong within a profession; see also ethics (Ch. 12).

**ethics** defined in terms of what is morally right and wrong; ethics will differ from person to person; often defined by a code or creed as in the Code of Ethics from the American Association of Medical Assistants (AAMA) (Ch. 8).

**etiquette** manners, politeness, proper behavior (Ch. 12).

**exclusive provider organization (EPO)** a closed-panel PPO plan where enrollees receive no beneifts if they opt to receive care from a provider who is not in the EPO (Ch. 18).

**exit interview** opportunity for departing employees to provide their positive and negative opinions of the position and facility (Ch. 23).

**expenses** decreases in the owner's equity in a business caused by transactions involving asset outflows (Ch. 20).

**expert witness** individual with highly specialized knowledge and skills in a particular area who testifies to a standard of care (Ch. 7).

**explanation of benefits (EOB)** insurance report that is sent with claim payments explaining the reimbursement of the insurance carrier (Ch. 18, 19).

**expressed contract** written or verbal contract that specifically describes what each party in the contract will do (Ch. 7).

**externship** transition stage between the classroom and actual employment; may also be referred to as internship or practicum (Ch. 1, 22).

**facial expressions** various aspects of facial anatomy that send nonverbal messages (Ch. 4).

**facilitate** to make an action or process easier (Ch. 1).

**Fair Debt Collection Practice Act** 1977 federal law that outlines collection practices (Ch. 20).

**fax (facsimile)** machine that sends documents from one location to another by way of telephone lines (Ch. 12).

**feedback** receiver's way of ensuring that the message that was understood is the same as the message that was sent (Ch. 4).

**field** basic data category within the database. Fields can be either numeric (numerals), alphanumeric (letters and numerals), logical, or memo (Ch. 11).

**financial accounting** provides information for entities external to the practice; e.g., the federal government (Ch. 21).

**firewall** software protection built into a computer system to prevent unauthorized access or hacking into a computer system and files (Ch. 11).

**first aid** immediate (or first) care provided to persons who are suddenly ill or injured; first aid is typically followed by more comprehensive care and treatment (Ch. 9).

**fiscal intermediary** local administrator for Medicare (Ch. 18).

**fixed cost** cost that does not vary in total as the number of patients vary (Ch. 21).

**flag** method of identifying a blank space or a question regarding dictator's meaning by attaching a note or marker to indicate the question (Ch. 16).

**floppy disk** portable read-write data storage device. It is storable and transferable between computers. Capacity is approximately 1.4 megabytes of data. Data is stored permanently until overwritten. Floppy drive unit is required to read-write data from disk (Ch. 11).

**fluent** facility in the use of a language (Ch. 12).

**footer** page formatting feature that allows for the bottom of all pages to be marked with keyed-in data. While the data is keyed in only once, it appears on every page in the document (Ch. 11).

**form letter** letter containing the same content in the body but sent to different individuals (Ch. 15).

**fractures** break in a bone. There are several types of fractures, but all are classified as either open fractures or closed fractures (Ch. 9).

**fraud** deliberate misrepresentation of facts (Ch. 19).

**freelance MTs** self-employed medical transcriptionists (Ch. 16).

**fringe benefit** benefit above and beyond salary to which an employee may be entitled. Examples include health and life insurance, paid vacation, sick days, personal days, and tuition reimbursement for courses related to employment (Ch. 2, 22).

**full block letter** major letter style in which all lines begin flush with the left margin. This style is suggested for offices desiring a contemporary-looking, efficient letter (Ch. 15).

**functional resume** resume format used to highlight specialty areas of accomplishment and strengths (Ch. 25).

**genetic engineering** alteration, manipulation, replacement, or repair of genetic material (Ch. 8).

**gestures/mannerisms** movement of various body parts while communicating (Ch. 4).

**gigabyte** 1,000 megabytes of data (Ch. 11).

**goal** result or achievement toward which effort is directed (Ch. 5).

**"going bare"** said of a physician who does not carry professional liability insurance (Ch. 22).

**Good Samaritan laws** laws designed to protect individuals from legal action when rendering emergency medical aid, without compensation, within the areas of their training and expertise (Ch. 12).

**graphics software** applications software used to create pictorial representations (Ch. 11).

**guide** device on file folders used to separate sections of file folders (Ch. 14).

**hacker** person who uses sophisticated software to gain unauthorized access to computer systems and files. Hacker gains access through use of a linked computer or a computer connected to the Internet (Ch. 11).

**hard disk** read-write data storage device permanently attached to the computer cabinet containing the CPU. Data is stored permanently until overwritten. Capacity is approximately 20 gigabytes or more of data (Ch. 11).

**hardware** physical equipment used by the computer system to process data (Ch. 11).

**HCFA Common Procedure Coding System (HCPCS)** standardized coding system used to process Medicare claims (Ch. 19).

**header** page formatting feature that allows the top of a page to be printed with identifying information. The data is only keyed in once, but appears on all pages in the document (Ch. 11).

**Health Care Financing Administration (HCFA)** the national administrator of Medicare (Ch. 18).

**health maintenance organization (HMO)** type of managed care operation that is typically set up as a for-profit corporation with salaried employees. HMOs "with walls" offer a range of medical services under one roof; HMOs "without walls" typically contract with physicians in the community to provide patient services for an agreed-upon fee (Ch. 2, 18).

**Heimlich maneuver** abdominal thrusts designed to overcome breathing difficulties in patients who are choking (Ch. 9).

**hemophilia** hereditary blood disease characterized by the blood's failure to clot, causing abnormal bleeding (Ch. 8).

**hierarchy** the order of significance or control; ranking of importance (Ch. 22).

**hierarchy of needs** needs that are arranged in a specific order or rank; sequential arrangement. Associated with Abraham Maslow (Ch. 4).

**history and physical examination report (H&P)** report of patient's history and physical examination to document reason for visit (Ch. 16).

**history of present illness (HPI)** the chronological description of the development of the patient's illness (Ch. 16).

**holistic** in medicine, used to identify a specific approach that treats the "whole" body, mind, and spirit (Ch. 2).

**home-based MTs** medical transcriptionists employed by transcription services (Ch. 16).

**human immunodeficiency virus (HIV)** AIDS virus; it is a retrovirus that ultimately destroys immune system cells (Ch. 6).

**hypothermia** extremely dangerous cold-related condition that can result in death if the individual does not receive care and if the progression of hypothermia is not reversed. Symptoms include shivering, cold skin, and confusion (Ch. 9).

**identification label** marking label placed on either the top or side edge of a file folder to indicate the proper designation for filing purposes (Ch. 14).

**implied consent** consent assumed by the health care provider, typically in an emergency that threatens the patient's life. Implied consent also occurs in more subtle ways in the health care environment; e.g., when a patient willingly rolls up the sleeve to receive an injection (Ch. 7).

**implied contract** contract indicated by actions rather than words (Ch. 7).

**improvise** to make, invent, or arrange in an offhand manner (Ch. 1).

**income statement** financial statement showing net profit or loss (Ch. 21).

**incompetence** legally, a person who is insane, inadequate, or not an adult (Ch. 7).

**independent physician association (IPA)** independent network of physicians in private practice who contract with the association to treat patients for an agreed-upon fee (Ch. 2).

**index counter** measures the length of dictation on a cassette cartridge (Ch. 16).

**indexing** selecting the name, subject, or number under which to file a record and determining the order in which the units should be considered (Ch. 14).

**indirect statements** means of eliciting a response from a patient by turning a question into a statement of interest (Ch. 4).

**information retrieval system** system that allows electronic access to very large databases for the retrieval of information; e.g., Medlais and Medline (Ch. 11).

**informed consent** consent given by the patient who is made aware of any procedure to be performed, its risks, expected outcomes, and alternatives (Ch. 7).

**inner-directed people** people who decide for themselves what they want to do with their lives (Ch. 5).

**inspect** to look carefully at the item to be filed to identify the key name, business, and subject the information relates to (Ch. 14).

**insurance abuse** incidents or misrepresentations that are inconsistent with acceptable practice of medicine and lead to improper reimbursement, treatment that is not medically necessary for a disorder, or procedures that are harmful and/or of poor quality (Ch. 19).

**integrate** to incorporate into a larger unit; to form or blend into a whole (Ch. 1).

**integrated delivery system** a health care organization of affiliated provider sites combined under a single ownership that offers the full spectrum of managed health care (Ch. 18).

**integrative medicine** bringing together of two or more treatment modalities so they function as a harmonious whole; as seen in alternative forms of health care (Ch. 2).

**International Classification of Diseases, 9th Revision, Clinical Modification (ICD-9-CM)** standard diagnosis codes used to identify a patient's medical problem. Used by most ambulatory care settings in encoding the claim form and recognized by most insurance carriers (Ch. 18, 19).

**Internet** worldwide computer network available via modem that connects universities, government laboratories, companies, and individuals around the world (Ch. 11, 15, 22).

**internship** transition stage between classroom and employment (Ch. 1).

**interview** meeting in which you and the interviewer discuss employment opportunities and strengths you can contribute to the organization (Ch. 25).

**interview techniques** methods of encouraging the best communication between professionals and the patient (Ch. 4).

**introjection** identification with another person or with some object (Ch. 4).

**involuntary dismissal** termination of employment based on poor job performance or violation of office policies (Ch. 23).

**itinerary** detailed written plan of a proposed trip (Ch. 22).

**jargon** words, phrases, or terminology specific to a profession (Ch. 12).

**Jaz® disk** read-write data storage device. It is storable and transferable between computers. Capacity is approximately 1 to 2 gigabytes of data. Data is stored permanently until overwritten. Jaz drive unit is required to read-write data from the disk (Ch. 11).

**job description** outline of tasks, duties, and responsibilities for every position in the office (Ch. 23).

**Joint Commission on Accreditation of Healthcare Organizations (JCAHO)** commission established to improve the quality of care and services provided in organized health care setting through a voluntary accreditation process (Ch. 16).

**key (keyed)** to input data by keystrokes on a computer, word processor, or typewriter (Ch. 15).

**key unit** first indexing unit of the filing segment (Ch. 14).

**kinesics** study of body language (Ch. 4).

**labyrinthitis** inflammation of inner ear or labyrinth (Ch. 9).

**lackluster** dull, lacking in sheen (Ch. 9).

**ledger** record of charges, payments, and adjustments for individual patient or family (Ch. 17).

**letter of reference** letter usually written by an employee's past employer describing the employee's performance, attitude, or qualifications. This letter is presented to a potential employer when applying for a new job (Ch. 23).

**letter of resignation** letter informing the current employer of the employee's decision to resign from a current position (Ch. 23).

**liabilities** debts and financial obligations for which one is responsible (Ch. 21).

**liability** legal responsibility (Ch. 22).

**libel** false and malicious writing about another constituting a defamation of character (Ch. 7).

**libido** sexual drive (Ch. 6).

**license** permission by competent authority (the state) to engage in a profession; permission to act (Ch. 1).

**licensure** granting of licenses to practice a profession (Ch. 1).

**litigation** court action (Ch. 7).

**litigious** prone to engage in lawsuits (Ch. 1).

**living will** document allowing a person to make choices related to treatment in a life-threatening illness (Ch. 6).

**long-range goals** achievements that may take three to five years to accomplish (Ch. 5).

**macro** a series of keystrokes that has been saved under a separate file name to be used and inserted repeatedly into a document or documents (Ch. 11).

**mainframe computer** large computer system capable of processing massive volumes of data (Ch. 11).

**major medical insurance** insurance that covers catastrophic expenses from illness or injury (Ch. 18).

**malpractice**    professional negligence (Ch. 7, 22).

**managed care**    strategies designed to reduce the cost of health care by managing an insured's health care benefits (Ch. 2).

**managed care operation**    any health care setting or delivery system that is designed to reduce the cost of care while still providing access to care (Ch. 2).

**managed care organization (MCO)**    a health insurance organization that adheres to the principles of strong dependence on selective contracting with providers, the use of PCPs, prospective and retrospective utilization management, use of treatment guidelines for high cost chronic disorders, and an emphasis on preventive care, education, and patient compliance with treatment plans (Ch. 18).

**managed competition**    medical care in which physicians and hospitals compete for patients (Ch. 2).

**managerial accounting**    generates information to enable more efficient internal management (Ch. 21).

**mandate**    formal order to obey certain rules and regulations (Ch. 7).

**masking**    attempt to conceal or repress true feelings or the message (Ch. 4).

**matrix**    to establish an appointment matrix, a physician's unavailable time slots are marked with an X. Patients are not scheduled during those times (Ch. 13).

**medical transcription**    process that traditionally consisted of one person dictating and another writing the words in shorthand. Today, physicians typically dictate into a machine or recording device for transcription into a hard copy at a later time (Ch. 16).

**medical transcriptionist certification commission (MTCC)**    credentialing program of the American Association for Medical Transcription (Ch. 16).

**medical transcriptionist (MT)**    one who transcribes dictation into written documents (Ch. 16).F

**Medicare allowable**    the maximum amount Medicare will pay for each procedure or service performed (Ch. 18).

**Medicare assignment**    in exchange for accepting Medicare assignment, those physicians participating receive direct payment from Medicare and the physician agrees to write off any amount in excess of the Medicare Fee Schedule (Ch. 18).

**Medicare Part A**    benefits covering inpatient hospital and skilled nursing facilities, hospice care, and blood transfusion (Ch. 18).

**Medicare Part B**    benefits covering outpatient hospital and health care provider services (Ch. 18).

**medigap policy**    an individual plan covering the patient's Medicare deductible and copay obligations that fulfills the federal government standards for Medicare supplemental insurance (Ch. 18).

**megabyte**    one million bytes of data (Ch. 11).

**memorandum**    interoffice correspondence, usually referred to as a memo (Ch. 15).

**menses**    menstruation (Ch. 22).

**mentor**    person assigned or requested to assist in training, guiding, or coaching another (Ch. 23).

**merge operation**    word processing operation designed to produce form letters (Ch. 11).

**message**    content being communicated (Ch. 4).

**microcomputer**    personal or desktop computer. Also, a handheld or laptop model (Ch. 11).

**minicomputer**    one of the four categories of computers based on size: larger than a microcomputer and smaller than a mainframe (Ch. 11).

**minor**    person who has not reached the age of majority, usually 18 years (Ch. 7).

**minutes**    written record of topics discussed and actions taken during meeting sessions (Ch. 15, 22).

**modes of communication**    speaking, listening, gestures, or body language, and writing. Also called channels of communication (Ch. 4).

**modified block letter, indented**    modified letter style with indented paragraphs. Paragraphs in this style of letter may be indented five spaces (Ch. 15).

**modified block letter, standard**    major letter style where all lines begin at the left margin with the exception of the date line, complimentary closure, and keyed signature. The exceptions usually begin at the center position or a few spaces to the right of center (Ch. 15).

**modified wave**    scheduling system where multiple patients are scheduled at the beginning of each hour, followed by single appointments every 10 to 20 minutes the rest of the hour (Ch. 13).

**modulated**    speech that varies in pitch and intensity (Ch. 12).

**money market account**    bank accounts that pay the highest interest rate (money-market rate) and permit writing a limited number of checks (Ch. 17).

**monthly billing**    method that sends all bills at the same time each month, usually on or around the 25th of the month (Ch. 20).

**motherboard**    printed circuit board upon which the CPU, ROM, and RAM chips and other electronic circuit elements of a digital computer are frequently located (Ch. 11).

**moxibustion**    ancient Chinese method of treatment that uses a powdered plant substance on the skin to raise a blister (Ch. 3).

**National Board of Medical Examiners (NBME)**    consultants for the certification examination (Ch. 24).

**negligence**    failure to exercise a certain standard of care (Ch. 7, 22).

**networking**    process in which people of similar interests exchange information in social, business, or professional relationships (Ch. 23).

**network interface**    software, servers, and cable connections used to link computers (Ch. 11).

**new patient**    patient being seen for the first time in a medical office, on whom the office staff has not obtained a complete current medical history (Ch. 13).

**nonavailability statement**    preauthorization for nonemergency civilian health care issued by the base commander when medical care required for a CHAMPUS eligible is not available at a government medical treatment facility within the patient's catchment area (Ch. 18).

**noncompliant**    failure to follow a required command or instruction (Ch. 7).

**nonconsecutive filing**    numeric filing method where numbers are considered in ascending order using subsets of figures within a number, e.g., in the number 574 19 2863: 2863 is unit 1, 19 is unit 2, 574 is unit 3 (Ch. 14).

**no-show**    patient who fails to keep an appointment without canceling the appointment with the office (Ch. 13).

**not current status** effective January 2003, all CMAs employed or seeking employment must have current certified status to use the CMA credential (Ch. 24).

**notary (notary public)** someone with the legal capacity to witness and certify documents; can take depositions (Ch. 17).

**obfuscation** making things clouded or confused (Ch. 12).

**occlusion** closure of a passage (Ch. 9).

**on-line** actively working on the Internet (Ch. 15).

**open-ended questions** questions that encourage verbalization and response; questions that seek a response beyond a simple yes or no (Ch. 4).

**open hours** scheduling system where patients are assigned a timeframe, e.g., 9:00 A.M. to 11:00 A.M., for arrival. They are then seen on a first-come, first-served basis within that time frame (Ch. 13).

**optical character reader (OCR)** United States Postal Service's computerized scanner that reads addresses printed on letter mail. If the information is properly formatted, then the OCR will find a match in its address files and print a bar code on the lower right edge of the envelope (Ch. 15).

**optical disk** portable and transferable read-write or read-only data storage device. Sometimes called a CD-ROM, CD-RW, or compact disk. Capacity is 1 to 8 gigabytes of data. Optical drive unit is required to read-write data from the disk (Ch. 11).

**orphan** in typesetting, a term describing the situation in which a new paragraph begins on the last line of a printed page or column (Ch. 11).

**outer-directed people** people who let events, other people, or environmental factors dictate their behavior (Ch. 5).

**out guide or sheet** card, folder, or slip of paper inserted temporarily in the files to replace a record that has been retrieved from the files (Ch. 14).

**overtime** money paid at a rate of not less than one and one-half times the regular rate of pay after a forty-hour work week is completed (Ch. 23).

**owner's equity** amount by which business assets exceed business liabilities. Also called net worth, proprietorship, and capital (Ch. 21).

**pagers** also known as beepers. One-way paging systems often used inside hospitals and by physicians on call. Pagers only receive signals (Ch. 12).

**paradigm** internalized example or pattern that may influence your perspective (Ch. 22).

**parasympathetic nervous system** part of the autonomic nervous system that returns the body to its normal state after stress has subsided (Ch. 5).

**partnership** in this text, the collaboration of two or more physicians who share the costs and liabilities of a medical practice (Ch. 2).

**password** a code word or number unique to a specific user. It is used to identify the user to authorize access to a database or specific computer system. The system administrator initially issues the password. Passwords must be changed frequently to prevent them from becoming known by unauthorized persons (Ch. 11).

**patch** modification to software to fix deficiencies in the software. Frequently downloaded from the software supplier's web site or from floppy disks provided by the supplier (Ch. 11).

**payee** person named on check who is to receive the amount indicated (Ch. 17).

**pegboard system** most commonly used manual medical accounts receivable system (Ch. 17).

**perception** conscious awareness of one's own feelings and the feelings of others (Ch. 4).

**personal computer** also known as microcomputer (Ch. 11).

**petty cash** small sum kept on hand for minor or unexpected expenses (Ch. 17).

**petty cash voucher** form used to record individual petty cash transactions (Ch. 17).

**pharmacopeia** book describing drugs and their preparation or a collection or stock of drugs (Ch. 3).

**physician-hospital organization (PHO)** a business entity in which the hospital and selected physicians form a health care network for the purpose of contracting with managed care organizations (Ch. 18).

**physician's directive** another name for a living will (Ch. 6).

**plaintiff** person bringing charges in litigation (Ch. 7).

**pluralistic (pluralism)** society where there are several distinct ethnic, religious, or cultural groups that coexist with one another (Ch. 3).

**point-of-service (POS) device** device allowing direct communication between a medical office and the health care plan's computer (Ch. 19).

**portfolio** notebook or file containing examples of materials commonly used (Ch. 15).

**position** physical stance of two individuals while communicating (Ch. 4).

**posting** recording financial transactions into a bookkeeping or accounting system (Ch. 17).

**posture** relates to the position of the body or parts of the body; the pose taken while communicating (Ch. 4, 12).

**power verbs** action words used to describe your attributes and strengths (Ch. 25).

**practice-based** determined by the type of practice; a system of scheduling unique to the type of medical care provided (Ch. 13).

**practicum** transitional stage providing opportunity to apply theory learned in the classroom to a health care setting through practical, hands-on experience (Ch. 1, 22).

**preauthorization** obtaining an insurance carrier's consent to proceed with patient care and treatment. Unless authorization is obtained, insurance carriers may not pay benefits for specific problems (Ch. 18).

**pre-existing condition** illness, disease, or injury that occurred before the inception of the policy (Ch. 18).

**preferred provider organization (PPO)** organization of physicians who network together to offer discounts to purchasers of heath care insurance (Ch. 2, 18).

**preferred provider** physician who has signed a contract with a particular insurance carrier or HMO to provide care for a reduced rate in exchange for direct payment from the insurer (Ch. 18).

**prejudice** opinion or judgment that is formed before all the facts are known (Ch. 4).

**primary care physician (PCP)** primary care physician for a patient; all care is coordinated through the PCP (Ch. 18).

**privileged** confidential information that may only be communicated with the patient's permission or by court order (Ch. 16).

**probate court** court that administers estates and validates wills (Ch. 20).

**probation** period of time during which the employee and supervisory personnel may determine if both the environment and the position are satisfactory for the employee (Ch. 23).

**problem-oriented medical record (POMR)** a type of patient chart recordkeeping that uses a sheet at a prominent location in the chart to list vital identification data. Patient medical problems are identified by a number that corresponds to the charting; e.g., bronchitis is #1, a broken wrist is #2, and so forth (Ch. 4).

**procedure code** numerical code signifying a specific medical procedure; codes found in CPT code book (Ch. 18, 19).

**procedures manual** manual providing detailed information relative to the performance of tasks within the job description (Ch. 22).

**professional liability insurance** insurance policy designed to protect assets in the event a claim for damages resulting from negligence is filed and awarded (Ch. 22).

**profit sharing** sharing in the financial profits, gains, and benefits of an organization (Ch. 22).

**progress notes** (also called chart notes) physician's formal or informal notes about presenting problem, physical findings, and plan for treatment for a patient examined in the office, clinic, acute care center, or emergency department (Ch. 16).

**projection** act of placing one's own feelings upon another (Ch. 4).

**pronunciation** saying words correctly (Ch. 12).

**proofread** to read a document to verify the accuracy of content and that correct grammar, spelling, punctuation, and capitalization were used (Ch. 15, 16).

**proprietary** privately owned and managed facility, a profit-making organization (Ch. 1).

**prospective payment** method of flat-fee pricing (Ch. 18).

**psychomotor retardation** slowing of physical and mental responses; may be seen in depression (Ch. 6).

**purging** method of maintaining order in the files by separating active from inactive and closed files (Ch. 14).

**quality assurance (QA)** process to provide accurate, complete, consistent healthcare documentation in a timely manner while making every reasonable effort to resolve inconsistencies, inaccuracies, risk management issues, and other problems (Ch. 16).

**random access memory (RAM)** a type of computer memory that can be written to and read from. The word *random* means that any one location can be read at any time. RAM commonly refers to the internal memory of a computer. RAM is usually a fast, temporary memory area where data and programs reside until saved or until the power is turned off (Ch. 11).

**rationalization** act of justification, usually illogically, that one uses to keep from facing the truth of the situation (Ch. 4).

**read-only memory (ROM)** permanently stored computer data that cannot be overwritten without special devices. Stores instructions required to start up the computer. Located on the motherboard (Ch. 11).

**receiver** recipient of the sender's message (Ch. 4).

**recertification** documentation admitted to support continued education for maintaining a professional credential (Ch. 16, 24).

**record** related fields, grouped together and organized in the same order (Ch. 11).

**references** individuals who have known or worked with you long enough to make an honest assessment and recommendation regarding your background history (Ch. 25).

**registered medical assistant (RMA)** credential awarded for successfully passing the AMT examination (Ch. 1, 24).

**regression** moving back to a former stage to escape conflict or fear (Ch. 6).

**release mark** symbol, usually in the form of initials, a code, or a stamp, which indicates that material is ready to be filed (Ch. 14).

**repression** coping with an overwhelming situation by temporarily forgetting it; temporary amnesia (Ch. 4).

**rescue breathing** performed on individuals in respiratory arrest, rescue breathing is a mouth-to-mouth (using appropriate protective equipment) or mouth-to-nose procedure that provides oxygen to the patient until emergency personnel arrive (Ch. 9).

**resource-based relative value scale (RBRVS)** basis for the Medicare fee schedule (Ch. 18).

**resume** written summary data sheet or brief account of qualifications and progress in your chosen career (Ch. 23, 25).

**retrovirus** common name for some viruses that contain reverse transcriptase (Ch. 8).

**revalidation** maintaining current RMA status (Ch. 24).

**review of systems (ROS)** inquires about the system directly related to the problems identified in the history of the present illness (Ch. 16).

**ribonucleic acid (RNA)** nucleic acid in all living cells; sometimes takes the place of DNA in certain viruses (Ch. 8).

**risk management** techniques adhered to in the ambulatory care setting that keep the practice, its environment, and its procedures as safe for the patient as possible. Proper risk management also reduces the possibility of negligence that leads to torts and malpractice suits (Ch. 7, 16, 22).

**ROA** standard abbreviation meaning Received On Account (Ch. 17).

**roadblocks (to communication)** verbal or nonverbal messages that block the communication cycle (Ch. 4).

**salary review** informing the employee of their revised base pay rate (Ch. 23).

**screen** in the medical office, determining who is calling and the reason for the call (Ch. 12).

**search engine** specialized computer program designed to find specific information on the Internet (Ch. 22).

**self-actualization** being all that you can be; developing your full potential and experiencing fulfillment (Ch. 5, 22).

**sender** the individual beginning the communication cycle (Ch. 4).

**septicemia** invasion of pathogenic bacteria into the bloodstream (Ch. 3).

**serum** liquid portion of blood obtained after blood has been allowed to clot (Ch. 9).

**server** computer with massive hard drive capacity that is used to link other computers together so that data can be shared by multiple users. A computer system in an ambulatory care facility are likely to be linked or networked with a central server (Ch. 11).

**shadow** follow a supervisor or delegated subordinate in order to learn facility protocol (Ch. 22).

**shingling** method of arranging charts in which sheets of paper are "shingled" up or across the page, with the most recent report placed on top of the previous one, giving access to the most current information first (Ch. 14).

**shock** condition in which the circulatory system is not providing enough blood to all parts of the body, causing the body's organs to fail to function properly (Ch. 9).

**short-range goals** long-range goals are dissected and reassembled into smaller, more manageable time segments (Ch. 5).

**simplified letter** major letter style recommended by the Administrative Management Society that omits the salutation and complimentary closure. All lines are keyed flush with the left margin. In medical offices, this style is most often employed when sending a form letter (Ch. 15).

**slack time** in the medical office, unscheduled time (Ch. 13).

**slander** false and malicious words about another constituting a defamation of character (Ch. 7).

**slang** nonstandard, often arbitrarily coined words used in casual speech (Ch. 12).

**SOAP** acronym for patient progress notes based on subjective impressions (S), objective clinical evidence (O), assessment or diagnosis (A), and plans for further studies (P) (Ch. 14).

**software** equivalent of a computer program or programs (Ch. 11).

**sole proprietorship** medical practice that is owned by only one individual (Ch. 2).

**sort** frequently used data processing operation that arranges data in a particular sequence or order (Ch. 11).

**source-oriented medical record (SOMR)** a type of patient chart record keeping that includes separate sections for different sources of patient information, such as laboratory reports, pathology reports, and progress notes (Ch. 14).

**spamming** sending the same message to hundreds or thousands of e-mail addresses (Ch. 15).

**splint** any device used to immobilize a body part. Often used by EMS personnel (Ch. 9).

**split keyboard** ergonomic keyboard; slanted to accommodate the natural position of the hands and support the wrists (Ch. 16).

**sprain** injury to a joint, often an ankle, knee, or wrist, that involves a tearing of the ligaments. Most sprains are minor and heal quickly; others are more severe, include swelling, and may not heal properly if the patient continues to put stress on the sprained joint (Ch. 9).

**spreadsheet software** computer applications packages that act as "number crunchers" because of their mathematical processing capabilities (Ch. 11).

**standard precautions** precautions developed in 1996 by the Centers for Disease Control and Prevention (CDC) that augment universal precautions and body substance isolation practices. They provide a wider range of protection and are used any time there is contact with blood, moist body fluid (except perspiration), mucous membranes, or nonintact skin. They are designed to protect all health care providers, patients, and visitors (Ch. 9).

**STAT** abbreviation for the Latin *statim*, meaning immediate (Ch. 16).

**statute** law enacted by a legislative body (Ch. 7).

**statute of limitations** statute that defines the period of time in which legal action can take place (Ch. 20).

**strain** injury to the soft tissue between joints that involves the tearing of muscles or tendons. Strains often occur in the neck, back, or thigh muscles (Ch. 9).

**stream** scheduling system where patients are seen on a continuous basis throughout the day, e.g., at 15-, 30-, or 60-minute intervals, each patient having a distinct appointment time (Ch. 13).

**stress** body's response to change; can be manifested in a variety of ways, including changes in blood pressure, heart rate, and onset of headache (Ch. 5).

**stressors** demands to change that cause stress (Ch. 5).

**sublimation** redirecting a socially unacceptable impulse into one that is socially acceptable (Ch. 4).

**subordinate** in an organization, a person under the direction of (reporting to) a person of greater authority (Ch. 22).

**subpoena** written command designating a person to appear in court under penalty for failure to appear (Ch. 7).

**subrogation** right of an insurer to collect monies it has paid out on behalf of its insured from another party (Ch. 18, 19).

**superbill** billing the patient receives from the physician at the time of service delineating the visit, tests, diagnoses, charges, and when to return. See also **charge slip** (Ch. 17, 19).

**supercomputer** fastest, largest, and most expensive of the four classes of computers currently being manufactured (Ch. 11).

**surrogate** substitute; someone who substitutes for another (Ch. 8).

**sympathetic nervous system** large part of the atuonomic nervous system that prepares the body for fight-or-flight (Ch. 5).

**syncope** fainting (Ch. 9).

**systems software** software that provides instructions to the computer hardware; the operating system is the most common systems software (Ch. 11).

**targeted resume** resume format utilized when focusing on a clear, specific job target (Ch. 25).

**task force for test construction** committee of professionals whose responsibility is to update the CMA examination annually to reflect changes in medical assistants' responsibilities and to include new developments in medical knowledge and technology (Ch. 24).

**teamwork** persons synergistically working together (Ch. 22).

**territoriality** represents the distance at which we feel comfortable while communicating with others (Ch. 4).

**therapeutic communication** use of specific and well-defined professional communication skills to create a feeling of comfort for patients even when difficult or unpleasant information must be exchanged (Ch. 4).

**tickler file** system to remind of action to be taken on a certain date (Ch. 14).

**tort** wrongful act that results in injury to one person by another (Ch. 7).

**touch** physically making contact with others (Ch. 4).

**transcriber** device that makes it possible to transform voice recordings into a transcript or printed documents (Ch. 16).

**traveler's check** often used in place of cash when traveling; available in denominations of $10 to $100; requires a signature at place of purchase as well as signature at the time the check is used (Ch. 17).

**triage** process to determine and prioritize patients' needs and the likely benefit from immediate medical attention. From the French *trier*, meaning "to sort" (Ch. 2, 9, 12, 13).

**Truth-in-Lending Act** also known as the Consumer Credit Protection Act of 1968; an act requiring providers of installment credit to state the charges in writing and to express the interest as an annual rate (Ch. 20).

**typhus (typhoid)** acute infectious disease that causes severe headache, rash, high fever, and progressive neurologic involvement. Prevalent where conditions are unsanitary and congested (Ch. 3).

**Uniform Bill 92 (UB92)** unique billing form used extensively by acute care facilities for processing inpatient and outpatient claims (Ch. 19).

**uniform resource locator (URL)** Web address that identifies and displays a particular Web page (Ch. 15).

**unit** each part of a name (business or person), words, or numbers that will be indexed and coded for filing (Ch. 14).

**universal emergency medical identification symbol** identification sometimes carried by individuals to identify health problems they may have (Ch. 9).

**usual, customary, and reasonable (UCR)** fee schedule often used by Medicare and some insurance carriers. *Usual* refers to the fee typically charged by a physician for certain procedures; *customary* is based on the average charge for a specific procedure by all physicians practicing the same specialty in a defined geographic region; and *reasonable* refers to the midrange of fees charged for this procedure (Ch. 17, 18).

**utilization review organization** responsible for authorization of treatment, payment of claims, and performance of retrospective utilization review for an insurance plan (Ch. 18).

**utilization review (UR)** review of medical services before they can be performed (Ch. 21).

**V codes** ICD-9-CM codes representing either factors that influence a person's health status or legitimate reasons for contacting the health facility when the patient has no definitive diagnosis or active symptom of any disorder (Ch. 19).

**variable cost** cost that varies in direct proportion to volume (Ch. 21).

**voucher check** check with detachable form used to detail reason check is drawn; commonly used in payroll checks (Ch. 17).

**waiting period** length of time defined in the insurance policy before the policy will begin to pay benefits for a pre-existing condition (Ch. 18).

**watermark** design incorporated in paper during the papermaking process that is visible when the paper is held up to the light (Ch. 15).

**wave** scheduling system where patients are scheduled for the first half hour of every hour and then seen throughout the hour (Ch. 13).

**Web site** a remote computer that stores World Wide Web documents consisting of Web pages (Ch. 22).

**widow** in typesetting, a term describing the situation in which a line of text that is the end of a paragraph ends on a new page or column of printed text (Ch. 11).

**word processing software** computer application that allows the user to format and edit documents before printing (Ch. 11).

**work history** outline of previous employment positions, employers, positions, duties, and responsibilities. Listed with the most recent position first (Ch. 23).

**work statement** concise description of the work you plan to accomplish (Ch. 22).

**World Wide Web (WWW)** commonly known as the Web; composed of computers called servers that contain Web pages that may include text, pictures, sound, video, and links to other Web pages (Ch. 15).

**wound** a break in the continuity of soft parts of body structures caused by violence or trauma to tissues. In an open wound, skin is broken as in a laceration, abrasion, avulsion, or incision. In a closed wound, skin is not broken as in contusion, ecchymosis, or hematoma (Ch. 9).

**wrist rest** device used with flat keyboard to support the wrists (Ch. 16).

**write-it-once system** another name used to refer to the pegboard system (Ch. 17).

**yellow fever** acute infectious disease where a person develops jaundice, vomits, hemorrhages, and has a fever; caused mostly by mosquitoes (Ch. 3).

**ZIP+4** standard Zip code including four additional digits that identify a postal delivery area. Mail will be processed more efficiently and effectively with the use of the ZIP+4 code in the address (Ch. 16).

**Zip® disk** portable read-write data storage device. It is storable and transferable between computers. Capacity is approximately 250 megabytes of data. Data is stored permanently until overwritten. Zip drive unit is required to read-write data from disk (Ch. 11).

# INDEX

**Note:** Page references in **bold type** refer to boxes, procedures, figures, and tables.

## A

AAMA *See* American Association of Medical Assistants
AAMT *Model Job Description*, 243, 244
Abbreviations
    correspondence, **229**
Abdominal thrust, 111–112
Abortion
    ethical issues concerning, 89–90
Abrasions, 100
Absorption
    poison, 108
Abuse
    child, 77
    elderly, 77
    ethical issues concerning, 88
    insurance, 306
Accomplishment statements, 391–392
Accounting
    computerized, 323
    double-entry, 323
    function, 323
    pegboard system, 322
    single-entry systems, 322
Accounts
    aging, 313–314
    past-due, 313
    payable, 268, 327
    receivable, 260
    ratio, 327
Accreditation, American Association of Medical Assistants and, 8
Accuracy, resumes and, 392
Accurate medical record, 248
Acidosis, **110**
Acquired immunodeficiency syndrome. *See* AIDS
Acupuncture, **25**, 30
ADA (Americans with Disabilities Act), 77, 78–79
    office design/environment and, 133–134
Adolescents
    ethical issues concerning, **85**

Adults
    CPR (cardiopulmonary resuscitation) for, **123–124**
    ethical issues concerning, **85**
    Heimlich maneuver
        on conscious, **114**
        on unconscious, **114–116**
    rescue breathing for, **120**
Advertising, ethics and, 87
Aging accounts, accounts, 313–314
AIDS, 77
    ethical issues concerning, 90
    patients with, therapeutic response to, 62–63
Alarm, adaptation to stress and, 52
Allied health professionals, **21–22**
Allopathic medicine, 30
Alphabetic filing, 201
Alpha-Z filing system, 199
Alternative health care therapies, role of, 24
AMA (American Medical Association)
    Code of Ethics, fee payments and, 260
    confidentiality guidelines, **148**
    ethical guidelines, 87–89
    patient confidentiality and, **148**
    Policy E5-07, 147
    Principles of Medical Ethics, 84, 85, **86**
Ambulatory health care, settings, 4, 16–18
American Association of Medical Assistants (AAMA)
    accreditation and, 8
    certification and, 8–9
    certification examination, 378
        format/content of, 379–380
        preparing for, 378–379
    Code of Ethics, 84, 85, **86**
        keys to, 86–87
    continuing education verification form, **383**
    creed, **86**
    examination, application process, 380
    founding of, 7–8
    liability insurance and, 349
    Role Delineation Chart, 9, 12, Appendix C

American Association of Medical Transcription
    history of, 243
    membership in, 243
American Diabetes Society, 109
American Medical Association (AMA)
    confidentiality guidelines, **148**
    ethical guidelines, 87
    patient confidentiality and, 147
    policy E5-07, 147
    Principles of Medical Ethics, 84, 85, **86**
American Medical Technologists Institute for Education (AMTIE), 383
Americans with Disabilities Act (ADA), 77, 78–79
    office design/environment and, 133–134
AMTIE (American Medical Technologists Institute for Education), 383
Anesthesia
    insurance coding, 297
Anesthesiologist assistant, **21**
Answering services/machines, 168
Applicants
    interviewing, 360–362
        questions, **361**
Application employment form
    cover letters, 396
    completing, 396, 398
Application software, 141
Appointment
    books, 183
        establishing, 184
    cancellations/changes, 182
        computer, 182–183
        procedure, **186–187**
    cards, 184
    guidelines, 180–183
    matrix, 184
        establishing, **187**
    reminder systems, 183
    scheduling guidelines, 180–183
    sheets, 183–184
Artificial insemination/surrogacy, ethical issues concerning, 90
ARU (Automatic routing units), 168

Asepsis
    reducing infection risk using, 32
Assignment of benefits, 287
Athletic trainer, **21**
Attitude, 5
Attributes, of professionals, 4–7
Automatic routing units (ARU), telephone, 168
Avulsion, 100

**B**

Balance sheet, 324–326
Bandages
    emergencies and, 101
Bank statement, **270**
    reconciling, 269
        procedure for, **277–278**
Banking
    accounts
        checking, 267
        savings, 267
    checks, 267
    deposits, 267–268
Bankruptcy, patient, 317
Banting, Frederick G., 33
Barrier-free accommodations, 78
Battery, 73–74
Behavior, ethical, 7
Beneficiary, defined, 284
Benefits, managing, 348
Best, Charles, 33
Biases, 40
Billing
    cycle, 312–313
    monthly, 312
    procedures, 310–311
Billing efficiency report, 310–311
Bioethics
    defined, 85
    dilemmas concerning, 89
Biofeedback, **25**
Biomedical databases, 208–209
Birthday rule, defined, 285
Blackwell, Elizabeth, 31
Bleeding
    control of, **112–113**
    external, 109
    internal, 110
Block operations, word processing, 142–143
Blood
    disease transmission and, 97
    stroke and, 110
Body fluids
    disease transmission and, 97
Body language, 42–44
Bond, defined, 349
Bones
    fractures of, 106
    injuries to, 107
Bookkeeping
    adjustment, 264
    computer service bureaus, 323
    computerized, 323
    computerized systems, 265–266
    day sheets, 261–262
        balancing, 264–265
    double-entry, 323
    ledger cards, 262–263
    month-end, 265
    patient accounts, 260–261
    pegboard system, 261–262, 322
    recording information, 264
    single-entry systems, 322

Breach of confidentiality, 305
Breathing
    emergencies, 111–112
Budgetary needs analysis, personal, 390
Buffer words, 48
Burnout
    assessing risk of, **55**
    combating, 55
    described, 54
    preventing, 55
    workplace, 54
Burns, 101–102
    caring for, 103
    degrees of, 102
    electrical, 105
    first aid for, 104, **104–105**
    solar radiation and, 105
Business
    letter, components of, 219–221
    record, filing, 196–197

**C**

CAAHEP (Committee on Accreditation of Allied Health Education Programs), 341–342
Captions, file, 194–195
Carbon copy, 220
Cardiopulmonary resuscitation (CPR), 111, 112
    for adults, **123–124**
    for children, **125**
    for infants, **126**
Cardiovascular technologist, **21**
Carpal tunnel syndrome, 246
Cashier's check, 267
Catchment area, 290
CC (Chief complaint), 249
CDC (Centers for Disease Control and Prevention)
    standard precautions and, 97
CE. *See* Continuing education, 246
Cellular telephones, 168–169
Centers for Disease Control and Prevention (CDC)
    standard precautions and, 97
Central processing unit (CPU), 139
Cerebral vascular accident (CVA), 110
Certification
    American Association of Medical Assistants (AAMA), 8–9
        examination, 378–380
    Certified medical assistant (CMA), examination, 380–383
Certified check, 267
Certified medical assistant (CMA), 8
    certification examination, 380–383
Certified medical transcriptionist (CMT), 243
CEUs (Continuing education units), CMA (Certified medical assistant), 382
CHAMPUS, 290
CHAMPVA, 290
Channels, communication, 40–41
Charge slips, 263–264, 311
Charges, ethical issues concerning, 88
Charisma, management and, 337
Chart notes, 249
Charts
    arranging, 205–206
Checking accounts, 267
Checking in, patients, 181
Check-out system, 204–205

Checks
    accepting, 268
    lost/stolen, 268
    payroll, preparing, 347–348
    types of, 267
    writing, rules for, 269
    writing/recording, 268
Cherokee, attitudes toward illness of, 31
Chief complaint (CC), 249
Children
    abuse of, 77
        ethical issues concerning, 85
    CPR (cardiopulmonary resuscitation) for, **125**
    Heimlich maneuver
        on conscious, **116**
        on unconscious, **114–115**
    rescue breathing for, **121**
Choking, Heimlich maneuver and, 111–112
Chronological
    arrangement of medical records, 206
    resume, 393
Civil law, 69
Civil Rights Act of 1964, 368
Claim
    computerized, 305
    defined, 285
    Explanation of Benefits, 305
    following up on, 305
    form, coding, 301
    HCFA-1500 form, 285–287
    insurance carriers role in, 305
    overseeing processing, 304–305
    register, maintaining, 304–305
Clinical databases, 208–209
Clinical laboratory
    scientist, **21**
    technician, **21**
Clinical notes, 205
Closed
    files, 207
    questions, 47
    wounds, 100
Closing, business letter, 219
Clustering
    nonverbal communication and, 44
    scheduling, 177
CMA. *See* Certified medical assistant
COB (Coordination of benefits), defined, 285
Code of Ethics
    American Association of Medical Assistants, 84, 85
    Association of Medical Assistants (AAMA), **86**
    keys to, 86–87
*Code of Medical Ethics*, 87–88
Coding
    claim form, 301
    errors, 306
    procedure, 296–299
    systems, insurance, 296–299
Coinsurance, defined, 284
Cold-related illnesses, 107
Collection
    agency, 310
        use of, 315, 317
    estates and, 317
    letters, 315, **315–316**
    patient bankruptcy and, 317
    process, 313
    ratio, 327
    small claims court and, 317

statute of limitations, 317
techniques, 314–315
tracing "skips," 317
Collection policies, 311
Colles fracture, 106
Color coding
filing systems and, 198
customized, 199–200
Coma, diabetic, **110**
Comminuted fracture, 106
Committee on Accreditation of Allied
Health Education Programs
(CAAHEP), 341–342
Communicate, ability to, 7
Communication
congruency in, 44–45
cultural influence on, 39–40
cycle, 40–41
envelopes, **233–234**
folding letters for, **235–236**
facial expression and, 43
five Cs of, 41–42
importance of, 39
legal/ethical considerations, 230
modes of, 40–41
nonverbal, 42–44
position and, 44
posture and, 43–44
roadblocks to, 45–46
skills, as management quality, 335
technology and, 45
territoriality and, 43
verbal, 41–42
written
business letter components,
219–221
fax preparation/sending, **237–238**
letter styles, 221–224
meeting agendas, 226
meeting minutes, 227
memoranda, 226
preparing outgoing, **237**
preparing/composing, **232–233**
proofreader's marks, 219
proofreading, 218
spelling and, 217–218
supplies for, 224–226
writing tips, 217
Compensation, as defense mechanism,
46
Complaint
chief, 249
Complete medical record, 248
Compliance, healthcare, 306–307
Complimentary closing, business letter,
219
Compound fracture, 106
Computer service bureaus, 323
Computer-Based Patient Records Institute
(CPRI), 147
Computers
bookkeeping systems, 265–266
components of, 139–141
confidentiality and, 210
databases and, 144–146
documentation for, 141
electrical surges and, 141
e-mail, 168
graphics and, 144
information retrieval systems, 146
medical records, 208–210
archival storage, 209
office applications, word processing,
142–144

patient
confidentiality and, 146–147
records using, 266
power outage and, 141
safe use of, 149, 152
scheduling patients using, 181
cancellations, 182–183
software and, 141
office applications, 141–146
spreadsheets and, 144
static discharge protection devices, 141
types of, 139
virus protection for, 146
Confidentiality
breach of, 305
computers and, 210
ethical issues concerning, 87–88
law, 76
telephone calls and, 167
transcriptionist and, 252
*Confidentiality—Computers*, 147
Conflict resolution, 371
Congruency, communication and, 44–45
Consent
implied, 75
informed, 74–75
form, **75**
Consultation reports, 249
transcriptionist and, **250**
Continuation page heading, 220–221
Continuing education
American Association of Medical Assistants and, 9
medical transcriptionist, 246
units (CEUs), 382
verification form, **383**
Continuous Speech Recognition (CSR),
252–253
Contracts, in law, termination of, 71
Coordination of benefits (COB), defined,
285
Copayment, defined, 285
Corporations, described, **17**
Correspondence, 205
business letter, 219–221
envelopes, folding letters for, **235–236**
fax preparation/sending, **237–238**
filing procedures for, 207–208
incoming, 207
legal/ethical considerations, 230
letter styles, 221–224
meeting
agendas, 226
minutes, 227
memoranda, 226
outgoing, 207
preparing
composing, **232–233**
outgoing, **237**
proofreading, 218
spelling and, 217–218
supplies for, 224–226
transcriptionist and, **251**
writing tips, 217
written, envelopes, **233–234**
Cost
accounting, 323
analysis, 324
ratio, 327
Costs
fixed, 324
variable, 324
Cover letters, employment application, 396,
**397**

CPR (cardiopulmonary resuscitation), 111,
112
for adults, **123–124**
for children, **125**
for infants, **126**
CPT (*Current Procedural Terminology*), 296
CPU (Central processing unit), 139
Credit arrangements, 260
policies concerning, 311
Crepitation, defined, 106
Criminal law, 69
Crosswait, C. Bruce, 41
CSR (Continuous Speech Recognition),
252–253
Cultural
heritage in medicine, 30
Culture
defined, 60
life-threatening illness and, 60–61
*Current Options of the Council on Ethical and
Judicial Affairs of the American Medical
Association*, 87–88
*Current Procedural Terminology* (CPT), 296
Customary fee, defined, 259, 289
CVA (Cerebral vascular accident). *See* Cere-
bral vascular accident (CVA), 110
Cycle billing, 312–313
Cytotechnologist, **21**

**D**
DACUM Competencies, 9
Daily worksheets, 184
Data
importing/exporting, 144
input devices, 139–140
locating missing, 205
output devices, 140
storage
devices, 140–141
memory, 140
services, 141
transfer of, 210
Database management systems (DBMS), 144
Databases, computer, 144–146, 208–209
structuring/defining, 144–146
Date line, business letter, 219
Day sheets, 261–262
balancing, 264–265
procedure for, **275–276**
posting, **272–273**
DBMS (Database management systems), 144
Da Vinci, Leonardo, 31
Death and dying
ethical issues concerning, 90
Deductible, defined, 284
Defamation of character, 74
Defendant, in law, 69
Defense mechanisms, 46–47
Dementia
ethical issues concerning, **85**
Denial, as defense mechanism, 46
Dependability, 5
Deposits
bank, 267–268
posting, procedure for, **277**
Depressed fracture, 106
Designation of health care surrogate, 78
Desktop publishing, 144
Diabetes mellitus, 109
Diabetic
coma, causes/symptoms of, **110**
Diagnostic
ultrasound, insurance coding, 297

Diagnostic medical sonographer, **22**
Diagnostic related groups (DRGs), 291
Diagnostics, insurance coding, 299
Diary
    claim, maintaining, 304–305
Digital
    photography, transcriptions and, 253
Direct payment, 287
Disbursement accounts, 269
Disease transmission
    blood, body fluids and, 97
Displacement, as defense mechanism, 46–47
Doctrines, negligence and, 73
Documentation, computer, 141
Domestic violence, 77
Double booking scheduling, 177
Dressings
    emergencies and, 101
DRGs (Diagnostic related groups), 291
Drug abuse
    injections and, 108
Drug formulary, 287
Drug screening, 76–77
Durable power of attorney, 61, 78
Dying and death, ethical issues concerning, 90

**E**

E codes, 300
Editing, transcriptions, 248
Education
    medical, 31
    medical assistant, 9–10
    office personnel and, 370–371, **373**
Egypt, medical treatment in ancient, 32
Elderly
    abuse, 77
    ethical issues concerning, **85**
Elective, procedures, defined, 285
Electrical
    burns, 105
    surges, computers and, 141
Electroneurodiagnostic technologist, **22**
Electronic mail, 168
    correspondence and, 230–231
E-mail, 168
    correspondence and, 230–231
Emancipated minor, 75
Emergency, 95
    arm splint, applying, **113**
    bleeding, 109–110
        control of, **112–113**
    blood, body fluids, disease transmission
        and, 97
    breathing, 111–112
    burns and, 101–102
    cerebral vascular accident (CVA), 110
    choking, infant back blows/chest thrusts
        for, **117–119**
    common, 99–100
        shock, 99–100
    CPR (cardiopulmonary resuscitation)
        for adults, **123–124**
        for children, **125**
        for infants, **126**
    diabetes, 109
    dressings/bandages, 101
    fainting, 109
    Good Samaritan laws and, 97
    heart attack, 110–111
    heat/cold related illnesses, 107
    Heimlich maneuver
        for conscious adult, **114**

    for conscious child, **116**
    for unconscious adult/child, **114–115**
    hemorrhage, 109–110
    insect stings, 108
    musculoskeletal injuries, 105–107
    poisoning, 107–108
    preparation for, medical crash tray/cart,
        98–99
    preparing for, 97–99
    recognizing an, 95
    rescue breathing
        for adults, **120**
        for children, **121**
        for infants, **122–123**
    responding to, 95–96
        primary survey, 96
    seizures, 109
    sudden illness, 108–109
    telephone calls, 163–164
    tourniquets and, 100–101
    using
        emergency medical services system, 97
        telephone no. 911, 97
    wounds, 100–105
Emergency medical technician, **22**
Empathy, 5
Employee
    supervising, 338–340
Employee Eligibility Verification Form, **369**
Employment strategies
    application/cover letters, 396, **397**
    budgetary needs analysis, 390
    contact tracker, 390
    interview process, 399–400
    job analysis/research, 388–390
    look of success, 398
    resume, preparation of, 391–396
    self-assessment, 388
Enclosure notation, business letter, 220
Enunciation, defined, 157
Envelopes, 225–226, **233–234**
    folding letters for, **235–236**
Epilepsy, 109
Epistaxis, 109
Equal Pay Act of 1963, 368
Equipment
    management, 348–349
    purchasing, 269–271
    verifying received, 271
Ergonomics
    medical transcriptionist and, 246–247
Eskimos, attitudes toward illness by, 31
Estates, collecting fees from, 317
Ethics
    abortion, 89–90
    abuse, 88–89
    advertising, 87
    AIDS, 90
    American Medical Association (AMA),
        code of ethics, 87–89
    artificial insemination/surrogacy, 90
    Association of Medical Assistants
        (AAMA), code of ethics, 86–87
    behavior and, 7
    bioethics
        defined, 85
        dilemmas, 89
    confidentiality, 87–88
    defined, 84
    dying and death, 90
    fetal tissue research, 89–90
    genetic engineering/manipulation, 90
    HIV (Human immunodeficiency virus), 90
    issues concerning, **85**

    media relations, 87
    medical
        records, 88
        resources allocation, 89
    professional
        fees/charges, 88
        rights/responsibilities, 88
    telephone calls and, 167
Evaluation, insurance coding, 297
Examination. *See* Physical examination
Exclusions, defined, 285
Exhaustion, adaptation to stress and, 53
Expenses, 327
Expert witness, defined, 72
Expressed contract, 69
External
    bleeding, 109–110
    referrals, telephone calls, 162–163, **163**
Externship, preparation for, 10

**F**

Facial expression, communication and, 43
Facilities management, 348–349
Facility environment
    Americans with Disabilities Act and,
        133–134
    closing, 135
    opening, 134–135
    reception area, 132
    receptionist's role and, 134
Facsimile (fax) machines, 168
    correspondence and, 229–230
    transcriptionist and, 247
Fainting, 109
Fair Debt Collection Practice Act, 314
Fairmindedness, as management quality,
    335
Fax machines, 168
    correspondence and, 229–230
    transcriptionist and, 247
Federal Drug Abuse Prevention, Treatment,
    and Rehabilitation Act, 76–77
Federal Wage Garnishment Law, 317
Feedback, 41
Fees
    adjustment of, 259–260
    bookkeeping and, patient accounts,
        260–261
    credit arrangements for, 260
    discussion of, 259
    ethical issues concerning, 88
    patient, determining, 258–260
    payment planning, 260
    usual, customary, and reasonable, 259
Fetal tissue research, ethical issues con-
    cerning, 89–90
Fight-or-flight, adaptation to stress and, 53
File
    folders, 194
        out guides, 195
    guides, 194
    units, movable, 193–194
Files
    closed, 207
    inactive, 207
    locating missing, 205
    retention/purging, 206–207
    *see also* Medical records
Filing
    alphabetic, 201
    alpha-Z system, 199
    business/organizational records, 196–197
    chart data, 205

color coding, 198
    customized, 199–200
correspondence, 207–208
identical names, 196
indexing units, 195
numeric, 201
patient charts, 195–196
rules of, 195–197
subject, 201–202
systems, choosing, 202–208
tab-alpha system, 198
techniques, 198–203
Financial
    accounting, 323
    management, 345–348
    ratios, using, 326–327
    records, 324–326
Financial practices
    banking procedures, 268
        account types, 266–267
        checks, 267–269
        deposits, 267–268
        purchasing supplies/equipment,
            269–271
    bookkeeping
        adjustments, 264
        balancing day sheets, 264–265
        charge slips, 263–264
        computerized systems, 265–266
        day sheets, 261–262
        ledger cards, 262–263
        month-end, 265
        patient accounts, 260–261
        pegboard system, 261–262
        receipts, 263
    credit arrangements, 260
    expenses, 327
    patient fees, determining, 258–260
    ratios, 326–327
Firewalls, patient confidentiality and, 146
First aid, purpose of, 95
First-degree burns, 102–103
    response guide for, **104**
Fiscal intermediary, HCFA (Health Care
        Financing Administration) and, 289
Fixed costs, 324
Flexibility, 5
Floppy disks, 140
Follow-up
    by telephone, 401
    letter, 400–401
Formulary, drug, 287
Fractures, 106
Fraud
    defined, 305
    examples of, 305–306
Freelance MTs, 245
Fringe benefits, defined, 348
Frostbite, 107
Full block letter, 221–222
Functional resume, 394

**G**

GAS (Hans Selye's General Adaptation
        Syndrome), 52, **53**
Genetic engineering/manipulation
    ethical issues concerning, 90
Gestures, communication and, 44
Goals
    defined, 56
    long-range/short-range, 56–57
    relieving stress through setting, 55–57
"Going bare," defined, 349

Good Samaritan law, 77
    emergencies and, 97
Goods, verifying received, 271
Graphics, computer, 144
Greeks, attitudes toward illness by, 31
Greenstick fracture, 106
Group medical practices, 16–17
Guides, file, 194

**H**

Hans Selye's General Adaptation Syndrome
        (GAS), 52, **53**
Hard disks, 140
Hardware, computer, 139
HCFA (Health Care Financing Administra-
        tion), 285, 289, 323
HCFA (Health Care Financing Administra-
        tion) Common Procedure Coding
        System (HCPCS), 298
HCFA-1500, 285
    completing, 301–304
HCPCS (Common Procedure Coding Sys-
        tem, 298
Health Care Financing Administration
        (HCFA), 285, 289, 323
Health care professionals
    allied, **21–22**
    role of, 19
Health care providers, regulation of,
        11–12
Health care specialties, **21**
Health care surrogate, 78
    form, **79**
Health care team, 18–25
Health care therapies, role of integrative or
        alternative, 24
Health information administrator, **22**
Health information technician, **22**
Health maintenance organizations (HMOs),
        17–18
Health unit coordinator (HUC), 23
Healthcare compliance, 306–307
Heart
    attacks, 110–111
Heat
    cramps, 107
    exhaustion, 107
    stroke, 107
Heat-related illnesses, 107
Heimlich maneuver, 111–112
    on conscious
        adult, **114**
        child, **114–116**
Hierarchy of needs, 45
Hippocrates, 33
Hippocratic Oath, 33, **34**
History and physical examination (H&P
        report), 249
History of present illness (HPI), 249
HIV (Human immunodeficiency virus), 62
    ethical issues concerning, 90
    informed consent and, 77
HMOs (Health care organizations), 17–18
Holism, **25**
Home-based MTs, 244
Homeopathy, **25**
HPI (History of present illness), 249
HUC (Health unit coordinator), 23
Human immunodeficiency virus (HIV),
        62, 77
Human resources manager
    conflict resolution and, 371
    discrimination and, 370

office personnel
    chemically dependent/emotionally ill,
        370
    dismissing, 366–368
    interviewing applicants, 360–362, **373**
    orienting/training new, 363
    performance evaluation of, 363–366
    providing training/education to,
        370–371, **373**
    recruiting, 359
    salary review, 366
    selecting, 362–363
    temporary, 368, 370
personnel laws, complying with, 368
personnel records and, 368
smoking policy, 370
tasks of, 358–359
*see also* Managers
Hypnotherapy, **25**
Hypothermia, 107

**I**

ICD-9-CM, 291, 296
Idea-oriented personality, as management
        style, 336
Identification labels, 194
Illness
    attitudes toward, 31–32
    life-threatening, 60–61
    sudden, 108–109
Immigration Reform Act, 368
Impacted fracture, 106
Implied
    consent, 75
    contract, 69
Inactive files, 207
Incisions, 100
Income statement, 324, **325–326**
Incompetence, 75
Incomplete
    fracture, 106
Independent physician association (IPA), 18
Index, insurance coding, 298
Indirect statements, 47
Individual medical practices, 16
Infants
    conscious/choking, back blows/chest
        thrusts for, **117**
    CPR (cardiopulmonary resuscitation) for,
        **126**
    ethical issues concerning, **85**
    rescue breathing for, **122–123**
    unconscious, back blows/chest thrusts for,
        **118–119**
Information retrieval systems, 146
Informational brochure, **185**, 186
Informed consent, 74–75
    form, **75**
    HIV (Human immunodeficiency virus)
        and, 77
Ingestion, poison, 107
Inhalation
    poison, 107–108
Initiative, 5
Injections
    drug abuse, 108
Injury, preventing computer, **149–150**
Inner-directed people, stress and, 55
Input devices, data, 139–140
Insect stings, 108
Inside address, business letter, 219
Insulin
    shock, **110**

Insurance
  abuse, 306
  carriers, correspondence with, 314
  coding
    accuracy of, 300
    claim form, 301
    systems, 296–299
  coverage, types of, 287–291
  diagnostic related groups (DRGs), 291
  evolution of medical, 283–284
  healthcare compliance, 306–307
  legal/ethical considerations, 291, 305–306
  liability, 349
  Medicaid, 290
  Medicare, 289–290
  payment systems, 291
  screening for, 283–284
  self, 291
  terminology
    insurance carriers, 285–287
    to policies, 284–285
  traditional vs. managed care policies, **288**
  Workers' Compensation, 290–291
Integrated delivery systems, 288
Integrative health care therapies, role of, 24
Internal
  bleeding, 110
  referrals, telephone calls, 162, **163**
Internal Revenue Service (IRS), scheduling
    books and, 179
*International Classification of Diseases, 9th
    Revision, Clinical Modification*, 291,
    296
International mail, 229
Interpersonal skills, scheduling and, 180
Interview
  employment, 399–400
    follow-up, 400–401
  techniques, 47
Introjection, as defense mechanism, 46
Invasion of privacy, 74
Inventories, managing, 348
Invoice, preparing for payment, 271
IPA (Independent physician association), 18
IRS (Internal Revenue Service), scheduling
    books and, 179
Itinerary, travel, 340–341

**J**

Jaz® drive, 141
Jenner, Edward, 32
Job
  analysis/research, 388–390
  descriptions, 359–360
Joints, injuries to, 107
*Journal of Continuing Education Topics &
    Issues*, 383

**K**

Keyboards, 247
Keyed signature, business letter, 220
Kinesics, 42
Koch, Robert, 32–33

**L**

Laboratory
  reports, insurance coding, 205, 298
Lacerations, 100
Lateral files, open-shelf, 193
Law
  abuse and, 77

Americans with Disabilities Act, 77,
    78–79
  battery, 73–74
  confidentiality, 76
  contracts in, 69, 71
  criminal/civil, 69
  defamation of character, 74
  emancipated minor, 75
  Good Samaritan law, 77
  incompetence, 75
  medical records and, 74–76
  minor, 75
  patient rights, 69, **70**
  public duties and, 76–77
  standard of care and, 72
  statute of limitations, 76
  subpoenas, 75
  torts, 72–73
Leaders
  described, **337**
  managers versus, **337**
Learning, desire for, 6
Ledger cards, 262–263
Ledger, computerized patient, 266
Leonardo da Vinci, 31
Letterhead, correspondence, 224–225
Libel, 74
License, described, 11
Licensed practical nurse (LPN), 23
Licensure, comparison of requirements, **11**
Life-threatening illness, 60–61
  choices in, 61–62
  cultural perspective on, 60–61
  medical assistant and, 63
Listening skills, 41
Lister, Joseph, 32
Living will, 61, 78
  form, **78**
Long-range goals, 56–57
LPN (Licensed practical nurse), 23
LPT (Phlebotomist), 24

**M**

Macros, word processing, 143
Mail, processing, 228–229
Mainframe computers, 139
Malpractice, defined, 72, 349
Managed care, operations, 17–18
Managed care organizations (MCOs),
    287–289
  computers and, 323
  impact of operations of, 18
Management
  insurance coding, 297
  medical practice, **17**
Managerial accounting, 323
Managers
  benefits management and, 348
  described, **337**
  facility/equipment management, 348–349
  figuring taxes, 348
  leaders versus, **337**
  liability coverage/bonding, 349
  marketing functions, 343–344
  medical assistant. *See* Medical assistant
  payroll processing and, 347
  procedures manual and, 342–343
  qualities of, 335–336
  records/financial management, 345–348
  risk management and, 349
  student practicums and, 341–342
  styles of, 336–337
  supervising people, 338–340

  time management and, 342
  travel arrangements and, 340–341
  *see also* Human resources manager
Mannerisms, communication and, 44
Marketing
  brochures, 344
    office, 344–345
  defined, 343
  managers and, 343–345
  newsletters, 345
  press releases and, 345
  seminars, 343–344
  special events and, 345
  tools, **344**
Masking, defined, 44
Maslow, Abraham, 45
Maslow's hierarchy of needs, 45
Matrix
  appointment, 184
    establishing, **187**
MCOs (Managed care organizations),
    287–289
  impact of operations of, 18
Media
  ethical issues concerning, 87
Medicaid, 290
Medical assistant, **22**, 358–359
  career opportunities for, 11
  education of, 9–10
  life-threatening illness and, 63
  Role Delineation Chart, 9, 11,
    Appendix C
  role of, 18–19
  value of, 25
  *see also* Human resources manager;
    Managers
Medical assisting
  definition of, 8
  historical perspective of, 7–8
Medical crash tray/cart, 98–99
Medical education, 31
Medical illustrator, **22**
Medical insurance. *See* Insurance, **278**
Medical laboratory. *See* Laboratory
Medical laboratory technologist (MLT), 23
*The Medical Manager*, 184
Medical office, computerizing the, 147, 149
Medical practice, management, **17**
Medical records, 74–76
  computer
    archival storage, 209
    computers and, 208–210
  equipment/supplies, 193–195
  ethical issues concerning, 88
  filing
    documentation in, 198
    techniques/systems, 198–208
  importance of, 193
  retention/purging, 206–207
  *see also* Files
Medical reports, 248–249
Medical resources, allocation of, 89
Medical specialists, 30–31
Medical transcriptionist
  attributes of, 243–244
  certification of, 245–246
  employment opportunities, 244–245
  history of, 243
  job description, 244
  recertification, 246
Medical Transcriptionist Certification
    Commission (MTCC), **243**
Medical treatments, 32–33
Medicare, 289–290

Medicine
  cultural heritage in, 30
  insurance coding, 298
  new frontiers in, 34
  significant contributions to, 33
Medigap policies, 289
Meeting
  agendas, 226, **339**
    preparing, **350**
  minutes, 227
Meetings, staff, 339–340
Memoranda, 226
Merge operations, word processing, 143
Message, in communications, 40–41
Michelangelo, 31
Microcomputers, 139
Minicomputers, 139
Minor, defined, 75
MLT (Medical laboratory technologist), 23
Modified block letter, 222, **223**
Modified wave scheduling, 177
Modifiers, insurance coding, 298
Monthly billing, 312
Movable file units, 193–194
Moxibustion, 30
MTCC (Medical Transcriptionist Certification Commission), 243
Multicolumn output, word processing, 144
Muscles
  injuries to, 107
Musculoskeletal injuries, 105–107

**N**
Names, filing identical, 196
National Board of Medical Examiners (NBME), 380
Native Americans
  attitudes toward illness by, 31
Naturopathy, **25**
Navaho, attitudes toward illness by, 31
NBME (National Board of Medical Examiners), 380
Neat medical record, 248
Negligence, defined, 72, 349
Newsletters, marketing and, 345
Nonavailability statement, 290
Nonverbal communication, 42–44
Nosebleed, 109
NP (Nurse practitioner), 23
Nuclear medicine
  insurance coding, 297
Nuclear medicine technologist, **22**
Numeric filing, 201
  procedures, **210**
Nurse practitioner (NP), 23
Nurses, 23

**O**
Objectivity, as management quality, 336
Occlusion, stroke and, 110
Occupational Safety and Health Act, 368
Occupational therapist, **22**
Occupational therapy assistant, **22**
Office applications, software for, 141–146
Office brochures, 344–345
Office design/environment, 133
Office of Inspector General (OIG), 306
Office personnel
  chemical dependencies/emotional problems and, 370
  interviewing applicants, 360–362, **373**

orienting/training new, 363
performance evaluation of, 363–366
personnel records and, 368
providing training/education to, **373**
selecting applicants, 362–363
smoking policy and, 370
temporary, 368, 370
Office policy manual, 359
  preparing, **372**
Office surgery
  salary review, 366
OIG (Office of Inspector General), 306
Omnibus Budget Reconciliation Acts of 1986, 306
Open hours scheduling, 177
Open wounds, 100
Open-ended questions, 47
Open-shelf lateral files, 193
Ophthalmic medical technician/technologist, **22**
Optical disks, 141
Organization skills, as management quality, 336
Organizational records, filing, 196–197
Orthotist, **22**
Out guides, 195
Outer-directed people, stress and, 55
Output devices, data, 140
Overtime, defined, 368

**P**
Page
  formatting, word processing, 143
  heading, continuation, 220–221
Paging systems, 169
Pain
  cultural perspective on, 61
Paramedic, **22**
*Parliamentary Procedure*, 339
Partnerships, described, **17**
Passwords, patient confidentiality and, 146–147
Past-due accounts, 313
Pasteur, Louis, 32
Pathology, insurance coding, 298
Patient
  fees. *See* Fees
  scheduling. *See* Scheduling
Patient accounts, computerized systems, 265–266
Patient confidentiality, computers and, 146–147
Patient Self-Determination Act, 61–62
Patients
  AIDS, therapeutic response to, 62–63
  analysis of flow of, 178–179
  charts, filing, 195–196
  check-in, 181
    procedure, **186**
  discharged by physician, 71
  education brochures, 344
  no longer needs treatment, 72
  physician withdraws from, 71
  recording information about, 180–181
  waiting time, 179
Patient's Bill of Rights, 69, **70**
Patients rights, 69, **70**
Payee, 268
Payments
  at time of service, 311
  received
    requiring a receipt, **274**
    through the mail, **275**

Payroll, 327
  processing, 347–348
PC (Personal computer), 139
Pegboard bookkeeping system, 261–262
People skills, managers, 335
People-oriented personality, as management style, 336
Perception, communication and, 45
Performance review, office personnel, 363–366
Personal computer (PC), 139
Personalities, management style and, 336–337
Personnel records, maintaining, 368
Peter, Laurence, 55
*The Peter Principle*, 55
Petty cash, 272
  balancing, procedure for, **278**
Pharmacist (RPh), 23–24
Phlebotomist (LPT), 24
PHO (Physician-hospital organization), 287
Photocopy machines, transcriptionist and, 247
Photography, digital, transcriptions and, 283
Physical attributes, of professionals, 6
Physical examination
  reports, 249
Physical therapist (PT), 24
Physical therapy assistant (PTA), 24
Physician assistant, **22**
Physician, telephone calls referred to, 162
Physician-assisted suicide, ethical issues concerning, **85**
Physician-hospital organization (PHO), 287
Physician's directives, 61, 78
  form, **78**
Plaintiff, in law, 69
POE (Proof of eligibility), 283
Point-of-service (POS) device, 304
Poisoning, 107–108
Policy manual, preparing, **372**
POMR (Problem-oriented medical record), 205–206
POS (Point-of-service) device, 304
Position, communication and, 44
Postal classes, 228–229
Posting day sheets, **272–273**
Posture
  communication and, 43–44
  telephone personality and, 157–158
Power outages, computers and, 141
Power verbs, **391–392**
PPO (Preferred provider organization), 18, 287
Practice, scope of, 11–12
Practice-based scheduling, 178
Preauthorization, defined, 285
Pre-existing condition, defined, 285
Preferred provider organization (PPO), 18, 287
Pregnancy tests
  urine and, 32
Prejudices, 40
Press releases, 345
Principles of Medical Ethics, American Medical Association (AMA), 84, 85, **86**
Problem-oriented medical record (POMR), 205–206
Problems, using teams to solve, 338
Problem-solving skills
  as management quality, 336

Procedures
  billing, 310–311
  coding, 296–299
  day sheets, balancing, **275–276**
  deposits, posting, **277**
  interviewing job applicants, **373**
  job description, preparing, **372**
  meeting agendas, preparing, **350**
  numeric filing system, **210**
  patient check in, **186**
  petty cash, balancing, **278**
  policy manual, developing/maintaining, **372**
  posting day sheets, **272–273**
  procedures manual, developing/maintaining, **352–353**
  receiving payments
    requiring a receipt, **274**
    through the mail, **275**
  recording, charges/payments on charge slips, **273–274**
  student practicums, supervising, **351–352**
  subject filing system, **211**
  telephone calls
    incoming, **169–170**
    placing outside, **172**
    problem calls, **171**
  travel arrangements, making, **350–351**
Procedures manual, 342–343
  developing/maintaining, **352–353**
*Professional Development*, 41
Professional fees, ethical issues concerning, 88
Professional liability insurance, 349
*The Professional Medical Assistant* (PMA), 383, 389
Professional rights/responsibilities, ethical issues concerning, 88
Professionals, attributes of, 4–7
Progress notes, 249
Projection, as defense mechanism, 46
Pronunciation, defined, 157
Proof of eligibility (POE), 283
Proofreader's marks, 219
Proofreading, 218
  transcriptions, 247–248
Prospective payment, 291
Prosthetist, **22**
Psychological suffering, range of, 62
PT (Physical therapist), 24
PTA (Physical therapy assistant), 24
Public duties, 76–77
Punctures, 100
Purchase orders, **271**
  preparing, 270–271
Purging records, 206–207

Q
Quickbooks™, 268

R
Radiation therapist, **22**
Radiographer, **22**
Radiology, insurance coding, 297
RAM (Random access memory), 140
Random access memory (RAM), 140
Rationalization, as defense mechanism, 46–47
RBRVS (Resource-based relative value scale), 289
RD (Registered dietitian), 23
Read-only memory (ROM), 140
Reasonable fee, defined, 259, 289

Receipts, 264
Receiver, in communications, 41
Reception area, 132
  office design/environment, 133
Receptionists, role of, 134
Recertification
  CMA (Certified medical assistant), 382
  medical transcriptionist, 246
Reconciling
  bank statements, 269
    procedure for, **277–278**
Records management, 345–348
Records retention, 206–207
Records. *See* Medical records
References, for resumes, 392
Referral appointments, 180
Registered dietitian (RD), 23
Registered medical assistant (RMA), 9
  examination, format/content of, 379–380
Registered nurse (RN), 23
Registration, comparison of requirements, **11**
Regression, as defense mechanism, 46
Release marks, 204
Repression, as defense mechanism, 46
*Res ipsa loquitur*, 73
Rescue breathing, 112
  for adults, **120**
  for children, **121**
  for infants, **122–123**
Resource-based relative value scale (RBRVS), 289
Respiratory therapist, **22**
Respiratory therapy technician, **22**
*Respondeat superior*, 73
Resume
  power verbs, **391–392**
  preparation of, 391–396
  vital information on, 396
Return-to-normal, adaptation to stress and, 53
Review of systems (ROS), 249
Risk management, 73, 349
  transcriptionist and, 252
RMA (Registered medical assistant), 9
RN (Registered nurse), 23
*Robert's Rules of Order*, 339
Role
  ambiguity, burnout and, 54
  conflict, burnout and, 54
  overload, burnout and, 54
Role Delineation Chart, 9, 11, Appendix C
ROM (Read-only memory), 140
Romans, attitudes toward illness by, 31
ROS (Review of systems), 249
RPh (Pharmacist), 23–24

S
Salutation, business letter, 219
Savings accounts, 267
Scheduling
  appointment
    cancellations/changes, 182
    guidelines, 180–183
  cancellations/changes, procedure, **186–187**
  computers use for, 181
  flexibility, 179
  interpersonal skills and, 180
  legal issues concerning, 179
  materials, 183–184
  patient flow analysis, 178–179
  reminder systems, 183
  representatives, 183

  types of, 177–178
  waiting time, 179
Scope of practice, 11–12
Second-degree burns, 102–103
  response guide for, **104**
Second sheets, correspondence, 225
Seizures, 109
Self-assessment, 388
  worksheet, **389**
Self-insurance, 291
Seminars, marketing, 343–344
Semmeweis, Phillipp, 32
Sender, communication, 40
Senior adults. *See* Elderly, **85**
Shingling, 206
Shipments, processing, 228–229
Shock, 99–100
  insulin, **110**
  signs/symptoms of, 99
  treatment of, 100
  types of, 99
Short-range goals, 56–57
Signature, business letter, 220
Simple
  fracture, 106
Simplified letter, 222, 224
"Skips," tracing, 317
Slack time, defined, 178
Slander, 74
Small claims court, collections and, 317
Smoking policy, 370
Social Security Act, Title 18, 289
softFLEX Computer Gloves™, 246
Software
  computer, 141
  fundamental operations of, **143**
  office applications, 141–146
Solar radiation, burns from, 105
Sole proprietorships, described, **17**
SOMR (Source-oriented medical record), 206
Sorting, word processing, 143
Source-oriented medical record (SOMR), 206
Spell check, word processing, 143
Spelling, correspondence and, 217–218
Spiral fracture, 106
Split keyboards, 247
Sprains, 105
Spreadsheets, 144
St. Benedict of Nursia, 31
Staff meetings, 339–340
Staff members, supporting, 340
Standard of care, negligence and, 72
*Standards and Guidelines for an Accredited Education Program for the Medical Assistant*, 8, 10
State Industrial Insurance, 290–291, **292**
Statements
  components of, 311–312
  computerized, 312
Static discharge protection, computers, 141
Statute of limitations, 76, 317
Storage
  devices, data, 140–141
Strains, 105–106
Stream scheduling, 177–178
Stress
  adaptation to, 52–53
  coping with, 53–54
  described, 52
  goal setting to relieve, 55–57
Stroke, 110

Student practicums
  managers and, 341–342
  supervising, **351–352**
Subject filing, 201–202
  procedures, **211**
Subject line, business letter, 219
Sublimation, as defense mechanism, 46
*Subpoena duces tecum*, 75
Subpoenas, 75
Sudden illness, 108–109
Suicide, physician assisted, ethical issues
    concerning, **85**
Sunburn, 105
Superbills, 263–264, 311
Supercomputers, 139
Supplementary health factors, V codes, 300
Supplies
  purchasing, 269–271
  verifying received, 271
Surgeon's assistant, **22**
Surgical
  specialties, 19–20
Surgical technologist, **22**

**T**

Tab-alpha filing system, 198
Targeted resume, 395
Task Force for Test Construction, 380
Taxes, figuring, 348
Teamwork, importance of, 337–338
Technical expertise, as management quality,
  336
Technology, communication and, 45
Telephone
  answering services/machines, 168
  automatic routing units (ARU), 168
  cellular, 168–169
  collections, 314–315
  courtesies, **159**
  directories, using, 166
  documentation, 166
  etiquette, 158
  legal/ethical considerations, 167
  paging systems, 169
  personality, 157–158
  reference check, **362**
  techniques, 47
  technology, 167–169
Telephone calls
  angry callers, 164
  elderly callers, 164
  emergency, 163–164
  ending, 161
  English as a second language caller, 164
  incoming, 159–161

  long distance, 165–166
  long-distance carriers, 166
  placing outside, 165
  procedure for handling
    incoming calls, **169–170**
    placing outside calls, **172**
    problem calls, **171**
  referred to physician, 162
  screening, 159–160
  special consideration, 162–164
  taking message from, 160
  transferring, 160
  types of, 161–162
Temporary employees, 368, 370
Terminal illness. *See* Life-threatening
    illness, 32
Territoriality, 43
Therapeutic
  communication, cultural influence on,
    39–40
  touch, **25**
Therapies, health care, role of, 24
Things-oriented personality, as management
    style, 336
Third degree burns, 103
  response guide for, **105**
Tickler files, 204
Time management, 342
Time zones, long distance telephone calls
    and, 165–166
Title VII of the Civil Rights Act, 368
Torts, 72–73
Touch, communication and, **44**
Tourniquets
  use of, 100–101
Traditional insurance, 287
Training
  office personnel and, 370–371, **373**
Transcription
  Continuous Speech Recognition (CSR),
    252–253
  defined, 242
  digital photographs and, 253
  equipment/supplies, 246
  ergonomics and, 246–247
  fax machines and, 247
  guidelines, 247
  legal/ethical considerations, 252
  proofreading/correcting, 247–248
  turnaround time, 249, **252**
Travel
  making arrangements for, 340–341, **350**
  via the Internet, **351**
Traveler's checks, 267
Treatments, medical, 32–33
Triage calls, 180

Triage, described, 95
Truthfulness, as management quality, 335
Truth-in-Lending Act, 311

**U**

UB92 (Uniform Bill), 303
Uniform Bill 92 (UB92), 303
Uniform Resource Locators (URLs), 231
Urgent care centers, 17
Urine
  pregnancy testing and, 32
URLs (Uniform Resource Locators), 231
Usual, customary, and reasonable fees, 259,
  289
Usual fee, defined, 259, 289
Utilization review organizations, 289

**V**

V codes, 300
Variable costs, 324
Verbal communication, 41–42
Vertical files, 193
Viruses
  protecting computers from, 146
Voluntary compliance program, 306–307
Voucher check, 267

**W**

W-2 form, **347**
W-4 form, **346**
Waiting time, patients, 179
Watermark, defined, 224
Wave scheduling, 177
Web address, 231
Wilkes, Mary, 41
Williams, Maxine, first AAMA
    president, 7
Word processing, 142–144
Words
  frequently misspelled, **217**
  frequently misused, **218**
Work habits, importance of good, 261
Workers' Compensation, 290–291, **292**
Wounds, 100–105
  closed, 100
  open, 100
Wrist rests, 247
Write-it-once bookkeeping system,
  261–262

**Z**

Zip® drive, 141

## Set-Up Instructions

1. Insert disk into CD-ROM player. The CD should start automatically. If it does not, go to step 2.
2. From *My Computer,* double click the **MedAssisting** folder.
3. Double click the **medAssist.exe** file to start the program.

## System Requirements

166 MHz Intel Pentium processor or greater

Microsoft® Windows® 95, 98, NT4, 2000

32 MB of installed RAM

100 MB of available disk space

256-color monitor capable of 800 × 600 resolution

CD-ROM drive

Microsoft® Windows® compatible sound card

## License Agreement for Delmar Thomson Learning Educational Software/Data

You, the customer, and Delmar Thomson Learning incur certain benefits, rights, and obligations to each other when you open this package and use the software/data it contains. BE SURE YOU READ THE LICENSE AGREEMENT CAREFULLY, SINCE BY USING THE SOFTWARE/DATA YOU INDICATE YOU HAVE READ, UNDERSTOOD, AND ACCEPTED THE TERMS OF THIS AGREEMENT.

Your rights:

1. You enjoy a non-exclusive license to use the software/data on a single microcomputer in consideration for payment of the required license fee (which may be included in the purchase price of an accompanying print component), or receipt of this software/data, and your acceptance of the terms and conditions of this agreement.

2. You acknowledge that you do not own the aforesaid software/data. You also acknowledge that the software/data is furnished "as is" and contains copyrighted and/or proprietary and confidential information of Delmar Thomson Learning or its licensors.

There are limitations on your rights:

1. You may not copy or print the software/data for any reason whatsoever, except to install it on a hard drive on a single microcomputer and to make one archival copy, unless copying or printing is expressly permitted in writing or statements recorded on the disk(s).

2. You may not revise, translate, convert, disassemble or otherwise reverse engineer the software/data except that you may add to or rearrange any data recorded on the media as part of the normal use of the software/data.

3. You may not sell, license, lease, rent, loan, or otherwise distribute or network the software/data except that you may give the software/data to a student or and instructor for use at school or temporarily at home.

Should you fail to abide by the Copyright Law of the United States as it applies to this software/data, your license to use it will become invalid. You agree to erase or otherwise destroy the software/data immediately after receiving note of Delmar Thomson Learning termination of this agreement for violation of its provisions.

Delmar Thomson Learning gives you a LIMITED WARRANTY covering the enclosed software/data. The LIMITED WARRANTY follows this License.

This license is the entire agreement between you and Delmar Thomson Learning interpreted and enforced under New York law.

This warranty does not extend to the software or information recorded on the media. The software and information are provided "AS IS."

Any statements made about the utility of the software or information are not to be considered as express or implied warranties. Delmar Thomson Learning will not be liable for incidental or consequential damages of any kind incurred by you, the consumer, or any other user.

Some states do not allow the exclusion or limitation of incidental or consequential damages, or limitations on the duration of implied warranties, so the above limitation or exclusion may not apply to you. This warranty gives you specific legal rights, and you may also have other rights which vary from state to state. Address all correspondence to Delmar Thomson Learning, Box 15015, Albany, NY 12212 Attention: Technology Department.

**LIMITED WARRANTY**

Delmar Thomson Learning warrants to the original licensee/purchaser of this copy of microcomputer software/data and the media on which it is recorded that the media will be free from defects in material and workmanship for ninety (90) days from the date of original purchase. All implied warranties are limited in duration to this ninety (90) day period. THEREAFTER, ANY IMPLIED WARRANTIES, INCLUDING IMPLIED WARRANTIES OF MERCHANTABILITY AND FITNESS FOR A PARTICULAR PURPOSE, ARE EXCLUDED. THIS WARRANTY IS IN LIEU OF ALL OTHER WARRANTIES, WHETHER ORAL OR WRITTEN, EXPRESS OR IMPLIED.

If you believe the media is defective, please return it during the ninety-day period to the address shown below. Defective media will be replaced without charge provided that it has not been subjected to misuse or damage.

This warranty does not extend to the software or information recorded on the media. The software and information are provided "AS IS." Any statements made about the utility of the software or information are not to be considered as express or implied warranties.

Limitation of liability: Our liability to you for any losses shall be limited to direct damages and shall not exceed the amount you paid for the software. In no event will we be liable to you for any indirect, special, incidental, or consequential damages (including loss of profits) even if we have been advised of the possibility of such damages.

Some states do not allow the exclusion or limitation of incidental or consequential damages, or limitations on the duration of implied warranties, so the above limitation or exclusion may not apply to you. This warranty gives you specific legal rights, and you may also have other rights which vary from state to state. Address all correspondence to Delmar Thomson Learning, Box 15015, Albany, NY 12212 Attention: Technology Department.